MATERNAL–FETAL TOXICOLOGY

MEDICAL TOXICOLOGY

Editor

GIDEON KOREN, M.D., A.B.M.T., F.R.C.P.C.

The Motherisk Program
The Hospital for Sick Children
and The University of Toronto
Toronto, Ontario, Canada

Additional Volumes in Preparation

MATERNAL–FETAL TOXICOLOGY

A Clinician's Guide

Second Edition, Revised and Expanded

Edited by

GIDEON KOREN

The Motherisk Program
The Hospital for Sick Children
Toronto, Ontario, Canada

Marcel Dekker, Inc.   New York•Basel•Hong Kong

Library of Congress Cataloging-in-Publication Data

Maternal–fetal toxicology: a clinician's guide / edited by Gideon
Koren. — 2nd ed., rev. and expanded.
    p. cm. — (Medical toxicology ; 2)
  Includes bibliographical references and index.
  ISBN 0-8247-8841-9
    1. Fetus—Effect of drugs on. 2. Fetus—Effect of chemicals on.
  3. Fetus—Effect of radiation on. 4. Fetus—Abnormalities-
-Etiology. 5. Developmental toxicology. I. Koren, Gideon.
  II. Series: Medical toxicology (New York, N.Y.) ; 2.
  [DNLM: 1. Fetus—drug effects. 2. Pregnancy—drug effects.
  3. Abnormalities, Drug-Induced. 4. Drug Therapy—in pregnancy.
  5. Teratogens. W1 ME5275N v. 2 1994 / QS 679 M425 1994]
  RG627.6.D79M37 1994
  618.3'2—dc20   93-45786
  DNLM/DLC   CIP

The publisher offers discounts on this book when ordered in bulk quantities.
For more information, write to Special Sales/Professional Marketing at the
address below.

This book is printed on acid-free paper.

MARCEL DEKKER, INC.
270 Madison Avenue, New York, New York 10016

Current printing (last digit):
10 9 8 7 6 5 4 3

PRINTED IN THE UNITED STATES OF AMERICA

Series Introduction

Our generation is characterized by an increased awareness of the effects of xenobiotics and environmental agents on humans. The introduction of unique but toxic medications, the development of novel methods of estimating short- and long-term adverse effects, and tighter regulatory demands have all contributed to new insights in the area of medical toxicology.

At present, the main sources of information in the field of medical toxicology are reviews of original research and textbooks. Reviews of research generally address a narrow aspect of one issue, whereas textbook reviews need to generalize, within a limited space, which often results in decreased quality.

This new series of books aims at filling a gap between these two sources of information. I have aimed at in-depth reviews of areas of interest in medical toxicology, recruiting leading international scientists to discuss the themes.

The planned volumes address issues in acute poisoning, chronic adverse drug reactions, regulatory aspects, and so on. We hope to bring new frontiers of medical toxicology to the clinical and scientific communities in a way that will improve the understanding of the complex relationships between xenobiotics and human health.

Gideon Koren

Foreword

Almost all mothers will do everything they can to ensure that their babies have the healthiest possible start in life. Although birth defects or congenital malformations have been reported in the earliest recordings of history, *teratology*, the study of environmentally induced birth defects, did not develop into a modern science until the middle of the 20th century. Although *congenital malformations* were considered to be serious medical problems, they were thought to be unpreventable and untreatable.

With the discovery in the 1940s that certain environmental factors (iodine deficiency and rubella virus) could cause congenital malformations, many embryologists developed an active interest in substances called *teratogens* that could induce or increase the incidence of human congenital malformations. The occurrence of the thalidomide tragedy in the late 1950s attracted worldwide interest. The publicity accorded this tragedy increased the awareness of the public and the medical and legal professions that some human birth defects are caused by drugs, chemicals, and radiation. It was not long before women, and some medical practitioners, viewed every drug, chemical, and virus as a reproductive hazard.

As revealed in this book, many pregnant women exposed to drugs and chemicals that are known not to be teratogenic believe that they have a high risk of having a malformed baby. For a woman who has been exposed to a possible teratogen, obtaining accurate information about the risk involved, if any, is of utmost concern. Information available from newspapers, magazines, and popular books is often frightening and misunderstood. Most physicians and other health professionals receive insufficient training to answer all the questions pregnant women ask about the effects of chemical, physical, or infectious agents on the developing human embryo or fetus.

Over a decade ago, teratogen information programs were established in major health centers to respond to pregnant women's inquiries about teratogens, and to advise physicians and other health professionals who are responsible for their care.

The second edition of *Maternal–Fetal Toxicology: A Clinician's Guide* will be greatly appreciated by all who desire to learn about the teratogenic risks of the many environmental factors that women are exposed to during pregnancy. The main purpose of this book is to present those who counsel women with accurate, up-to-date estimates of the teratogenic risks of exposure to drugs, chemicals, viruses, and radiation during pregnancy. This information is very important to women making a decision to continue or terminate a pregnancy.

For many years there has been a need for a practical book on teratogens that can be used in health-care programs for pregnant women. This book describes current teratogen information programs and the process of counseling for teratogenic risk. I strongly recommend this book to all who share my enthusiasm for the developing human and my desire to see every one of them have the best possible chance of developing normally.

Keith L. Moore, Ph.D., F.I.A.C.
Professor of Anatomy
The University of Toronto
and President
American Association of Clinical Anatomists
Toronto, Ontario, Canada

Preface

Approximately one fetus is aborted for every child born in Western countries. Since the thalidomide disaster over three decades ago, medicine has been practiced as if every drug were a potential human teratogen. Women exposed to nonteratogens commonly believe they have a high teratogenic risk. Their physicians often encourage them to terminate their pregnancies, yet only about 20 drugs and chemicals have been proven to be teratogenic.

Every year scores of new drugs and hundreds of new chemicals are introduced into the market. In neither case are human reproductive effects known. Furthermore, according to different studies, between 40 and 90% of pregnant women consume one or more medications during gestation. Finally, despite hundreds of scientific studies published yearly on reproductive effects of xenobiotics, little has been done in the past to crystallize a clinical approach to deal with these issues.

No single medical specialty is equipped to deal with the complex issues of reproductive toxicology. While geneticists commonly deal with congenital malformations, it is unlikely that they have the experience of pharmacologists in tailoring alternative therapy. Neither group is trained to evaluate such factors as occupational exposures. A multidisciplinary team of pharmacologists, toxicologists, geneticists, obstetricians, neonatologists, occupational and addiction specialists, drug information specialists, psychologists, sonographers, and epidemiologists is needed.

In September of 1985 we counseled the first patient in the Motherisk clinic in Toronto. This program was designed to inform, counsel, and follow up pregnant women exposed to drugs, chemicals, or radiation in pregnancy. In order to perform these tasks, new approaches and clinical tools had to be developed by our multidisciplinary team; these are presented in this volume.

Much of the confusion surrounding the counseling process stems from the well-understood "do not use in pregnancy" statements commonly found in the *Physicians' Desk Reference*, *Compendium of Pharmaceuticals and Specialties*, or their equivalents. Since many women are inadvertently exposed to medications *before* finding out they have conceived, the "do not use in pregnancy" statements are easily translated into "harmful" or "teratogenic." While the exact rate of pregnancy termination due to fears of adverse fetal effects of xenobiotics is not known, there is indirect evidence that this is not uncommon. Similarly disturbing are the many cases where women are exposed to drugs and chemicals known to adversely affect the fetus without being appropriately informed.

The goal of this book is to assist the large number of health professionals who are asked by women and their families to provide answers on potential reproductive effects of xenobiotics and radiation. These include general physicians, obstetricians, poison control specialists, geneticists, occupational specialists, pediatricians, pharmacologists, toxicologists, pharmacists, nurses, and others. With increasing public awareness of environmental toxins, it is likely that concerns surrounding reproductive toxicology will increase over the next few decades. We hope that an appropriate clinical approach will help put the issue in its correct perspective, by avoiding both understatements and ambiguity.

In the four years that have elapsed since the first edition of *Maternal–Fetal Toxicology: A Clinician's Guide*, the field of teratology information has seen an exponential growth, both in terms of quantity and quality of knowledge. The Motherisk Program in Toronto, in collaboration with several American services, has initiated and brought to completion large-scale, prospective studies on the safety of drugs in pregnancy, some of which are presented in this volume. In addition to revising and updating most chapters, we have added several novel aspects, such as the maternal–fetal toxicology of medicinal plants, developmental risk assessment, and biological markers of intrauterine exposure to drugs of abuse. This revised and expanded edition also includes clinical cases at the beginning of most chapters, with answers at the end. It is hoped that this idea will enhance the clinical relevance of this book as well as increase its educational value.

Finally, I wish to thank the members of the Motherisk team, my students, fellows, and colleagues for being active in generating new knowledge in the field of maternal–fetal toxicology.

Gideon Koren

Contents

Contributors

Deborah Czuchta Altmann, B.A., D.C.S. Department of Psychology Research, The Hospital for Sick Children, Toronto, Ontario, Canada

Peter Ashby, M.D. Department of Neurology, Toronto Hospital, Western Division, Toronto, Ontario, Canada

Stan Ashby, M.D. Department of Psychology, The Hospital for Sick Children, Toronto, Ontario, Canada

Yedidia Bentur, M.D. Israel Poison Information Center, Rambam Medical Center, Technion–Israel Institute of Technology, Haifa, Israel

James B. Besunder, D.O. Department of Pediatrics, Metro Health Medical Center, and Case Western Reserve University School of Medicine, Cleveland, Ohio

Jeffrey L. Blumer, M.D., Ph.D. Department of Pediatrics, Rainbow Babies and Children's Hospital, and Case Western Reserve University School of Medicine, Cleveland, Ohio

Monica Bologa, M.D. Motherisk Program, Division of Clinical Pharmacology and Toxicology, Department of Pediatrics, The Hospital for

Sick Children, and The Upjohn Company of Canada, Toronto, Ontario, Canada

Shirley Chan Department of Pharmacology, The University of Toronto, Toronto, Ontario, Canada

Gerald F. Chernoff, Ph.D. Office of Environmental Health Hazard Assessment, California Environmental Protection Agency, Sacramento, California

David Chitayat, M.D. The Prenatal Diagnosis Program, Division of Clinical Genetics, Department of Genetics, The Hospital for Sick Children, Toronto, Ontario, Canada

John Chu Department of Pharmacology, The University of Toronto, Toronto, Ontario, Canada

Ronald G. Davidson, M.D. Professor Emeritus, Faculty of Health Sciences, McMaster University, Hamilton, Ontario, Canada

Jill E. Dolgin, Pharm.D. Western New York Regional Poison Center, Children's Hospital of Buffalo, Buffalo, New York

Alan Donnenfeld, M.D. Department of Obstetrics and Gynecology, Pennsylvania Hospital, Philadelphia, Pennsylvania

Thomas R. Einarson, Ph.D. Motherisk Program, Division of Clinical Pharmacology and Toxicology, Department of Pediatrics, The Hospital for Sick Children, Toronto, Ontario, Canada

Frank F. Fassos, B.Sc., M.Sc. Division of Clinical Pharmacology and Toxicology, Department of Pediatrics, The Hospital for Sick Children, Toronto, Ontario, Canada

Annette Feigenbaum, M.B., Ch.B. Division of Clinical Genetics, Department of Pediatrics, The Hospital for Sick Children, Toronto, Ontario, Canada

Marcia Feldkamp, M.S. University of Utah, Salt Lake City, Utah

Yaacov Feldman, M.D. Motherisk Program, Division of Clinical Pharmacology and Toxicology, Department of Pediatrics, The Hospital for Sick Children, Toronto, Ontario, Canada

Rachel Forman Motherisk Program, Division of Clinical Pharmacology and Toxicology, Department of Pediatrics, The Hospital for Sick Children, Toronto, Ontario, Canada

H. Allen Gardner, M.D. Genetic Services, Oshawa General Hospital, Oshawa, Ontario, Canada

Lorne K. Garrettson, M.D.   Department of Pediatrics, Emory University, Atlanta, Georgia

David Gladstone, B.Sc.   Faculty of Medicine, University of Toronto, Toronto, Ontario, Canada

Richard Gladstone, M.D.   Department of Neurology, North York Medical Arts Building, Willowdale, Ontario, Canada

Susan Goldberg, M.D.   Department of Psychology, The University of Toronto, Toronto, Ontario, Canada

Ron Gonen, M.D.   Department of Obstetrics and Gynecology, Faculty of Medicine, B'nai Zion Medical Center, Technion, Haifa, Israel

Karen Graham, M.D.   Department of Psychiatry, McMaster University, Hamilton, Ontario, Canada

R. Kelly Hill, Jr., M.D.   Hyperbaric Medicine, Our Lady of the Lake Regional Medical Center, Baton Rouge, Louisiana

Kathy A. Hodgkinson, B.Sc., M.Sc.   The Prenatal Diagnosis Program, The Toronto Hospitals, Toronto, Ontario, Canada

Shinya Ito, M.D.   Motherisk Program, Division of Clinical Pharmacology and Toxicology, Department of Pediatrics, The Hospital for Sick Children, Toronto, Ontario, Canada

Sheila Jacobson, MBB.ch.   Division of General Pediatrics, Department of Pediatrics, The Hospital for Sick Children, Toronto, Ontario, Canada

Ken Jones, M.D.   Division of Dysmorphology and Teratology, Department of Pediatrics, University of California, San Diego, San Diego, California

Arlene King, M.D.   Fairview Health Complex, Fairview, Alberta, Canada

Julia Klein, M.Sc.   Division of Clinical Pharmacology, The Hospital for Sick Children, Toronto, Ontario, Canada

Gideon Koren, M.D.   Motherisk Program, Division of Clinical Pharmacology and Toxicology, Department of Pediatrics, The Hospital for Sick Children, Toronto, Ontario, Canada

Warif Laila, M.D.   Motherisk Program, Division of Clinical Pharmacology and Toxicology, Department of Pediatrics, The Hospital for Sick Children, Toronto, Ontario, Canada

J. Steven Leeder, Pharm.D., Ph.D. Division of Clinical Pharmacology and Toxicology, The Hospital for Sick Children, Toronto, Ontario, Canada

Marsha Leen-Mitchell University of Utah, Salt Lake City, Utah

Beatrix Lutiger, M.D. Motherisk Program, Division of Clinical Pharmacology and Toxicology, Department of Pediatrics, The Hospital for Sick Children, Toronto, Ontario, Canada

Stuart M. MacLeod, M.D., Ph.D. St. Joseph's Health Center, Hamilton, Ontario, Canada

Laura Magee, M.D. Motherisk Program, Division of Clinical Pharmacology and Toxicology, Department of Pediatrics, The Hospital for Sick Children, Toronto, Ontario, Canada

Michael McCormack, Ph.D. University of Medicine and Dentistry of New Jersey, Camden, New Jersey

Michael McGuigan, M.D. Ontario Regional Poison Information Centre, The Hospital for Sick Children, Toronto, Ontario, Canada

Vanessa Milich Department of Pharmacology, The University of Toronto, Toronto, Ontario, Canada

Irena Nulman, M.D. Motherisk Program, Division of Clinical Pharmacology and Toxicology, Department of Pediatrics, The Hospital for Sick Children, Toronto, Ontario, Canada

Anne Pastuszak, B.Sc. Motherisk Program, Division of Clinical Pharmacology and Toxicology, Department of Pediatrics, The Hospital for Sick Children, Toronto, Ontario, Canada

Elizabeth M. Pellegrini Motherisk Program, Division of Clinical Pharmacology and Toxicology, Department of Pediatrics, The Hospital for Sick Children, Toronto, Ontario, Canada

My-Khanh Phan, B.Sc. Motherisk Program, Department of Clinical Pharmacology, The Hospital for Sick Children, Toronto, Ontario, Canada

Izhar ul Qamar, M.D. Motherisk Program, Division of Clinical Pharmacology and Toxicology, Department of Pediatrics, The Hospital for Sick Children, Toronto, Ontario, Canada

Samuel Randor, M.D. Motherisk Program, Division of Clinical Pharmacology and Toxicology, Department of Pediatrics, The Hospital for Sick Children, Toronto, Ontario, Canada

Michael J. Rieder, M.D., Ph.D. Department of Pediatrics, Pharmacology and Toxicology, and Department of Medicine, The University of Western Ontario and the Children's Hospital of Western Ontario, London, Ontario, Canada

Mark Rorem, M.D. Geisinger Medical Center, Danville, Pennsylvania

Joanne Rovet, Ph.D. Department of Pediatrics, The Hospital for Sick Children, Toronto, Ontario, Canada

Ivan Samson, M.D. Community Group Health Centre, St. Catherines, Ontario, Canada

Betsy Schick, M.S.N. Department of Obstetrics and Gynecology, Pennsylvania Hospital, Philadelphia, Pennsylvania

Joyce F. Schneiderman, M.D. The Addiction Research Foundation and The University of Toronto, Toronto, Ontario, Canada

Dennis Scolnik, M.D. Motherisk Program, Division of Clinical Pharmacology and Toxicology, Department of Pediatrics, The Hospital for Sick Children, Toronto, Ontario, Canada

Teresa Sharav, M.D. Motherisk Program, Division of Clinical Pharmacology and Toxicology, Department of Pediatrics, The Hospital for Sick Children, Toronto, Ontario, Canada

Kathleen Shilalukey, B.Sc., MB.Ch.B. Motherisk Program, Division of Clinical Pharmacology and Toxicology, Department of Pediatrics, The Hospital for Sick Children, Toronto, Ontario, Canada

Jerry Shime, M.D. Department of Obstetrics and Gynecology, Women's College Hospital, Toronto, Ontario, Canada

Joanne Smith, B.Sc. Pharm. Drug Information Service, Department of Pharmacy, The Hospital for Sick Children, Toronto, Ontario, Canada

Stephen P. Spielberg, M.D., Ph.D. Merck Research Laboratories, West Point, Pennsylvania

Anna Taddio, B.Sc. Division of Clinical Pharmacology and Toxicology, Department of Pediatrics, The Hospital for Sick Children, Toronto, Ontario, Canada

Milton Tenenbein, M.D. Departments of Pediatrics and Pharmacology, Winnipeg Children's Hospital, University of Manitoba, Winnipeg, Manitoba, Canada

Rosanna Weksberg, M.D., Ph.D.   Department of Genetics, The Hospital for Sick Children, Toronto, Ontario, Canada

Philip R. Wyatt, M.D., Ph.D.   Department of Genetics, North York General Hospital and Children's Centre, Toronto, Ontario, Canada

Eli Zalzstein, M.D.   Department of Cardiology, Soroka Medical Center, Beer-Sheva, Israel

Susan Zeesman, M.Sc.   Section of Laboratory Medicine, Department of Pathology, Chedoke-McMaster Hospitals, Hamilton, Ontario, Canada

Carol Zuber, M.S.N.   University of Medicine and Dentistry of New Jersey, Camden, New Jersey

MATERNAL–FETAL
TOXICOLOGY

Part I

Drugs in Pregnancy

1

Changes in Drug Disposition in Pregnancy and Their Clinical Implications

Gideon Koren
The Hospital for Sick Children, Toronto, Ontario, Canada

Clinical Case

One of your patients, a G1 P0 epileptic woman (65 kg in late gestation) who was maintained on 400 mg/d of phenytoin taken in two equal doses every 12 hours has just had her first and only grand mal seizure during pregnancy at 26 weeks of gestation. Upon arrival to the emergency room her phenytoin level was 5 mg/L 10 hours after her evening dose. Three trough levels taken before, at various times during pregnancy, were between 12 and 17 mg/L. What are your thoughts about the mechanism leading to this seizure?

INTRODUCTION

While the potential hazards to the unborn baby from medications administered to the pregnant woman are a major concern, one should be very careful not to neglect the maternal part of the fetomaternal unit. It has been universally agreed that the well-being of the mother should dictate her need for drug therapy and that one should not subject pregnant women to suboptimal therapy that may endanger them.

Pregnancy is associated with a plethora of physiological changes that may affect the natural course of diseases, the way the body handles drugs, or both. This chapter summarizes major changes in the pharmacokinetics of drugs in pregnancy and their clinical implications. Whereas Chapter 26 deals with the effects of maternal diseases on the reproductive outcome, this chapter focuses on the possible need for alterations in drug therapy in pregnancy to deal with pharmacokinetic and pathophysiological changes.

PHARMACOKINETICS OF THE MATERNAL–FETAL UNIT

Several pharmacokinetic models have been used to describe the movement of different drugs between the maternal and fetal circulations (1). In general, two principal groups of changes characterize pregnancy with respect to drug disposition.

Alterations in Drug Kinetics Due to Maternal Changes

There is a gradual increase in renal function in pregnancy. This will result in an augmented elimination rate of agents that are excreted by the kidney (e.g., ampicillin, gentamicin, amikacin, digoxin) (2–5). Distribution volume may be altered during pregnancy because of increases to 50% in blood (plasma) volume and 30% in cardiac output (6–8). A parallel 50% increment in renal flow and a substantial increase of uterine blood flow to 600–700 mL/min also take place. During pregnancy there is a mean increase of 8 L in body water: 60% of it is distributed to the placenta, fetus, and amniotic fluid, and 40% is distributed to maternal tissues (6,9–11). Consequently, a decrease in the serum concentrations of many drugs has been documented. It is very likely that lower serum concentrations in pregnancy will be noted, especially with drugs having a relatively small distribution volume which corresponds to water compartments. During pregnancy there is a well-documented fall in the protein binding of drugs, partially because of the decrease in serum albumin concentrations (12). Consequently, the unbound (free) fraction is increased, resulting in larger distribution volumes because it is the unbound drug that is free to move into various tissue compartments.

Of potential clinical importance, the protein binding of several antiepileptic drugs including phenytoin, diazepam, and valproic acid has been shown to decrease significantly toward the last trimester of pregnancy (13). These drugs are discussed later in this chapter.

Changes in hepatic elimination patterns during pregnancy are less consistent. Hepatic blood flow appears to be unchanged during pregnancy (1). However, there is evidence that the elimination rate of clindamycin, which is metabolized by the liver, is increased during pregnancy (3), suggesting a possible increase in hepatic clearance. It is possible that the faster elimination of trimethoprim/sulfamethoxazole observed during pregnancy is due to higher liver clearance, although increased renal clearance may be the major determinant of this change (14).

The decrease in drug-protein binding discussed previously may also account for higher clearance rates of drugs in pregnancy, as it is the free fraction which is accessible to the metabolizing systems. Studies in epileptic women have shown an increase in the clearance of phenytoin during pregnancy, accounting for lower serum concentrations (13).

As shown in Table 1, the above-mentioned changes in the pharmacokinetics of many drugs administered during pregnancy result in a decrease in serum concentrations when compared to levels measured in nonpregnant women. Thus, the standard dose schedule may result in lower concentrations in pregnancy and, as discussed later, these changes may have important implications in treating the pregnant woman.

The Effects of the Placental–Fetal Compartment

Almost all drugs have been shown to cross the placenta and to appear in measurable concentrations in the fetal blood. Several determinants govern the movement of drugs across the placental barrier and determine the materno-fetal ratio of concentrations. In general, the ratio between drug concentration in the fetus versus the mother is different from (in most cases less than) unity (Table 2).

Differences in Protein Binding

Fetal protein appears to bind less avidly various drugs, including ampicillin and benzylpenicillin (33). Conversely, no differences between maternal and

Table 1 Selected Drugs Having Lower Serum Concentrations During Pregnancy and Relevant Pharmacokinetic Changes (3,4,13,15–21)

Drug	Elimination half-time	Vd	Clearance	Protein binding
Amikacin	↓			
Ampicillin	↓	↑	↑	↓
Cephalosporins	↓	↓		
Erythromycin				
Gentamicin	→			
Kanamycin	→			
Methicillin	↑			
Nitrofurantoin				
Oxacillin		↑	↑	
Phenobarbitol			↑	↓
Phenytoin		↑	↑	↓

Table 2 Fetomaternal Concentration Ratio
of Antibiotics (3,22–32)

Drug	Fetomaternal ratio
Ampicillin	0.38–0.87
Cephalosporins	0.13–1.0
Clindamycin	0.4–0.5
Dicloxacillin	0.07–0.27
Gentamicin	0.21–1.0
Methicillin	0.83–1.43
Penicillin G	0.06–0.7

fetal protein binding were found for methicillin and dicloxacillin (30). Salicylates, on the other hand, appear to have a more extensive binding to fetal than to maternal protein (34).

During pregnancy there is a gradual decrease in the concentrations of maternal albumin and an increase in the concentrations of fetal albumin. Consequently, at different times during pregnancy, different fetal/maternal ratios of albumin occur. At term, it appears that fetal albumin concentrations are equal or even higher than in the mother. The degree of protein binding of a drug is an important determinant of its movement across the placenta. The least protein-bound drugs (e.g., digoxin, ampicillin, 20%) reach higher concentrations in the fetus and in the amniotic fluid. Drugs with high protein binding (e.g., dicloxacillin, 96%) achieve higher maternal and lower fetal concentrations because only the free fraction of the drug crosses the placental barrier. Since, however, additional determinants other than protein binding may play an important role in placental passage, drugs such as sulfisoxazole reach therapeutic concentrations in the fetus in spite of their high protein binding.

Differences in pH

Fetal blood pH is slightly lower than the maternal. The pH gradient may influence the movement of drugs according to their pK_a; weak bases, with a pK_a value close to the blood pH, will be mainly nonionized and consequently will easily cross the placenta, since nonionized molecules penetrate biological membranes more quickly than ionized molecules. However, after crossing the placenta and making contact with the more acidic fetal blood, these molecules are ionized because the fetal pH is less close to their pK_a. This results in an apparent fall in fetal concentrations of nonionized drugs and leads to a concentration gradient, leading to net movement from maternal to fetal systems (35). This mechanism is commonly referred to as "ion trapping." In contrast to weak bases, ion trapping induced from fetal to maternal circulations is likely to occur with weak acids.

Other Effects

Other important determinants of drug transport across the placenta are water/lipid solubility, molecular weight, and the surface available for diffusion. A good example of the different effects on placental passage is the higher concentrations of trimethoprim in the fetus than in the mother, corresponding to its relatively low protein binding (42–46%), pK_a of 6.6, and poor water solubility. Sulfamethoxazole, on the other hand, has good water solubility at physiological pH and therefore has more difficulties in crossing the lipid-placental barrier. Both drugs appear to reach the amniotic fluid, and their concentration ratio there closely corresponds to that in the fetal serum (36).

Following repeated doses of drugs, concentrations measured in the fetus appear to be higher than following a single dose (37). Repeated high bolus injections of ampicillin or gentamicin yield higher concentrations in fetal serum and amniotic fluid than a similar pattern of transplacental transfer, and after a single intravenous dose a peak umbilical concentration is achieved within 30–60 min.

Fetoplacental Drug Elimination

Drug metabolism has been documented by the fetal liver as early as 7–8 weeks of pregnancy. Virtually all enzymatic processes, including phase 1 (oxidation, dehydrogenation, reduction, hydrolysis, etc.) and phase 2 (glucuronidation, methylation, acetylation, etc.) have been documented in the fetal liver (39). However, the degree of activity is very low in most cases when compared to the adult liver. Similarly, drug-metabolizing activity has been demonstrated in human placental tissue. In summary, the placentofetal unit contributes only marginally to the total elimination capacity of drugs by the maternal body. As pregnancy progresses, higher amounts of antimicrobials are excreted into the amniotic fluids through fetal urine. This process depends upon maturation of the fetal kidney.

In general, metabolites are more polar than their parent compounds and are therefore less likely to cross the placental barrier. As a result, metabolites may accumulate in various tissues of the fetus or may be recovered from the amniotic fluid. It has been shown that thiamphenicol achieves higher concentrations in the umbilical vein than in the umbilical artery, reflecting some degree of extraction of the drug by the fetus, probably by renal excretion (32).

CLINICAL IMPLICATIONS

As reflected in the preceding discussion, a variety of drugs appear to achieve lower serum concentrations during pregnancy. For agents that maintain good correlation between serum concentrations and pharmacological effects, this may mean that during pregnancy patients may be at a higher risk of suboptimal therapy.

Anticonvulsants

As discussed above, there is good evidence that the serum concentrations of phenytoin, phenobarbital (40), ethosuximide (41), and carbamazepine (42) decrease as pregnancy progresses. Some authors observed an increase in the frequency of seizures as phenytoin clearance increased in pregnancy and plasma levels fell (40). A variety of reasons have been put forward to explain this fall in drug concentrations in pregnancy:

1. Increase in extracellular fluid and tissue volume, leading to increase in distribution volume of the drug.
2. Decreased plasma-protein binding, leading to more free drug available for biotransformation. It should be mentioned, however, that higher free drug concentration may secure antiepileptic effect even in the presence of lower total drug level, as it is the free drug that reaches the brain.
3. Folate supplementation, given to the pregnant woman, may increase liver metabolism of phenytoin (41).
4. Increase in glomerular filtration rate (GFR), leading to faster clearance rates of drugs eliminated by the kidney.

The question of whether epilepsy is worsened during pregnancy is of extreme importance; current evidence, however, is inconclusive: Schmidt reviewed 2162 pregnancies and could not detect a clear pattern, as some 23% reported improvement, 53% no change, and 24% worsened (43). Yet, other studies suggest that epilepsy with at least one seizure per month is likely to worsen in pregnancy (44).

Changes in seizure frequency in pregnancy may stem from fluid and sodium retention, hyperventilation, a rise in estrogen levels, emotional and psychological problems, and of course the tendency of drug levels to fall (13). Although presently no research has addressed the contribution of each factor, there are well-documented cases to prove the importance of adequate serum concentrations during pregnancy (13,41).

Caring for the pregnant epileptic patient must, therefore, incorporate careful monitoring of serum concentrations and appropriate adjustment of the antiepileptic dose. After pregnancy, most women will need lower dosages, and failure to adjust their schedule may lead to drug toxicity.

Lithium

The antidepressant lithium is eliminated almost entirely by the kidney. The pregnancy-induced increase in the GFR is consistent, therefore, with lower serum concentrations of lithium reported sporadically during pregnancy (45). Because in many cases lithium exerts its pharmacological effects at nearly toxic levels, the drop in serum concentrations may lead to suboptimal therapy.

After birth, with the return of the GFR to its prepregnancy values, patients may need reduction of their doses.

Some lithium is reabsorbed by the renal tubule, and this process is in competition with sodium reabsorption. Pregnant patients with toxemia are kept on a restricted sodium intake, and therefore they may experience higher levels of lithium owing to higher renal reabsorption of the cation.

Digoxin

Similar to lithium, digoxin is eliminated in humans mainly by renal excretion and therefore is expected to maintain lower steady-state concentrations in pregnancy. When measured at term, digoxin serum concentrations were found in five pregnant women to be almost twofold lower than 1 month later (5).

Ampicillin

Since ampicillin is one of the most widely used antibiotics, knowledge of its pharmacokinetics in pregnancy may yield valuable information about the dose requirement during gestation. Philipson, who studied the disposition of ampicillin once during and again after pregnancy, found the plasma concentration to be 50% lower during gestation owing to both the larger distribution volume and faster clearance rate (2). Similar to digoxin and lithium, ampicillin is eliminated mainly through the kidney, and the twofold decrease in its levels is consistent with that described for digoxin.

Other Drugs

Similar observations have been documented with cephalosporins, clindamycin, erythromycin, kanamycin, amikacin, tobramycin, nitrofurantoin, and sulfamethoxazole-trimethoprim (37). In all instances, the lower serum concentrations during pregnancy could be attributed to pharmacokinetic changes.

SUMMARY

It is conceivable that for many drugs not yet studied the same pattern of higher clearance rates and, therefore, lower steady-state concentrations prevails in pregnancy.

Drugs for which levels are monitored routinely are summarized in Table 3, along with their therapeutic range of serum concentrations. In monitoring chronic drug therapy in pregnancy it is important to repeat measurements more often than routinely, since toward the end of pregnancy the physiological

Table 3 Therapeutic Serum Concentrations of Drugs Commonly Monitored in Clinical Practice, and Documented Changes in Pregnancy

Drug	Units of therapeutic concentration		Documented changes in drug concentration during pregnancy
	Metric	SI[a]	
Amikacin	Peak < 20–30 μg/mL		↓
	Trough < 5–10 μg/mL		
Amiodarone	< 2.5 μg/mL		
Carbamazepine	4–12 μg/mL	17–51 μM	↓
Chloramphenicol	< 25 μg/mL		
Cyclosporin	< 200–250 ng/mL		
Digoxin	0.5–2 ng/mL	0.7–2.6 nM	↓
Disopyramide	3–5 μg/mL	9–15 μM	
Ethosuximide	40–100 μg/mL	285–710 μM	↓
Gentamicin	Trough < 2–3 μg/mL		↓
	Peak < 8–10 μg/mL		
Lidocaine	1.5–5.0 μg/mL	6–21 μM	
Lithium		0.8–1.0 mM	↓
Methotrexate		< 5 μM 24 h after high dose	
Phenobarbitol	15–40 μg/mL	65–172 μM	↓
Phenytoin	10–20 μg/mL	39–79 μM	↓
Primidone	5–12 μg/mL	23–55 μM	
Procainamide	4–10 μg/mL	15–37 μM	
Quinidine	2.3–5.0 μg/mL	7–15 μM	
Theophylline	10–20 μg/mL	55–110 μM	
Tobramycin	Trough < 2–3 μg/mL		
	Peak < 8–10 μg/mL		
Valproic acid	50–100 μg/mL	347–693 μM	
Vancomycin	Trough < 10 μg/mL		
	Peak < 45 μg/mL		

[a]M = 1 mol/L.

changes leading to lower serum concentrations are at their maximum. Decisions concerning increases of daily doses should incorporate the clinical status and the course of the disease, and they are best performed by the physician familiar with the woman's condition. It is important to remember not to "treat numbers"; while some patients have good control of their illness with low serum concentrations, others do not achieve favorable effects even at supratherapeutic drug levels. Concentrations of most drugs are not measured routinely in clinical practice; the general pattern delineated above should be borne in mind, since a higher clearance rate would mean that some pregnant women may need higher doses, especially if the regular (prepregnancy) schedule fails to produce the expected effects.

Answer

Epileptic women tend to have more seizures during pregnancy. After ruling out preeclampsia-eclampsia, electrolyte changes, and hypoalbuminemia, you should consider increased clearance rate of phenytoin as a cause for lower levels and the resulting seizures. To that end, you need to rule out decrease in compliance (i.e., the patient had not been taking her medications as before).

REFERENCES

1. Krauer B, Krauer F. Drug kinetics in pregnancy. In Handbook of Clinical Pharmacokinetics (Gibaldi M, Prescott L, eds), Section II, ADIS, New York, 1983, pp 1-17.
2. Philipson A. Pharmacokinetics of ampicillin during pregnancy. J Infect Dis 1977; 136:370-376.
3. Weinstein AJ, Gibbs RS, Gallagher M. Placental transfer of clindamycin and gentamicin in term pregnancy. Am J Obstet Gynecol 1976; 124:688-691.
4. Bernard B, Abate M, Thielen PF, Attar H, Ballard CA, Wehnle PF. Maternal fetal pharmacological activity of amikacin. J Infect Dis 1977; 135:925-932.
5. Rogers ME, Willerson JT, Goldblatt A, et al. Serum digoxin concentrations in the human fetus, neonate and infant. N Engl J Med 1972; 287:1010-1013.
6. Hytten FE, Leitch T. The Physiology of Pregnancy. Blackwell, Oxford, 1971.
7. Pizani BBK, Campbell DM, McGillivray T. Plasma volume in normal pregnancy. J Obstet Gynecol 1973; 80:884-887.
8. Walters WAW, Lengling Y. Blood volume and haemodynamics in pregnancy. In Obstetrics and Gynecology, Vol 2. Saunders, London, 1975, pp 301-302.
9. Davidson JM, Hytten FE. Glomerular filtration during and after pregnancy. J Obstet Gynecol 1974; 81:588-595.
10. Young IM. The placenta: Blood flow and transfer. In Modern Trends in Physiology, Butterworth, London, 1972, pp 214-244.
11. Kerr MG. Cardiovascular dynamics in pregnancy and labour. Br Med Bull 1968; 24:19-24.

12. Rebound P, Groulade J, Groslambert P, Colomb M. The influence of normal pregnancy and the postpartum state on plasma proteins and lipids. Am J Obstet Gynecol 1963; 86:820-828.
13. Perucca E, Richens A. Antiepileptic drugs, pregnancy and the newborn. In Clinical Pharmacology in Obstetrics (Lewis P, ed), Wright PSG, Bristol, England, pp 264-287, 1983.
14. Ylikorkala O, Sjostedt E, Jarvinen PA, Tikkanen R, Raines T. Trimethoprim-sulfonamide combination administered orally and intravaginally in the first trimester of pregnancy: Its absorption into serum and transfer to amniotic fluid. Acta Obstet Gynecol Scand 1973; 52:229-234.
15. Bray RE, Boe RW, Johnson WL. Transfer of ampicillin into fetus and amniotic fluid from maternal plasma in late pregnancy. Am J Obstet Gynecol 1966; 96: 938-942.
16. Bernard B, Barton L, Abate M, Ballard CA. Maternal fetal transfer of cefazolin in the first twenty weeks of pregnancy. J Infect Dis 1977; 136:377-;382.
17. Philipson A, Saboth LD, Charles D. Erythromycin and clindamycin absorption and elimination in pregnant women. Clin Pharmacol Ther 1976; 19:68-77.
18. Good RG, Johnson G. The placental transfer of kanamycin in late pregnancy. Obstet Gynecol 1971; 38:60-62.
19. MacAuley MA, Berg SR, Charles D. Placental transfer of methicillin. Am J Obstet Gynecol 1973; 115:58-65.
20. Amon K, Amon I, Huller H. Verteilung und Kinetik von Nitrofurantoin in der Fruhschwangerschaft. Int J Clin Pharmacol Ther Toxicol 1972; 63:218-222.
21. Bastert G, Muller WG, Wallhauser KH, Hebauf H. Pharmacokinetishe Untersuchungen zum Ubertriff von Antibiotika in das Fruchtwasser am Enter der Schwangerschaft. 3. Oxacillin. Geburtschilfe Perinatol 1975; 179:346-355.
22. Hirsch HA, Dreher E, Perrochet A, Schmid E. Transfer of ampicillin to the fetus and amniotic fluid during continuous infusion (steady state) and by repeated single intravenous injections to the mother. Infection 1974; 2:207-212.
23. Croft I, Forster TC. Materno-fetal cephadine transfer in pregnancy. Antimicrob Agents Chemother 1978; 14:924-926.
24. Barr W, Graham RM. Placental transmission of cephaloxidine. J Obstet Gynecol 1947; 74:739-745.
25. Hirsch HA, Herbet S, Lang R, Dettli L, Goblinger A. Transfer of a new cephalosporin antibiotic to the fetus and the amniotic fluid during a continuous infusion (steady state) and single repeated intravenous injections to the mother. Anz Fonsch 1974; 24:1474-1478.
26. MacAuley MA, Abou-Sabe M, Charles D. Placental transfer of dicloxacillin at term. Am J Obstet Gynecol 1968; 102:1162-1168.
27. Forreres L, Paz M, Martin G, Gobernado M. New studies on placental transfer of fosfomycin. Chemotherapy 1977 (suppl 1):175-179.
28. Daubenfeld O, Modde H, Hirsch HA. Transfer of gentamicin to the foetus and amniotic fluid during a steady state in the mother. Arch Gynecol 1974; 217: 233-240.
29. Yoshioka H, Monma T, Matsudo S. Placental transfer of gentamicin. J Pediatr 1972; 80:121-123.

30. Depp R, Kind AC, Kirby WMM, Johnson WL. Transplacental passage of methicillin and dicloxacillin into the fetus and amniotic fluid. Am J Obstet Gynecol 1970; 107:1054–1057.
31. Charles D. Placental transmission of antibiotics. J Obstet Gynecol 1954; 61: 790–797.
32. Plomp TA, Moes RAA, Thiery M. Placental transfer of thiamphenicol in term pregnancy. Eur J Obstet Gynecol Reprod Biol 1977; 7:383–388.
33. Tucker GT, Boyes RN, Bridenbaugh PO. Binding of anilide-type local anesthetics in human plasma. II. Implications in vivo, with special reference to transplacental distribution. Anesthesiology 1970; 33:304–314.
34. Levy G. Salicylate pharmacokinetics in the human neonate: In Basic and Therapeutic Aspects of Perinatal Pharmacology (Morselli P, Garattini C, Sereni Y, eds), Raven Press, New York, 1975, pp 319–330.
35. Asling JH, Way EL. Placental transfer of drugs. In Fundamentals of Drug Metabolism and Drug Disposition (La Du, Mandel, Way Y, eds), Williams & Wilkins, Baltimore, 1972, p 88.
36. Walter AM, Heilmeyer L. Antibiotika-Fibel, Vol 4. Auflage. Thieme, Stuttgart, 1975.
37. Philipson A. Pharmacokinetics of antibiotics in pregnancy and labour. Clin Pharmacokinet 1979; 4:297–309.
38. Chow AW, Jewesson PJ. Pharmacokinetics and safety of antimicrobial agents during pregnancy. Rev Infect Dis 1985; 7:287–313.
39. Juchau MR, Chao ST, Omiecinski CJ. Drug metabolism by the human fetus. In Handbook of Clinical Pharmacokinetics (Gibaldi M, Prescott L, eds), Section II, ADIS, New York, 1983, pp 58–78.
40. Dam M, Mygind KJ, Christiansen J. Antiepileptic drugs: Plasma clearance during pregnancy. Epileptology 1976; Jan.3 179–183.
41. Eadie MJ, Lander CM, Tyrer JH. Plasma drug level monitoring in pregnancy. In Handbook of Clinical Pharmacokinetics (Gibaldi M, Prescott L, eds), Section IV, ADIS, NY, 1983, pp 53–62.
42. Dam M, Christiansen J, Munck O, Mygind KI. Antiepileptic drugs: Metabolism in pregnancy. Clin Pharmacokinet 1979; 4:53–62.
43. Schmidt D. The effect of pregnancy on the natural history of epilepsy. In Epilepsy, Pregnancy and the Child (Janz D, Bossi L, Dam M, eds), Raven Press, New York, 1981, pp 3–14.
44. Knight AH, Rhind EG. Epilepsy and pregnancy: A study of 153 pregnancies in 59 patients. Epilepsia 1975; 16:99–110.
45. Schou M, Amidsen A, Steenstrup DR. Lithium and pregnancy. II: Hazards to women given lithium during pregnancy and delivery. Br Med J 1973; 2: 137–138.

2

Developmental Risk Assessments

Gerald F. Chernoff
California Environmental Protection Agency, Sacramento, California

INTRODUCTION

For those on the front line communicating risk information to pregnant women, one of the more frustrating questions that can be asked regards the risk of exposures to occupational chemicals and environmental hazards. Whereas information about pharmaceuticals is available from central sources such as the *Catalog of Teratogenic Agents* (1), information on occupational and environmental exposures is often available only from government agencies such as the U.S. Environmental Protection Agency (2). The information provided by these agencies can be quite limited, consisting of only permissible emission levels (PELs), maximum concentration limits (MCLs), acceptable daily intakes (ADIs), or some other regulatory number derived from a formal risk assessment. What is a risk assessment? What do the regulatory numbers mean? How can they be used in the risk communications process?

Originally presented as a workshop at the Fifth International Conference of Teratogen Information Services, March 1992.

The material presented in this chapter represents the views of the author, and does not necessarily reflect the policy of the Office of Environmental Health Hazard Assessment.

In this chapter we investigate some of these questions. The intent is not to provide a formula for instant expertise on risk assessments, but rather to broaden the reader's appreciation for how these assessments can be used and misused in counseling concerned individuals. To accomplish this task, we review briefly the basic principles of each of the four steps in the risk assessment process: hazard identification, reference dose determination or dose-response assessment, exposure assessment, and risk characterization (3). After each step has been reviewed, a database of fictional studies on the imaginary chemical AVOID is presented. This database will help illustrate the types of study available for risk assessments and will provide an opportunity to apply the principles of risk assessment to representative data. Finally, questions germane to the evaluation of the AVOID data are listed, and the issues that generate the most controversy are discussed briefly.

HAZARD IDENTIFICATION

Principles

1. The purposes of hazard identification are to identify the types of adverse health effect that may be associated with exposure to an agent and to characterize the quality and strength of evidence supporting this identification. For the purpose of this exercise only developmental (teratogenic) adverse effects induced by AVOID are considered.
2. Human studies are generally considered to be the best source of information, since ultimately it is the human population that we are attempting to protect. Unfortunately, for most chemicals of concern, good human studies are lacking, and even when data do exist, establishing a causal link between the exposure and developmental endpoint is seldom possible. Human developmental studies can generally be divided into two categories, descriptive and analytical (4).
   a. Descriptive studies, which are useful for generating hypotheses, include case reports, surveillance systems, and ecological and cluster studies.
   b. Analytical studies, which test a hypothesis to examine cause-effect relationships, include case control, cohort, and human experimental studies.
3. Studies with experimental animals are often the best source of information for hazard identification. These studies can be either regulatory or experimental.
   a. Regulatory studies are those that are prescribed or recommended by agencies such as the U.S. Environmental Protection Agency and the Food and Drug Administration; they include single and multigeneration reproductive studies, continuous breeding studies, and develop-

mental studies with exposure in the embryonic and fetal periods, or in the perinatal period (5–10). These studies have the advantage of consistent protocols, with full reporting of all the collected data. Unfortunately, they apply to only a limited spectrum of agents, and they are generally not reported in the open scientific literature.

b. Experimental studies are those conducted to investigate a hypothesis of interest to the investigator, and as such, they do not conform to any one protocol. The results of these studies are reported in the open literature and often are your only source of information for hazard identification.

4. In evaluating the individual human and animal studies, several important factors should be taken into consideration.

   a. Exposure parameters such as the route, time, and duration of exposure, and the actual or estimated dose of exposure should be well defined; for animal studies, these should be within the realm of expected human exposures.

   b. The endpoints evaluated should be described, and the methodology used in the evaluation should be appropriate.

   c. The presence of maternal toxicity should be evaluated (11).

   d. Appropriate statistical procedures should be used to demonstrate the significance of the adverse effect (12). For human studies, the strength of the association and study power should be discussed (13–15).

   e. The results should be evaluated for the presence of a dose-response relationship.

   f. The quality of each paper should be assessed using the foregoing considerations.

5. The evaluation of each individual study should lead to one of three conclusions.

   a. The study provides data indicative of an adverse effect.

   b. The study provides data indicative of no adverse effect. For a chemical to be placed in this category, it is essential that the study design be adequate to detect an adverse effect if one is present.

   c. The study provides inconclusive data. The reasons for placing a study in this category are many but usually involve inadequate or inappropriate study designs or incomplete reporting of the data.

6. After the individual studies have been evaluated, it is necessary to assess the total body of evidence. This is usually accomplished by evaluating the animal data separately from the human data. The following factors should be taken into consideration.

   a. Consistent adverse findings in two or more studies that use different study designs and populations are generally regarded as evidence of a causal relationship.

b. The evidence that an agent is a developmental toxicant may be strengthened by demonstrating biological plausibility of a causal relationship. This is an especially important consideration in evaluating a group of epidemiological studies.

c. Pharmacokinetic and pharmacogenetic differences that may account for differences between studies should be evaluated.

d. Structural relationships and other evidence for chemical similarity may in some cases be useful in drawing inferences of potential developmental toxicity.

7. The final step in hazard identification is a weight of evidence determination. Different agencies use different schemes, which range from the very simple to the very complex (16,17). Most of these schemes can be reduced to three basic categories:

a. *Sufficient human evidence*: data from human studies provide sufficient evidence for the scientific community to judge that a causal relationship is or is not supported. Supporting animal data may or may not be available.

b. *Sufficient experimental animal evidence/limited human data*: data from experimental animal studies and/or limited human data that provide sufficient evidence for the scientific community to judge that the potential for developmental toxicity does or does not exist.

c. *Insufficient evidence*: data are not available; or the data that are available are based on human or experimental animal studies that are flawed in design.

Database

Eight studies on AVOID, three in humans and five in animal, make up the database available for the hazard identification step. Each study is briefly summarized below.

Study 1

There have been a series of anecdotal reports from the union health and safety committee at the formulation and packaging facility, as well as from rural health clinics, suggesting that pregnant workers exposed to AVOID experience a high incidence of spontaneous abortions. These reports have not been published or reviewed in any scientific forum.

Study 2

A paper on accidental and purposeful poisoning with AVOID was recently published in a reputable peer-reviewed medical journal. Forty cases were described, and six involved women who were estimated to be in their first trimester of pregnancy at the time of the poisoning. The poisoning was attributed to unsuccessful suicide attempt by AVOID ingestion in five of the cases and to attempted homicide with AVOID-poisoned food in one case. The clinical symptoms recorded at the time of admission to the emergency room for the poisoning, and the pediatrician's evaluation of each newborn in the perinatal period are shown in Table 1.

Study 3

An epidemiological study was conducted in a plant where AVOID was formulated and packaged. The study, which was conducted for the plant owners by investigators from Cosmic University, has never been published. The study population consisted of women who had worked in the packaging section of the plant for at least 6 months between 1981 and 1985. Over this 4-year period, the mean combined dose of AVOID from respiration and dermal absorption was estimated to be less than 0.07 mg/kg/d in the packaging department. The highest combined dose during this same period was estimated at 0.26 mg/kg/d. The control group consisted of female clerical staff who worked in plant offices, where it was assumed that there was no exposure to AVOID. After identifying the study and control populations, the investigators sent each woman a questionnaire regarding any pregnancies she may have had while working at the plant. Included were questions on each respondent's length of time working in the plant, her work location, and the outcome of pregnancy. Response rates to the questionnaire were 37% for the study group, and 42% for the controls. Table 2 gives the major results as reported by the investigative team.

Study 4

In an unpublished study conducted for the manufacturer of AVOID, groups of 20 C57 mated mice were administered AVOID in their diets at doses of

Table 1 Clinical Symptoms and Newborn Evaluations Reported in Study 2

Case	Clinical symptoms	Newborn evaluation
1	Sweating, tremors	Normal physical and growth
2	Sweating, tremors	Normal physical and growth
3	Sweating, tremors	Spina bifida with myeloschisis
4	Sweating, tremors, convulsions	Normal physical; pre- and postnatal growth retardation
5	Sweating, tremors, convulsions	Fetal alcohol syndrome
6	Sweating, tremors, coma	Normal physical and growth

Table 2 Summary of Major Results Reported in Study 3

Group	Study	Control
Respondents	56	48
Pregnancies	110	86
Abortions		
Therapeutic	10 (9%)	1 (1%)
Spontaneous	10 (9%)	9 (10%)
Stillbirths	1 (1%)	0
Live births	89 (81%)	76 (88%)
Normal	85 (96%)	74 (97%)
Abnormal	4 (4%)	2 (3%)
Anencephaly	1	0
Extra finger	1	0
Heart defect	1	1
Holoprosencephaly	1	0
Trisomy 21	0	1

0, 25, or 75 mg/kg/d from days 6–18 of gestation. At the high dose tested there was a significant decrease in maternal food consumption between days 6 and 12, and several of the females exhibited convulsions. Fetal resorptions and exencephaly were significantly increased. At the middose, there was a nonsignificant increase in cleft palate. Major study results are summarized in Table 3.

Table 3 Summary of Major Results Reported in Study 4

	Number of cases per dose (mg/kg/d) group		
	0	25	75
Mated	20	20	20
Pregnant	15	13	20
Resorbed litters	0	0	10[a]
Live litters	15	13	10
Live fetuses	125	99	52[a]
Resorbed fetuses	7	6	37[a]
Abnormal fetuses	4	9	42[a]
Delayed ossification	4	3	7
Cleft palate	1	7	0
Exencephaly	0	0	38[a]
Anophthalmia	0	0	2

[a]Significantly different from control ($p < 0.05$).

Study 5

A meeting abstract reported that groups of five C3H mice administered AVOID by intraperitoneal injection at 5 mg/kg/d on days 10, 11, and 12 of gestation exhibited a significant increase in cleft palate (86%) compared to controls. No mention was made of maternal toxicity or the presence of any other malformations in the treated group.

Study 6

In an unpublished teratology study conducted for the manufacturer of AVOID, groups of 20 pregnant SD rats were administered AVOID in their diets at doses sufficient to provide 0, 0.2, 2.0, or 20 mg/kg/d from days 6–20 of gestation. At the high dose, several females died between days 10 and 18 of gestation; between days 7 and 15, maternal food consumption and weight gain were significantly depressed, and a statistically significant increase in fetal resorptions and exencephaly was noted. At 2.0 mg/kg/d there was a significant increase in microphthalmia and wavy ribs. Wavy ribs were also noted at 0.2 mg/kg/d, but the incidence did not reach statistical significance. The key results of this study are summarized in Table 4.

Study 7

In an unpublished study conducted for the manufacturer, groups of 20 pregnant CR rats were exposed to AVOID by inhalation at doses of 0, 0.16, 0.3, or 0.64 mg/m^3 for 6 hours per day, from days 6–20 of gestation. At the high

Table 4 Summary of Major Results Reported in Study 6

	Number of cases per dose (mg/kg/d) group			
	0	0.2	2.0	20
Mated	20	20	20	20
Pregnant	19	20	18	20
Resorbed litters	1	0	0	6[a]
Live litters	18	20	18	6[a]
Live fetuses	175	182	179	32[a]
Resorbed fetuses	10	5	7	38[a]
Abnormal fetuses	6	13	27[a]	32[a]
Delayed ossification	4	5	3	32[a]
Wavy ribs	4	7	15[a]	5
Exencephaly	1	0	0	29[a]
Microphthalmia	1	0	12[a]	2

[a]Significantly different from controls ($p < 0.05$).

dose there was a slight decrease in maternal food consumption between days 6 and 7 of gestation, and a significant increase in microphthalmia. No significant findings were reported at the other doses tested. The key results of this study are summarized in Table 5.

Study 8

The final animal study was an unpublished report using groups of 20 NZW rabbits administered AVOID by oral gavage at doses of 0, 0.2, 20, or 200 mg/kg/d from days 7–19 of gestation. Maternal toxicity was observed at the high dose, with a significant decrease in body weight and increase in liver weight. At this dose there was also a statistically significant increase in resorptions and exencephaly. No significant findings were reported at any of the other dose levels tested.

Questions to Ask When Evaluating Hazard Identification Data

1. How do these data conform (or not conform) to the principles used in hazard identification?
2. What is the most sensitive endpoint of potential teratogenicity in the animal and in the human studies?
3. Should the wavy ribs in rodents be considered relevant to low exposure risks to humans?
4. Should the data obtained by IP injection treatment be considered relevant to human exposure?

Table 5 Summary of Major Results Reported in Study 7

| | Number of cases per dose (mg/m^3) group | | | |
	0	0.16	0.3	0.64
Mated	20	20	20	20
Pregnant	20	17	17	20
Resorbed litters	1	0	2	0
Live litters	19	17	16	20
Live fetuses	193	180	169	198
Resorbed fetuses	7	9	4	5
Abnormal fetuses	7	10	3	25[a]
Delayed ossification	3	2	3	4
Wavy ribs	7	5	0	3
Microphthalmia	1	4	0	21[a]

[a]Significantly different from controls ($p < 0.05$).

5. Should the evidence for maternal toxicity at high doses in the animal studies negate considering the adverse effects seen in the fetuses as true developmental effects?
6. From the data given, is there any way to determine whether responses in humans are likely to be similar to those of the experimental animals?
7. Do the data provide sufficient evidence to convince you that AVOID should be considered to be a teratogen?

There are no simple or straightforward answers to these questions, and the underlying issues continue to be debated. One area of lively controversy is the role of maternal toxicity in interpreting study results (11,18–20). Can a 20% decrease in maternal weight gain in the early part of organogenesis negate the finding of a high incidence of cleft palate or decreased fetal weight? These issues remain unresolved. Similarly, the importance of skeletal variations such as wavy ribs or partially ossified sternebra remains controversial, and as yet, unresolved (21–23).

At the conclusion of the hazard identification step in the risk assessment process, a choice must be made. It must be decided which of the following conclusions the data support: (1) AVOID is teratogenic in humans; (2) it is highly likely that AVOID is a teratogen in humans; (3) AVOID is a potential human teratogen; or (4) AVOID is not classifiable as to human teratogenicity.

REFERENCE DOSE DETERMINATION

Principles

1. The reference dose (RfD) is defined as an estimate (with uncertainty spanning perhaps an order of magnitude) of a daily exposure to the human population (including sensitive subgroups) that is assumed to be without appreciable risk of deleterious developmental effects (24).
2. The RfD is usually derived from the "no observed adverse effect level" (NOAEL) or the "lowest observed adverse effect level" (LOAEL).
3. The most appropriate NOAEL is determined from the body of evidence examined in the hazard identification stage.
   a. Dose-response data from human studies are generally preferred over animal data, provided the human data are sufficiently quantitative.
   b. Data on the most sensitive relevant endpoint should be used.
4. To calculate the RfD, the NOAEL is divided by an overall uncertainty factor (UF), ranging from 10 to 10,000 (25). The total UF is calculated by multiplying together appropriate individual UFs of 10:
   a. UF for intraspecies variability = 10
   b. UF for interspecies variability = 10

   c. UF for different exposure scenarios = 10

   d. UF when using the LOAEL rather than NOAEL = 10

5. The RfD may be further reduced by applying a modifying factor greater than zero but less or equal to 10, which may be used to reflect qualitative professional judgments about scientific uncertainties such as the completeness of the overall database and the number of species and animals tested.

Database

The data to be used in this section consist of the same eight studies used in the hazard identification step.

Questions to Ask When Evaluating Reference Dose Data

1. What study is the most appropriate for deriving a no observed adverse effect level (NOAEL) for AVOID?
2. What do you consider to be the appropriate NOAEL?
3. Is the observed NOAEL from the studies a true "no-effect" level? Could it simply reflect the fact that in experiments with relatively small numbers, the failure to observe a statistically significant increase in adverse developmental effects is an artifact of the experimental design, not a true absence of biological effect?
4. What uncertainty factors should be applied to the NOAEL for AVOID?
5. What is the appropriate reference dose (RfD) for AVOID?
6. Does the RfD adequately account for the uncertainties associated with the NOAEL?
7. Is it appropriate to use an RfD derived from a study using one route of exposure for all routes of exposure?
8. Is the RfD a reliable indicator of human risk? Are there any other conditions that should be applied to this number?

Again, there are no simple or straightforward answers to these questions. Of greatest controversy is the use of NOAELs and safety factors (26). It is now generally recognized that the determination of a NOAEL is highly dependent on the sample size and dose levels used. Methods using various mathematical models that are less sensitive to sample size and utilize the full dose-response curve have been proposed as alternatives to the NOAEL/UF approach (27–31). No one method has yet gained favor, and the majority of risk assessment still utilize the NOAEL-derived RfD.

After completing the RfD determination step in the risk assessment process, you may conclude that the RfD you calculated, and the NOAEL from which it was derived, are sufficient to determine the developmental risks associated with exposure to AVOID. Alternatively, you may wish to conclude that RfDs are of little value and in fact create a false sense of precision in an area involving tremendous uncertainty. A third possible conclusion is that while risks from developmental toxicants cannot be quantified, they should be described in qualitative terms.

EXPOSURE ASSESSMENT

Principles

1. An exposure assessment serves to identify the magnitude of human exposure to an agent, the frequency and duration of that exposure, and the routes by which humans are exposed (32). It may be useful to identify the number of exposed people along with other characteristics of the exposed population such as age, genetic history, and exposure to (other) known teratogens.
2. Exposure may be based on quantitative or qualitative measurements in various media such as air, water, or food.
   a. Daily intake of individual and combined media exposures should be determined.
   b. When individuals may be exposed by contact with several media, it is important to consider total intake from all media.
   c. Daily intake under different conditions of activities in different locations should be determined.
3. Sampling and monitoring of individual exposures is usually conducted by contractors for either the responsible parties or regulatory bodies.
4. Usually only a limited amount of monitoring, and only a limited number of samples of various media, can be taken for measurement.
   a. The representativeness of measured values is usually uncertain.
   b. The degree to which data for a given medium are representative of that medium should be estimated.
5. When data are incomplete or lacking, mathematical models may be used to estimate air and water concentrations. The validity of the model should be checked in context of the exposure scenario.
6. Standard average values and ranges for human intake of various media are available and are generally used, unless data on specific agents indicate that such values are inappropriate (33).
   a. Adults drink approximately 2 liters of water per day.
   b. The average adult inhales 23 cubic meters of air per day.

Database

Four monitoring studies have been conducted on AVOID: two were conducted in workplace settings, one on air, and one on water. A brief description is provided below.

Study 1

In conjunction with the epidemiology study reported earlier, a 3-day study was conducted in the plant, during which time workers packaging AVOID were monitored for exposure via the inhalation and dermal routes. The data collected were used to estimate the mean combined dose, which was calculated to be 0.07 mg/kg/d. The highest dose received by a single worker on any one day was 0.26 mg/kg.

Study 2

A study was conducted by a state regulatory agency that used passive dosimetry to monitor field worker exposure to AVOID. From the data collected, the absorbed dosage was calculated. The relative contributions of the inhalation and dermal routes of exposure were back-calculated from the total absorbed dosage, assuming that a certain proportion of AVOID exposure was through inhalation. This proportion was based on measured concentrations of AVOID in the air, standard respiratory rate and retention, and 100% absorption. The calculated absorbed exposure dosage for a 70 kg body weight person expressed micrograms per kilogram per day is shown in Table 6.

Study 3

An air monitoring study was conducted in four rural communities near fields where AVOID was being used. Twenty-four-hour collections were conducted over three 4-day periods in 1987. The mean concentrations (ng/m^3) of airborne AVOID over the 12 sampling days, along with the range of values, were published in a reputable peer-reviewed journal and are shown in Table 7.

Study 4

A water monitoring study was conducted using samples collected from the major river that runs through the agricultural area and past several metro-

Table 6   Exposure Levels Reported in Study 2

Workers	Route of exposure	
	Dermal	Inhalation
Pilots	0.50	1.13
Aerial mix/load	0.02	0.53
Flagger	0.53	1.73
Ground mix/load	0.05	0.85
Ground applications	0.02	0.37
Combined mix/load/applications	0.10	1.77
Gofer	0.03	0.70

Table 7 Sampling Results Reported in Study 3

	Location			
	1	2	3	4
Mean	62	132	152	630
Range	2–142	<1.4–280	76–415	145–1720

politan areas downstream. Samples were collected near each of the metropolitan areas, one per month from May through September of 1989. The results of the study, which appear in a government report, indicate that only trace amounts of AVOID were detected. The validity of this study has been challenged by several environmental advocacy groups.

Questions to Ask When Evaluating Exposure Data

1. Do the monitoring data adequately describe exposures to AVOID in all possible media? If not, what additional media need to be considered, and why?
2. Should the different types of exposure data be treated the same for purposes of characterizing human risk?
3. Is the mean concentration in the various media the appropriate summary statistic to use to characterize human exposure? Should the upper range or statistical upper confidence limit be used as an alternative?
4. Are the various assumptions about human intake and average exposure to various media valid?
5. Should exposure and risk to workers at the production facility be considered in the same context as field workers, or residents in exposed communities?

It should come as no surprise that there are no simple or straightforward answers to these questions. Debate continues on the use of various models for estimating exposures, but generally, the issue of greatest concern is the method of extrapolating from one route of exposure to another (34,35). This is typified by the debate over the various routes of exposure following an animal whole-body versus nose-only exposure. With whole-body exposure, it must be decided how much of the agent enters via the respiratory route, how much via the dermal route, and how much via ingestion from grooming behavior and contaminated food. The rates of absorption for these various routes may differ rather dramatically. With nose-only exposures, the majority of the exposure is considered to be respiratory, but dermal adsorption from the nose area and ingestion by swallowing cannot be ruled out.

After the exposure assessment step in the risk assessment process has been completed, you may conclude that although different exposure estimates are based on different data and assumptions, they are all adequate and sufficient for assessing risks. Alternatively, you may wish to conclude that none of the exposure data are adequate for use in risk assessment and that no quantitative risk assessment should be developed until better information is available.

RISK CHARACTERIZATION

Principles

1. The purpose of risk characterization, the final step of the risk assessment, is to integrate the information collected and analyzed in the first three steps to characterize the excess risk to humans.
2. An explicit numerical RfD should be included in the characterization.
3. Compare the exposures experienced or expected for different groups of individuals.
4. Estimate the margin of exposure (MOE) for each group by dividing the NOAEL from the critical study used to estimate the RfD by the exposure for each group.
5. Describe risks qualitatively for each population group.
6. Describe the statistical and biological uncertainties in estimating the extent of adverse health effects.

Database

The data used in the risk characterization step are those accumulated in the preceding steps of the risk assessment process.

The risk characterization can be thought of as the conclusion of the risk assessment, summarizing the information from the preceding steps (hazard identification, RfD determination, and exposure assessment). As such, the issues of controversy discussed earlier also apply to this final step.

CONCLUSION

Having gained some appreciation of risk assessments, we can now consider how they can be used in the risk communication process. Paul Peters (personal communications) has observed that there are two types of risk information: "ready made" and "tailor made." The RfDs developed in the risk assessment process are applicable to all individuals in the population, and as such, represent "ready made" information. They serve as a powerful public health tool in defining the exposure level below which it can be assumed that no adverse developmental effects will occur. In contrast, individual risk counseling requires "tailor made" information. Typically, this information is based on interpreting the results of human and animal studies in the context of a pregnant woman's age, parity, genetic background, and exposure to other chemicals of concern.

The "ready made" information from the risk assessment can have value beyond the public health perspective. While using an RfD as the sole basis for individual risk counseling is never appropriate, the studies that served as the basis for obtaining the NOAEL on which the RfD is based can serve as the starting material for crafting the "tailor made" information needed to communicate risk information to individual pregnant women.

ACKNOWLEDGMENTS

I am indebted to the U.S. Environmental Protection Agency's Workshop on Risk and Decision Making, which served as a model for the workshop on which this chapter is based. I am also grateful to Linda Chernoff and Dr. Paul Peters for their help and insight in planning this project, and to Dr. Gideon Koren for his encouragement to complete the project.

REFERENCES

1. Shepard TH. Catalog of Teratogenic Agents, 6th ed. Johns Hopkins University Press, Baltimore, 1989.
2. U.S. Environmental Protection Agency. Integrated Risk Information Service (IRIS). Online. Office of Health and Environmental Assessment, Washington, DC, 1991.
3. National Research Council. Risk Assessment in the Federal Government: Managing the Process. Committee on the Institutional Means for the Assessment of Risks to Public Health. Commission on Life Sciences, National Research Council. National Academy Press, Washington, DC, 1983, pp 17–83.
4. Erickson JD. Epidemiology and developmental toxicology. In Developmental Toxicology (Kimmel CA, Buelke-Sam J, eds), Raven Press, New York, 1981, pp 289–301.
5. U.S. Environmental Protection Agency. Pesticide assessment guidlines, subdivision F. Hazard evaluation: Human and domestic animals, EPA-540/9-82-025. Office of Pesticides and Toxic Substances, Washington, DC, 1982. Available from NTIS, Springfield, VA.
6. U.S. Environmental Protection Agency. Toxic Substances Control Act test guidelines; final rules. Fed Reg 1985; 50:39426–39428 and 39433–39434.
7. U.S. Environmental Protection Agency. Pesticide Assessment guidelines, subdivision F. Hazard evaluation: Human and domestic animals, EPA 540/09-91-123. Addendum 10: Neurotoxicity, series 81-83. Office of Pesticides and Toxic Substances, Washington, DC, 1991. Available from NTIS, Springfield, VA.

8. Organization for Economic Cooperation and Development. Guidelines for Testing of Chemicals' Teratogenicity. OECD, 1981.
9. U.S. Food and Drug Administration. Guidelines for reproduction and studies for human use. Bureau of Drugs, Rockville, MD, 1966.
10. U.S. Food and Drug Administration. Advisory Committee on Protocols for Safety Evaluation. Panel on reproduction—Studies in the safety evaluation of additives and pesticide residues. Toxicol Appl Pharmacol 1970; 16:264-296.
11. Kimmel GL, Kimmel CA, Francis EZ, eds. Evaluation of maternal and developmental toxicity. Teratogenesis Carcinog Mutagen 1987; 7:203-338.
12. Kimmel CA, Kimmel GL, Frankos V, eds. Interagency Regulatory Liaison Group Workshop on Reproductive Toxicity Risk Assessment. Environ Health Perspect 1986; 86:193-221.
13. Bloom AD. Guidelines for reproductive studies in exposed human populations. Report of Panel II. In Guidelines for Studies of Human Populations Exposed to Mutagenic and Reproductive Hazards (Bloom AD, ed), March of Dimes Birth Defects Foundation, White Plains, NY, 1981, pp 37-110.
14. Stein Z, Kline J, Shrout P. Power in surveillance. In Occupational Hazards and Reproduction (Hemminki K, Sorsa M, Vaninio H, eds). Washington, DC, Hemisphere, 1985, pp 203-208.
15. Greenland S. Quantitative methods in the review of epidemiologic literature. Epidemiol Rev 1987; 9:1-30.
16. U.S. Environmental Protection Agency. Guidelines for developmental toxicity risk assessment. Fed Reg 1991; 56:63798-63826.
17. California Department of Health services. Draft guidelines for hazard identification and dose-response assessment of agents causing developmental and/or reproductive toxicity, 1991. Available from Office of Environmental Health Hazard Assessment, Sacramento, CA.
18. Schardein JL. Approaches to defining the relationship of maternal and developmental toxicity. Teratogenesis Carcinog Mutagen 1987; 7:255-271.
19. Johnson E, Christian M. When is a teratology study not an evaluation of teratogenicity? J Am Coll Toxicol 1984; 3:431-434.
20. Black DL, Marks TA. Role of maternal toxicity in assessing developmental toxicity in animals: A discussion. Regul Toxicol Pharmacol 1992; 16:189-201.
21. Kimmel CA, Wilson JG. Skeletal deviations in rats: Malformations or variations? Teratology 1973; 8:309-316.
22. Chernoff N, Rogers JM, Turner CI, Francis BM. Significance of supernumerary ribs in rodent developmental toxicity studies: Postnatal persistence in rats and mice. Fundam Appl Toxicol 1991; 17:448-453.
23. Palmer AK. Incidence of sporadic malformations, anomalies and variations in random-bred laboratory animals. In Methods in Prenatal Toxicology (Neubert D, Merker HJ, Kwasigroch TE, eds), Thieme, Stuttgart, 1977, pp 52-71.
24. Barnes DG, Dourson M. Reference dose (RfD): Description and use in health risk assessments. Regul Toxicol Pharmacol 1988; 8:471-486.
25. Dourson M, Stara J. Regulatory history and experimental support of uncertainty (safety) factors. Regul Toxicol Pharmacol 1983; 3:224-238.

26. Gaylor DW. Incidence of developmental defects at the no observed adverse effect level (NOAEL). Regul Toxicol Pharmacol 1992; 15:151–160.
27. Crump KS. A new method for determining allowable daily intakes. Fundam Appl Toxicol 1984; 4:854–871.
28. Gaylor DW. Quantitative risk analysis for quantal reproductive and developmental effects. Environ Health Perspect 1989; 79:243–246.
29. Kimmel C, Gaylor D. Issues in qualitative and quantitative risk analysis for developmental toxicology. Risk Anal 1988; 8:15–20.
30. Kodell RL, Howe RB, Chen JJ, Gaylor DW. Mathematical modeling of reproductive and developmental toxic effects for quantitative risk assessment. Risk Anal 1991; 11:583–590.
31. Ryan L. The use of generalized estimating equations for risk assessment in developmental toxicity. Risk Anal 1992; 12:439–447.
32. U.S. Environmental Protection Agency. Guidelines for exposure assessment. Fed Reg 1986; 51:34042–34054.
33. U.S. Environmental Protection Agency. Exposure Factors Handbook, EPA-600/8-89-043. Office of Health and Environmental Assessment, Washington, DC, 1989. Available from NTIS, Springfield, VA.
34. Sachsse K, Zbinden K, Ullman L. Significance of mode of exposure in aerosol inhalation toxicity studies: Head-only versus whole-body exposure. Arch Toxicol Suppl 1980; 4:305–311.
35. Iwasaki M, Yoshida M, Ikeda T, Tsuda S, Shirasu Y. Comparison of whole-body versus snout-only exposure in inhalation toxicity of fenthion. Jpn J Vet Sci 1988; 50:23–30.

3

Teratogenic Drugs and Chemicals in Humans

Gideon Koren and Irena Nulman
The Hospital for Sick Children, Toronto, Ontario, Canada

Clinical Case

A 28-year-old epileptic woman, treated for 6 years with valproic acid, reports amenorrhea of 12 weeks. Pregnancy test is positive, and the patient, who had tried unsuccessfully to conceive for several years, is very happy. What would you advise her?

INTRODUCTION

Since the thalidomide disaster, drugs and chemicals have been scrutinized carefully for their potential human teratogenicity. However, despite valiant efforts in this direction, several objective limitations hinder our ability to detect human teratogens.

1. Most birth defects occur rarely; therefore, even an increased risk posed by a teratogen may not be easily identified. While thalidomide caused more than 20% of major malformations following first-trimester exposure, most suspected teratogens increase the baseline risk of major malformations very slightly (1-3%), even when significantly increasing the risk of a specific pattern. For example, valproic acid increases 200-fold the risk for neural tube defects (NTDs); yet its impact on the overall risk for major malformations is less than 0.5% (1). Consequently, a woman exposed to valproic acid may still have better than a 95% chance of having a healthy baby.

As a result, it may be necessary to study large numbers of infants exposed in utero to a certain drug to prove or disprove its teratogenic potential. Most studies are limited in their statistical power because their numbers are not large enough.

2. For obvious reasons, pharmaceutical manufacturers warn the public not to use drugs in pregnancy owing to a lack of information about their safety. Consequently, the accumulation of data on a specific drug is often sketchy and uncontrolled. While most manufacturers try to record and follow up voluntary reports of exposures in pregnancy, it has to be recognized that such data are incomplete and may be biased. For example, it is conceivable that disproportionately high numbers of families having malformed children will report their drug exposure to the manufacturer or to the regulatory agencies, whereas families with healthy babies are less likely to do so. This tendency was recently documented in a large study on the teratogenicity of retinoic acid: in the prospective section of that cohort, 38% of the infants were malformed, whereas 80% of those reporting retrospectively had major malformations. This means that a large number of families having normal children after first-trimester exposure to retinoic acid did not report voluntarily to either the manufacturer or the Centers for Disease Control (CDC) (2,3).

3. As part of the regulatory process, the teratogenic potential of drugs has to be tested in animals. The failure of animal models to detect the teratogenicity of thalidomide before the human disaster occurred has resulted in a growing feeling that we cannot extrapolate from animal studies to humans. Differences in pharmacokinetics, metabolism, embryology, target organ sensitivity, and other factors may account for such discrepancies. Yet, almost all known human teratogens have been shown to cause similar effects in animals, coumadin being the exception (4). Moreover, in the case of retinoic acid (Accutane), the most potent human teratogen currently available, animal data clearly prevented a postmarketing disaster similar to that of thalidomide (5).

CASE REPORTS

Cases associating in utero exposure to a certain drug or chemical with an adverse outcome may be either most helpful or useless, depending on the following statistical considerations.

In a case of a drug that is rarely used in pregnancy, a small number of cases showing the same pattern of malformation may be most indicative, since these cases may already exceed manyfold the baseline risk for the occurrence of such malformations. For example, if a new drug has been reported to cause 10 cases of cleft palate out of the total 100 known cases of first-trimester exposure, then it has a 10% risk of causing cleft palate. This calculated risk exceeds by 100-fold the known risk of cleft palate, which is 0.1%. Based on this approach, several human teratogens, including coumadins and retinoic acid, were incriminated long before prospective studies confirmed these associations.

At the other extreme, it will be impossible to prove teratogenicity based on case reports when the drug is commonly used (e.g., salicylates) and the malformation is not rare. Salicylates are consumed by thousands of pregnant women every year; therefore, based on statistical chance only, one would expect to find within this group offspring with any described malformation.

Bendectin (the combination of pyridoxin and doxylamine) was for decades one of the most widely used antiemetic drugs to cope with pregnancy-associated morning sickness. The drug was wrongly incriminated as causing congenital malformations based on case reports: hundreds of thousands of pregnant women were exposed to this drug, 1–3% of their offspring would have had major malformations, just because of their baseline risk. Subsequently, controlled studies (both case control and prospective) failed to confirm an association between Bendectin and human teratogenicity; however, the American manufacturer withdrew the drug from the market owing to excessive insurance costs (see Chapter 32). In Canada, this antiemetic is available under the trade name Diclectin, and recently the Canadian Health Protection Branch has specifically labeled it as an antiemetic appropriate for use in pregnancy.

EPIDEMIOLOGICAL STUDIES

Several approaches are commonly employed in studying the potential reproductive effects of drugs and chemical.

The retrospective study tries to identify women exposed in pregnancy to the drug in question and to evaluate the outcome of the exposed offspring. A variety of methodological problems may complicate the interpretation of such data.

It may not be possible to identify and assess all cases, and it is conceivable that cases with an adverse outcome will be overrepresented. For example, the Danish lithium registry is a voluntary reporting system of exposure to the drug in pregnancy. Of its 300 cases reported by 1983, about 10% represented cardiac malformation; however, it is probable that parents of healthy babies born after such exposures had less motivation to report to the registry than those with an adverse outcome (6).

Another major disadvantage of such cohorts, owing to the rare occurrence of most congenital anomalies, is the need for very large numbers of individuals exposed to the drug. To overcome this shortcoming, the case control study focuses on offspring with a specific malformation and tries to assess maternal exposure to the drug in question. The percentage of maternal use is then compared to a group of mothers of infants not having the tested malformation. A major problem with all retrospective studies, both cohorts and case control, is the need to rely on maternal recall of drug exposure (i.e., time and dose). In a recent study, mothers we had interviewed first at the time of their exposure in pregnancy tended not to remember significant parts of this information when questioned again after giving birth

(7). Mitchell has significantly improved the reliability of case control studies by developing questionnaires that reduce the effect of maternal recall characteristic of the previously used open-ended questionnaires (8).

In prospective studies, the information about exposure and other possible pregnancy risk factors is collected at the time of exposure or soon after it. Although this is likely to be the most accurate approach to assess potential teratogenicity, such studies are lengthy and costly because very large numbers of test subjects are needed to overcome the rareness of most congenital malformations.

Whereas full discussion of methodological problems associated with each approach is beyond the scope of this chapter, it is clear that proving the teratogenicity of a specific drug in humans may be a complex process, demanding a high degree of scrutiny. In many cases evidence is accumulated through several different approaches (e.g., case reports, case control, and prospective studies).

The combination of increased awareness to human teratogenicity with the above-mentioned difficulties in differentiating normal background from slightly increased rates of malformations has led to unjustified incrimination of useful medications, which were later found out to be nonteratogenic. These include oral contraceptive hormones, diazepam, Bendectin, and spermicides. Typically, a devastating potential, as reflected above in the case of Bendectin, may result from wrong incrimination of a nonteratogen, as many women may terminate an otherwise wanted pregnancy.

Presently, it is felt that several criteria must be met before an agent is incriminated as a human teratogen (9):

An abrupt increase in the frequency of a particular defect or association of defects (syndrome)

Coincidence of this increase with a known environmental change, such as widespread use of a new drug or sudden exposure to a chemical

Known exposure to the environmental change early in pregnancy yielding characteristically defective infants

Absence of other factors common to all pregnancies yielding infants with the characteristic defect(s)

COUNSELING WOMEN ABOUT KNOWN TERATOGENS

Table 1 presents details of drugs and chemicals known to be teratogenic in humans with a major reference for each.

When a clinician confronts an exposure of a pregnant patient to a known teratogen, it is important to convey the available information to the family in a way that will prevent both understatements and ambiguity. An accurate estimate of the risk for an adverse outcome should be provided because pregnant women tend to have an unrealistically high perception of teratogenic risk even when exposed to nonteratogens (see Chapter 29).

Table 1 Drugs and Chemicals Proven to Be Teratogenic in Humans

Drug/chemical	Fetal adverse effects	Relative risk for teratogenicity	Clinical intervention	Ref.
Alcohol	*Fetal alcohol syndrome:* mental retardation, microcephaly, poor coordination, hypotonia, hyperactivity, short upturned nose, micrognathia or retrognathia (infancy) or prognathia (adolescence), short palpebral fissures, hypoplastic philtrum, thinned upper lips, microphthalmia, antenatal/postnatal growth retardation, occasional pathologies of eyes, mouth, heart, kidneys, gonads, skin, muscle, and skeleton	In alcoholic women consuming above 2 g/kg/d ethanol over first trimester: two- to threefold higher risk for congenital malformations (about 10%).	To calculate accurate dose of alcohol: *Prospective:* to discontinue exposure; if woman is alcoholic, refer to addiction center *During pregnancy:* to alleviate fears in mild or occasional drinkers who may terminate pregnancy based on unrealistic perception of risk, level 2 ultrasound to rule out visible malformation	10
				11,12
Alkylating agents (busulfan, chlorambucil, cyclophosphamide, mechlorethamine)	Growth retardation, cleft palate, microphthalmia hypoplastic ovaries, cloudy corneas, agenesis of kidney, malformations of digits, cardiac defects, multiple other anomalies.	Based on case reports, between 10 and 50% of cases were malformed for different drugs. It is possible that adverse outcome was overrepresented.	Level 2 ultrasound to rule out visible malformations. Supplement folic acid to women receiving antifolates (e.g., methotrexate).	4

Table 1 Continues

Table 1 Continued

Drug/chemical	Fetal adverse effects	Relative risk for teratogenicity	Clinical intervention	Ref.
Antimetabolite agents (aminopterin azauridine, cytarabine, 5-FU, 6-MP, methotrexate)	Hydrocephalus, meningoencephalocele, anencephaly, malformed skull, cerebral hypoplasia, growth retardation, eye and ear malformations, malformed nose and cleft palate, malformed extremities and fingers	Based on case reports 7–75% of cases were malformed. It is possible that adverse outcome was overrepresented.	Level 2 ultrasound to rule out visible malformations	4
	Aminopterin syndrome: Cranial dysostosis, hydrocephalus, hypertelorism, anomalies of external ear, micrognathia, posterior cleft palate			13
Carbamazepine	Increased risk for neural tube defects (NTDs)	NTDs estimated at 1% with carbamazepine.	Periconceptional folate; maternal and/or amniotic α-fetoprotein; ultrasound to rule out NTD.	14
Carbon monoxide	Cerebral atrophy, mental retardation, microcephaly, convulsions, spastic disorders, intrauterine or postnatal death	Based on case reports, when mother is severely poisoned, high risk for neurological sequelae; no increased risk in mild accidental exposures.	Measure maternal carboxyhemoglobin levels. Treat with 100% oxygen for 5 h after maternal carboxyhemoglobin returns to normal because fetal equilibration takes longer. If hyperbaric chamber available, should be used, as elimination $T_{1/2}$ of CO is more rapid.	15–16

Coumadins	*Fetal warfarin syndrome:* nasal hypoplasia, chondrodysplasia punctata, branchydactyly, skull defects, abnormal ears, malformed eyes, CNS malformations, microcephaly, hydrocephaly, skeletal deformities, mental retardation, optic atrophy, spasticity, Dandy Walker malformations	16% of exposed fetuses have malformations; another 3% hemorrhages; 8% stillbirths.	Fetal monitoring by an obstetrician; sonographic follow-up. *Prospective:* switch to heparin for the first trimester. Deliver by a cesarean section. Women should be followed up in a high-risk perinatal unit.	17
Diethylstilbestrol (DES)	*Female offspring:* clear cell vaginal or cervical adenocarcinoma in young female adults exposed in utero (before 18th week): irregular menses (oligomenorrhea), reduced pregnancy rates, increased rate of preterm deliveries, increased perinatal mortality and spontaneous abortion *Male offspring:* cysts of epididymis, cryptorchidism, hypogonadism, diminished spermatogenesis	Exposure before 18 weeks of gestation: ≤1.4/1000 of exposed female with carcinoma. Congenital morphological changes in vaginal epithelium in 39% of exposures.	*Diagnosis:* direct observation of mucosa and Shiller's test. *Treatment:* mechanical excision or destruction in relatively confined area. Surgery and radiotherapy for diffused tumor.	18

Table 1   Continues

Table 1 Continued

Drug/chemical	Fetal adverse effects	Relative risk for teratogenicity	Clinical intervention	Ref.
Lead	Lower scores in developmental tests	Higher risk when maternal lead is above 10 μg/dL.	*Maternal lead levels > 10 μg/dL:* investigate for possible source of contamination. *Levels > 25 μg/dL:* consider chelation.	19
Lithium carbonate	Possibly higher risk for Ebstein's anomaly; no detectable higher risk for other malformations		Women who need lithium should continue therapy, with sonographic follow-up. Patients may need higher doses because of increased clearance rate.	6
Methyl mercury, mercuric sulfide	Microcephaly, eye malformations, cerebral palsy, mental retardation, malocclusion of teeth	Women of affected babies consumed 9–27 ppm mercury; greater risk when ingested at 6–8 gestational months. Relative risk was not elucidated, but 13/220 babies born in Minamata, Japan, at time of contamination had severe disease.	Good correlation between mercury concentrations in maternal hair follicles and neurological outcome of the fetus. Hair mercury content above 50 ppm was used successfully as a cut point for termination. In acute poisoning, the fetus is 4–10 times more sensitive than the adult to methylmercury toxicity.	20,21
PCBs	*Stillbirth* *Signs at birth:* white eye discharge, 30% (32/108); teeth present, 8.7% (11/127); irritated/swollen	4% (6/159)–20% (8/39)	These figures, which are from cases poisoned by high consumption of PCB-contaminated rice oil, cannot be extrapolated to cases in which	22

	Findings	Risk/comments	Recommendations	Ref
	gums, 11% (11/99); hyperpigmentation ("cola" staining), 42.5% (54/127); deformed/small nails, 24.6% (30/122); acne, 12.8% (16/125) *Subsequent history:* bronchitis or pneumonia, 27.2% (30/124); chipped or broken teeth, 35.5% (38/107); hair loss, 12.2% (14/115); acne scars, 9.6% (11/115); generalized itching, 27.8% (32/1150) *Developmental:* do not meet milestones lower scores than unexposed controls evidence of CNS damage		maternal poisoning has not been verified. Women working near PCBs (e.g., hydroelectric facilities) should use effective protection.	
Penicillamine	Skin hyperelastosis	Few case reports; risk unknown.		23
Phenytoin	*Fetal hydantoin syndrome:* low nasal bridge, inner epicanthal folds, ptosis, strabismus, hypertelorism, low set or abnormal ears, wide mouth, large fontanels, anomalies and hypoplasia of distal phalanges and nails, skeletal abnormalities, micro-	5–10% of typical syndrome; about 30% of partial picture. Relative risk of 7 for offspring IQ ≤ 84 (see Chapter 4)	Neurologist should consider changing to other medications. Keep phenytoin concentrations at lower effective levels. Level 2 ultrasound to rule out visible malformations. Vitamin K to neonate. Epilepsy itself increases teratogenic risk.	24,25

Table 1 Continues

Table 1 Continued

Drug/chemical	Fetal adverse effects	Relative risk for teratogenicity	Clinical intervention	Ref.
Phenytoin (continued)	cephaly and mental retardation, growth deficiency, neuroblastoma, cardiac defects, cleft palate/lip			
Systemic retinoids (isotretinoin, etretinate)	Spontaneous abortions; deformities of cranium, ears, face, heart, limbs, liver; hydrocephalus, microcephalus, heart defects Cognitive defects even without dysmorphology	For isotretinoin: 38% risk: 80% of malformations are CNS.	Treated women should have an effective method of contraception. Pregnancy termination. If diagnosed too late, sonographic follow-up to rule out confirmed malformations.	2
Trimethadione	*Fetal trimethadione syndrome:* intrauterine growth retardation, cardiac anomalies,	Based on case reports: 83% risk; 32% infantile or neonatal death.	No need for this antiepileptic to date.	26

Drug	Effects	Risk	Comment	Ref
Thalidomide	microcephaly, cleft palate and lip, abnormal ears, dysmorphic face, mental retardation, tracheoesophageal fistula, postnatal death Limb phocomelia, amelia, hypoplasia, congenital heart defects, renal malformations, cryptorchidism, abducens paralysis, deafness, microtia, anotia	About 20% risk when exposure to drug occurs in days 34–50 of gestation.	Thalidomide is an effective drug for some forms of leprosy. Treated women should have an effective mode of contraception.	27
Tetracycline	Yellow, gray-brown, or brown staining of deciduous teeth destruction of enamel	From 4 months of gestation and on, occurs in 50% of fetuses exposed to tetracycline: 12.5% to oxytetracycline	If exposure before 14–16 weeks of gestation, no known risk.	28
Valproic acid	Lumbosacral spina bifida with meningomyelocele; CNS defects, microcephaly, cardiac defects	1.2% risk of neural tube defects.	Level 2 ultrasound and maternal α-fetoproteins or amniocentesis to rule out neural tube defects. Epilepsy itself increases teratogenic risk.	1

In the Motherisk Program, we find that the same estimated risk may be unacceptably high for some families, and reasonable for others. For example, epileptic women who are well controlled with phenytoin and have failed to have their epilepsy controlled with other anticonvulsants are often reluctant to change their medication in pregnancy. Conversely, we recently consulted the mother of three healthy children who was treated briefly with phenytoin following a single seizure. When it became apparent that she was pregnant again, an electroencephalogram was taken. The results were normal, and it was planned to discontinue the drug. For this patient, the teratogenic risk of phenytoin was perceived as unacceptable.

Not included in Table 1 are scores of drugs that cause direct fetal toxicity consistent with their pharmacological effects. These are detailed in Chapter 13.

Proven human teratogens are by no means a homogeneous group of compounds; however, they can be divided by several criteria into subgroups.

Obsolete Drugs

Diethylstilbestrol and trimetadion are currently unlikely to create a problem in pregnancy because they are not used clinically. Thalidomide, which was banned after the disaster three decades ago, is an important drug for some forms of leprosy. It is presently used in South America for leprosy in women who receive infectable forms of contraceptive hormone. However, recently there have been reports of a new wave of malformed children due to inappropriate use. Retinoic acid, which bears a rate of teratogenicity similar to that of thalidomide, is widely used, mostly for the treatment of cystic acne in adolescents and young adults, who are the most likely group to fail contraceptives. In fact, the U.S. Food and Drug Administration (FDA) is reevaluating conflicting reports on the number of pregnancies and birth defects associated with retinoic acid in order to decide the future of this drug in the American market.

Existence of Alternative Therapy

Several teratogenic drugs may have value as alternative therapies in pregnancy; however, each case is characterized by unique problems.

Although there are alternatives to lithium carbonate (e.g., tricyclics) for manic-depressive disorders, some patients may not respond to favorably replacement drugs. Moreover, recent evidence suggests lithium to be safe during pregnancy (6). The same argument is valid for phenytoin and valproic acid, and in each case the physician caring for the woman planning pregnancy should evaluate other alternatives. Heparin, which does not cross the placenta, may substitute coumadin during the first trimester; the former has to be injected, however, and compliance may become a major problem.

From a pharmacological standpoint, very few human teratogens do not have an alternative drug: retinoic acid, however, appears to be very efficacious in complicated types of acne, and no other compound shares the same mechanisms of action. This is a strong argument in favor of not removing the drug from the market despite its known teratogenic risk—thousands of patients would be deprived of an irreplaceable therapy. Clearly, this drug is completely contraindicated in pregnancy.

Alkylating agents and antimetabolites (azathioprine, chlorambucil, etc.) represent a specific therapy that may need to be continued uninterrupted. Their main teratogenic effects are associated with first-trimester exposure; current analysis done by us in Toronto reveals that in most cases when cancer is diagnosed in early pregnancy, the women choose to terminate the pregnancy. However, to date there is increasing use of some of these agents in collagen diseases, nephritis, and postorgan transplants, and it is likely that the number of women seeking prospective advice on these drugs will increase.

Magnitude of the Public Health Issue

Alcohol is undoubtedly the most common human teratogen. Because 10 million Americans are alcoholics, large numbers of fetuses are exposed to the amount of alcohol associated with the fetal alcohol syndrome (FAS). It has been estimated that one baby in every 2500 live births has FAS, which means 1600 new cases in the United States per year (10). Clearly the number of consumers of this teratogen is several orders of magnitude larger than for any other teratogenic compound. With increasing public awareness of the adverse fetal outcome associated with alcohol, many women and families fear the potential adverse effects of alcohol consumed before conception was realized, even when much smaller amounts than that associated with FAS are involved. Although there is some preliminary evidence of a dose-response relationship of alcohol teratogenicity in humans (11), even two drinks a day during embryogenesis has not been associated with increased morphological or developmental risks (12). The problem of verifying the degree of drinking is major. Recently, for example, we documented that women who have had an adverse outcome of their pregnancy tend to decrease the amount of alcohol reported postnatally compared to their initial report during pregnancy (7).

Phenytoin is undoubtedly another drug which through its common use creates a public health issue. It has been estimated by Hanson et al. (22) that between 5 and 10% of fetuses exposed in utero to the drug will exhibit the full picture of fetal hydantoin syndrome (FHS). Since 0.5% of pregnant women are epileptic, and about half of them are treated with phenytoin, the rate of FHS should be somewhere between 0.019% and 0.025% of births (23). This means that with an annual birthrate of 4 million in the United States, every year between 500 and 1000 newborns suffer from this serious syndrome.

Retinoic acid, evolving as a commonly used drug for acne in young adults, has the potential of becoming a similar public health issue, if not a worse one. However, no peer-reviewed data have been published on the number of pregnancies occurring while women are being treated with Accutane. Unlike phenytoin, which may be essential in pregnancy, the use of retinoic acid is absolutely contraindicated in pregnancy, and treatmeı.t of acne can be postponed without risk to the mother.

Environmental Contamination

The common denominator of methyl mercury, carbon monoxide, and polychlorinated biphenyls (PCBs) is that their human teratogenic effect has been shown only following maternal exposure to excessive amounts. Extrapolation from these exposures to the background amounts of carbon monoxide or PCBs in the environment is not justified. Yet, because the lower part of the dose-response curves has not been described, it is possible that moderate exposure may have clinical implications: heavy smokers, for example, have a carboxyhemoglobin level of 10% and even more; such levels have been shown to be associated with lower birth weights, and according to preliminary reports, with a less favorable developmental outcome (29).

Environmental lead may differ from the compounds above; recent studies suggest adverse developmental effects even with levels within the subtoxic range (above 10 μg/dL but below 25 μg/dL) (19).

Answer

Valproic acid causes neural tube defects (NTDs) in about 2% of first-trimester exposures. Maternal α-fetoproteins and ultrasound at 16 weeks of gestation are accepted as the screening test. Positive cases are tested by determinations of amniotic fluid α-fetoproteins. With these diagnostic means, NTDs are detected in almost 100% of cases.

REFERENCES

1. Fabro S, Brown NA, Scialli AR. Valproic acid and birth defects. Reprod Toxicol 1983; 2:9–11.
2. Lammer EJ, Chen DT, Hoar RM, et al. Retinoic acid embryopathy. N Engl J Med 1985; 313:837–841.
3. Koren G. Retinoic acid embryopathy. N Engl J Med 1986; 315:262.
4. Schardein J. Chemically Induced Birth Defects. Marcel Dekker, New York, 1985.
5. Rosa FW, Wilk AL, Kelsey FO. Vitamin A congeners. In Teratogen Update (Sever JL, Brent RL, eds), Liss, New York, 1986, pp 61–70.

6. Jacobson SJ, Jones K, Johnson K, et al. A prospective multicenter study of pregnancy outcome following lithium exposure during the first trimester of pregnancy. Lancet 1992; 339:530-533.
7. Feldman Y, Koren G, Mattice D, Shear H, Pellegrini E, MacLeod SM. Determinants of recall and recall bias in studying drug effects in pregnancy. Teratology 1989; 40:37-46.
8. Mitchell AE, Cottler LB, Shapiro S. Effect of questionnaire design on recall of drug exposure in pregnancy. Am J Epidemiol 1986; 123:670-676.
9. Wilson JG. Environmental and Birth Defects. Academic Press, New York, 1973, p 58.
10. Rosett HZ, Weiner L. Alcohol and the Fetus. Oxford University Press, New York, 1984.
11. Graham JM, Hanson JW, Darby BL, Barr HM, Streissguth AP. Independent dysmorphology evaluation at birth and 4 years of age for children exposed to varying amounts of alcohol in utero. Pediatrics 1988; 81:772-778.
12. Mills JL, Graubard BI. Is moderate drinking during pregnancy associated with an increased risk of malformations? Pediatrics 1987; 80:309-314.
13. Emerson DJ. Congenital malformations due to attempted abortion with aminopterin. Am J Obstet Gynecol 1982; 84:356-357.
14. Rosa FW. Spina bifida in infants of women treated with carbamazepine during pregnancy. N Engl J Med 1991; 324:674-676.
15. Longo LD. The biological effects of carbon monoxide on the pregnant woman, fetus and newborn infant. Am J Obstet Gynecol 1977; 129:69-103.
16. Koren G, Sharav T, et al. A multicenter prospective study of reproductive outcome following carbon monoxide poisoning in pregnancy. Reprod Toxicol 1991; 5:397-403.
17. Iturbe-Alessio J, Fonseca MDC, Mutchiniko Santos MA, Zafarias A, Salazar E. Risks of anticoagulant therapy in pregnant women with artificial heart valve. N Engl J Med 1986; 315:1390-1393.
18. Herbst AL, Uffelder H, Posbanzer DC. Adenocarcinoma of the vagina. Association of maternal stilbestrol therapy with tumor appearance in young girls. N Engl J Med 1971; 284:878-881.
19. Bellinger D, et al. Longitudinal analyses of prenatal and postnatal lead exposure and early cognitive development. N Engl J Med 1987; 316:1037-1043.
20. Amin-Zakil, Majeed MA, Greenwood MR, El Hassani SB, Clarkson TW, Doherty DA. Methylmercury poisoning in the Iraqi suckling infant: A longitudinal study over five years. J Appl Toxicol 1981; 1:210-214.
21. Harada M. Congenital Minamata disease: Intrauterine methyl mercury poisoning. Teratology 1978; 18:285-288.
22. Rogan WJ, Gladen BC, Kun-Long H, Koong SL, Shih LY, Taylor JS, Wu YC, Yang D, Ragan B, Hsu CC. Congenital poisoning by polychlorinated biphenyls and their contaminants in Taiwan. Science 1988; 241:334-336.
23. Rosa FW. Teratogen update: Penicillamine. Teratology 1986; 22:127-131.
24. Ehrenbard LT, Chaganti RSK. Cancer in the fetal hydantoin syndrome. Lancet 1981; 2:97.

25. Hansen JW. Fetal hydantoin syndrome. Teratology 1976; 13:185–188.
26. Goldman AS, Zachai EH, Yaffe SJ. Fetal trimethadione syndrome. Teratology 1978; 17:103–106.
27. Newman CGH. Clinical aspects of thalidomide embryopathy—A continuing preoccupation. Teratology 1985; 32:133–144.
28. Cohlan SQ. Tetracycline staining of the teeth. Teratology 1977; 15:127–130.
29. Sexton MJ, Fox NL, Hebel JR. The effects of neonatal exposure to tobacco on behavioral outcomes in three-year-old children. Teratology 1988; 37:491.

4

The Effects of Phenytoin and Carbamazepine Monotherapy on Infants' Development

Dennis Scolnik, Irena Nulman, Joanne Rovet, Deborah Czuchta Altmann, Thomas R. Einarson, and Gideon Koren
The Hospital for Sick Children, Toronto, Ontario, Canada

H. Allen Gardner
Oshawa General Hospital, Oshawa, Ontario, Canada

David Gladstone
University of Toronto, Toronto, Ontario, Canada

Richard Gladstone
North York Medical Arts Building, Willowdale, Ontario, Canada

Peter Ashby
Toronto Hospital, Western Division, Toronto, Ontario, Canada

Clinical Case

An epileptic woman treated for many years with phenytoin wishes to know whether the bad things she has heard about the drug in pregnancy are right and if yes, what to do.

INTRODUCTION

Maternal epilepsy has been associated with offspring malformation rates higher than those found in the general population (1). While it is generally agreed that women at risk of seizures during pregnancy should be treated with effective antiepileptic therapy, several drugs commonly used in epilepsy have been documented to be human teratogens. In 1976 Hanson and Smith described the fetal hydantoin syndrome (FHS), characterized by major malformations and developmental delay, in babies exposed in utero to phenytoin (DPH) (2). The exact rate of this syndrome among babies exposed to the

49

drug is not known, but it has been estimated to be between 6 and 30% (3). However, children with phenotypic characteristics of FHS have been also reported in untreated epileptics and also in some women using barbiturates (1). Valproic acid, a potent antiepileptic drug, has been documented to cause neural tube defects in an estimated 2% of exposed fetuses (4).

During the last two decades, carbamazepine (CBZ) has been documented to be an effective antiepileptic agent for seizures of various types. Preliminary reports of its use in pregnancy were controversial, with both no (5,6) and adverse (7) fetal effects described. However, similar to studies with phenytoin, these reports were not controlled for a variety of confounders that may affect pregnancy outcome. In recent consensus guidelines (8) the participants could not define, based on available data, which of the four major antiepileptics (DPH, CBZ, valproate, and phenobarbital) is the most teratogenic.

The assessment of risk/safety of antiepileptic drugs in pregnancy is complicated by a variety of issues. It has been suggested that even when not exposed to medication, babies of mothers with epilepsy have higher rates of malformations than the general population (1,3). Moreover, mothers with epilepsy are often treated with more than one medication, and there is evidence that fetuses exposed to polytherapy have higher rates of malformations (1). In addition, assessments of neurobehavioral outcome often fail to control for such determinants as maternal IQ, socioeconomic status (SES), and age, which may affect offspring outcome (9). Any comparison between children of mothers exposed to an antiepileptic medication and children in a control group must therefore address the potential impact of such confounders. The present study is aimed at prospectively comparing pregnancy outcome of either phenytoin or carbamazepine monotherapy to the general population with particular emphasis on cognitive function of offspring.

PATIENTS AND METHODS

The protocol was approved by the Human Subject Review Committee of The Hospital for Sick Children in Toronto. The study groups were comprised of panels of prospectively collected pregnant women treated with either phenytoin (DPH) or carbamazepine (CBZ) monotherapy and their offspring born after these pregnancies. The women were recruited either by the Motherisk Program, by neurologists at North York General Hospital and the Toronto Hospital (Western Division), or by Genetic Services, Oshawa General Hospital. In these participating centers, all women prospectively collected (i.e., before the outcome of the index pregnancy was known) were followed, even in the few cases of women who moved from the Toronto area (see below).

The following details were recorded for each woman: age, medical and obstetric history, clinical diagnoses, last menstrual period, time and dose of the antiepileptic drug before and during pregnancy, and cigarette smoking and alcohol drinking before and during pregnancy. Serum concentrations of either DPH or CBZ were recorded whenever available. Details on pregnancy course, mode of delivery, and pregnancy outcome were retrieved from the medical records. Birth weight, neonatal course and complications, and attainment of developmental milestones were obtained by interviewing the mothers and by a report from the children's pediatricians.

Each mother exposed to DPH or CBZ was matched by age (± 4 years), gravidy (± 1), parity (± 1), and socioeconomic status (± 2 points on Hollingshead scale) (10) to the next woman attending our clinic for counseling following gestational exposure to nonteratogens (e.g., penicillins, acetaminophen), thus ensuring similar ages of the offspring. Women attending the Motherisk Clinic are advised during the consultation that we may wish to study them and their offspring postnatally, and a letter explaining this goal is sent to their physicians. All studies described above for women and children exposed to DPH and CBZ were performed on the control mother-child pairs.

Between January 1991 and March 1992 all but three participating mothers and their children were studied in our laboratory by a team comprised of pediatricians, neurologists, psychometrists, and a psychologist. Complete physical and neurological examination of the children was performed, followed by neurobehavioral testing of both mothers and offspring. Maternal IQ was assessed by the Wechsler Adult Intelligence Scale (revised) (11). Socioeconomic status was assessed by Hollingshead Four-Factor Index of Social Status (10). In three cases, mothers residing originally in Toronto who later moved to other Canadian cities were located by us; these women and their children were tested in a similar protocol by physicians and psychologists in their respective areas.

Children between 18 and 30 months of age were tested using the Bayley Scales of Infant Development (12) and above that age with the McCarthy Scales (13). All children were tested also with the Reynell Developmental Language Scales (14). The three psychometrists who performed the evaluations were blinded to the nature of maternal illness, to drug therapy, and to the assignment of the mother-child pairs to the study or control groups, as was the psychologist who oversaw and supervised the assessment.

STATISTICAL ANALYSIS

Women and their offspring exposed to either DPH or CBZ were compared to their matched controls in a large number of values using the Student's *t*-test for paired data or the chi-square test whenever appropriate. Subsequently, we also performed multivariate analysis to verify whether children's global IQ was affected by a possible confounder (maternal age, IQ, SES) or only by prenatal exposure to DPH. Correlations between values were studied by least-squares regression analysis. Data are reported as mean plus or minus standard deviation.

Sample Size Considerations

The primary endpoint of our study was children's global developmental quotient measured by the Bayley MDI or McCarthy GCI. Power analysis indicated that to detect an 8-point decrease (0.5 SD) in IQ of children exposed to DPH or CBZ compared to their matched controls with power of 80% and α of 0.05, a sample size of 30 would be needed for each group.

RESULTS

A total of 36 mother-child pairs exposed to CBZ and 34 exposed to DPH were studied and compared to an equal number of matched controls. All women treated with DPH had epilepsy except for one, who was receiving the drug for postcraniotomy prophylaxis. Six women in the CBZ group were not epileptic and were treated with the drug for other conditions (bipolar affective disorder, $n = 3$; glossopharyngeal neuralgia, $n = 1$; trigeminal neuralgia, $n = 1$; postcraniotomy prophylaxis, $n = 1$). None of the women in either group received concomitantly any other antiepileptic drugs during the index pregnancy. All women were treated with DPH or CBZ during the first trimester; 29 women took DPH throughout pregnancy and 30 women continued CBZ. Most women on either DPH ($n = 27$) or CBZ ($n = 26$) were treated for generalized tonic clonic seizures. A few were treated for partial complex seizures (7 DPH and 2 CBZ), or petit mal (4 DPH and 2 CBZ).

Mothers using DPH or CBZ were similar to their matched controls in a large number of characteristics, including age at conception, gravity, parity, number of miscarriages, and proportions of women smoking cigarettes and consuming alcohol. None of these women drank heavily or smoked more than 10 cigarettes per day. Similarly, they had comparable scores of IQ and of Hollingstead Four-Factor Index of Social Status (Table 1). The mean maternal dose of DPH was 346 $\pm$ 97 mg/d, (5.9 $\pm$ 1.9 mg/kg/d) and of CBZ 531 $\pm$ 268 mg/d, (8.9 $\pm$ 4.7 mg/kg/d). Of the 34 offspring exposed to DPH, 20 were males and 14 females; in their matched control groups there were 18 boys and 16 girls [not significant (NS)]. Of the 36 offspring exposed to CBZ, there were 17 males and 19 females; their controls comprised of 20 males and 16 females (differences NS).

Table 1 Maternal Characteristics: Comparison of Women Exposed to DPH Versus Their Controls, and Women Exposed to CBZ and Their Controls

	DPH	DPH-control	CBZ	CBZ-control
Age at conception, y	27.2 ± 4	27.3 ± 4	30.2 ± 5	30.3 ± 5
Gravida	1.8 ± 0.9	1.7 ± 0.8	2.2 ± 1.0	2.3 ± 1.3
Parity	0.6 ± 0.7	0.3 ± 0.5	0.8 ± 0.9	0.8 ± 0.9
Number of miscarriages	0.2 ± 0.5	0.3 ± 0.5	0.24 ± 0.5	0.4 ± 0.9
Maternal IQ	90 ± 12.2	93.9 ± 11.4	96.5 ± 14	96 ± 14.5
SES, total score	40.8 ± 13	40.9 ± 13.8	44.7 ± 14.6	46.1 ± 12.9
Daily dose, mg/kg/d	5.9 ± 1.9		8.9 ± 4.7	

Offspring exposed to DPH or CBZ were similar to their controls in a large number of neonatal and infancy characteristics, including gestational ages, birth weights, and proportions of modes of delivery (Table 2), as well as neonatal course and time of attainment of developmental milestones according to the Denver Scale (data not shown).

Of the 34 children exposed to DPH, 21 had the Bayley test and 13 the McCarthy test, as dictated by their ages. Of the 36 children exposed to CBZ, 28 had the Bayley test and 8 the McCarthy test. The matched control children had the same tests as the study cases. Children exposed in utero to DPH

Table 2 Comparison of Offspring Characteristics: Children Exposed to DPH or CBZ Versus Their Matched Controls

	DPH	DPH-control	CBZ	CBZ-control
Gestational age, wk	40 ± 1.9	39.6 ± 1.6	39 ± 2.5	39.6 ± 1.4
Birth weight, y	3526 ± 592	3374 ± 519	3427 ± 685	3290 ± 575
Mode of delivery				
Normal vaginal	16	15	21	22
Complex vaginal[a]	8	7	5	7
Cesarean section	10	12	10	7
Major malformations	2[b]	0	2[c]	1[d]
Major perinatal	3[e]	5[f]	4[g]	5[h]

[a]Forceps, vacuum.
[b]Cleft palate and hypospadias (1); last joint of right index finger missing and nail hypoplasia (1).
[c]Hypospadias (1); meningomyelocele and hydrocephalus (1).
[d]Pulmonary atresia (1).
[e]Pulmonary atresia and fetal distress (3).
[f]Fetal distress (5).
[g]Fetal distress (4); adrenal bleeding (1); pneumothorax (1).
[h]Fetal distress (4); meconium aspiration (1).

had a significantly lower mean score of global IQ than their controls. A similar trend emerged when the children tested by the Bayley test and those tested with McCarthy test were looked at separately (Bayley 113 ± 13 vs. 103 ± 17; McCarthy 117 ± 12 vs. 100 ± 33). Conversely, children exposed in utero to CBZ had global IQ similar to their controls (Table 3). Seven children in the DPH group and only one among their matched controls had global a IQ 1 SD or more below the mean of this test (a score ≤ 84) ($P < 0.01$), yielding a relative risk of 7.0 (95% confidence interval, 2.5–12.2). Three children exposed to CBZ and one of their matched control had a global IQ of 84 or less (NS). Subsequent multivariate analysis revealed that maternal IQ, maternal SES, and maternal age did not contribute to lowering children's global IQ in the DPH group compared to their matched controls.

There was no correlation between the daily dose per kilogram of either DPH or CBZ and global IQ of the exposed children; the seven DPH-exposed children with IQ ≤ 84 were exposed to maternal doses (6.1 ± 2.6 mg/kg/d) not significantly different from the mean of the group (5.9 ± 1.9 mg/kg/d). Only one DPH-treated mother of the seven having a child with an IQ of 84 or less had herself IQ lower than 84; two of the three CBZ-treated mothers who had children with an IQ of 84 also had IQs in the same range. Similar to the intelligence test findings, children exposed to DPH achieved significantly lower on the Reynell Developmental Language Scales (in both Expressive and Comprehension scales).

Maternal serum concentrations of DPH were available in 3 mothers giving birth to children with IQs of 84 or less and in 15 mothers whose children had IQs exceeding 84. Levels did not differ between these two subgroups (30.4 ± 22.5 μM and 31.6 ± 19.6 μM). CBZ-exposed children did not differ from matched children in either language component (Table 3).

DISCUSSION

Concerns about potential adverse morphological and neurobehavioral effects of antiepileptic drugs on the exposed fetus have long been raised (1,3,

Table 3 Neurobehavioral Development of Children Exposed In Utero to DPH or CBZ Versus Their Matched Controls

	DPH	DPH-controls	CBZ	CBZ-controls
Global IQ	103.1 ± 25.2[a]	113.4 ± 13.1[a]	111.5 ± 19.7	114.9 ± 13.3
Reynell	0.2 ± 1.6[a]	1.1 ± 0.95[a]	0.72 ± 1.4	1.05 ± 0.81
Verbal comprehension				
Expressive language	−0.47 ± 1.2[a]	0.2 ± 0.96[a]	0.05 ± 0.9	0.26 ± 0.9

[a]$P < 0.05$ when DPH compared to DPH control for the same test.

15), and there have been a relatively large number of studies trying to address the safety/risk of these drugs. Such studies, however, have been criticized for not accounting for factors in addition to the drugs themselves that may adversely affect the fetus (1,3). It has been argued that babies of women with epilepsy who are not on anticonvulsant therapy have a higher risk for major malformations (1,3). Moreover, in comparing offspring of epileptic women to babies not exposed to these drugs, it is crucial to account for factors such as maternal IQ and SES, which are known to correlate with children's achievements in cognitive tests. This is especially important because epileptics tend to have lower IQs (9). Finally, most studies have not addressed the risks of polytherapy versus monotherapy in women with epilepsy.

Since the inception of the Motherisk Program, an antenatal counseling service for women exposed to drugs, chemicals, radiation, and infection in pregnancy, it has become apparent to us that the lack of authoritative data on the relative risk/safety of antiepileptic drugs is causing confusion among patients and physicians alike. In particular, families are concerned about potential long-term damage to the central nervous system, which may cause children not to achieve their intellectual potential. The potential damage of phenytoin in causing the fetal hydantoin syndrome has been known for almost two decades; yet the relative risk of the syndrome has not been assessed through well-controlled studies.

In planning the present study we addressed potential problems that have made earlier investigations difficult to interpret (1,3). It was deemed important to collect pregnant women with epilepsy prospectively, before the outcome of pregnancy was known. This facet of study design was aimed at solving the well-known reporting bias typical of retrospective analyses: it is more likely that adverse events will be reported than normal outcome. Prospective collection of information allows a complete account of exposure data in terms of the drug in question, but also with respect to other potential risk factors such as drugs, alcohol, smoking, and substance abuse. We have recently documented that women interviewed a year after their gestational exposures show major flaws in recall, as well as recall bias (16).

We compared children exposed in utero to either DPH or CBZ to controls matched for maternal characteristics. Data on the controls were collected in an identical manner from a pool of women attending the Motherisk Program for nonteratogenic exposures. The primary end-point of our study was the cognitive function of children exposed in utero to DPH or CBZ. It was therefore important to measure maternal IQ and SES, both of which are known to impact on young children's achievements in testing of global intelligence. It was important that the psychometrists testing the children be blinded to the nature of intrauterine exposure, to obviate the risk of tester bias.

Our study confirms the neurotoxic effects of DPH, first described by Hanson in 1976 (2). Children exposed in utero to DPH monotherapy achieved on average 10 IQ points lower than their matched controls, and there was a similar decrease in both aspects of the Reynell language test. These differences could not be accounted for by differences in other factors, such as maternal obstetric history, course of pregnancy, maternal IQ, or the family's SES, all of which were similar between the DPH group and its control group.

Clinicians often find it difficult to relate to differences in means of IQ scores between two groups, especially when attempting to put these differences in their clinical context (i.e., "statistical significance" vs. "clinical significance"). It is therefore worth noting that children exposed in utero to DPH had increased risk of having an IQ of 84 or less. Subanalysis of the seven children (IQs ≤ 84) has failed to show more prevalent lower maternal IQs or SES, suggesting that maternal genetic/socioeconomic mechanisms did not cause the fetal impairment.

It has been suggested that reduction of DPH dose may decrease its teratogenic risk (1). Our study has failed to show such an association when the drug was used in its recommended dose range. It is worth remembering that levels of DPH tend to decrease during pregnancy as a result of increases in both body weight and clearance rate (3). Further decrease in dose may expose the pregnant woman to increased risk of seizures. Our results do not show dose-response neurotoxicity, and they agree with the pharmacogenetic theory of phenytoin teratogenesis: there is increasing evidence that genetically susceptible fetuses, possibly those suffering from lack of epoxide hydrolase, may be at increased risk for the fetal hydantoin syndrome (17). In idiosyncratic reactions such as this, the dose of the drug generally does not play a major role.

During the last two decades CBZ has gained acceptability in the treatment of seizure disorders of various types. After the fetal hydantoin syndrome had been described, various authorities suggested CBZ as a drug of choice for seizure control in pregnancy (5). However, several studies have suggested that the drug may not be safe. In particular, Jones and colleagues reported on several children with lower than one standard deviation achievement in the Bayley Scales (18). This study was open and unblinded, and it did not control for key confounders such as maternal IQ and SES.

The present study has failed to find differences in cognitive function between children exposed in utero to CBZ and their matched controls. These subjects did not differ in either global IQ or expressive and receptive language characteristics. Subanalysis of the three exposed children with global IQ of 84 or less revealed that two of the mothers had also lower IQ and lower SES, both of which could account for the children's low IQ score. One of these three children had neural tube defect.

In 1991 Roza described an association between first-trimester exposure to CBZ and neural tube defects (NTDs) (19), and presently Motherisk recommends that women on CBZ undergo definitive tests to rule out NTD. Because a combination of maternal blood or amniotic fluid α-fetoprotein and ultrasound can detect NTDs with very high sensitivity and specificity, it is likely that a case like our NTD (which was part of Roza's initial cohort) will be diagnosed in the future before 20 weeks of gestation.

In summary, our study suggests the existence of a clinically important adverse effect of DPH on neurobehavioral development, independent of maternal or environmental factors, causing a substantial number of children to have lower cognitive abilities. No similar effects could be shown following gestational use of CBZ. It is recommended that switching therapy from DPH to CBZ be considered whenever such a change is clinically possible.

Answer

Our study verifies the neurotoxicity of phenytoin. The child of a woman treated with this drug may have abnormally low levels of cognitive achievement. The neurologist should consider a switch to carbamazepine if this drug is appropriate to the patient's seizure disorder. If she is being switched, neural tube defects should be ruled out. In addition, folic acid supplements should be prescribed before conception occurs.

ACKNOWLEDGMENTS

The authors are grateful to Joanne Rudolph and Donna Sarbara for their assistance in testing, and to Niki Tsoukalis for preparing the manuscript.

This study was supported by the Motherisk Research Fund, the Ontario Ministry of Health, Ciba Geigy Canada, and the Institute of Medical Sciences, University of Toronto.

REFERENCES

1. Schardein J. Chemically Induced Birth Defects. Marcel Dekker, New York, 1985, pp 142–189.
2. Hanson JW, Smith DW. The fetal hydantoin syndrome. J Pediatr 1975; 87:285–290.
3. Kaneko S. Antiepileptic drug therapy and reproductive consequences: Functional and morphologic effects. Reprod Toxicol 1991; 5:179–198.
4. Robert E, Guibaud P. Maternal valproic acid and congenital neural tube defects. Lancet 1983; 2:937.
5. Saunders M. Epilepsy in women of childbearing age. If anticonvulsants cannot be avoided, use carbamazepine. Br Med J 1989; 299–581.

6. Gaily E, Kantola-Sorsa E, Granstrom MZ. Specific cognitive dysfunction in children with epileptic mothers. Dev Med Child Neurol 1990; 32:403–414.
7. Bertollini R, Kallen M, Mastroiocovo P, Robert E. Anticonvulsant drugs in monotherapy: Effects on the fetus. Eur J Epidemiol 1987; 3:164–171.
8. Delgado Escueta AV, Janz D. Consensus guidelines: Preconception counseling, management, and care of the pregnant woman with epilepsy. Neurology 1992; 42 (suppl 5):149–160.
9. Vining EPG. Cognitive dysfunction associated with antiepileptic drug therapy. Epilepsia 1987; 28:S18–S22.
10. Hollingshead AB, Redlich FC. Social class and mental illness. A community study. New York, Wiley, 1958.
11. Wechsler D. Wechsler adult intelligence scale (revised). New York, Psychological Corp., 19   .
12. Bayley N. Bayley Scales of infant development. New York, Psychological Corp, 1969.
13. McCarthy D. The McCarthy scales of children's abilities. New York, Psychological Corp, 1972.
14. Reynell JK. The Reynell development language scales (revised). Windsor, England, National Foundation for Educational Research, 1977.
15. Vorhees CV. Developmental effects of anticonvulsants. Neurotoxicology 1986; 7:235–244.
16. Feldman Y, Koren G, Mattie D, Shear H, Pellegrini E, MacLeod SM. Determinants of recall and recall bias in studying drug and chemical exposure in pregnancy. Teratology 1989; 40:37–46.
17. Strickler SM, Miller MA, Andermann E, Dansky LV, Seni M, Spielberg SP. Genetic predisposition to phenytoin induced birth defects. Lancet 1985; 2:746–479.
18. Jones KL, Lacro RV, Johnson KA, Adams J. Pattern of malformation in the children of women treated with carbamazepine during pregnancy. N Engl J Med 1989; 320:1661–1666.
19. Roza FW. Spina bifida in infants of women treated with carbamazepine during pregnancy. N Engl J Med 1991; 324:674–676.

5

The Safety of Antidepressants in Pregnancy

Gideon Koren, Anne Pastuszak, and Sheila Jacobson
The Hospital for Sick Children, Toronto, Ontario, Canada

Betsy Schick and Alan Donnenfeld
Pennsylvania Hospital, Philadelphia, Pennsylvania

Marcia Feldkamp and Marsha Leen-Mitchell
University of Utah, Salt Lake City, Utah

Carol Zuber and Michael McCormack
University of Medicine and Dentistry of New Jersey, Camden, New Jersey

Ken Jones
University of California, San Diego, San Diego, California

H. Allen Gardner
Oshawa General Hospital, Oshawa, Ontario, Canada

Clinical Case

A woman with manic-depressive disorder, dependent on lithium, has just found out she is pregnant. She considers termination of pregnancy, a move that was supported by two other doctors. What should be your advice?

INTRODUCTION

A substantial number of women of reproductive age need antidepressant therapy, and many of the conditions represented cannot be well controlled without such medications during pregnancy. The information available on the reproductive safety of the major classes of antidepressants has been sparse. Recently, two large prospective studies, the result of collaboration by several teratogen information services have shed light on pregnancy outcome following first-trimester exposure to lithium, tricyclic antidepressants, and fluoxetine. This chapter reviews the results of these studies and their practical implications.

LITHIUM IN PREGNANCY

It is estimated that 0.1% of pregnant women use lithium (1). This drug crosses the placenta, and concentrations are much the same in maternal and cord serum. Therapeutic and supratherapeutic doses of lithium have caused craniofacial defects in rodents (2), but malformations have not been demonstrated in primates (3). Since 1970, isolated instances of congenital anomalies (specifically Ebstein's anomaly) as well as normal outcomes have been reported in association with lithium exposure during pregnancy (4-6).

In 1968 the Danish Registry of Lithium Babies was established to obtain further information about infants and children who had been exposed to lithium during the first trimester of pregnancy. Data collected by a voluntary retrospective reporting system included cases from Scandinavia, Canada, and the United States. Of a total of 225 cases reported by 1983, 25 (11%) had major congenital malformations (7). Eighteen (72%) of these patients had cardiac anomalies; of these, a third were Ebstein's anomaly, which is a rare congenital heart defect with an incidence of 1 in 20,000 in the general population. On the basis of this information, lithium has become widely regarded as a human teratogen.

Voluntary, retrospective reports of reproductive outcome have many serious methodological shortcomings. In particular, there is evidence that bias toward reporting of adverse outcomes is common (8). With an unknown denominator (total number of exposures), an increased risk cannot be defined. Furthermore, two case control studies (1,9) have not demonstrated increased use of lithium in mothers giving birth to children with Ebstein's anomaly [although one of them reported Ebstein's anomaly after exposure to lithium (9)], and a retrospective study (10) of 350 women with major affective disorders showed no difference in outcome between infants exposed to lithium and those who had been exposed to other psychotropic drugs, although four cardiac defects were seen in 59 lithium-exposed infants, and none in the 38 controls (10).

To evaluate the teratogenic potential of lithium in pregnancy, we conducted a controlled, prospective study of women using lithium who contacted teratogen information services in two American and two Canadian university programs (11).

Patients and Methods

We enrolled 148 women who called one of four teratogen information services to obtain information about the potential risks of therapeutic drugs during pregnancy: these centers were Motherisk (Toronto), the California

Teratogen Information Service (CTIS) (San Diego), the Philadelphia Pregnancy Healthline, and Fetal Risk Assessment from Maternal Exposure (FRAME) (London, Ontario).

The prospective collection of the study and follow-up data were consistent between centers. Motherisk and FRAME referred patients to a weekly clinic, where at interview a physician obtained information about drugs or other chemicals taken during or before pregnancy, including indication, dose, toxicity of the drug and its toxic effects, and monitoring. A medical and obstetric history was also elicited, as well as occupational exposures and family history. At this visit advice was offered and appropriate referrals were made. After the expected date of delivery, each woman was telephoned and a follow-up history of the pregnancy was obtained. The mother was asked for details about pregnancy outcome, perinatal complications, birth weight, physical findings, and developmental milestones. In addition, the physician caring for the baby was contacted to confirm this information and to provide a written report of the delivery and health status of the child. The CTIS and the Philadelphia Pregnancy Healthline obtained all initial information by telephone interview. In San Diego, postnatal follow-up was done by one of the investigators in the clinic, who collected details of delivery and postnatal course. The Philadelphia Pregnancy Healthline obtained all follow-up data by telephone; detailed records from physicians caring for the babies were also obtained. Patient enrollment into the study began with the initiation of each program: CTIS, 1979; Philadelphia Pregnancy Healthline, 1984; Motherisk, 1985; FRAME, 1989 until February 1991.

All pregnant women who called and reported lithium ingestion during part or all of their first trimester were prospectively enrolled. Lithium exposures as early as 3 weeks' gestation were included, since the half-life of lithium is long (2.4 days) in patients receiving long-term therapy (11). Thus detectable serum concentrations can still be present 2 weeks after cessation of treatment. All patients were offered fetal echocardiography at 18 weeks' gestation, to rule out cardiac anomalies. If prenatal echocardiography had not been done, infants were referred for postnatal echocardiographs. Patient enrollment was as follows: CTIS, 101; Motherisk, 25; Philadelphia Pregnancy Healthline, 19; and FRAME, 3.

Controls were women who were seen at the Motherisk clinic for counseling about drugs that are not known or suspected to be teratogenic. Each study patient was matched with a woman of similar age (to within 2 years). Prenatal and postnatal evaluation was the same as described for the Motherisk program. Echocardiography was not done in this group, since this procedure was not deemed to be medically or ethically justifiable.

We used Marden's definition of major anomaly: that is, one that has an adverse effect on either the function or social acceptability of the individual (13).

We used chi-square analysis to compare the frequency of malformations in study and control groups and the frequency of smoking in the two groups. We calculated risk ratios and 95% confidence intervals (Taylor series) to establish the relation between lithium exposure and malformations. These statistics were obtained first for all congenital malformations, then for cardiac malformations and Ebstein's anomaly. Birth weight, gestational age, and developmental milestones were compared with Student's t-test for paired data. Correlations between values were studied by least-squares regression analysis.

Results

Ten of the 148 subjects were lost to follow-up postnatally; however, they were included in part of the analysis because all had had prenatal echocardiography. A total of 68 patients had echocardiographs (46%). Maternal age ranged from 15 to 40 years (mean 30, SD 5 years). All patients were receiving lithium for major affective disorders. The mean daily lithium dose was 927 (SD 340) mg; the range was 50–2400 mg.

Pregnancy outcome did not differ between patients and controls with respect to the total number of live births, frequency of major anomalies, spontaneous or therapeutic abortions, ectopic pregnancy, and prematurity (Table 1). Three major congenital malformations occurred in each group: 2.8% of live births in the lithium group and 2.4% in controls. The 10 pregnancies for which final outcome was not known were not included in this part of the analysis. There were four sets of twins in the lithium group; one pair was born at 23 weeks' gestation, and both infants died shortly after

Table 1   Pregnancy Outcome[a]

Outcome	Lithium ($n = 138$)	Control ($n = 148$)
Normal live births	105 (76%)	123 (83%)
Full term	99 (72%)	116 (78%)
Premature (<36 weeks)	6 (44%)	7 (5%)
Congenital defects	3 (3%)	3 (2%)
Spontaneous abortion	13 (9%)	12 (8%)
Therapeutic abortion[b]	15 (10%)	9 (6%)
Stillbirth	1	0
Ectopic pregnancy	1	1
Unknown	10 (7%)	0

[a]Ectopic pregnancies and spontaneous and therapeutic abortions are expressed as percentages of all outcomes ($n = 148$). Stillbirths and normal live births are expressed as percentages of known outcomes ($n = 138$). Congenital defects are expressed as a percentage of all live births.
[b]One therapeutic abortion because of Ebstein's anomaly diagnosed in utero.

birth as a result of complications of prematurity. There was one set of twins in the control group.

Two children in the lithium group had neural tube defects: one had hydrocephalus and meningomyelocele and had also been exposed to carbamazepine during the first trimester; the other had spina bifida and tethered cord. A third infant (a twin) was born at 23 weeks, had meromelia, and died shortly after birth. One fetus in the lithium group had a severe form of Ebstein's anomaly, which was diagnosed at 16 weeks' gestation, and this pregnancy was terminated. This fetus had also been exposed to fluoxetine, trazodone, and L-thyroxine in the first trimester. In the controls, one child had a ventricular septal defect, one had congenital hip dislocation, and one had cerebral palsy and torticollis.

The risk ratio for all congenital defects was 1.2 (95% confidence interval 0.2–5.7) when only live births were compared. When the case of Ebstein's anomaly was included (since this pregnancy probably would have gone to term if the anomaly had not been detected), the risk ratio became 1.5 (0.4–6.7). The risk ratio for cardiac anomalies was 1.1 (0.1–16.6).

The mean age at which postnatal follow-up was done in the lithium-exposed group was 61 (SD 87.5) weeks (range, 1 week to 9 years). Lithium-exposed infants weighed a mean of 92 g more than controls ($p = 0.01$) at birth (Table 2). Gestational age and frequency of prematurity did not differ between the groups. Because all controls were enrolled in Toronto, we examined whether the difference in birth weight was related to geographic factors in the various study groups. However, when the Motherisk data were analyzed separately, the difference in birth weight persisted and remained significant ($p = 0.018$). There was no correlation between maternal lithium dose and birth weight. There were more cigarette smokers among the women using lithium than among the controls (31.8% vs. 15.5%; $p = 0.002$).

Data on attainment of major developmental milestones (smiling, lifting head, sitting, crawling, standing, talking, and walking) were available for 21 lithium-exposed patients enrolled by Motherisk and 1 patient enrolled by

Table 2 Comparison of Sample Characteristics in Lithium-Exposed and Control Groups: Mean (SD) and Range

	Lithium group	Control group	p
Birth weight, g	3475 (660) (539–5024)	3383 (566) (950–4896)	0.025
Gestational age, wks	39.1 (3.0) (23–42.5)	39.2 (2.5) (26–43)	0.562
Maternal age, y	30.0 (5.3) (15–40)	29.8 (5.3) (16–40)	0.614

FRAME. Study and control groups did not differ in age of attainment of any of the milestones (data not shown).

Discussion

Discontinuation of lithium therapy can have devastating results for the mental and physical health of young women with major affective disorders. On the other hand, many women who inadvertently conceive while on lithium therapy choose to terminate pregnancy because of a perception of teratogenic risk based on the unfounded retrospective reports. As far as we are aware, this is the first prospective study of infants exposed to lithium during the first trimester of pregnancy. The recent establishment of teratogen information services has provided a very good opportunity to investigate large numbers of patients exposed to substances of interest within short periods. Our service is uniquely designed to counsel pregnant women, and we are contacted directly by those exposed to lithium, almost invariably at the time of exposure. Accurate information about time of exposure and drug dosage is crucial to assess any causal relation between any xenobiotic and outcome. Moreover, information about other risk factors such as illicit drugs and smoking is obtained prospectively.

Case control studies rely on maternal recall, which can be poor and is subject to bias (14). Our results accord with those of earlier prospective cohort and case control studies (1,9,10), suggesting that the risk of congenital defects in babies after lithium exposure is lower than that reported by the Danish Registry of Lithium Babies. The registry investigators claim that lithium is associated with a 10% incidence of cardiac malformations and a 3% incidence of Ebstein's anomaly; they believe that the drug is a major teratogen. Because the registry is a voluntary, retrospective database, neither the number of cases not reported nor the number of unreported normal outcomes of lithium exposure is known.

Our results cannot rule out an association between lithium and major anomalies, even though there was no difference in the number of anomalies between the study and control groups. Since Ebstein's anomaly is very rare, a much larger sample size would be needed to define the real risk of this abnormality. That the single cardiac malformation in our study group was Ebstein's anomaly indicates that lithium as a cause of this disorder is rare.

Since fewer than half our patients had echocardiographs, some cardiac malformations might have been missed, including milder forms of Ebstein's anomaly. This might also be true for the control group, in which no echocardiographs were done. Since all patients were examined by a physician, however, it is unlikely that clinically significant lesions were missed.

The infant with hydrocephalus and meningomyelocele who was exposed to lithium in utero had also been exposed during the first trimester to carbamazepine, a drug that has been associated with an increased incidence of neural tube defects (14). The fetus that had Ebstein's anomaly was also exposed in the first trimester to several other drugs, none of which has been associated with cardiac anomalies; lithium remains the most likely causative factor.

The teratogenicity of lithium might be dose-related, as has been shown in animals (2). The doses used at the time the Danish registry data was obtained could have been higher than present recommended doses. This could explain the discrepancy between their results and ours. However, there is no evidence that lithium doses have changed during this time (16). In addition, lithium has a very narrow therapeutic window, above which toxic effects are common. Most patients are prescribed the highest dose they can tolerate that will maintain serum concentrations in the therapeutic range (15). We therefore believe that a dose relation does not account for the different findings of the two studies. The probable reason is the different methods of data collection used by the two groups.

Although the difference in the number of elective abortions was not statistically significant between the groups, the rate was higher in the lithium group than in the controls (10% vs. 6%). The increased trend to voluntary termination might have been due to the perceived teratogenic risk of lithium, since women who believe that they are at such risk are more likely to terminate their pregnancies (17). Counseling provided by the teratogen information services and referral for appropriate screening tests such as echocardiography might have reduced the perception of teratogenic risk of lithium. As a result, the number of terminations in our study was probably lower than it would have been, and thus the figures for elective abortion are higher than ours in centers where no such counseling is provided; American Medicaid data indicate termination rates exceeding 50% in women exposed to lithium during pregnancy (F. Rosa, personal communication).

The babies exposed to lithium were heavier than controls, and fetal macrosomia has been associated with lithium therapy (18,19). Yoder (19) proposed that lithium may have an insulinlike effect on carbohydrate metabolism. We did not find that demographic variations contributed to the difference in weight between the groups, and the proportion of diabetic patients did not differ. In addition, the proportion of cigarette smokers in the lithium group was twice that in the controls. One would therefore expect the babies in the lithium group to be smaller than the controls. Hence, the effect of the drug on birth weight might be even larger than is evident in this study. Although only a few babies were assessed for development milestones, no differences were seen, which is consistent with findings of earlier reports (20). We conclude on the basis of our results and those of others (1,9,10) that lithium is not a major human teratogen. We believe that women with major affective disorders who wish to have children may continue lithium during pregnancy and do not need to terminate pregnancy, provided level 2 ultrasound and fetal echocardiography are done to rule out the presence of major cardiac anomalies.

FLUOXETINE AND TRICYCLIC ANTIDEPRESSANTS DURING THE FIRST TRIMESTER

Fluoxetine (Prozac) is a new antidepressant that causes selective inhibition of neuronal serotonin (5-HT) uptake. Presently, the drug is used by millions of patients with major depression in North America. The manufacturer (Eli Lilly Ltd.) suggests that the drug not be given to women of childbearing potential, since the safe use of fluoxetine during human pregnancy has not been conclusively established. In rats and rabbits treated with 9 and 11 times the maximum daily human dose, fetal morphology and pregnancy outcome were not shown to be compromised (21).

Experiential data have so far been limited to voluntary reports collected by the manufacturer. In a retrospective analysis of 38 women who reported first-trimester exposure to fluoxetine there were 16 normal live births, 8 elective abortions, 3 miscarriages, 9 cases that were lost to follow-up, 1 infant born with hepatoblastoma, and 1 twin pregnancy with 1 miscarriage. In a postmarketing report summarizing the outcome of 226 prospective spontaneous reports of pregnant patients exposed to fluoxetine, outcome data were available for only 113 babies. There were 64 normal live births, 8 premature births, 18 elective abortions, 16 miscarriages, 3 twin pregnancies, and 1 infant born with transposition of the great arteries, although fluoxetine exposure occurred in the second trimester, well after embryological formation of the arteries (22).

Voluntary reports collected by manufacturers regarding gestational exposures to drugs are fraught with major methodological problems. The original sources of these data are unknown and are not compared to appropriate control groups. Moreover, the quality of ascertainment and follow-up is often poor, and as documented above (22), there is almost 50% loss of follow-up data. There is ample evidence that abnormal outcome is more likely to be reported voluntarily and thus, in the absence of a denominator of all pregnant women treated with fluoxetine, it is impossible to ascertain the frequency of defects associated with this drug and compare them with the baseline risk in the general population.

The recommendation that women of reproductive age not conceive while on fluoxetine totally ignores that almost half the pregnancies in North America are unplanned. Indeed, during the last few years, teratology information services throughout North America have received hundreds of calls by pregnant women who conceived in an unplanned manner while on fluoxetine therapy. Following the success of the first collaboration by teratology information services which investigated the first-trimester use of lithium (11), we undertook to collect prospectively and compare pregnancy outcome following fluoxetine in the first trimester to two control groups, one exposed to tricyclic antidepressants and the other to nonteratogens.

Patients and Methods

Our prospective collaborative study enrolled pregnant women who contacted one of four teratogen information services (TIS) requesting counseling about the teratogenic potential of fluoxetine. The participating centers were Motherisk (Toronto), Pregnancy Healthline (Pennsylvania), Pregnancy and Risk Information Service (New Jersey), and Pregnancy RiskLine (Utah). All women contacting these services during pregnancy were included. Prospective collection of information and follow-up data was consistent between centers, although collection was performed in different manners. Motherisk referred all women concerned about first-trimester fluoxetine exposure to a weekly clinic, during which information was obtained in an interview with a team physician regarding indication, dose, toxicity, and dates of initiation and discontinuation. Four women were referred to Motherisk by a geneticist outside Toronto who collected the cases prospectively in a similar manner. In addition, obstetrical, medical, genetic, and drug exposure history was obtained from both the mother and biological father of the fetus. Approximately 8–12 months after the expected date of delivery, all patients were contacted by telephone and asked details about the outcome of pregnancy, birth weight, presence or absence of birth defects, and perinatal and neonatal complications. All follow-up information was corroborated by written documentation from the child's physician. Pregnancy Hotline, Pregnancy and Risk Information Service, and Pregnancy RiskLine recorded maternal information similar to Motherisk by telephone interviews. Postnatal follow-up data, similar to those collected in Toronto, were obtained by telephone in Pennsylvania, Utah, and New Jersey. The Pennsylvania Service also used follow-up cards received in the mail.

Photocopies of each center's fluoxetine cases were sent to Toronto for matching and statistical analysis, after all names and addresses had been deleted. Each woman exposed to fluoxetine during the first trimester was age-matched (± 2 years) to two controls, closest in date to the date of consultation of the fluoxetine case. The first control group consisted of pregnant women who voluntarily sought counseling at Motherisk after first-trimester exposure to tricyclic antidepressants and the second control group consisted of pregnant women who voluntarily sought counseling at Motherisk regarding exposure to a nonteratogen. A nonteratogen is defined as a medication or environmental agent which has been proven in large studies not to increase the baseline teratogenic risk (e.g., acetaminophen, penicillins, dental x-rays). Both control groups were selected from our computerized database. Although the primary outcome of interest was the rate of birth defects in pregnancies exposed to fluoxetine as compared to the tricyclic and nonteratogen groups, maternal characteristics (age, obstetrical history, alcohol and cigarette use), pregnancy outcome (maternal weight gain, method of delivery, use of forceps, rates of live births, elective abortions, and miscarriages) and offspring characteristics (gestational age and birth weight) were also compared. Chi-square analysis and Fisher's exact test were used to compare proportions, Student's t-test was employed to compare paired data (two groups) and analysis of variance (three groups) to compare continuous data. Wilcoxon sign-rank (two groups) and Kruskal-Wallis (three groups) were used to compare data that did not follow normal distribution. Data are expressed as mean plus or minus standard deviation.

Results

A total of 128 pregnant women treated with fluoxetine for depression during the first trimester were followed prospectively by the participating centers (45 in Toronto, 44 in Philadelphia, 21 in New Jersey, and 18 in Utah). The mean daily maternal dose of fluoxetine was 25.8 ± 13.1 mg (range, 10–80 mg/d) ($n = 122$), and mean weight-adjusted dose (for 75 cases where maternal weight was available) was 0.19 ± 0.1 mg/kg. The drug was taken during the first trimester by all 128 women, during the first and second trimesters by 2, and throughout the pregnancy by 6 women. Because of the limited number of tricyclic antidepressant cases in the Motherisk database suitable for matching (within 2 years of maternal age), our reported data are divided into comparisons between 128 fluoxetine cases and 128 age-matched nonteratogen controls (NTC), and comparisons among 74 fluoxetine cases, 74 age-matched tricyclic antidepressant (TCA) cases, and 74 age-matched nonteratogen controls. There were no differences in any of the characteristics of the women using fluoxetine across the four participating centers.

There was no difference in the rate of major birth defects when the live births exposed to fluoxetine were compared to the NTC live births (2% vs. 1.8%, $p = 0.38$) or when the smaller fluoxetine group was compared to both of its controls [3.4% vs. 0% (TCA) vs. 3% (NTC), $p = 0.8$] (Table 3).

Table 3 Pregnancy Outcome in Cases (Fluoxetine-Exposed) and Age-Matched Controls (TCA and NTC)

Characteristics	Fluoxetine (n = 128)	NTC (n = 128)	p	Fluoxetine (n = 74)	TCA (n = 74)	NTC (n = 74)	p
Outcome							
Live birth	98/128	110/128	0.14[a]	58/74	60/74	67/74	0.34[a]
Elective abortion	11/128	8/128		6/74	5/74	2/74	
Spontaneous abortion	19/128	10/128	0.1[b]	10/74	9/74	5/74	0.31[b]
Major congenital anomalies	2/98	2/110	0.3[b]	2/58	0/60	2/67	0.3[b]
Weight gain, kg	17.8 ± 6.3	16.3 ± 6.0	0.69	17.2 ± 6.2	16.8 ± 5.8	15.9 ± 5.3	0.53
Gestational age, wks	39.4 ± 1.7	39.4 ± 1.8	0.96	39.4 ± 1.6	39.1 ± 2.3	39.6 ± 1.9	0.40
<37 wks	6/85	7/85	0.22[b]				
>42 wks	1/85	2/85	0.38[b]				
Birth weight, g	3459.7 ± 660.2	3421.1 ± 563	0.68	3421.9 ± 664.1	3515.9 ± 672.3	3408.6 ± 602.2	0.62
>4000 g	15/84	9/81	0.08[b]				
Forceps used	8/38	9/83	0.13	4/23	6/42	5/41	0.85
Delivery							
Vaginal	61/82	62/83	0.04	32/42	32/43	31/41	0.43
Emergency C/S	9/82	17/83		4/42	5/43	8/41	
Repeat C/S	12/82	4/83		6/42	6/43	2/41	

[a]Chi-square for 2 × 3 table.
[b]Fisher (2 group) and chi-square (3 group) (miscarriages vs. live birth, excluding elective abortions).

69

Table 4 details all major and minor birth defects as well as neonatal complications. There was no statistical difference in pregnancy outcome, maternal weight gain during pregnancy, gestational age at delivery, birth weight, or use of forceps at delivery, whether the fluoxetine group was compared to NTC only or to both age-matched control groups (Table 3). Conversely, however, there was a tendency for a higher percentage of miscarriages in the 128 fluoxetine patients compared with NTC, but it did not reach statistical significance [14.8% vs. 7.8% reported rate (RR), 1.9; 95% confidence interval (CI), 0.92–3.92]. A similar trend was observed in the smaller sample size, although the TCA also had a miscarriage rate similar to the fluoxetine group (13.5% vs. 12.2% vs. 6.8%). There was no statistical difference between rates of vaginal or cesarean section deliveries between the fluoxetine group and age-matched controls. Infants born to depressive women of both groups (fluoxetine and TCA) tended to have more neonatal complications, although when looked at individually, none of those recorded was significantly more common (Table 4).

Because one patient from Utah was gravida 33 (para 9, miscarriages 23, likely as a result of diagnosed maternal trisomy 8), obstetrical history data deviated from a normal, Gaussian distribution and consequently, nonpara-

Table 4 Major Malformations and Neonatal Complications

	Fluoxetine	Tricyclic antidepressants	Nonteratogens
Major malformations	Jejunal obstruction Ventricular septal defect	None	Pulmonary atresia Ventricular septal defect
Neonatal complications[a]	Jaundice needing therapy (2) Shoulder dystocia and apnea (1) Patent ductus arteriosus and cyanosis (1) Sepsis and seizures (1) Hemangioma (2) Lacrimal stenosis (1) Aspiration pneumonia (1) Club feet (1) Congenital dislocation of hip (1)	Metatarsus adductus (1) Congenital dislocation of hip (1) Slight hypotonia (1) β-Hemolytic *streptoccus* (1) Apnea (1) Hydrocele (1) Respiratory distress syndrome (1) Meconium aspiration and sepsis (1) Metatarsus varus (1)	Jaundice (1) Clipped tongue (1)

[a]Number of infants with the complication indicated in parentheses.

Table 5 Maternal Characteristics of Cases (Fluoxetine-Exposed) and Age-Matched Controls (TCA and NTC)

Characteristics	Fluoxetine (n = 128)	NTC (n = 128)	p	Fluoxetine (n = 74)	TCA (n = 74)	NTC (n = 74)	p
Maternal age, y	31.6 ± 5.7	31.2 ± 4.9	0.51	31.7 ± 5.2	31.6 ± 5	31.0 ± 4.3	0.66
Gestational age at first consultation, wk				8.5 ± 4.9	8.6 ± 6.3	8.9 ± 5.8	0.93[a]
Obstetrical history							
Gravidity	2.9 ± 3.2	2.1 ± 1.3	0.01[b]	2.5 ± 1.6	2.3 ± 1.7	2.0 ± 1.2	>0.05[c]
Parity	0.9 ± 1.1	0.6 ± 0.8	0.01[b]	0.9 ± 0.9	0.7 ± 1	0.7 ± 0.8	>0.05[c]
Elective abortions	0.5 ± 0.9	0.3 ± 0.7	0.3[b]	0.5 ± 0.8	0.4 ± 0.8	0.3 ± 0.6	>0.05[c]
Spontaneous abortions	0.5 ± 2.5	0.2 ± 0.7	0.13[b]	0.2 ± 0.6	0.4 ± 0.8	0.2 ± 0.4	>0.05[c]
Ethanol							
Abstainers	62/109	68/125	0.31	41/62	35/72	40/73	0.12
<2.5 drinks/wk	35/109	49/125	0.8[d]	14/62	32/72	27/73	0.02[d]
≥2.5 drinks/wk	12/109	8/125		7/62	5/72	6/73	
Tobacco							
Abstainers	74/105	93/125	0.42	42/61	46/73	52/73	0.38
<0.5 package/d	17/105	21/125	0.61[e]	11/61	19/73	15/73	0.55[e]
<1 package/d	11/105	6/125		6/61	7/73	2/73	
≥1, <1.5 packages/d	3/105	5/125		2/61	1/73	4/73	

[a] Analysis of variance.
[b] Wilcoxon sign-rank analysis.
[c] Kruskal-Wallis analysis.
[d] Chi-square analysis: abstainers versus admitted drinkers.
[e] Chi-square analysis: abstainers versus admitted smokers.

71

metric analysis was performed. Excluding this patient from the statistical analysis did not alter the results in any way. There was no statistical difference in gravidity, parity, and previous elective and previous spontaneous abortions between the three groups, although comparison of the fluoxetine and NTC groups revealed a higher mean gravidity and parity in the fluoxetine group (Table 5). There was a similar distribution of abstainers of ethanol and tobacco in all groups (Table 5).

Discussion

Many women of reproductive age suffer from depression, which necessitates chronic therapy with antidepressants. According to O'Hara et al., as many as 10% of pregnant women meet the criteria for major or minor depression (23). Exposing any fetus to drugs is perceived by most women as being associated with an increase in teratogenic risk (24), and women with psychiatric disorders are likely to be more prone to emotional instability due to unfounded perceptions of teratogenic risk following such exposures. While manufacturers and health providers often suggest that depressed women not be treated during gestation, such practice may endanger their health, hence the safety of their pregnancies. This reality, coupled with the fact that half of North American pregnancies are unplanned, implies that there is urgent need for credible data on the safety/risk ratio of antidepressant use in pregnancy. This need is in sharp contradistinction to the complacency exhibited by many pharmaceutical manufacturers in helping to collect such data and many of the regulatory agencies in enforcing such collection.

Presently, systematic collection of postmarketing data on pregnancy exposure to drugs is not mandatory, and many manufacturers feel that their duties responsibilities are met by disclaiming their product's use in pregnancy, thus often orphaning pregnant women from essential drugs. Our study, similar to the earlier lithium project (11), demonstrates the ability of TIS to prospectively collect and ascertain large cohorts of women exposed during the first trimester to specific medications. Because pregnant women contact these services at the time of exposure, complete documentation of exposure and other potential confounders is possible, as well as prospective follow-up of pregnancy.

We have chosen to compare pregnant women exposed to fluoxetine to two control groups: one comprised of women treated with tricyclic antidepressants, the selection of which was intended to control for potential effects of depression, and a second group of women who were exposed to nonteratogens, a group that should represent healthy pregnant women. Drawing all three groups from pregnant women counseled by TIS attempted to obviate potential bias introduced by different referral patterns.

Prospective collection of pregnant women exposed to the drug in question and detailed ascertainment of the outcome of pregnancy have allowed us to construct a meaningful denominator and subsequently to calculate and compare rates of outcome measurements between the fluoxetine and control groups. Although this study is based on maternal reports, the Motherisk program routinely corroborates these reports with physicians' written reports; the former have been found to be very accurate. Because the elimination half-life of fluoxetine ranges between 2 and 6 days, it is likely that many women were still exposed to the drug into their second trimester (e.g., 5 half-lives or 30 days after cessation of therapy). The rate of major malformations in live births exposed to fluoxetine during the first trimester was within the expected normal range (1–3%) and comparable to the two control groups. Although the strength of this study to rule out minimal increased risk above baseline is limited ($n = 128$), it is very unlikely that fluoxetine is a major human teratogen. The similar rate of major malformations to the control group indicates that the power of a much larger cohort would not likely be sufficient to identify a different trend. The sample size of this prospective cohort would have the power to detect a fourfold increased risk of major malformations, assuming a baseline risk of 2% in the NTC group, with a power of 80% and an α of 0.05.

When compared to control women not exposed to teratogens, the fluoxetine group had a tendency for a higher rate of reported miscarriages which did not reach statistical significance (14.8% vs. 7.8%, RR 1.9, 95% CI 0.92–3.92). Our cohort has a limited power to show that an RR of 1.9 is significant; for such an RR to be statistically significant, more than 700 women would be needed in each group. The three group comparison reveals that women exposed to TCA also had a similar tendency for a higher rate of reported miscarriages, which suggests that this tendency may be associated with the depression and/or the emotional instability or other putative biological changes associated with these psychiatric conditions. Another possible explanation is that when questioned during follow-up interviews, some women reported a miscarriage when in fact they had chosen to terminate their pregnancy. Our methodology did not have means to corroborate their reports.

Our recent prospective study with lithium in pregnancy has shown similar miscarriage rates between the lithium and control groups (9.4% vs. 8.1%, respectively: Table 6), which is similar to our present control group, whereas women exposed to lithium tended to electively terminate more often. This may suggest that the report obtained by the present study is genuine and that either the depressive condition or some of its therapies (fluoxetine and TCA) are inducing higher rates of miscarriage. To date, no other studies address this potential association between depression or its therapies and reported rates of miscarriage. Comparison of gestational age at first consulta-

Table 6   Rates of Spontaneous Abortion and Live Births in Women with Depression Exposed to Fluoxetine, Tricyclic Antidepressants, or Lithium[a]

	Fluoxetine	Tricyclic antidepressants (TCA)	Nonteratogen controls (NTC)	Lithium	Controls
Miscarriages	10/74	9/74	5/74	13/138	12/148
	19/128		10/128		
Live births	58/74	60/74	67/74	105/138	123/148
	98/128		110/128		

[a]NTC (n = 128) versus lithium controls, p = 0.19 (Fisher's exact); fluoxetine (n = 74) versus TCA (n = 74) versus lithium, p = 0.76 (chi-square); fluoxetine (n = 128) versus lithium, p = 0.08 (Fisher's exact); TCA (n = 74) versus lithium, p = 0.17 (Fisher's exact).

tion revealed that the lower spontaneous abortion rate in the NTC group was not due to these patients contacting Motherisk later in gestation compared to the fluoxetine and the TCA groups; the stages in pregnancy were identical [8.5 ± 4.9 weeks (fluoxetine) vs. 8.6 ± 6.3 weeks (TCA) vs. 8.9 ± 5.8 weeks (NTC), p = 0.93] (Table 5). Very sparse published information exist on the potential teratogenicity of TCAs (25); the present prospective study failed to show this group as teratogenic. Women exposed to fluoxetine had an obstetric history as well as patterns of ethanol and tobacco use that were, in general, not different from the two control groups. Moreover, their characteristics are comparable to the general population of women contacting Motherisk. The mean dose of fluoxetine consumed by the participating women was within the recommended range, and therefore it is unlikely that the lack of evidence of teratogenicity is due to a suboptimal dose.

In summary, our study suggests that the use of fluoxetine during embryogenesis is not associated with an increased risk of major malformations. Women treated with both fluoxetine and tricyclic antidepressants had a tendency toward higher rates of miscarriage that the nonteratogen control group; further studies will be needed to confirm this observation and to separate the effects of the psychiatric condition from the associated drugs. Long-term studies will be warranted to rule out potential developmental teratology of this drug, which affects a central nervous system neurotransmittor.

Answer

The woman does not have an overall higher risk for major malformations. She may have a higher risk for the rare Ebstein's anomaly, and echocardiogram starting at 16 weeks may help to detect or rule out this condition.

REFERENCES

1. Zalstein E, Koren G, Einarson T, et al. A case-control study on the association between first trimester exposure to lithium and Ebstein's anomaly. Am J Cardiol 1990; 65:817–818.
2. Smithberg M, Dixet PK. Teratogenic effects of lithium in mice. Teratology 1982; 26:239–246.
3. Gralla EJ, McIlhenny HM. Studies in pregnant rats, rabbits and monkeys with lithium carbonate. Toxicol Appl Pharmacol 1972; 21:428–433.
4. Nora JJ, Nora AH, Toews WH. Lithium, Ebstein's anomaly, and other congenital heart defects. Lancet 1974; ii:594–595.
5. Long WA, Park WW. Maternal lithium and neonatal Ebstein's anomaly: Evaluation with cross-sectional echocardiography. Am J Perinatol 1984; 1:182–184.
6. Fries H. Lithium in pregnancy. Lancet 1970; i:1233.
7. Frankenberg FR, Lipinski JF. Congenital malformations. N Engl J Med 1983; 309:311–312.
8. Koren G, Retinoid embryopathy. N Engl J Med 1986; 315:262.
9. Kallen B. Comments on teratogen update: Lithium. Teratology 1988; 38:597–598.
10. Kallen B, Tandberg A. Lithium and pregnancy. Acta Psychiatr Scand 1983; 68:134–139.
11. Jacobson SJ, Jones K, Johnson K, Ceolin L, Kaur P, Sahn D, Donnenfeld AE, Rieder M, Santelli R, Smythe J, Pastuszak A, Einarson T, Koren G. Prospective multicentre study of pregnancy outcome after lithium exposure during first trimester. Lancet 1992; 339:530–533.
12. American Hospital Formulary Service. In (McEvoy GK, ed), American Society of Hospital Pharmacists, New York, 1989, p 1245.
13. Marden PM, Smith DW, McDonald MJ. Congenital anomalies in the newborn infant, including minor variations. J Pediatr 1964; 64:357–371.
14. Koren G. Teratogenic drugs and chemicals in humans. In Maternal-Fetal Toxicology, 1st ed (Koren G, ed), Marcel Dekker, New York, 1990, p 17.
15. Rosa F. Spina bifida in infants of women treated with carbamazepine during pregnancy. N Engl J Med 1991; 324:674–677.
16. Goodman L, Gilman A, eds. The pharmacological basis of therapeutics, 7th ed. Macmillan, New York, 1985, p 429.
17. Koren G, Bologa M, Pastuszak A. The way women perceive teratogenic risk: The decision to terminate pregnancy. In Maternal-Fetal Toxicology, 1st ed (Koren G, ed), Marcel Dekker, New York, 1990, pp 373–381.
18. Belik J, Yoder M, Pereira GR. Fetal macrosomia: An unrecognized adverse effect of maternal lithium therapy. Pediatr Res 1983; 17:304A.
19. Yoder MC, Belik J, Lannon RA, et al. Infants of mothers treated with lithium during pregnancy have an increased incidence of prematurity, macrosomia and perinatal mortality. Pediatr Res 1984; 18:404A.
20. Schou M. What happened later to the lithium babies? Acta Psychiatr Scand 1976; 54:193–197.
21. Byrd RA, Brophy GT, Markham JK. Developmental toxicology studies of fluoxetine hydrochloride administered orally to rats and rabbits. Teratology 1989; 39:444.

22. Goldstein DJ. Outcome of fluoxetine-exposed pregnancies. Proceedings of the Fourth International Conference of Teratogen Information Services, Chicago, April 18–20, 1991.

23. O'Hara MW, Neunober DJ, Zekoski GH. Prospective study of postpartum depression; prevalence and predictive factors. J Abnorm Psycholol 1984; 93:158–171.

24. Koren G, Pastuszak A. Prevention of unnecessary pregnancy terminations by counselling women on drug, chemical and radiation exposure during the first trimester. Teratology 1990; 41:657–661.

25. Cohen LS, Heller VL, Rosenbaum JF. Treatment guidelines for psychotropic drug use in pregnancy. Psychosomatics 1989; 30:25–33.

6

Prospective Assessment of Pregnancy Outcome Following First-Trimester Exposure to Benzodiazepines

Anne Pastuszak and Gideon Koren
The Hospital for Sick Children, Toronto, Ontario, Canada

Vanessa Milich, Shirley Chan, and John Chu
The University of Toronto, Toronto, Ontario, Canada

Clinical Case

Your obstetrician colleague asks you to attend a complicated birth of a G2, P4 woman who was maintained throughout pregnancy on valium (20 mg/d) for panic attacks. He wishes to know what kinds of risk the baby may have.

INTRODUCTION

Benzodiazepines (BDZs) are used for diverse clinical indications because of their anxiolytic, anticonvulsant, muscle relaxant, and sedative-hypnotic properties. Therefore, thousands of pregnant women may need them to reduce anxiety, to induce sedation or muscular relaxation, or to treat eclampsia or preeclampsia. Moreover, since half the pregnancies in North America are unplanned, a large number of women will expose their fetuses to BDZ before realizing that they have conceived. It has been estimated that 11% of American adults use some antianxiety medication annually (1), and up to 35% of pregnant women take some type of psychoactive drug during fetal development (2). Maternal use near term may cause decreased neonatal respiratory rate and withdrawal (3,4), hypotonia (5), and detectable pharmacological activity in the newborn for up to 8–10 days. Some have postulated that these medications cause cleft lip and/or palate (6); however, prospective studies will be needed to confirm or refute the teratogenicity of BDZs.

Retrospective analyses using birth defect registry data have suggested that infants exposed in utero to diazepam are more likely to be born with both a cleft lip and palate but less likely to be born with cleft palate alone (7,8). However, in a subsequent retrospective case control analysis, which controlled for potential confounding factors, others were unable to corroborate such findings (9). Laegreid et al. reported that eight infants of mothers who regularly ingested high doses of either diazepam or oxazepam throughout pregnancy had a common pattern of dysmorphic features and abnormal neurology in the neonatal period (10), whereas in a survey based on four different epidemiological approaches, Czeizel reported no association between first-trimester BDZ exposure and abnormal fetal outcome (11).

Collectively, the data above are confusing in that lack of a consensus in the medical literature may cause a woman to terminate her pregnancy unnecessarily following first-trimester BDZ exposure. Obtaining maternal information regarding the timing of BDZ exposure after delivery may introduce recall bias (7,9), and retrospective studies have their limitations (11); it is probable that clinicians are more likely to report abnormal outcomes simply because they have less motivation to report a pregnancy with a normal outcome. Unless one prospectively ascertains first-trimester BDZ exposure and compares pregnancy outcome in this group to outcome in a control group, patient selection or referral and recall bias may result.

In the work reported here, we compared pregnancy outcome and rate of major birth defects in BDZ-exposed women and a control group. Both groups had voluntarily sought counseling through the Motherisk Program in Toronto.

PATIENTS AND METHODS

We included all women counseled in our clinic between September 1986 and September 1991 about first-trimester exposure to any BDZ, and we compared each BDZ case to a control temporally closest to the study case in our computerized database. The control cases sought counseling following exposure to nonteratogenic drugs: agents known to be safe in human pregnancy. A team physician obtained information about maternal drug history, as well as medical, genetic, obstetric, and occupational history in an interview at the hospital. A trained interviewer ascertained pregnancy outcome in a telephone interview with the mother, and the infant's physician corroborated this by sending a written report to the clinic.

The primary outcome of interest was the rate of birth defects in the live births in each group. Secondary outcome measurements included maternal age, gravidity, parity, rates of elective and spontaneous abortions, exposure to ethanol and tobacco, marital status, weight gain during pregnancy, use of forceps at delivery, presence of meconium, premature rupture of the membranes, gestational age, birth weight, and attainment of developmental milestones. We compared data expressed as a proportion using contingency table analysis and used Student's *t*-test to compare unpaired data expressed as mean plus or minus standard deviation. Values in parentheses represent 95% confidence intervals.

RESULTS

Pregnancy outcome was ascertained for 137 cases of BDZ exposure and their controls. The mean daily dose of BDZ ingested during gestation was 15.3 ± 39.9 mg/d (6.0, 24.6) (Fig. 1). Monotherapy was the norm, the majority (88.7%) of women consuming only one BDZ, the remainder (16/137) using two. The BDZ ingested by the 137 women, as ascertained during interviews, is given in Table 1; the indications for ingestion in and patterns of fetal exposure appear in Tables 2 and 3, respectively.

Ninety-three percent of women (127/137) consumed their BDZ in the first trimester only [which we defined as the time from the first day of the

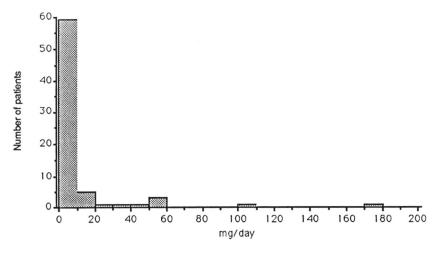

Figure 1   Frequency distribution of reported daily benzodiazepine dose ingested.

Table 1 Use of Benzodiazepines, as Reported by Patients

Benzodiazepine	Number[a]
Alprazolam	17
Bromazepam	7
Chlordiazepoxide	4
Clonazepam	13
Diazepam	43
Flurazepam	5
Lectopam	1
Lorazepam	33
Nitrazepam	1
Oxazepam	4
Temazepam	1
Triazolam	15

[a]Total of 144 greater than 137 patients because some women used more than one type of BDZ.

last menstrual period (LMP) to the end of the 13th week postconception] and 2% in the second trimester only (defined as the time from 14 to 26 weeks postconception). Seventeen percent of women consumed their BDZ throughout the entire pregnancy. Although the majority of women consumed BDZ as the only psychopharmacological agent, there were 13 women (9.5%) who concurrently ingested tricyclic antidepressants: amitriptylline (3), clomipramine (2), desipramine (3), fluoxetine (1), imipramine (3), and trazadone (1). We included such women in the comparative analysis because we have recently established that the family of tricyclic antidepressants do not increase the baseline rate for major malformations (12). The three most common voluntarily reported indications for BDZ use were anxiety and stress, insomnia, and depression; the most preferred BDZ was diazepam ($n = 43$), followed by lorazepam ($n = 33$) and alprazolam ($n = 17$).

There was no statistical difference in the rates of major birth defects among the two groups. In the BDZ-exposed group, there was a single case of epiblepharon; in the control group, there were two cardiac anomalies, one ventricular septal defect, one atrial septal defect with pulmonary valve stenosis, and an additional case of imperforate anus (Table 4). There was no statistical difference in the number of live births, the number of elective abortions, or the number of reported miscarriages. Analysis of maternal characteristics is displayed in Table 5 and Figures 2 and 3. Women exposed to BDZ tended to be significantly older and had been pregnant more times than those in

Table 2 Reported Indications for Benzodiazepine Use

Indication	Number
Agoraphobia	2
Anxiety and/or stress	47
BDZ abuse	1
Car accident	1
Cardiovascular	
Palpitations	1
Mitral valve prolapse	2
Depression	11
Drug rehabilitation therapy	1
Headache/migraine	6
Heartburn	1
Hiatal hernia	1
Insomnia	22
Nervous breakdown	2
Obsessive-compulsive disorder	1
Panic attacks	8
Procedures	
General anesthesia	1
Tooth extraction	2
Surgery	1
Myelogram	1
Intravenous pyelogram	1
Psychosis	1
Seizures	2
Sore jaw	1
Weight loss therapy with metamphetamine	1
Unknown/not given	19
Total	137

the control group. The two groups were similar in other characteristics compared in Table 5.

Of the cases of live births, there were no intergroup differences in maternal weight gain, gestational age at delivery, birth weight, type of delivery (vaginal vs. cesarean section), or neonatal complications (Table 6, Figure 4); we did, however, observe that our control group had forceps-assisted delivery more often than those exposed to BDZ (40% vs. 20%, $p = 0.04$).

Table 3 Gestational Age at Exposure to Various Benzodiazepines

Fetal exposure	Number (%)[a]
First day of LMP to 13 weeks	127/137 (93%)
14–26 weeks only	3/137 (2.2%)
First day of LMP to delivery	23/137 (17%)
First day of LMP to 14 weeks	2/137 (1.4%)
First day of LMP to 16 weeks	1/137 (0.7%)
First day of LMP to 20 weeks	1/137
First day of LMP to 25 weeks	1/137
First day of LMP to 28 weeks	1/137
First day of LMP to 31 weeks	1/137
First day of LMP to 33 weeks	1/137
16 to 39 weeks	1/137

[a]Percentages add to more than 100 because some women took more than one BDZ during more than one time period during pregnancy.

Table 4 Pregnancy Outcome in BDZ-Exposed and Control Patients

	Benzodiazepine-exposed (n = 137)	Non-teratogen-exposed (n = 137)	p
Pregnancy outcome			
Live births	106/137 = 77.4%	115/137 = 83.9%	0.2
Miscarriages	19/137 = 13.9%	10/137 = 7.3%	0.1
Elective abortions	12/137 = 8.8%	12/127 = 8.8%	
Major congenital malformations	1/106 = 1%[a]	3/115 = 2.6%[b]	0.69
	Epiblepharon	Ventricular septal defect Atrial septal defect, pulmonary valve stenosis Imperforate anus	

[a]Information not available for 5 cases.
[b]Information not available for 2 cases.

Table 5 Characteristics of BDZ-Exposed and Non-Teratogen-Exposed Women: Data Presented as Mean ± Standard Deviation; *95% Confidence Intervals*

	Benzodiazepine-exposed (*n* = 137)	Non-teratogen-exposed (*n* = 137)	*p*
Maternal age	32.4 ± 5 (*31.5, 33.2*)	30.4 ± 5.1 (*29.5, 31.2*)	0.002
Obstetrical history			
Gravidity	2.4 ± 1.5 (*2.1, 2.6*)	1.9 ± 1.1 (*1.7, 2.1*)	0.01
Parity	0.8 ± 1 (*0.6, 1*)	0.6 ± 0.8 (*0.5, 0.8*)	0.07
Previous elective abortion	0.4 ± 0.6 (*0.3, 0.5*)	0.2 ± 0.6 (*0.1, 0.4*)	0.09
Previous miscarriage	0.2 ± 0.7 (*0.1, 0.4*)	0.2 ± 0.4 (*0.1, 0.3*)	0.7
Tobacco			
Abstainers[a]	89/132 = 66.9%	96/125 = 76.8%)	0.1
Cigarettes smoked by those who admit smoking	17 ± 11.1 (*13.6, 19.9*)	14.5 ± 6.5 (*12.3, 17.4*)	0.3
Ethanol			
Abstainers[a]	55/124 = 43.5%	69/124 = 55.6%	0.08
<1 drink per day	61/124 = 49.2%	48/124 = 38.7%	0.1
≥1, <2 drinks per day	6/124 = 4.8%	5/124 = 4%	1
≥2 drinks per day	3/124 = 2.3%	2/124 = 1.6%	1
Marital status			
Single	9/104 = 8.6%	9/103 = 8.7%	0.8
Married	95/104 = 91.3%	94/103 = 91.3%	

[a]Abstainers versus those who admitted ingesting.

DISCUSSION AND CONCLUSION

Safra and Oakley reported that infants exposed in utero to benzodiazepines had an increased risk for both cleft lip and cleft palate (7). Other researchers, however, could not confirm this observation (9,11). Accepting only prospective data in the evaluation of rare outcomes may be falsely reassuring (13), since it is often difficult to obtain a large enough sample size to detect a statistically significant elevation in the rate of that rare event. However, much of the discrepancy regarding BDZ use in pregnancy stems from physician-prompted concern regarding the issue of oral clefts following maternal BDZ use. It is encouraging that we did not find a single case of cleft lip and/or palate following corroboration of neonatal well-being by the infant's physician in our 106 patients.

Recently, Laegreid et al. reported abnormal growth and neurodevelopment of 17 children born to mothers who used BDZ in therapeutic doses

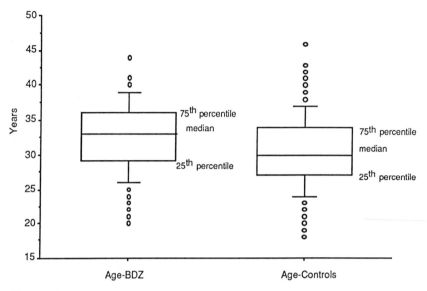

Figure 2 Box plots of 25th, 50th, and 75th percentiles and outlying values (open circles) for maternal age in BDZ-exposed and control groups.

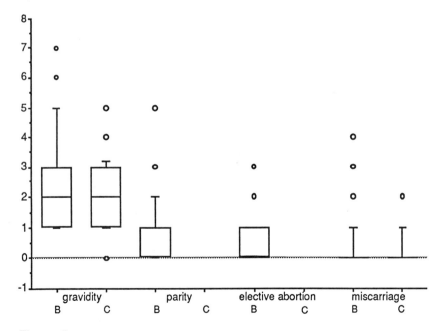

Figure 3 Box plots of 25th, 50th, and 75th percentiles and outlying values (open circles) for obstetrical parameters in BDZ-exposed (B) and control (C) groups.

Table 6 Comparison of Offspring Characteristics from BDZ-Exposed and Non-Teratogen-Exposed Patients: Nonproportion Data Presented as Mean ± Standard Deviation; *95% Confidence Intervals*

	Benzodiazepine-exposed (*n* = 137)	Non-teratogen-exposed (*n* = 137)	*p*
Maternal weight gain, kg	15.8 ± 6.3 (*14.5, 17.0*)	16.6 ± 6.1 (*15.3, 17.8*)	0.4
Gestational age, wk	39.2 ± 2.6 (*38.6, 39.7*)	38.7 ± 2.7 (*38.2, 39.2*)	0.2
Birth weight, g	3396.3 ± 710 (*3256.2, 3536.5*)	3304.6 ± 603.3 (*3203.8, 3429*)	0.3
Delivery method			
Vaginal[a]	72/101 = 71.3%	81/110 = 73.6%	0.8
C/S (type undefined)	19/101 = 18.8%	21/110 = 19.1%	
Repeat C/S	4/101 = 4.2%	2/110 = 1.8%	
Emergency C/S	6/101 = 5.9%	6/110 = 5.4%	
Forceps used			
Yes	11/55 = 20%	21/53 = 39.6%	0.04
No	44/55 = 80%	32/53 = 60.4%	
Meconium			
Yes	3/54 = 5.6%	10/84 = 11.9%	0.3
No	51/54 = 94.4%	74/84 = 88.1%	
Premature rupture of the membranes			
Yes	17/95 = 20%	14/85 = 16.5%	0.7
No	68/95 = 80%	71/85 = 83.5%	

[a]Vaginal delivery compared to all cesarean deliveries.

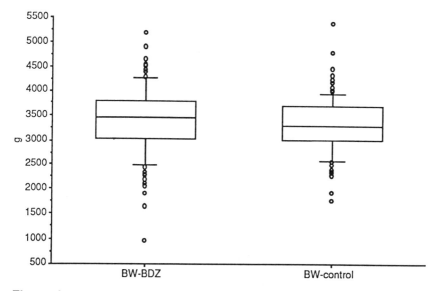

Figure 4 Box plots of 25th, 50th, and 75th percentiles and outlying values (open circles) for birth weight (BW) in BDZ-exposed and control groups.

as their only psychotropic drug in pregnancy (14). Gross motor development that was slow at 6 and 10 months became normal by 18 months, but fine motor functions were found to be impaired on all study occasions. Infants attained developmental milestones, as defined by the Denver Developmental Scale (ages at first smile, lifting of head, unaided sitting, crawling, stand, speech, walk), at the appropriate ages (Table 7). Such discrepancy among these studies may reflect that the patients in the Swedish study constantly used high doses of BDZ (e.g., 75–105 mg oxazepam/d and 30 mg diazepam/d), whereas women counseled by Motherisk used relatively low doses of BDZ (mean dose, 15.3 ± 39.9 mg/d). If geographic differences within the same country demonstrate striking differences in intake habits of BDZ during pregnancy (15), one can only imagine how difficult it would be to relate such conclusions to an entirely different group of patients, who most likely represent the "typical" user of benzodiazepines.

Our results are more similar to those of a study by Bergman et al., which used the Michigan Medicaid database to establish that of 64 live-born infants whose mothers received more than 10 BDZ prescriptions throuoghout pregnancy, 50 (78%) showed no developmental abnormalities (16). Only 8 infant records were consistent with developmental teratogenicity. This study, however, was a computerized retrieval of health claims files, which did not incorporate validation of medical records or contact with patients or physicians, and one must assume that prescription documentation reflects drug ingestion. Strengths of our study include the patients' reports of drug exposure soon after starting therapy and the corroboration of infant outcome and health status by physician reports and, in some cases, by neonatal assessment forms.

The elimination from the newborn infant of benzodiazepines, which are lipid soluble and highly protein bound, is slow due to immaturity of liver

Table 7 Age (Months) of Attainment of Developmental Milestones for BDZ-Exposed and Control Infants

Milestone	Benzodiazepine-exposed	Non-teratogen-exposed	*p*
First smile	1.7 ± 1, *n* = 81	1.6 ± 0.9, *n* = 98	0.6
First lifted head	2.3 ± 1.4, *n* = 67	1.9 ± 1.1, *n* = 87	0.08
First sat unaided	5.8 ± 1.5, *n* = 60	5.6 ± 1.2, *n* = 82	0.5
First crawled	7.1 ± 1.5, *n* = 58	7.2 ± 2.5, *n* = 76	0.6
First stood	8.5 ± 1.9, *n* = 53	8.5 ± 2.6, *n* = 71	0.8
First word spoken	8.2 ± 2.8, *n* = 42	8.5 ± 2.7, *n* = 62	0.5
First walked unaided	11 ± 2.2, *n* = 37	11.3 ± 2, *n* = 41	0.5

metabolism. In addition, increased serum benzodiazepine concentrations and an immature blood–brain barrier may increase neonatal sensitivity to these compounds. Our failure to observe neonatal complications shortly after birth may reflect the low maternal dose (15.3 ± 39.9 mg/d; range, 0.07–202 mg/d) or inconsistency of maternal drug use (i.e., drug use did not continue to term for every case).

The rate of major birth defects in the BDZ-exposed group was no higher than the 1–3% which one would expect in the general population. The present study failed to detect an increased risk for major defects following first-trimester exposure to benzodiazepines as a class. Presently, benzodiazepines are one of the most widely prescribed classes of drugs in the world.

Because almost 50% of North American pregnancies are unplanned, thousands of fetuses are exposed inadvertently to these agents. Implicating BDZ as major human teratogens may cause women to abort an otherwise wanted pregnancy. Clinicians faced with the dilemma of prescribing benzodiazepines for their pregnant patients for a variety of conditions may find our results encouraging. Although our sample has limited power of proving some small increase in teratogenic risk, we find it encouraging that 105 out of 106 exposed babies did not have major malformations.

Answer

It is unlikely that the infant will have more congenital malformations than those expected in the general population, and no specific malformation has been attributed to benzodiazepines. However, depending on the time of the last administration of valium, the baby may not be alert and may even be floppy. Later on, the infant may exhibit a neonatal withdrawal syndrome.

REFERENCES

1. Uhlenhuth EH, DeWit H, Balter MB, Johanson CE, Mellinger GD. Risks and benefits of long-term benzodiazepine use. J Clin Psychopharmacol 1988; 8(3): 161–167.
2. Kerns LL. Treatment of mental disorders in pregnancy. A review of psychotropic drug risks and benefits. J Nerv Ment Dis 1986; 174:652–657.
3. Finnegan LP. Outcome of children born to women dependent on narcotics. Adv Alcohol Subst Abuse 1982; 1:55–97.
4. Kreek MJ. Opioid disposition and effects during chronic exposure in the perinatal period in man. Adv Alcohol Subst Abuse 1982; 1:21–54.
5. Gilberg C. Floppy infant syndrome and maternal diazepam. Lancet 1977; 2:244.
6. Nahas C, Goujard J. Phenothiazines, benzodiazepines and the fetus. Rev Perinatol Med 1978; 243:280.

7. Safra MJ, Oakley GP Jr. Association between cleft lip and/or palate and prenatal exposure to diazepam. Lancet 1975; 2:478-480.
8. Saxén I, Saxén L. Association between cleft lip with or without cleft palate and prenatal exposure to diazepam. Lancet 1975; 2:498.
9. Rosenberg L, Mitchell AA, Parsells JL, et al. Lack of relation of oral clefts to diazepam use during pregnancy. N Engl J Med 1983; 309(21):1282-1285.
10. Laegreid L, Olegard R, Wahlström J, Conradi N. Abnormalities in children exposed to benzodiazepines in utero. Lancet 1987; 1:108-109.
11. Czeizel A. Lack of evidence of teratogenicity of benzodiazepine drugs in Hungary. Reproduct Toxicol 1988; 1(3):183-188.
12. Pastuszak AL, Schick-Boschetto B, Zuber C, Feldkamp M, Pinelli M, Sihn S, Donnenfeld A, McCormack M, Leen-Mitchell M, Woodland C, Gardner A, Koren G. Pregnancy outcome following first trimester exposure to fluoxetine (Prozac). JAMA 1993; 269(17):2246-2248.
13. Cordero JF, Oakley GP Jr. Drug exposure during pregnancy: Some epidemiologic considerations. Clin Obstet Gynecol 1983; 26:418–428.
14. Laegreid L, Hagberg G, Lundberg A. Neurodevelopment in late infancy after prenatal exposure to benzodiazepines – A prospective study. Neuropediatrics
15. Bergman U, Boethius G, Swartling PG, Isacson D, Smedby B. Teratogenic effects of benzodiazepine use during pregnancy. J Pediatr 1990; 116(3):490.
16. Bergman U, Rosa FW, Baum C, Wiholm B-E, Faich GA. Effects of exposure to benzodiazepine during fetal life. Lancet 1992; 340:694-696.

7

Drugs and Chemicals Most Commonly Used by Pregnant Women

Monica Bologa
The Hospital for Sick Children and The Upjohn Company of Canada, Toronto, Ontario, Canada

Gideon Koren, Frank F. Fassos, and Michael McGuigan
The Hospital for Sick Children, Toronto, Ontario, Canada

Michael J. Rieder
The University of Western Ontario and the Children's Hospital of Western Ontario, London, Ontario, Canada

Clinical Case

A woman with repeated miscarriages tells you that she was found to have lupus antibodies and a specialist in the university hospital put her on low-dose aspirin for the rest of this pregnancy. She has heard bad things about salicylates in pregnancy.

INTRODUCTION

The thalidomide tragedy of the late 1950s has resulted in medical practitioners often viewing every drug and chemical as a reproductive hazard to the pregnant woman. The reality is that only a few compounds have been proven to be teratogenic in humans (see Chap. 3), whereas the vast majority probably do not pose a reproductive hazard.

In a recent analysis, we demonstrated that pregnant women exposed to drugs and chemicals known not to be teratogenic assigned themselves an unrealistically high teratogenic risk of 25. This assigned risk is comparable to the risk associated with thalidomide (1). There is a clear need for authoritative information and consultation services to assist pregnant women and their physicians in understanding fetal risks. The advice provided should

                                     Bologa et al.

Table 1 Most Common Antenatal Exposures Consulted in the
Motherisk Clinic in Toronto

1. Antibiotics
    $n = 55$ (12.8%)
    Erythromycin: 16
    Ampicillin: 12
    Penicillin: 9
    Trimethoprim-sulfamethoxazole: 9
    Tetracycline: 6
    Cephalosporins: 3
2. Analgesic-anti-inflammatory medication
    $n = 37$ (8.6%)
    Acetaminophen: 22
    ASA: 6
    Percocet, Tylenol #3: 3
    Percodan 222, 282: 3
    Codeine: 3
3. Paints, organic solvents
    $n = 34$ (7.9%)
    Water-based: 11
    Oil-based: 10
    Unspecified: 10
    Lead: 3
4. Cold medications
    $n = 32$ (7.5%)
    Sympathomimetic action (decongestants): 6
    Antihistamines: 11
    Sympathomimetic + antihistaminic action: 8
    Antitussives (dextromethorphan) + throat antiseptics: 7
5. Environmental pesticides
    $n = 28$ (6.5%)
    Unspecified: 16
    Organophosphates: 7
    Carbamates: 5
6. Cosmetic products for hair care
    $n = 24$ (5.6%)
    Dye: 10
    Permanent wave solution: 4
    Both: 7
    Bleach: 3
7. Video display terminals: 20 (4.7%)
8. Antiasthmatic medications
    $n = 17$ (4%)
    Adrenergic stimulants (Ventolin, Berotec): 9
    Corticosteroid (Beclovent, Beconase): 5
    Theophylline: 3

Table 1 (Continued)

9. X-rays: 17 (4%)
10. Pediculocides
    $n = 13$ (3%)
    Chlorinated insecticides (Lindane): 5
    Pyrethrins-piperonyl butoxide (R&C shampoo): 4
    Unspecified: 4
11. Anxiolytic medications
    $n = 11$ (2.6%)
    Diazepam and related drugs: 7
    Chlordiazepoxide: 4
12. Corticosteroids: 10 (2.3%)
13. Oral contraceptives: 8 (1.9%)
14. Rubella vaccine: 7 (1.6%)
15. Sugar substitutes: 6 (1.4%)
16. Local anesthesia (usually for dental work): 5 (1.1%)
17. H_2-receptor antagonists (ranitidine, cimetidine): 5 (1.1%)
18. Antihelmintic medications: 5 (1.1%)
19. Antifungal medications: 4 (0.9%)
20. Antitrichomonal medications (metronidazole): 4 (0.9%)
21. Laxatives: 4 (0.9%)
22. Antiemetics (Gravol): 4 (0.9%)
23. Mercury compounds: 4 (0.9%)
24. Ammonia: 4 (0.9%)
25. Natural gas (gas furnace and fuel gas): 4 (0.9%)
26. Antimalarial medications: 3 (0.7%)
27. General anesthesia: 3 (0.7%)

be based on unbiased, up-to-date information on the reproductive effects of drugs, chemicals, and radiation.

In September 1985, we started a consultation program for women concerned about antenatal exposure to drugs, chemicals, and radiation as well as exposure during lactation. A detailed description of the Motherisk Program appears elsewhere (2,3). Initially, all the women who contacted us were seen in our weekly clinic. Subsequently, because of the increase in the number of women and families seeking advice and the repetition of some of the questions posed by women and their physicians, we started a telephone information service for certain drug and chemical exposures. Calls are answered by a staff physician or a postgraduate fellow from the Motherisk team. During the telephone interviews, data are collected on special forms, which include the information deemed necessary, as well as a summary of the advice given (see Chapter 30).

A summary of the data from the first 6 months of telephone consultations (total = 450) appears in Table 1, which lists, in descending order of occurrence, the most common drugs and chemicals concerning women who called the Motherisk Program. The available information about the most common exposures during pregnancy is reviewed by the Motherisk team in an attempt to provide health professionals with the necessary information to answer such questions. By being prepared to answer questions about the listed exposures, the health professional is likely to cover more than 80% of the common exposures during pregnancy.

In most cases this chapter references a representative article for each exposure. For more information, the reader may wish to consult one of several textbooks (4–7).

ANTIBIOTICS AND ACYCLOVIR

For *erythromycin*, one initial animal study showed an association with congenital malformations (8), which was not confirmed by subsequent studies in animals or humans (9). Erythromycin estolate is contraindicated in pregnancy because the risk of cholestatic hepatitis appears to be increased in pregnant women (10).

Penicillin and *ampicillin* are commonly used antibiotics in pregnancy. Neither animal nor human studies provided evidence that either antibiotic is harmful to the fetus (11–13).

Trimethoprim has been shown to cross the placenta, and fetal concentrations are comparable to maternal concentrations (14), but the drug has not been incrimated as a teratogen (15,16).

Sulfonamides have been shown to cross the placenta at all stages of gestation (14). Large studies have not incriminated these substances as agents of teratogenesis in humans (15). Acute hemolytic anemia may occur in fetuses with glucose-6-phosphate dehydrogenase (G6PD) deficiency. When used during late pregnancy, sulfonamides may cause neonatal hyperbilirubinemia owing to displacement of bilirubin from albumin binding sites (17).

The main risk from *tetracycline* is a yellow-brown discoloration of teeth due to deposition of the antibiotic in calcifying teeth (18,19). The risk exists only later than 4–5 months of gestation, when the deciduous teeth begin to calcify. As for other malformations, large studies are contradictory or negative. Some authors could not demonstrate an increase in malformations associated with tetracycline (20,21). Others found a statistical association with minor malformations (inguinal hernia, hypospadias) (7). It is generally felt that tetracyclines are embryotoxic (in their effect on teeth), rather than teratogenic (22,23).

Cephalosporins have not demonstrated teratogenic potency in humans or animals (13,24,25).

ANALGESIC ANTI-INFLAMMATORY MEDICATION

Acetaminophen is believed to be nonteratogenic at therapeutic doses (26, 27). However, the effect of very high doses has not been assessed. There is a case report of a woman who consumed 1.3 g of acetaminophen daily throughout pregnancy for headache and nausea. She also developed severe anemia, which required several transfusions. During the fifth month, polyhydramnios developed; eight amniocenteses recovered 16 L of fluid. The infant died from severe renal insufficiency (28). The association between the drug intake and infant anomalies cannot be established on the basis of a single case report, however.

Aspirin is one of the most frequently ingested drugs in pregnancy (29). The intake of aspirin in the first trimester has not been associated with adverse effects (26). Aspirin intake in late pregnancy, especially within 1 week of delivery, may affect neonatal coagulation and may cause premature closure of the ductus arteriosus. There are reports ranging from no apparent effect in the newborn to minor hemorrhagic phenomena to neonatal purpura with depressed platelet function (30). An increased incidence of intraventricular hemorrhage (IVH) in premature or low birth weight infants has been associated with maternal aspirin intake: 12 out of 17 aspirin-exposed newborns (71%) developed IVH, compared to 41 out of 91 non-aspirin-exposed infants (41%) (31).

Aspirin consumption late in pregnancy may also produce adverse effects in the mother: antepartum and/or postpartum hemorrhage, prolonged gestation, and prolonged labor, resulting from the inhibition of prostaglandin synthetase (32).

Codeine is a widely used narcotic analgesic. It has not been associated with an increased risk of malformations (33). The use of large doses of codeine near term may result in a neonatal narcotic withdrawal syndrome (34–36).

PAINTS, ORGANIC SOLVENTS

Organic solvents are ubiquitous in the industrialized environment, appearing as individual agents or in complex associations. These compounds are volatile, and their vapors may gain access to the maternal and fetal circulations. While the most common site of toxicity is the central nervous system (CNS), the wide structural diversity of organic solvents results in potentially different teratogenic effects (37).

Many industrial solvents are teratogenic in laboratory *animals*. While malformations depend on the specific solvent and animal species, described animal malformations include poor fetal development, hydrocephalus, exencephaly, liver abnormalities, blood changes, and skeletal and cardiovascular defects. In vitro studies show that some organic solvents are weak mutagens (38).

Chronic exposure to benzene induces chromosomal changes in human hematopoietic cells and may lead to an increased risk of leukemia or aplastic anemia. This compound is teratogenic or embryolethal in some animal species (39).

Induction of birth defects in *humans* by industrial solvents is controversial. A widely quoted case control study claimed increased exposure to organic solvents among mothers of children with CNS malformations when compared to mothers of normal controls (40). Several epidemiological studies have demonstrated that women who work in laboratories or other industrial environments have an increased risk of miscarriage (37,41,42) or gastrointestinal malformations, such as omphalocele, gastroschisis, and esophageal stenosis or atresia (39). Another study reports that exposure to organic solvents can induce menstrual disturbances or decreased fertility (the latter in males as well) (43).

Most pregnant women who use oil-based paints apply them to one or more rooms of their home, generally in preparation for the new child. It is unlikely that such a brief, low dose exposure will cause any of the conditions that may be associated with occupational exposure throughout pregnancy.

Water-based paints, or latex paints, pose no increased reproductive risk because they have low volatility.

Lead is a common constituent in glass-staining materials. It is teratogenic in laboratory animals, causing skeletal and CNS defects, oral clefts, and fetal death (37,44).

In humans, lead is known to induce abortions; however, no increase in teratogenic risk has been described. Because of its abortifacient properties, there are occupational regulations for women's exposure to lead (45). In a study of 71 pregnancies in women working with lead, 11% ended in miscarriages and neonatal mortality was almost 40% (46). When the course of 253 pregnancies of women residing in America's "lead belt" was compared with an equal number of pregnancies occurring elsewhere, there were more cases of premature rupture of membranes and more preterm babies in the first group. Malformations were not reported (47). One infant with a high blood lead level and erythrocyte protoporphyrin at birth developed neurological disability at 13 months of age (48). A recent study pointed to a possible association between umbilical lead above 10 μg/dL and slightly lower scores in the Bailey test (49).

Pregnant women who may have occupational exposure to lead during pregnancy shold be referred to a reproductive toxicologist or other health professionals with similar expertise.

COLD MEDICATIONS

Decongestants

Phenylephrine and *pseudoephedrine* as well as other sympathomimetic agents have not been shown to increase the risk of teratogenicity in humans (50). An association was found between the intake of sympathomimetic drugs in the first trimester of pregnancy and minor malformations, like inguinal hernia and clubfoot (7), but this was not confirmed by other studies. However, sympathomimetic amines are teratogenic in some animal species (51).

Antihistamines

Most of the antihistamine compounds available in over-the-counter preparations have not been implicated as bearers of untoward effects. A large prospective study of antihistamine exposure in pregnancy showed that only with brompheniramine was there a statistically significant association with teratogenicity: out of 65 cases of first-trimester exposures (in the Collaborative Perinatal Project: CPP), 10 had malformed offspring (7). However, a recent meta-analysis failed to show teratogenicity of brompheniramine (52).

Diphenhydramine, despite an initial report of possible association with an increased incidence of oral clefts, is now considered to have no significant teratogenic potential.

The use of antihistamines in the first trimester does not increase the risk for major birth defects (53).

Antitussives

Dextromethorphan has not been implicated as a potential teratogen.

ENVIRONMENTAL PESTICIDES

Increasing interest in the reproductive toxicity of pesticides and other agricultural chemicals arose after the extensive use during the Vietnam War of the defoliant Agent Orange, which was believed to be associated with an increased incidence of spontaneous abortions, stillbirths, and malformations (45). However, current data do not reveal strong evidence of fetotoxicity unless the dose was excessive.

Insecticides are basically divided into organophosphates, aromatic carbamate esters, and chlorinated compounds. Many of them have teratogenic potential in laboratory animals, inducing various structural abnormalities (skeletal and brain defects) (54–56).

Organophosphates are commonly used insecticides with irreversible cholinesterase-inhibiting properties (56). In animal studies, dose levels that were not maternally lethal did not produce fetotoxicity, fetal lethality, or malformations (57). *Malathion* is a common household organophosphate insecticide that is also used topically for the treatment of lice. There are no reports of human teratogenicity from the use of malathion, and animal studies were negative (58).

Carbamates exert a reversible cholinesterase-inhibiting activity (56). In animal studies, neither *propoxur* nor *carbofuran* caused fetal lethality or developmental abnormalities at dose levels that were not maternally lethal (57). *Methyl benzimidazole carbamate* (MBC) has a demonstrated capacity to interfere with mitosis in different species (fungi, viruses, bacteria, cells of bovine brain). Although the studies concluded that MBC was a potential teratogen, a study in rats and rabbits revealed some degree of embryolethality but no visceral or skeletal malformations (60). Although the cholinesterase inhibitors are commonly used, there is a lack of human reports on their reproductive effects.

Very few of the women consulting the Motherisk Clinic with concerns about environmental pesticides had been exposed to toxic amounts of these compounds; rather, they had been in the area where pesticides were sprayed and consequently could smell them. It is conceivable that in the absence of symptomatic maternal toxicity, such short exposure will not cause embryonal or fetal damage. Whenever a woman exposed to these chemicals experiences any degree of clinical toxicity, she and her fetus should be closely monitored by a physician.

COSMETIC PRODUCTS FOR HAIR CARE

Dyes

The numerous hair dye formulations available on the market can be classified into five groups:

1. Hair restorers
2. Vegetable hair dyes
3. Temporary dyes
4. Semipermanent dyes
5. Permanent/oxidation dyes

The most frequent consultations to the Motherisk Clinic involved the "permanent" formulations. These are complex compounds of a variety of chemical classes, which may include phenylenediamine, toluenediamine, resorcinol, aminophenol, naphthol, 1-methyl-[^{20}H]aminobenzene, nonoxynol, oleic acid, isopropyl alcohol, ammonium hydroxide, trisodium acetate ascorbic acid, sodium sulfite, and sodium hydroxide (61).

Questions about the safety of hair products were raised as a result of some studies showing mutagenic activity in the Ames test (62). Recently, a study of 13 Chinese hair dyes showed negative Ames test results (63).

There are no *human* studies available on these substances. Studies in laboratory *animals* (rats, rabbits) are available for some of them, and no teratogenicity has been shown for most. Some compounds (phenylenediamine and toluene compounds, possibly animophenol and resorcinol) are considered to be potentially mutagenic and teratogenic (61,63).

As to the potential toxicity of the substances, aromatic nitro and amino compounds can become cyanogenic at toxic levels, thus theoretically raising the possibility that the fetus will be affected, as well. However, documentation of these potentially toxic effects has involved cases of industrial intoxication, with digestive absorption of large amounts of chemicals (61). The transcutaneous absorption of these substances is not well defined, but probably the amount of hair coloring agents entering the systemic circulation is small (64).

In a study of 12 hair dye formulations tested for systemic toxicity by topical application to rabbits, no clinical or histomorphological evidence of systemic effects was found. These formulations (three semipermanent formulations and nine oxidation dyes) were also tested for teratogenic effects following dermal application to pregnant rats. The course of pregnancy was not significantly affected, and no biologically significant soft tissue or skeletal changes were noted (62).

In another study, five oxidation dyes were administered by gavage to pregnant rats. No signs of toxicity were observed during the treatment period. Even after administration of doses exceeding 110-fold the human exposure, there were no significant changes in fetal development and structure (65), but a significant decrease in the mean maternal weight gain was recorded.

Permanent Wave Solutions

Permanent waves in hair are produced by the use of two solutions: the *waving fluid*, which is an alkaline thioglycolate solution (e.g., ammonium thioglycolate, thioglycerol), and the *fixation/neutralization* solution, which is an acid hydrogen peroxide solution.

The waving solution may have irritant properties; the ammonium thioglycolate may cause respiratory symptoms owing to immediate-type hypersensitivity. No teratogenicity has been implicated in the use of these products in animals. The hydrogen peroxide, which has a local irritant effect, is rapidly degraded to water and oxygen, and does not cause systemic effects (64).

Bleach

Hair bleaching formulas contain *hydrogen peroxide* and *"per-" salt*, such as ammonium persulfate, which may cause contact allergy and rhinitis or serious respiratory symptoms owing to immediate-type hypersensitivity (64). In general, most exposures involve low dose levels. If there should be evidence of apparent toxicity, the pregnant woman should be seen by a physician. There are no reports of reproductive effects in either humans or animals.

VIDEO DISPLAY TERMINALS

The suspicion that the use of video display terminals (VDTs) had adverse effects on the embryo and fetus started after several clusters of miscarriages and malformations were reported (66). However, investigation reconfirmed that video display terminals do not emit x-rays, microwaves, or other radiation at levels that would be harmful (67,68). Current data indicate that VDTs do not increase the risk to either the pregnant woman or the fetus (67,68).

ANTIASTHMATIC MEDICATIONS

None of the medications used for the treatment of acute asthmatic attacks has been incriminated as a teratogen.

Salbutamol has not been shown to be teratogenic in animals. There are no human studies on the first-trimester use of salbutamol. The drug may cause fetal tachycardia and maternal hyperglycemia, which results in increased serum insulin and potential postnatal hypoglycemia (69,70). The use of inhaled β-adrenergic agonists during pregnancy does not cause any significant increase in incidences in fetal defects or labor complications (71–73).

Theophylline has not been associated with an increased teratogenic risk (7) or stillbirths (74) in humans. In asthmatic pregnant patients at risk for premature delivery, theophylline was suggested to reduce perinatal death and respiratory distress syndrome frequencies (75).

Systemic *corticosteroids* have been shown to induce cleft palate and lip in numerous animal species (76,77). However, reports of more than 1100 pregnancies have failed to demonstrate teratogenicity in humans (7,78). The systemic bioavailability of corticosteroids is poor, and thus it is very unlikely that they would cause an untoward effect (72,79). The current approach is to treat optimally asthmatic attacks during pregnancy, since the complications of untreated asthma far outweigh unproven reproductive effects (64, 79) associated with the medications. It is believed that corticosteroids can be used safely in pregnancy (72,79).

X-RAYS

Exposure to radiation doses less than 5 rad is not associated with an increase in congenital malformations (80). In the dose range of 5–15 rad, there may be an increased teratogenic risk. For dosages of more than 15 rad, there appears to be a two- to threefold increase in the incidence of major malformations (81,82). The normal exposure for diagnostic x-rays generally should be far below the teratogenic range. In any case, the radiologist involved should be contacted to estimate the apparent dose of exposure.

PEDICULOCIDES

There are no reports of an increased incidence of malformations associated with the topical use of antilouse medication.

Lindane (γ-benzene hexachloride) is a chlorinated insecticide. Animal studies showed no teratogenicity associated with the use of this drug (4). The manufacturer recommends caution in pregnancy, although there are no reports of congenital defects in humans. Lindane is potentially neurotoxic (83). Therefore, percutaneous absorption should be minimized by decreasing the concentration of the solution (< 1%) and the duration of exposure (few minutes), since the substance is readily absorbed (84).

Pyrethrins with piperonyl butoxide are poorly absorbed and their potential toxicity is lower than for lindane. Therefore, they are generally considered safer in pregnancy (85).

Sulfur compounds are often used as alternative scabicides in children, pregnant women, and patients with massively excoriated skin. Approximately 1% of the topically applied sulfur compound is absorbed, but it does not appear to cause systemic toxicity. There are no reports of teratogenicity from sulfur compounds. In animal studies, despite some evidence of adverse reproductive effects, sulfur compounds had no developmental toxicity (86).

ANXIOLYTIC MEDICATIONS

Initial studies reported a three- to fourfold increased risk of cleft palate in the offspring of women exposed to *diazepam* (87,88). This would increase the specific risk to 3–4 per 1000 in the general population. (When compared to the general population baseline, teratogenic risk of 1–5 per 100, the figures are not alarming.) Conversely, other studies did not confirm this finding (89,90). In surveys, no such association was detected (91,92). A large single dose (> 30 mg) or sustained prenatal diazepam use can lead to the "floppy infant syndrome" (93), in which the infant demonstrates hypotonia, respiratory embarrassment, difficulty in suckling, and hypothermia (93,94).

Chlordiazepoxide is a benzodiazepine compound. Initial studies associated its use in early pregnancy with an increased malformation rate (95). A case control study suggested a higher usage by mothers of children with congenital heart disease (96). Animal studies (mice and hamsters) showed a higher risk of cleft palate and multiple malformations (97). The Collaborative Perinatal Project did not detect an increased risk in 257 cases of exposure in the first trimester (7). More recently, studies have confirmed the findings of the project (91,92). At present, chlordiazepoxide is not considered to significantly increase the occurrence of malformations (93).

CORTICOSTEROIDS

Corticosteroids are indicated for a variety of conditions that occur during pregnancy, including asthma, arthritis, nephrotic syndrome, and inflammatory bowel disease (see discussion on corticosteroids under Antiasthmatic Medications, above).

ORAL CONTRACEPTIVES

The literature on the teratogenic effect of oral contraceptives is extensive. Although limb reduction defects, neural tube defects, cardiovascular lesions, and renal, anal, tracheal, and esophageal malformations from steroidal estrogens have been suggested (60%), a large number of studies contradict these reports (98–102). Most studies, both positive and negative, have been heavily criticized for their methodology. The current consensus of opinion is: "Oral contraceptives present no major teratogenic hazard" (102). Wilson and Brent have summarized recent data by saying that "the use of exogenous hormones during human pregnancy has not been proved to cause developmental abnormalities in non-genital organ and tissue . . ." (103). (For development of genital organs, see discussion of progesterone, which follows.)

Progesterone

Current literature on the teratogenic effects of progesterone is voluminous. Several synthetic progestins have been documented to cause female pseudohermaphroditism (104). Of the progestins reported, ethisterone and norethindrone are the most active and account for most of the 200 cases of masculinization reported to date. Natural progestin (i.e., progesterone) appears to be responsible for very few cases of sex changes. The overall risk appears to be 0.3–2.2%, with one early series describing 18% with norethrindrone (105). The small amount of progestogens present in oral contraceptives is unlikely to cause virilization of a female fetus (98).

It is currently believed that these hormones do not contribute measurably to the frequency of hypospadias (106).

RUBELLA VACCINE

Almost 1000 normal infants have been born to women who received rubella vaccine during pregnancy. In two cases, there were defects typical of rubella embryopathy (107,108). In one case, the mother was seronegative, and it was argued that teratogenic effects will be evident only in nonimmune women. However, 15% of the injected mothers are seronegative, and if this mechanism were responsible, many more should have had teratogenic effects. On the basis of two cases of adverse outcome versus 1000 with no problems, the pregnancy-related exposure to rubella vaccine cannot be considered to be significantly teratogenic.

SUGAR SUBSTITUTES

There is no strong evidence to indicate that the use of reasonable amounts of artificial or nonsugar sweetening agents has any adverse effect on human fetal development.

One study outlined an increased prevalence of behavior problems (hyperactivity, irritability, and nervousness, as well as mental retardation) and physical anomalies (deformities of bones) among offspring of mothers who were users of artificial sweeteners during pregnancy as compared to nonusers (109). However, the type of sweetening agent was not identified in the above-mentioned reports.

Saccharin was shown to have no teratogenic activity in a number of studies in mice, rats, and rabbits (110,111). Some commercially available by-products (e.g., the benzoic forms) were teratogenic in a few animal studies, inducing ocular and other developmental anomalies (111).

Aspartame is broken down in the small intestine into aspartic acid, methanol, and phenylalanine. *Aspartic acid* does not readily cross the placenta (112); *methanol* is oxidized to formaldehyde and subsequently to formic acid. However, the rate of formate synthesis does not exceed the rate of urinary excretion (113). Furthermore, the amount of methanol ingested per can of aspartame-sweetened beverage would be less than that from an equal volume of fruit juice (112). *Phenylalanine* is concentrated on the fetal side of the placenta but does not pose any risk to the fetus at the doses studied (113).

LOCAL ANESTHESIA

Teratogenicity (skeletal anomalies, cataracts) has been associated with the use of *lidocaine hydrochloride* in animals (114). In humans, lidocaine crosses the placenta and may cause some neonatal depression and neurobehavioral changes after maternal intravenous administration of doses slightly higher than the antiarrhythmic doses (84). Lidocaine does not cause malformations after topical administration or injection for local anesthesia (115).

H₂-RECEPTOR ANTAGONISTS

Ranitidine and *cimetidine* are very commonly prescribed, and there are no reports of teratogenicity from either of these two drugs. *Animal* studies were negative in the rabbit for ranitidine, and negative in the mouse, rat, and rabbit for cimetidine (116,117). Cimetidine crosses the placenta and has been used at term with antacids to prevent gastric acid aspiration and subsequent pneumonitis (Mendelson's syndrome). No adverse effects have been noted in the neonate in these studies (118,119). Transient liver impairment has been described in one newborn after cimetidine exposure at term (120).

Three women took ranitidine throughout their pregnancy for control of duodenal ulcers and no teratogenic effects on the offspring were detected (121). In a prospective study we failed to show teratogenicity of ranitidine and cimetidine in humans (119).

ANTIHELMINTHIC MEDICATIONS

Among the various drugs used for the treatment of helminthic infestations, the common ones used during pregnancy were *pyrantel pamoate, pyrvinium pamoate,* and *piperazine.* These drugs act within the gastrointestinal (GI) lumen, and their intestinal absorption is ideally small. Piperazine is readily absorbed from the GI tract, whereas for pyrantel pamoate and pyrvinium pamoate the absorption is low (< 15% for pyrvinium pamoate) (122).

Animal studies on piperazine (in rats and pigs) and on pyrantel pamoate (in rats, pigs, and goats) were all negative (123,124).

There are no data available on human exposure during pregnancy for pyrantel pamoate or pyrvinium pamoate.

In a prospective study of three mother–child pairs with first-trimester exposure to piperazine, no evidence was found that would suggest a relationship to malformations (7). In a case report, piperazine tartrate was effective and safe in eliminating a helminthic infection (125).

ANTIFUNGAL MEDICATIONS

Few of the antifungals have been proven to be teratogenic in animal studies. Systemic administration of flucytosine or griseofulvin has caused multiple malformations in different animals (126–128). In human studies, only systemic griseofulvin has been associated with congenital malformations. This positive association is limited to one report, in which three abortions and two congenital malformations were described (129).

Any *topical antifungal agent* can be used during pregnancy. Vaginal application should be avoided after the amniotic membranes have ruptured (84). *Clotrimazole* has been used topically in pregnancy, and no associations with congenital malformations have been reported (130). *Miconazole* has been associated with an increase in fetal mortality in different animal studies when administered during active organogenesis (131). In humans, there is no reported adverse effect of miconazole on the fetus (132). *Nystatin* is poorly absorbed, and its use has not been associated with teratogenesis (130,133).

ANTITRICHOMONAL MEDICATION

Metronidazole has not been incriminated as a teratogen in more than 800 pregnancies, including almost 300 with first-trimester exposure (134). Rats given up to five times the human dose showed no apparent adverse effect on either fertility or fetal development. Lifetime studies in hamsters were negative (135). Two infants with midline facial defects were reported whose mothers were treated with metronidazole during the first trimester for amebiasis (136). If a teratogenic risk exists with metronidazole use, it must be minimal.

LAXATIVES

Laxatives are among the most frequently used drugs during pregnancy, and there is no evidence to indicate adverse effects on human development from the most of them. Since their action is local, their absorption and, therefore, access to the fetus is minimal (122). Most animal studies were negative; however, a few cathartics or laxatives are teratogenic or embryotoxic in animals, inducing minor skeletal changes (137).

Docusate (sodium, potassium or calcium) is a common ingredient in many laxative preparations. A prospective study of 116 patients exposed to docusate sodium during pregnancy revealed no evidence of an association with malformations (7). Chronic use of large doses of the laxatives throughout pregnancy may cause hypomagnesemia in the mother and offspring (138). *Castor oil* may induce uterine contractions and therefore is contraindicated in pregnancy (122).

ANTIEMETICS

Dimenhydrinate is the chlorotheophylline salt of diphenhydramine. Two prospective studies (7,139) show no increased risk of teratogenicity from the use of dimenhydrinate. These data are consolidated by negative results in animals (140). Dimenhydrinate is not known to carry an increased risk of birth defects (141).

Bendectin is a combination of doxylamine and pyridoxine, developed as an antinauseant for use during pregnancy. Shortly after it came on the market, isolated case reports of limb reduction defects led to a large number of litigations against the manufacturer, although cohort and case control studies did not show a higher than baseline risk for malformations (141,142). The manufacturer removed the product from the American market in 1983 because of the exceedingly high costs of insurance. A company in Quebec now makes an identical product, which has been approved in Canada to be used in pregnancy.

MERCURY COMPOUNDS

In our survey, the concerns about mercury almost always involved the accidental ingestion of metallic (elemental) mercury in the form of dental amalgams or the contents of a thermometer. Swallowed elemental mercury is not absorbed to a significant degree from the GI tract and does not pose any risk for systemic toxicity.

Once absorbed, practically all mercury compounds are teratogenic in animals and humans (143). The most potent teratogen is *methyl mercury*, the causative agent of the well-defined Minamata disease (144).

Prolonged inhalation exposure to inorganic mercury may cause menstrual disturbances (45). This substance also reduces fertility and contaminates breast milk (145). In animals, inorganic mercury crosses the placenta and can be found in the fetal brain. Normal fetal development may be reduced (144). Metallic (mercuric) mercury, injected into pregnant rats, causes structural and functional damage to the mother's kidneys. It also causes fetal malformations, mainly brain defects. It is possible that the fetal defects result not from any direct action of mercury on the fetus, but from the inhibition of the transport of essential metabolites from the mother or from maternal kidney dysfunction (146). Because of potential adverse effects of inhaled mercury vapors, occupational levels should be zero to allow pregnant women to work in this environment.

AMMONIA

Ammonia vapors can cause respiratory tract irritation but no systemic toxicity (147).

The different halogenated ammonia compounds and ammonia salts have been associated with negative studies as well as some positive reports on developmental anomalies, which were most likely caused by the halogen, not by the ammonia (148).

NATURAL GAS

Natural gas is approximately 85% methane. In high concentrations *methane* is an asphyxiant, but it causes no systemic toxicity (149). Of more concern is the combustion product, *carbon monoxide.* Carbon monoxide is a known teratogen causing CNS abnormalities in the fetus (150). In pregnant women exposed to leaking or malfunctioning gas furnaces, the carboxyhemoglobin level should be determined and the patient should be referred to a specialized service.

Fuel gas, a mixture of methane, ethane, propane, and butane, is considered to be potentially teratogenic in animals. Pregnant mice exposed to 5–8% concentrations of fuel gas on day 8 of gestation produced offspring with hydrocephalus and exencephaly (151).

ANTIMALARIAL MEDICATION

Chloroquine and *hydroxychloroquine* are the drugs of choice for prophylaxis and treatment of sensitive malaria species during pregnancy (152). There was no evidence of teratogenicity in a study of 169 infants exposed to 300 mg of chloroquine base per week in utero (153) or in a study at the Motherisk Clinic, where 14 healthy babies were born to women exposed to either of the drugs in the first trimester of pregnancy (154). Currently these drugs are used for the treatment of systemic lupus erythematosus in doses much higher than those used for malaria prophylaxis. The safety of these higher doses has not been established.

The other antimalarials—quinine, primaquine, and pyrimethamine with dapsone (Maloprim) or with sulfadoxine (Fansidar)—have been incriminated as possible abortifacients and should be avoided during pregnancy (152).

GENERAL ANESTHESIA

There is no evidence that a single course of general anesthesia in early pregnancy is teratogenic. A recent study (115) supports the findings of a prospective study (155), demonstrating the safety of nitrous oxide. Similarly, thiopental, enflurane, and halothane were not shown to cause untoward embryonal or fetal effects (115,156,157). These results are different from occupational exposure to inhalational anesthetics, where cumulative exposure may be hazardous to the developing fetus (38) or may cause an increased risk for miscarriages (115).

GENERAL INSTRUCTIONS

When advising a pregnant woman over the telephone about the potential reproductive effect of drugs, chemicals, or radiation, the health professional should rule out other risk factors that may affect her pregnancy outcome. These factors include age; obstetrical and medical history; other exposure, including alcohol and smoking; genetic background; paternal exposures;

and medical history. Socioeconomic status also plays an important role in the normal nutrition and progress of a pregnancy.

The interviewer should advise the woman that in every pregnancy there is a 1–5% risk of major malformations and that even if her exposure does not appear to increase the teratogenic risk, such a risk still exists.

Answer

Salicylates, alone or combined with low-dose corticosteroids, have been shown to prevent repeated miscarriages in selected groups of women. The drug has not been shown to adversely affect the fetus. Theoretically, it may cause premature closure of fetal ductus arteriosus or bleeding complications, but these complications were not documented in small doses.

REFERENCES

1. Koren G, Bologa M, Long D, Feldman Y, Henderson K, Shear N. The perception of teratogenic risk by pregnant women exposed to drugs and chemicals during the first trimester. Am J Obstet Gynecol 1989; 160:1190–1194.
2. Koren G, Feldman Y, Shear N. Motherisk — A new approach to antenatal counselling of drug/chemical exposure. Vet Hum Toxicol 1986; 28:563–565.
3. Koren G, MacLeod SM. Monitoring and avoiding drug and chemical teratogenicity. Can Med Assoc J 1986; 125:1079–1081.
4. Schardein JL. Chemically Induced Birth Defects. Marcel Dekker, New York, 1985.
5. Briggs GC, Freeman RK, Yaffe SJ. Drugs in pregnancy and lactation, 2nd ed. Williams & Wilkins, Baltimore, 1986.
6. Sheppard TH. Catalog of Teratogenic Agents, 5th ed. Johns Hopkins University Press, Baltimore, 1986.
7. Heinonen OP, Slone D, Shapiro S. Birth Defects and Drugs in Pregnancy. PSG Publishing Company, Littleton, MA, 1977.
8. Miyoshi T. Experimental studies on the effects of toxicants on pregnancy of rats. J Osaka City Med Center 1959; 8:309–318.
9. Philipson A, Sabath LD, Charles D. Erythromycin and clindamycin absorption and elimination in pregnant women. Clin Pharmacol Ther 1976; 19:68–77.
10. McCormack WM, George H, Donner A, Kodgis LF, Albert S, Lowe EW, Kass EH. Hepatotoxicity of erythromycin estolate during pregnancy. Antimicrob Agents Chemother 1977; 12:630–635.
11. Wasz-Hockert O, Nummi S, Voupala S, Jarvinen P. Transplacental passage of azidocillin, ampicillin and penicillin G during early and late pregnancy. Acta Paediatr Scand 1970; 206(suppl):109–110.
12. Ceccarelli P, Rossi M, Cianti F, Domenici C. Use of amoxicillin in the obstetrical and gynecological field. Minerva Gynecol 1977; 29:137–142.
13. Cheung M. Counselling the pregnant patient. Cont Pract 1988; 15(2):7–14.

14. Reid DWJ, Caille G, Kaufmann NR. Maternal and transplacental kinetics of trimethoprim and sulfamethoxazole, separately and in combination. Can Med Assoc J 1975; 112:67S–72S.
15. Ochoa AG. Trimethoprim and sulfamethoxazole in pregnancy. JAMA 1971; 217:1244–1245.
16. Brumfitt W, Prusell R. Double-blind trial to compare ampicillin, cephalexin, cotrimoxazole, and trimethoprim in treatment of urinary infection. Br Med J 1972; 2:673–676.
17. Jamerot G, Into-Malmberg MB, Esbjorner E. Placental transfer of sulphasalazine and sulphapyridine and some of its metabolites. Scand J Gastroenterol 1981; 16:693–697.
18. Cohlan SQ. Tetracycline staining of teeth. Teratology 1977; 15:127–130.
19. Rubin P. Prescribing in pregnancy. Practitioner 1990; 234:556–560.
20. Culshaw JA. TTC and congenital limb abnormalities. Br Med J 1962; 2:924–927.
21. Elder HA, Santamarina BAG, Smith S, Kass EH. The natural history of asymptomatic bacteriuria during pregnancy. The effect of tetracycline on the clinical course and the outcome of pregnancy. Am J Obstet Gynecol 1971; 111:441–462.
22. Corcoran R, Castles JM. Tetracycline for acne vulgaris and possible teratogenesis. Br Med J 1977; 2:807–808.
23. Graham JM, Blanco JD. Chlamydial infections. Prim Care 1990; 17(1):85–93.
24. Hasegawa Y, Yoshida T, Kozen T. A teratological study on cefamandole in rats and rabbits. Chemotherapy 1979; 27(suppl 5): 658–681.
25. Chu Chen K, Sabeti S. L'evaluation clinique de la cephalexin orale. Int J Clin Pharmacol 1970; 2(suppl):124–128.
26. Rudolph AM. Effects of aspirin and acetaminophen in pregnancy and in the newborn. Arch Intern Med 1981; 141:358–363.
27. Levy G, Garretson LK, Soda DM. Evidence of placental transfer of acetaminophen. Pediatrics 1975; 55:895–899.
28. Char VC, Chandra R, Fletcher AB, Avery GB. Polyhydramnios and neonatal renal failure — A possible association with maternal acetaminophen ingestion. J Pediatr 1975; 86:638–639.
29. Corby DG. Aspirin and pregnancy: Maternal and fetal effects. Pediatrics 1978; 62(suppl):930–937.
30. Collins E, Turner G. Maternal effects of regular salicylate ingestion in pregnancy. Lancet 1975; 2:335–337.
31. Rumack CM, Guggenheim MA, Rumack BM, Peterson RG, Johnson ML, Braithwaite WR. Neonatal intracranial hemorrhage and maternal use of aspirin. Obstet Gynecol 1981; 58(suppl):525–565.
32. Wolff F, Berg R, Bolte A. Clinical study of the labor inhibiting effects and side effects of ASA. Geburtshilfe Frauenheilkd 1981; 41:96–100.
33. Little BB, Snell LM, Klein VR, Gilstrap LC, Knoll KA, Breckenridge JD. Maternal and fetal effects of heroin addiction during pregnancy. J Reprod Med 1990; 35:159–162.
34. Mangurten HH, Benawra R. Neonatal codeine withdrawal in infants of non-addicted mothers. Pediatrics 1980; 65:159–160.

35. Van Leeuwen G, Guthrie R, Strange F. Narcotic withdrawal reaction in a newborn infant due to codeine. Pediatrics 1965; 36:635–636.

36. Smith CG, Smith MT. Substance abuse and reproduction. Sem Reprod Endocrinol 1990; 8(1):55–64.

37. Taskinen HK. Effects of parental occupational exposures on spontaneous abortion and congenital malformations. Scand J Work Environ Health 1990; 16: 297–314.

38. Hemminki K, Sorsa M, Vainio H. Occupational Hazards and Reproduction. Hemisphere, Washington, DC, 1985.

39. Editorial. Is there a fetal solvent syndrome? A medical letter. Reprod Toxicol 1983; 2(5).

40. Holmberg PC. CNS defects in children born to mothers exposed to organic solvents during pregnancy. Lancet 1979; 2:177–179.

41. Huel G, Merlger D, Bowler R. Evidence for adverse reproductive outcomes among women microelectronic assembly workers. Br J Ind Med 1990; 47:400–404.

42. Lindbohm MJ, Taskinen H, Sallman M, Herminki K. Spontaneous abortions among women exposed to organic solvents. Am J Ind Med 1990; 17:449–463.

43. Wong O, Utidjian MD, Karten VS. Retrospective evaluation of reproductive performance of workers exposed to ethylene dibromide (EDB). J Occup Med 1979; 21:98–102.

44. Roeleveld N, Zielhuis GA, Gabreels F. Occupational exposure and defects of the central nervous system in offspring: Review. Br J Ind Med 1990; 47:580–588.

45. Barlow SM. Reproductive effects of occupation. In Drug and Chemical Action in Pregnancy (Fabro S, Scialli AR, eds), Marcel Dekker, New York, 1986, pp 353–373.

46. Rom WN. Effects of lead on the female and reproduction: A review. Mt Sinai J Med 1976; 43(5):542–551.

47. Fahim MS, Fahim Z, Hall DG. Effects of subtoxic lead levels on pregnant women in the state of Missouri. International Conference on Heavy Metals in the Environment, Toronto, 1975.

48. Singh N, Donovan CM, Hanshaw JB. Neonatal lead intoxication in a prenatally exposed infant. J Pediatr 1978; 93:1019–1021.

49. Bellinger D, Leviton A, Watermaux C, Needleman H, Rabinowitz M. Longitudinal analysis of prenatal and postnatal lead exposure and early cognitive development. N Engl J Med 1987; 316:1037–1043.

50. Smith CV, Rayburn WF, Anderson JC, Duckworth AF, Appell LL. Effect of a single dose of oral pseudoephedrine on uterine and fetal Doppler blood flow. Obstet Gynecol 1990; 76:803–806.

51. Loevy H, Roth BF. Induced cleft palate development in mice: Comparison between the effect of epinephrine and cortisone. Anat Rec 1968; 160:386–390.

52. Seto A, Einarson TR, Koren G. Evaluation of brompheniramine safety in pregnancy. Repro Tox 1993; 7:393–395.

53. Seto A. Meta-analysis of adverse neonatal effects due to maternal exposure to antihistamines. M Sc thesis, University of Toronto, 1993.

54. Kavlock RJ, Chernoff N, Gray LE, Gray JA, Whitehouse D. Teratogenic effects of benomyl in the Wistar rat and CD-1 mouse, with emphasis on the route of administration. Toxicol Appl Pharmacol 1982; 62:44–54.
55. Ottolenghi AD, Haseman JK, Suggs F. Teratogenic effects of aldrin, dieldrin, endrin in hamsters and mice. Teratology 1974; 9:11–16.
56. Banerjee J. Inhibition of human fetal brain acetylcholinesterase; marker effect of neurotoxicity. J Toxicol Environ Health 1991; 33:283–290.
57. Courtney KD, Andrees JE, Springer J, Dalley L. Teratogenic evaluation of the pesticides baygon, carbofuran, dimethoate, and EPN. J Environ Sci Health 1985; B20(4):373–406.
58. Kanja LW, Skaare JV, Ojwang SBO, Maitai CK. A comparison of organochlorine pesticide residues in maternal adipose tissue, maternal blood, cord blood, and human milk from mother/infant pairs. Arch Environ Contam Toxicol 1992; 22:21–24.
59. Dobbins PK. Organic phosphate insecticides as teratogens in the rat. J Fla Med Assoc 1967; 54:452–456.
60. Janardhan A, Sattur PB, Sisodia P. Teratogenicity of methyl benzimidazole carbamate in rats and rabbits. Bull Environ Contam Toxicol 1984; 33:257–263.
61. Gosselin RE, Smith RP, Hodge HC, Braddock JE. Clinical Toxicology of Commercial Products, 5th ed. Williams & Wilkins, Baltimore, 1984.
62. Burnett C, Goldenthal EI, Harris SB, Wazeter FX, Strausburg J, Kapp R, Voelker R. Teratology and percutaneous toxicity studies on hair dyes. J Toxicol Environ Health 1976; 1:1027–1040.
63. Wong L, Li SL, Qin YH, Xu FD, Wang ZS, Song XD, Li J. Studies on mutagenicity of hair dyes made in China. Biomed Environ Sci 1991; 4:310–316.
64. Nater JP, DeGroot AC. Unwanted Effects of Cosmetics and Drugs Used in Dermatology. Elsevier, Amsterdam, 1985.
65. DiNardo JC, Picciano JC, Schnetzinger RW, Morris WE, Wolf BA. Teratological assessment of five oxidative hair dyes in the rat. Toxicol Appl Pharmacol 1985; 78:163–166.
66. Aldridge JFL. Visual display units and health. Practitioner 1985; 229:539–545.
67. Schnorr TM, Grajewski BA, Hornung RW, Thun MJ, Egeland GM, Murray WE, Conover DL, Halperin WE. Video display terminals and the risk of spontaneous abortion. N Engl J Med 1991; 324:727–733.
68. Cluff S. Health hazards of video display terminals. Modern Med Can 1986; 41:501–509.
69. Hastwell G. Salbutamol aerosol in premature labour. Lancet 1975; 2:1212–1213.
70. Thomas DJB, Dove AF, Alberti KGMM. Metabolic effects of salbutamol infusion during premature labour. Br J Obstet Gynaecol 1977; 84:497–499.
71. Barsky HE. Asthma and pregnancy. Postgrad Med 1991; 89:125–132.
72. D'Alonzo GE. The pregnant asthmatic patient. Sem Perinatol 1990; 14:119–129.
73. Wellner A, Duncan SR. Update: Management of asthma. Compr Ther 1990; 16:24–33.
74. Neff RK, Leviton A. Maternal theophylline consumption and the risk of stillbirth. Chest 1990; 97:1266–1267.

75. Hadjigeorgiou E, Kitsiou S, Psarondakis A, Segos C, Nicolopoulos D, Kaskarelis D. Antepartum aminophylline treatment for prevention of the respiratory distress syndrome in premature infants. Am J Obstet Gynecol 1979; 135:257–260.
76. Walker BE. Effect of glucocorticoids on palate development in the rat. Anat Rec 1969; 163:281–285.
77. Walker BE. Induction of cleft palate in rats with anti-inflammatory drugs. Teratology 1971; 4:39–42.
78. Greenberger PA, Patterson R. Management of asthma during pregnancy. N Engl J Med 1985; 312:897–903.
79. Dunlap NE, Bailey WC. Corticosteroids in asthma. South Med J 1990; 83:428–432.
80. Bentur Y, Horlatsch N, Koren G. Exposure to ionizing radiation during pregnancy: Perception of teratogenic risk and outcome. Teratology 1991; 43:109–112.
81. Brent RL. Evaluating the alleged teratogenicity of environmental agents. Clin Perinatol 1986; 13:615–648.
82. Brent RL. The effects of embryonic and fetal exposure to x-rays, microwaves and ultrasound. In Clinics in Perinatology, Vol 13, Teratology (Brent RL, Beckman DA, eds). Saunders, Philadelphia, 1988, pp 301–330.
83. Sanmiguel GS, Ferrer AP, Alberich MT, Genaoui BM. Consideraciones sobre el tratamiento de la infancia y en el embarazo. Actas Dermosifilogr 1980; 71: 105–108.
84. Berkowitz RL, Constan DR, Mochizuki TK. Handbook for Prescribing Medications During Pregnancy. Little Brown, Boston, 1981.
85. Robinson DH, Shepherd DA. Control of head lice in school children. Curr Ther Res 1980; 27:1–6.
86. Palanker AL, Keating JW, Weinberg MS, Sheffner AL, Dean R. Reproductive teratogenic and egg production studies in animals fed SO_2-treated activated sewage sludge. Toxicol Appl Pharmacol 1973; 25:454–459.
87. Saxén I. Associations between oral clefts and drugs taken during pregnancy. Int J Epidemiol 1975; 4:37–44.
88. Safra JM, Oakley GP. Association between cleft lip with or without cleft palate and neonatal exposure to diazepam. Lancet 1975; 2:478–480.
89. Czeizel A. Diazepam, phenytoin and etiology of cleft lip and/or cleft palate. Lancet 1976; 1:810–811.
90. Rosenberg L, Mitchell AA, Parsells JL, Pashayan H, Lonik C, Shapiro S. Lack of relation of oral clefts to diazepam use during pregnancy. N Engl J Med 1983; 309:1282–1285.
91. Czeizel A. Lack of evidence of teratogenicity of benzodiazepine drugs in Hungary. Reprod Toxicol 1988; 1:183–188.
92. Bergman U, Boethius G, Swartling PG, Isacson D, Smedby B. Teratogenic effects of benzodiazepine use during pregnancy. J Pediatr 1990; 116:490–491.
93. Loudon JB. Psychotropic drugs. Br Med J 1987; 294:1.
94. Grimm NE. Diazepam and other benzodiazepines in pregnancy. In Neurobehavioral Teratology (Yanai J, ed). Elsevier, New York, 1984, pp 153–163.
95. Milkovich L, van den Berg BJ. Effects of prenatal meprobamate and chlordiazepoxide hydrochloride on human embryonic and fetal development. N Engl J Med 1974; 291:1268–1271.

96. Rothman KJ, Fyler DC, Golblatt A, Kreidberg MB. Exogenous hormones and other drug exposures of children with congenital heart disease. Am J Epidemiol 1979; 109:433–439.
97. Geber WF, Gill TS, Guran MS. Comparative teratogenicity of chlordiazepoxide, diazepam, amitriptyline and imipramine in the fetal hamster. Teratology 1980; 21:39A.
98. Simpson JL. Review: Relationship between congenital anomalies and contraception. Adv Contracept 1985; 1:3–30.
99. Simpson JL, Phillips OP. Spermicides, hormonal contraception and congenital malformations. Adv Contracept 1990; 6:141–167.
100. Katz Z, Lancet M, Skornick J, Chemke J, Mogilner BM, Klinberg M. Teratogenicity of progestogens given during the first trimester of pregnancy. Obstet Gynecol 1985; 65:775–780.
101. Yovich JL, Turner SR, Draper R. Medroxyprogesterone acetate therapy in early pregnancy has no apparent fetal effects. Teratology 1988; 38:135–144.
102. Bracken MB. Oral contraception and congenital malformations in offspring: A review and meta-analysis of the prospective studies. Obstet Gynecol 1990; 76:552–557.
103. Wilson JG, Brent RL. Are female sex hormones teratogenic? Am J Obstet Gynecol 1981; 141:567–580.
104. Roe TF, Alfi OS. Ambiguous genitalia in XX male children. Report of two infants. Pediatrics 1977; 60:55–59.
105. Jacobson BD. Hazards of norethindrome therapy during pregnancy. Am J Obstet Gynecol 1962; 84:962–968.
106. Kallen B, Mastroiacovo P, Lancaster PAL, Mutchinick O, Kringelbach M, Martinez-Frias ML, Robert E, Castilla EE. Oral contraceptives in the etiology of isolated hypospadias. Contraception 1991; 44:173–182.
107. Archer KA. Poland BJ. An embryo with developmental abnormalities in association with multiple maternal factors. Teratology 1975; 11:13A.
108. Colombo ML, Dogliani P. Rubella embryopathy caused by vaccination. A clinical case with unusual characteristics. Minerva Pediatr 1976; 28:2429–2436.
109. Stone D, Matalka E, Pulaski B. Do artificial sweeteners ingested in pregnancy affect the offspring? Nature 1971; 231:53–59.
110. Taylor JM, Friedman L. Combined chronic feeding and three-generation reproduction study of sodium saccharin in the rat. Toxicol Appl Pharmacol 1974; 29:154–158.
111. Lederer J. Saccharin, its by-products and their teratogenic effects. Louvain Med 1977; 96:495–501.
112. Pitkin RN. Aspartame ingestion during pregnancy. In Aspartame Physiology and Biochemistry (Stegink LD, Filer LJ Jr, eds). New York, Marcel Dekker, 1984, pp 555–563.
113. Sturtevant FM. Use of aspartame in pregnancy. Int J Fertil 1985; 30:85–87.
114. Zhivkov E, Atanasov L. Experiments in obtaining and preventing congenital cataracts in rats. Ophthalmologia 1965; 2:105–112.
115. Friedman JM. Teratogen update: Anesthetic agents. Teratology 1988; 37:69–77.

116. Brogden RN, Speight TM, Avery GS. Cimetidine: A review of its pharmacological properties and therapeutic efficacy in peptic ulcer disease. Drugs 1978; 15:93–131.
117. Tamura J, Sato N, Ezaki H. Teratological study on ranitidine hydrochloride in rabbits. J Toxicol Sci 1983; 8(suppl 1):141–150.
118. Crawford JS. Cimetidine in elective caesarian section. Anaesthesia 1981; 36: 641–642.
119. Koren G, Zemlickis DM. Outcome of pregnancy after first trimester exposure to H_2 receptor antagonists. Am J Perinatol 1991; 8(1):37–38.
120. Glade G, Saccar CL, Pereira GR. Cimetidine in pregnancy: Apparent transient liver impairment in the newborn. Am J Dis Child 1980; 134:87–88.
121. Cipriani S, Conti R, Vella G. Rantidine in pregnancy. Report on three cases. From the Manufacturer – Glaxo Canada Ltd, November 1986.
122. Goodman Gilman A, Goodman LS, Rale TH, Murad F. The Pharmacological Basis of Therapeutics, 7th ed. Macmillan, New York, 1985.
123. Owaki Y, Sakai T, Momiyama H. Teratological studies on pyrantel pamoate in rats and rabbits. Oyo Takuri 1970; 5:33–50.
124. Wilk AL. Relation between teratogenic activity and cartilage-binding affinity of norchlorcyclizine analogues. Teratology 1969; 2:272.
125. Young RL, Zund G, Mason BA, Faro S. Pelvic inflammatory disease complicated by massive helminthic hyperinfection. Obstet Gynecol 1989; 74:484–486.
126. Chaube S, Murphy ML. The teratogenic effects of 5-fluorocytosine in the rat. Cancer Res 1969; 29:554–557.
127. Jindra J, Anjezdska A, Janousek V. Embryotoxic effects of high doses of griseofulvin on the skeleton of the albino mouse. In Evaluation of Embryotoxicity, Mutagenicity and Carcinogenicity Risks in New Drugs. Proceedings of the Third Symposium on Toxicological Testing for Safety of New Drugs, Prague, 1979, pp 161–165.
128. Lecyk M. Toxicity of copper sulfate in mice embryonic development. Zool Pol 1980; 28:101–106.
129. Gotz H, Reichenberger M. Ergebrisse einer Fragebogenaktion bei 1670 Dermatologen der BD über Nebenwirkungen bei der Griseofulvin-therapie. Hautarzt 1972; 23:485–492.
130. Doering PL, Santiago TM. Drugs for treatment of vulvovaginal candidiasis: Comparative efficacy of agents and regimens. Drug Intell Clin Pharm 1990; 24:1078-1983.
131. Ito C, Shibutani Y, Taya K, Ohnishi H. Toxicological studies of miconazole. 3. Teratological studies of miconazole in rabbits. Jyakuhin Kenkyu 1976; 7: 377–381.
132. Wallenberg HCS, Wladimiroff JW. Recurrence of vulvovaginal candidiasis during pregnancy. Comparison of miconazole vs nystatin treatment. Obstet Gynecol 1976; 48:491–494.
133. Donders GGG, Moerman P, Caudron J, Van Assche FA. Intrauterine *Candida* infection: A report of four infected fetuses from two mothers. Eur J Obstet Gynecol Reprod Biol 1990; 38:233–238.
134. Morgan J. Metronidazole treatment in pregnancy. Int J Gynaecol Obstet 1978; 15:501–502.

135. Hammill HA. Trichomonas vaginalis. Obstet Gynecol Clin North Am 1989; 16(3):531–540.
136. Cantu JM, Carcia-Cruz D. Midline facial defect as a teratogenic effect of metronidazole. Birth Defects 1982; 18:85–88.
137. Asuzu IU, Shetty SN, Anika SM. Effects of chronic oral administration in mice of the gut-stimulating crystals *Croton penduliflorus* seed oil. J Ethnopharmacol 1990; 30:135–143.
138. Schindler AM. Isolated neonatal hypomagnesaemia associated with maternal overuse of stool softeners. Lancet 1984; 2:822.
139. Mellin GW, Katzenstein M. Meclozine and fetal abnormalities. Lancet 1963; 1:222–223.
140. McColl JD. Dimenhydrinate in pregnancy. Can Med Assoc J 1963; 88:861.
141. Zierler S, Rothman KH. Congenital heart disease in relation to maternal use of Bendectin and other drugs in early pregnancy. N Engl J Med 1985; 313: 347–352.
142. Einarson TR, Leeder JS, Koren G. A method for meta-analysis of epidemiological studies. Drug Intell Clin Pharm 1988; 22:813–824.
143. Koos BJ, Longo LD. Mercury toxicity in the pregnant woman, fetus and newborn infant. Am J Obstet Gynecol 1976; 126(3):390–409.
144. Roeleveld N, Zielhaus GA, Gabreels F. Occupational exposure and defects of the central nervous system in offspring: Review. Br Med J 1990; 47:580–588.
145. Hatch M, Stein ZA. Agents in the workplace and effects on reproduction. In Occupational Medicine, Vol 1, No 3. Hanley and Belfus, Philadelphia, 1986, pp 531–534.
146. Holt D, Webb M. The toxicity and teratogenicity of mercuric mercury in the pregnant rat. Arch Toxicol 1986; 58:243–248.
147. Close LG, Catlin FI, Cohn AM. Acute and chronic effects of ammonia burns of the respiratory tract. Arch Otolaryngol 1980; 106:151–158.
148. Livingstone CS. Neonatal goitre. Br Med J 1966; 2:50–54.
149. Windholz M, ed. The Merck Index, 9th ed. Merck, Rahway, NJ, 1976.
150. Longo LD. The biological effects of carbon monoxide in the pregnant woman, fetus and newborn infant. Am J Obstet Gynecol 1977; 129:69–103.
151. Kato T. Embryonic abnormalities of the CNS caused by the fuel-gas inhalation of the mother animal. Folia Psychiatr Neurol Jpn 1958; 11:301–324.
152. Recommendations for the prevention of malaria in travelers. MMWR 1988; 37:277–284.
153. Hart CW, Naunton RF. The ototoxicity of chloroquine phosphate. Arch Otolaryngol 1964; 80:407–412.
154. Levy M, Buskila D, Gladman DD, Urowitz MB, Koren G. Pregnancy outcome following first trimester exposure to chloroquine. Am J Perinatol 1991; 8(3): 174–178.
155. Crawford JS, Lewis M. Nitrous oxide in early human pregnancy. Anaesthesia 1986; 41:900–905.
156. Mellin GW. Comparative teratology. Anesthesiology 1968; 29:1–4.
157. Pope WD, Halsey MJ, Lansdown AB, Bateman PE. Lack of teratogenic dangers with halothane. Acta Anaesthesiol 1975; 23(suppl):169–173.

8

Drugs of Choice for Pregnant Women

Joanne Smith, Anna Taddio, and Gideon Koren
The Hospital for Sick Children, Toronto, Ontario, Canada

Clinical Case

A 25-year-old woman conceived during a course of ranitidine for an ulcer. She is very afraid of the effects on the unborn baby.

INTRODUCTION

While in many cases health professionals are asked by pregnant women to assess the reproductive risk of medications ingested inadvertently during pregnancy, a large number of prospective inquiries deal with safe use of drugs. In our experience, about one-third of Motherisk patients in Toronto are not pregnant upon coming to the Motherisk Clinic. Rather, they wish to identify drugs for chronic disorders that they may use safely during pregnancy. A second group of patients contact us upon starting therapy for an acute condition during pregnancy, such as urinary tract infection or allergic rhinitis. Hence, crystallizing an approach to drugs of choice in pregnancy is as important as informing women post factum about their reproductive risks.

Table 1 summarizes drugs on which there are sufficient data in humans to show that there is no increased reproductive risk. This does not, however, imply that drugs not listed here have been proven to be teratogenic in humans.

Clearly, the drug of choice should be decided by the physician and the patient, who are familiar with the nature and context of the patient's condition. It is our rule of thumb that if a pregnant women needs medication, she should discuss her options with her physician.

Readers who will be counseling women planning to be taking any medication(s) for the duration of their pregnancy may wish to consult Chapter 13 for possible neonatal toxicities that may have to be diagnosed and/or treated.

Table 1   Drugs of Choice in Pregnancy

Condition (Reference)	Drug(s) of choice	Alternative(s)	Comments
Acne (1)	Topical Erythromycin Clindamycin Benzoyl peroxide	Systemic Erythromycin Topical Tretinoin (vitamin A acid)	Isotretinoin is contra-indicated in pregnancy
Allergic rhinitis (1–3)	Topical Corticosteroids Cromolyn (sodium cromoglycate) Decongestants (use sparingly) Xylometazoline Oxymetazoline Naphazoline Phenylephrine Systemic Diphenhydramine Dimenhydrinate Tripelennamine	Immunotherapy	Limited experience with terfenadine and astemizole has not revealed a sub-stantial teratogenic risk
Anemia (3)			
Iron deficiency	Iron supplements		
Folic acid deficiency	Folic acid		Folic acid now rec-ommended for all pregnant women commencing before conception (4,5)
Vitamin B_{12} deficiency	Vitamin B_{12} PO/IM, multivitamins		
Pernicious	Vitamin B_{12} IM or vitamin B_{12} PO + intrinsic factor PO		
Hemolytic	Corticosteroids Iron supplements Blood transfusions		
Sickle cell (6)	Prophylaxis Penicillin Folic acid supple-ment Iron supplement Blood transfusions		Vaccinate with pneu-mococcal vaccine before pregnancy. Vaccinate during pregnancy only if patient at risk of contracting disease

Table 1   (Continued)

Condition (Reference)	Drug(s) of choice	Alternative(s)	Comments
Sickle cell (6) (continued)	Crisis Morphine Meperidine Sodium bicarbonate, O_2		
Anticoagulation (after prosthetic valve replacement) (1,7−11)	Heparin (1st trimester + prior to delivery) Aspirin	Warfarin (2nd + 3rd trimester; avoid at term) Dipyridamole Streptokinase (use for pulmonary embolism if heparin fails)	Avoid aspirin in 3rd trimester Streptokinase: risk of bleeding. If used at term, should be with cesarean section
Anxiety disorders (1,12,13)	Benzodiazepines		
Arrhythmias (7,8, 10,11,14,15)	Quinidine Digoxin	Procainamide Propranolol Lidocaine (late in pregnancy, short-term) Verapamil (late in pregnancy, short-term)	Amiodarone has been associated with adverse thyroid effects in neonates (16–18)
Asthma (1,8, 19–21)	Inhalational β-adrenergic agonists; salbutamol Corticosteroids Cromolyn (sodium cromoglycate) Ipratropium Systemic Theophylline Corticosteroids		Emergency treatment Epinephrine SC, IV
Cold sores (1,11)	Topical Heparin + zinc (Lipactin) Zinc sulfate	Acyclovir	
Constipation (1,3,22)	Bulk-forming agents Psyllium mucilloid Fibyrax, bran	Saline laxatives Magnesium citrate Fleet Enema	Avoid gastrointestinal stimulants if possible

(continued)

Table 1   (Continued)

Condition (Reference)	Drug(s) of choice	Alternative(s)	Comments
Constipation (1,3,22) (continued)	Stool softeners/ osmotic agents Docusate sodium, calcium Glycerin Sorbitol Lactulose Mineral oil Magnesium hydrox- ide (Milk of Magnesia)	Gastrointestinal stimulants Bisacodyl Phenolphthalein	
Cough (1)	Cough lozenges Diphenhydramine Codeine	Dextromethorphan	
Depression (1,12,13,23)	Tricyclic antidepres- sants Fluoxetine	Lithium	When lithium is used in 1st trimester, fetal echocardio- gram and level 2 ultrasound recom- mended owing to small risk of Eb- stein's anomaly
Dermatitis Atopic, contact (1,11)	Topical Wet dressings Normal saline Sodium bicar- bonate Aluminum acetate Calamine lotion Aveeno oatmeal or oilated bath Corticosteroids Moisterizing/emol- lient lotions or ointments Systemic Diphenhydramine Chlorpheniramine Hydroxyzine		
Diabetes mellitus (24,25)	Insulin, human	Insulin, beef or pork	Avoid hypoglycemics if possible

Table 1   (Continued)

Condition (Reference)	Drug(s) of choice	Alternative(s)	Comments
Diarrhea (3,8)	Oral rehydration solution Attapulgite (kaolin + pectin) Bulk-forming agents Methylcellulose Psyllium mucilloid		
Dyspepsia, heartburn (1,3,22)	Antireflux Alginic acid + antacids (Gaviscon) Antacids Magnesium hydroxide (Milk of Magnesia) Aluminum hydroxide Magaldrate Calcium carbonate Antiflatulants Simethicone	H_2 blockers (e.g., ranitidine, cimetidine)	Limited experience with H_2 blockers suggest that they are not human teratogens
Fever	Acetaminophen	Aspirin Ibuprofen	Avoid aspirin and ibuprofen in 3rd trimester
Headache (1,8,26)			
Tension	Acetaminophen	Aspirin/nonsteroidal anti-inflammatory drugs (NSAID) Benzodiazepines	Avoid aspirin and NSAIDs in 3rd trimester
Migraine	Treatment Acetaminophen Codeine Morphine Meperidine Dimenhydrinate	Prophylaxis β-adrenergic blocker Tricyclic antidepressants Treatment Butalbital/aspirin/codeine (Fiorinal ± codeine)	Ergotamine: limited experience has not revealed evidence of teratogenicity, but concerns of potent vasoconstriction
Cluster	Prophylaxis Corticosteroids Amitriptyline Propranolol Treatment Corticosteroids		

(continued)

Table 1   (Continued)

Condition (Reference)	Drug(s) of choice	Alternative(s)	Comments
Hiccups	Antacids Magnesium hydroxide (Milk of Magnesia) Aluminum hydroxide Magaldrate CO_2	Lidocaine, viscous PO Chlorpromazine	
Hypertension (1,3,8,10,27–29)	Methyldopa Hydralazine	β-adrenergic blockers (e.g., propranolol, labetalol) Prazocin Nifedipine (in later stages of pregnancy)	Angiotensin-converting enzyme (ACE) inhibitors should be avoided owing to cases of severe neonatal renal insufficiency (30)
Hyperthyroidism (8,31)	Propylthiouracil Methimazole	Symptomatic β-adrenergic blockers (e.g., propranolol)	Surgery may be required if patient uncontrolled with medications Maternal propylthiouracil doses > 200 mg may affect fetal thyroid
Hypothyroidism (8,31,32)	Levothyroxine Liothyronine	Dessicated thyroid	
Idiopathic thrombocytopenic purpura (ITP) (33)	Corticosteroids IV immunoglobulin Blood transfusions		
Infections (1,3, 34–37)			
Bacterial	Systemic Penicillins Cephalosporins Cotrimoxazole (sulfamethoxazole + trimethoprim) Erythromycin Clindamycin Nitrofurantoin Topical Polysporin	Aminoglycosides Metronidazole Trimethoprim Nalidixic acid	Try to avoid sulfonamides in late pregnancy Avoid metronidazole in 1st trimester if possible Avoid tetracycline during pregnancy

Table 1   (Continued)

Condition (Reference)	Drug(s) of choice	Alternative(s)	Comments
Viral	No agents have been proven definitely safe because numbers of patients have been limited	Acyclovir Amantadine Zidovudine Idoxuridine Trifluridine Vidarabine	
Tuberculosis	Isoniazid Ethambutal	Rifampin (especially for 1st trimester) Streptomycin	
Fungal	Nystatin: oral, topical, vaginal Miconazole: topical, vaginal Clotrimazole: topical, vaginal Econazole: vaginal Ketoconazole: topical	Ketoconazole PO: use only if absolutely necessary	
Protozoal Toxoplasmosis	Pyrimethamine + sulfadiazine Spiramycin		
Malaria (38–40)	Prophylaxis Chloroquine Treatment Chloroquine Quinine/quinidine Quinine + clindamycin	Alternative Pyrimethamine + dapsone/sulfadoxine	
Trichomonas (41)		Metronidazole Clotrimazole: vaginal Sulfonamide: vaginal	Metronidazole in single 2 g oral dose preferred
Inflammatory bowel disease (ulcerative colitis and Crohn's disease) (1,8,42)	5-Aminosalicylic acid (i.e., 5-ASA, mesalamine, mesalazine) Olsalazine Sulfasalazine Corticosteroid: oral, rectal, IV	Codeine Metronidazole Loperamide for severe diarrhea	

(continued)

Table 1 (Continued)

Condition (Reference)	Drug(s) of choice	Alternative(s)	Comments
Inflammatory bowel disease (1,8,42) (continued)	Antibiotics (see bacterial infections above) Vitamin supplements Calcium carbonate		
Insomnia (1)	Diphenhydramine Dimenhydrinate Benzodiazepines		
Lice (1,3,43)	Pyrethrins Permethrins (Nix) Petrolatum ointment to eyelashes	Lindane (GBH)	
Lichen planus (1)	Topical Corticosteroids Intralesional Corticosteroids Systemic Hydroxyzine (for itching) Corticosteroids		
Mania (12,13) (and bipolar affective disorder)	Lithium Antipsychotics Chlorpromazine Haloperidol	Depressive episodes: Tricyclic antidepressants Fluexitime	If lithium is used in 1st trimester, fetal echocardiogram and level 2 ultrasound recommended owing to small risk of Ebstein's anomaly
Myasthenia gravis (1,26)	Pyridostigmine Prednisone		
Nasal congestion	Nasal drops/spray Normal saline Xylometazoline Oxymetazoline Phenylephrine Naphazoline	Pseudoephedrine	
Nausea, vomiting, motion sickness (1,3,22)	Antihistamines Diclectin (doxylamine + pyridoxine) Diphenhydramine Dimenhydrinate Meclizine Cyclizine	Chlorpromazine Metoclopramide has been used safely in 3rd trimester	

Table 1 (Continued)

Condition (Reference)	Drug(s) of choice	Alternative(s)	Comments
Pain (1,22,44)	Systemic Acetaminophen Morphine Codeine Meperidine Topical Capsaicin Local anesthetics Salicylates	Aspirin NSAIDs	Avoid aspirin, salicylates and NSAIDs in 3rd trimester Opioids (e.g., morphine, meperidine, codeine) may cause neonatal withdrawal syndrome
Peptic ulcer disease (3)	Antacids Magnesium hydroxide (Milk of Magnesia) Aluminum hydroxide Magaldrate Calcium carbonate	Sucralfate H_2 blockers Bismuth subsalicylate (Pepto-Bismol)	Avoid salicylates in 3rd trimester
Pinworms (11,45)	Piperazine citrate, adipate	Pyrantel pamoate Pyrvinium pamoate	
Pruritis	Topical Moisterizing creams/lotions Wet dressings Aluminum acetate Aveeno oatmeal bath Zinc oxide cream/ointment Calamine lotion Corticosteroids Systemic Hydroxyzine Diphenhydramine Corticosteroids	Topical Local anesthetics	
Psoriasis	Topical Corticosteroids Salicylic acid Emollient ointments Calamine lotion (acute lesions)		Avoid salicylates in 3rd trimester Etretinate contraindicated in pregnancy

(continued)

Table 1 (Continued)

Condition (Reference)	Drug(s) of choice	Alternative(s)	Comments
Raynaud's phenomenon (11)	Vasodilators Prazocin Nitrates	Nifedipine (in later stages of pregnancy)	
Reflux esophagitis (22)	Alginic acid + antacids (Gaviscon) Antacids Magnesium hydroxide (Milk of Magnesia) Aluminum hydroxide Magaldrate Calcium carbonate		Position of patient sitting, sleeping, is important. Frequent, small meals may help
Rheumatoid arthritis (8,44, 46–48)	Aspirin NSAIDs Corticosteroids: systemic, intraarticular	Gold Chloroquine Hydroxychloroquine Azathioprine (after 1st trimester if necessary)	Avoid aspirin and NSAIDs in 3rd trimester Avoid cancer chemotherapeutic agents as much as possible
Rosacea (1,49)	Topical Erythromycin Benzoyl peroxide Metronidazole	Systemic Corticosteroids	Avoid metronidazole in 1st trimester if possible
Scabies (1,3,43)	Permethrins (Nix) Pyrethrins + piperonyl butoxide (Rid, R&C)	Crotamiton Lindane (GBH) Benzyl benzoate Sulfur 5% in petrolatum	
Schizophrenia (12,13)	Phenothiazines		
Seborrheic dermatitis	Salicyclic acid shampoo		Avoid salicylates in 3rd trimester
Seizures (8,26,50)	Benzodiazepines Carbamazepine Ethosuximide	Valproic acid Phenobarbital Primidone Phenytoin	Folic acid supplementation recommended. Carbamazepine and valproic acid are associated with a small risk of neural tube defects; level 2 ultrasound and α-fetoprotein monitoring recommended

Table 1 (Continued)

Condition (Reference)	Drug(s) of choice	Alternative(s)	Comments
Seizures (8,26,50) (continued)			Phenytoin causes the fetal hydantoin syndrome
Systemic lupus erythematosis (SLE) (1,46,47, 51)	Corticosteroids	Azathioprine (after 1st trimester if necessary) Chloroquine Hydroxychloroquine	Avoid cancer chemotherapeutic agents as much as possible
Thrombophlebitis, deep vein thrombosis (8,10)	Anticoagulants Heparin Warfarin (2nd + 3rd trimester; avoid at term) Antifibrinolytics Streptokinase		Streptokinase: risk of bleeding. If used at term, should be with cesarean section
Superficial vein thrombosis	Warm compresses Aspirin/NSAIDs		Avoid aspirin and NSAIDs in 3rd trimester
Trigeminal neuralgia		Carbamazepine Tricyclic antidepressants Phenothiazines	Carbamazepine is associated with a small risk of neural tube defects. Level 2 ultrasound and α-fetoprotein monitoring recommended
Urticaria	Topical Aveeno bath Moisterizing/emollient lotions Systemic Hydroxyzine Diphenhydramine		

Answer

At present there is only one prospective study on the issue, and it does not suggest increased teratogenic risk, although the power of this study is relatively weak because the cohort was limited (see p. 102).

REFERENCES

1. Motherisk Drug List. Toronto, 1993.
2. Marshall LB. Allergic rhinitis in pregnancy. Drug Intell Clin Pharm 1987; 21: 971–972.

3. Cheung M. Counseling the pregnant patient. On Cont Pract 1988; 15(2):7–15.
4. U.S. Centers for Disease Control. Recommendations for the use of folic acid to reduce the number of cases of spina bifida and other neural tube defects. MMWR 1992; 41(RR-14):1–7.
5. Kirke PN, Daly LE, Elwood JH. A randomized trial of low dose folic acid to prevent neural tube defects. Arch Dis Child 1992; 67:1442–6.
6. McLaughlin BN, Martin R, Morrison JC. Clinical management of sickle cell hemoglobinopathies during pregnancy. Clin Perinatol 1985; 12(3):551–69.
7. Lang R, Borow KM. Pregnancy and heart disease. Clin Perinatol 1985; 12(3): 551–569.
8. Rayburn WF, Lavin JP Jr. Drug prescribing for chronic medical disorders during pregnancy: An overview. Obstet Gynecol 1986; 155:565–569.
9. de Swiet M. Anticoagulants. In Prescribing in Pregnancy (Rubin PC, ed). British medical Journal, London, 1987, pp 87–95.
10. Lees KR, Rubin PC. Treatment of cardiovascular diseases. In Prescribing in Pregnancy (Rubin PC, ed). British Medical Journal, London, 1987, pp 80–86.
11. Briggs GG, Freeman RK, Yaffe SJ. Drugs in Pregnancy and Lactation, 3rd ed. Williams & Wilkins, Baltimore, 1990.
12. Csernansky JG, Hollister LE. Psychotropic medications: The risk of teratogenesis. Hosp Formul 1984; 19:718–723.
13. Loudon JB. Psychotropic drugs. In Prescribing in Pregnancy (Rubin PC, ed). British Medical Journal, London, 1987, pp 49–57.
14. Mitani GM, Steinberg I, Lien EJ, et al. The pharmacokinetics of antiarrhythmic agents in pregnancy and lactation. Clin Pharmacokinet 1987; 12:253–291.
15. Rotmensch HH, Rotmensch S, Elkayan U. Management of cardiac arrhythmias during pregnancy. Drugs 1987; 33:623–633.
16. Plomp TA, Vulsma T, de Vijlder JJM. Use of amiodarone during pregnancy. Eur J Obstet Gynecol Reprod Biol 1992; 43:201–207.
17. Tubman R, Jenkins J, Lim J. Neonatal hyperthryoxinaemia associated with maternal amiodarone therapy: Case report. Irish J Med Sci 1988; 157:243.
18. Laurent M, Betremieux P, Biron Y, et al. Neonatal hypothyroidism after treatment by amiodarone during pregnancy. Am J Cardiol 1987; 60:942.
19. Greenberger PA. Asthma in pregnancy. Clin Perinatol 1985; 12(3):571–584.
20. Gray JD. Cardiovascular and respiratory agents during pregnancy: Implications for fetal development. Clin Invest Med 1985; 8:339–344.
21. Chung KF, Barnes PJ. Treatment of asthma. In Prescribing in Pregnancy (Rubin PC, ed). British Medical Journal, London, 1987, pp 41–48.
22. Howden CW. Treatment of common minor ailments. In Prescribing in Pregnancy (Rubin PC, ed). British Medical Journal, London, 1987, pp 19–25.
23. Pastuszak A, Schick-Boschetto B, Zuber C, et al. A prospective multicenter study of pregnancy outcome following first trimester exposure to fluoxetine (Prozac). JAMA 1993; 269:2246–2248.
24. Vaughan NJA. Treatment of diabetes. In Prescribing in Pregnancy (Rubin PC, ed). British Medical Journal, London, 1987, pp 111–119.

25. Buchanan TA, Unterman TG, Metzger BE. The medical management of diabetes in pregnancy. Clin Perinatol 1985; 12(3):625–650.
26. Noronha A. Neurologic disorders during pregnancy and the puerperium. Clin Perinatol 1985; 12(3):695–713.
27. Lubbe WF. Hypertension in pregnancy: Pathophysiology and management. Drugs 1984; 28:170–188.
28. Naden RP, Redman CWB. Antihypertensive drugs in pregnancy. Clin Perinatol 1985; 12(3):521–538.
29. Knott C. The treatment of hypertension in pregnancy: Clinical pharmacokinetic considerations. Clin Pharmacokinet 1991; 21:233–241.
30. Rosa FW, Bosco LA, Graham CF, et al. Neonatal anuria with maternal angiotensin-converting enzyme inhibition. Obstet Gynecol 1989; 74:371–374.
31. Hague WM. Treatment of endocrine diseases. In Prescribing in Pregnancy (Rubin PC, ed). British Medical Journal, London, 1987, pp 68–79.
32. Mestman JH. Thyroid disease in pregnancy. Clin Perinatol 1985; 12(3):651–667.
33. Hoffman PC. Idiopathic thrombocytopenic purpura in pregnancy. Clin Perinatol 1985; 12(3):599–607.
34. Wise R. Antibiotics. In Prescribing in Pregnancy (Rubin PC, ed). British Medical Journal, London, 1987, pp 26–40.
35. Holdiness MR. Teratology of the antituberculous drugs. Early Hum Devel 1987; 15:61–74.
36. Marcus JC. Nonteratogenicity of antituberculous drugs. S Afr Med J 1967; II: 758–759.
37. Folb PI, Dukes MNG. Drug Safety in Pregnancy. Elsevier, Oxford, 1990, pp 199–210.
38. U.S. Centers for Disease Control. Recommendations for the prevention of malaria among travelers. MMWR 1990; 39(RR-3):1–10.
39. Keystone JS. Prevention of malaria. Drugs 1990; 39:337–354.
40. Panisko DM, Keystone JS. Treatment of malaria – 1990. Drugs 1990; 39:160–189.
41. Hammill HA. Trichomonas vaginalis. Obstet Gynecol Clin North Am 1989; 16: 531–540.
42. Hanan IM, Kirsner JB. Inflammatory bowel disease in the pregnant woman. Clin Perinatol 1985; 12(3):669–682.
43. Nix product monograph. Burroughs Wellcome, 1987.
44. Lee P. Anti-inflammatory therapy during pregnancy and lactation. Clin Invest Med 1985; 8:328–332.
45. Wise R. Antibiotics. In Prescribing in Pregnancy (Rubin PC, ed). British Medical Journal, London, 1987, pp 26–40.
46. Byron MA. Treatment of rheumatic diseases. In Prescribing in Pregnancy (Rubin PC, ed). British Medical Journal, London, 1987, pp 58–67.
47. Folb PI, Dukes MNG. Drug Safety in Pregnancy. Elsevier, Oxford, 1990, pp 205–210.

48. Klipple GL, Cecere FA. Rheumatoid arthritis and pregnancy. Rheum Dis Clin North Am 1989; 15:213–239.
49. Schmadel LK, McKevoy GK. Topical metronidazole: A new therapy for rosacea. Clin Pharm 1990; 9:94–101.
50. Hopkins A. Epilepsy and anticonvulsant drugs. In Prescribing in Pregnancy (Rubin PC, ed). British Medical Journal, London, 1987, pp 96–110.
51. Hayslett JP, Reece EA. Systemic lupus erythematosus in pregnancy. Clin Perinatol 1985; 12(3):539–550.

9

Periconceptional Folate and Neural Tube Defects

Time for Rethinking

Gideon Koren
The Hospital for Sick Children, Toronto, Ontario, Canada

Clinical Case

A patient of yours who is now 6 weeks into gestation has heard that maternal supplementation of folic acid may decrease the risk for neural tube defects. She wants you to recommend vitamin pills that will have enough folate. How much daily folate does she need?

INTRODUCTION

The Motherisk Program in Toronto evaluates and counsels pregnant women, their families, and health professionals on the teratogenic risks of drugs, chemicals, environmental agents, and infections. At present we deal with 60 inquiries a day, mainly from Ontario but also from other parts of Canada and the United States. In addition to performing follow-up of our own patients and conducting prospective studies, we continuously review and analyze new published studies. When important information becomes available, we feel it is our mandate to publicize such data, which may have a direct impact on the health of many unborn babies. We believe the new data on preconceptual folate supplementation qualify as such a major breakthrough.

THE PROBLEM

Neural tube defects (NTD) affect about 0.6–1.5/1000 born babies in Canada. Consisting mainly of anencephaly and meningomyelocele, NTDs are serious lethal or severely debilitating congenital malformations. It is estimated that the risk of a recurrence of NTD in a woman who has had a previous NTD is about 3–4% (1). During the last decade effective antenatal methods have been developed to diagnose NTD in utero, with second-trimester ultrasound combined with amniotic or maternal blood α-fetoprotein offering an almost 100% sensitivity in some centers (2). Presently, ultrasound is recommended at 16 and 19 weeks. In most centers, amniocentesis for raised α-fetoprotein is the diagnostic approach, whereas maternal α-fetoprotein and ultrasound are used for screening. However, these tests are not performed routinely on women with unknown risk for NTD (e.g., because of previous NTD or because they are receiving valproic acid, carbamazepine, or retinoids).

Evidence has been accumulated during the last two decades suggesting that low preconceptual consumption of folate and vitamins is associated with an increased risk of NTD. These retrospective studies could not separate between the potential effects of vitamins versus folate, however. The main criticism of these observational studies was that women consuming low amounts of folate and vitamins may have clustering of many other nutritional and socioeconomic risk factors, leading them to increased teratogenic risk (3). However, this controversy was laid to rest when the British Medical Research Council study, a multinational, double-blind, placebo-controlled effort, clearly proved the protection effect of pharmacological folate dose (4 mg/d) over placebo on the recurrence rate of NTD in women who had a previous NTD. Vitamins alone (without folate) had no protective effect (1).

It was subsequently argued that this protective effect may not be relevant to the prevention of the occurrence of a first NTD in the general population. However, a recently completed double-blind, placebo-controlled study from Hungary has clearly shown the protective effect of folate at 0.8 mg/d plus vitamins over placebo (4) in women with no previous history of NTD. It is probable that in a heterogeneous society such as that in Canada, different ethnic groups have different magnitudes of risk for NTD; however, this new evidence suggests that at least in part, NTDs are caused by folate deficiency. An association between folate deficiency and other malformations (e.g., cleft lip or palate) has been suggested, but has not been verified.

In Canada, the recommended dose of dietary folate for the general population was 0.2 mg/d. This recommendation stems from the concept that 0.2 mg/d of folate is high enough to prevent saturation of hepatic stores of folate. With the new data presented above, it is quite clear that this decrease in recommended dose of folate may increase the risk of NTD in Canada. Recently, the national Health and Welfare changed its recommendations to 0.4 mg/d.

There is recent evidence that large segments of North American women below or near poverty have median intakes of folic acid of 0.15 mg/d. Even

among those above poverty, many have very low folate intake (e.g., 25%
of women have average folic intake of only 0.142 mg/d) (5). Moreover,
insulin-dependent diabetic mothers and women with potentially low folate
levels, due to inflammatory bowel disease and other disease states, may be
at a higher risk than the normal population. At present it is not clear whether
0.4 mg/d of folate is inferior to the 0.8 mg/d tested in Hungary; however,
it is very probable that intake of 0.2 mg/d is below the preventive dose.

RETHINKING THE SOLUTION

Because NTDs are induced in the first 28 days of pregnancy, adequate maternal folate intake must start preconceptionally. Since, however, almost
half of all pregnancies in North America are unplanned, it is evident that
recommendations alone are not likely to reach many women and are very
likely to miss high-risk women of low socioeconomic status who tend to consume substantially less folate.

A variety of methods have been suggested to ensure that women of reproductive age receive adequate folate supplements (6). Educating women
to consume more fruits and vegetables might achieve that goal, but supplementation of basic food sources such as bread, salt, cereals, or milk might
turn out to be more efficacious because it does depend on changing the behavior patterns of women. The potential deleterious effects of incorporating
folic acid in basic food supplementation must be carefully reviewed, however. Some masking of B_{12} deficiency may occur in patients with combined
deficiencies of vitamin B_{12} and folic acid (7).

NTDs induced by folate deficiency are now proven to be preventable at
the primary level (versus secondary prevention by pregnancy termination).
This is an exciting opportunity, similar in magnitude to the prevention of
cretinism by means of iodine supplements.

The health community, in concert with the various governments, should
address these issues as soon as possible. Any delay in response will result
in unnecessary occurrence of NTDs, with immense suffering and cost to
the children, their families, and to the Canadian public at large.

Answer

*At 6 weeks of gestation supplementation of folate will not reverse an NTD
if it was already formed. The point here is that one needs to give folate peri-
conceptionally at a dose of 400 μg/d.*

REFERENCES

1. MRC Vitamin Study Research Group. Prevention of neural tube defects: Results of the Medical Research Council Vitamin Study. Lancet 1991; 338:131-137.
2. Nodel AS, Green NK, Holmes LB, Frigoletto FD, Benacerraf BR. Absence of need for amniocentesis in patients with elevated levels of maternal alpha fetoprotein and normal ultrasonographic examinations. N Engl J Med 1990; 323:557-561.
3. Mills JL, Rhoads GG, Simpson JL, et al. The National Institute of Child Health and Human Development Neural Tube Defect Study Group. N Engl J Med 1989; 321:430-435.
4. Czeizel A. Controlled studies of multivitamin supplementation on pregnancy outcome. In Maternal Nutrition and Pregnancy Outcome (Keen CL, Bendich A, Willhite CC, eds). New York Academy of Sciences, May 17-20, 1992, San Diego, CA.
5. Block G, Abrams B. Vitamin and mineral status of women of childbearing potential. In Maternal Nutrition and Pregnancy Outcome (Keen CL, Bendich A, Willhite CC, eds). New York Academy of Sciences, May 17-20, 1992, San Diego, CA.
6. Oakley G. Periconceptional folic acid supplementation for the prevention of spina bifida and anencephaly. In Maternal Nutrition and Pregnancy Outcome (Keen CL, Bendich A, Willhite CC, eds). New York Academy of Sciences, May 17-20, 1992, San Diego, CA.
7. Babior BM, Bunn HF. Megaloblastic anemias. In Harrison's Principles of Internal Medicine (Braunwald E, Isselbacher KJ, et al., eds). 1987, pp 1498-1504.

10

Drug Use During Lactation

Anna Taddio and Shinya Ito
The Hospital for Sick Children, Toronto, Ontario, Canada

Clinical Case

A woman who has just given birth to an apparently healthy baby asks you whether her amiodarone therapy is compatible with breastfeeding.

INTRODUCTION

This chapter reviews the safety of commonly used medications in lactating ambulatory care patients. These medications include antibiotics, analgesics, antihypertensives, and many others. Breastfeeding mothers may require drug therapy and must make informed decisions about the safety of possible drug consumption by their nursing infants. We hope to provide nursing mothers and their health care givers with some general guidelines for these situations. The mother's decision to breastfeed during drug therapy should be based on a reasonable understanding of any risks to her infant. The choice to avoid breastfeeding during drug therapy should be made when there is an unacceptable risk to the baby. In many cases, mothers may continue to breastfeed while on drug therapy with little risk to the child. In some situations of short-term courses of drug therapy, a mother may wish to temporarily suspend breastfeeding.

It is not known how many women stop breastfeeding because of their concern for drugs in their breastmilk. The use of medication, however, is believed to contribute to a mother's choice to bottle-feed. Other factors that affect this decision are the mother's parity, education level, social class, psychosocial factors, and socioeconomic class. The type of delivery and the presence of illness in mother or baby are also contributory factors (1,2).

Studies have shown that drug use in the postpartum period is high. One study reviewed medication use in 970 postpartum women in Norway in 1980. According to medical records, almost 98% of these women were breastfeeding when discharged from hospital. Ninety percent received at least one drug during the early postnatal period. The most frequently used drugs were analgesics (mainly codeine and dextropopoxyphene), hypnotics (mainly nitrazepam), and methylergometrine or ergometrine (3).

A similar study examined medication use in 2004 postpartum women in Northern Ireland in 1982. Thirty-three percent of these mothers were breastfeeding at the time of discharge from hospital. More than 99% of all postpartum women received at least one drug during the first week after delivery. The drugs used encompassed the following therapeutic classes: antibiotics, analgesics, psychotropics, antiepileptics, gastrointestinal drugs, cardiovascular drugs, antihistamines, steroids, hematinics and vitamins, and miscellaneous drugs. The most commonly prescribed medications included iron and vitamin preparations and analgesics. The pattern of prescribing was not much different between breastfeeding and bottle-feeding mothers except for the use of sedatives and iron and vitamins. The mothers who did not breastfeed used sedatives and iron/vitamin preparations more often (4).

The use of medication by breastfeeding women implies that nursing infants may be exposed to the medication through ingestion of breast milk. We discuss safety in terms of the magnitude of the risk to the baby from this practice, and we emphasize that safety needs to be evaluated in each patient's case. To assist in this decision, this chapter summarizes determinants of drug excretion into milk and the methods used to estimate a nursing infant's dose or exposure. An extensive summary of data obtained from selected studies on drug excretion into milk is provided. Some conclusions are made regarding the safety of these medications during lactation. The health professional should note that we do not recommend the use of any drug without the advice that each nursing infant be monitored for any adverse effects during maternal drug therapy. The intensity of this monitoring will vary with the potential risk and with the mother's own concerns.

BACKGROUND

Breastfeeding Patterns and Impact on Infant Health

Patterns of breastfeeding worldwide have been changing considerably over the past several decades. In the United States, the proportion of women breastfeeding their babies in the 1950s was measured at 30%. This proportion declined steadily, and by 1970 it had reached 25%. Then the trend reversed, and from 1971 to 1984 there was a positive trend in the incidence and duration of breastfeeding, with more than 60% of women initiating breastfeeding in 1984 (5). The results from surveys in Canada also showed increasing rates of breastfeeding in the early 1980s as compared to the 1960s (6). Recent data from the United States, however, showed a decrease in the incidence of breastfeeding from 1984 to 1989 (7).

Breastfeeding offers many health benefits over other methods of infant feeding and is the preferred method of infant feeding for the first 6 months of life. A review performed by a U.S. task force showed that breastfeeding is associated with decreased gastrointestinal disease (8). Others have found that breastfeeding is associated with decreased mortality rates, decreased respiratory illness, and decreased immunological and chronic disease (9). It has also been associated with natural child spacing (10) and economic savings. These factors should be considered whenever medications are required by nursing women, for in many cases, breastfeeding need not be interrupted during maternal drug use.

Breast Milk Production

Breast milk is synthesized in the mammary tissue. The alveolar cells make up the functional units of this gland and are responsible for secreting newly formed milk. A lactating breast can be compared to a cluster of grapes, with each grape consisting of a cluster of alveolar cells and a central lumen (11). Capillaries surround the alveolar cells (12). The alveolar cells discharge milk products into the lumen, where they are transported to the duct system. The ducts meet in channels of increasing size until the nipple is reached (11).

The process of lactogenesis is under the control of many hormones; principal among these are estrogen, progesterone, prolactin, and oxytocin. Estrogen and progesterone are necessary for the maturation of the mammary gland during pregnancy. These hormones, which are secreted under the control of the pituitary and placental follicle stimulating hormone (FSH) and luteotrophic hormone (LH), have an inhibitory effect on milk production. At the end of pregnancy, the alveolar cells are not completely developed and milk production is relatively slow. Just prior to parturition the levels of estrogen and progesterone decrease rapidly, removing the inhibitory effect of these hormones on prolactin (13). Prolactin is the major stimulus for milk production and secretion, and it is released from the pituitary gland under the stimulus of infant suckling (14). Regular milk production is stimulated by the actual nursing period by the infant and continues after the nursing episode. Breast emptying during nursing is prompted by oxytocin. Oxytocin promotes the contraction of the myoepithelial cells that surround the alveoli and ducts and causes the "milk ejection reflex" (13). Other supportive hormones are insulin, cortisol, thyroid-parathyroid hormone, and growth hormone (15).

Breast Milk Composition

Breast milk contains water, proteins, electrolytes, lipids, carbohydrates (mainly lactose), vitamins, minerals, and immune factors. Its composition changes over time during the course of lactation. Lactation can be divided into three periods according to these changes. Colostrum, the first milk produced by a lactating mother, is formed in the first 5 days postpartum. Transitional milk is produced after colostrum. Mature milk follows transitional milk, approximately 2–3 weeks postpartum (16). Mature milk contains higher concentrations of lactose and fat compared to colostrum, but protein and immunoglobulin content is lower (17). Water constitutes about 88% of mature milk, while lactose, lipids, protein, and mineral constituents comprise 7, 4, 1, and 0.2%, respectively (18). Although the overall composition of mature milk is not thought to vary significantly (19), concentrations of lipid-, fat-, and water-soluble vitamins in milk do change according to the mother's nutrient intake (20).

There is a correlation between blood flow and milk production (21). Milk volume is usually low during the first 2 days postpartum but increases rapidly and levels off by 5 days (22). Milk yields reach approximately 800 mL/d by 6 months (22) or more. The average daily intake by infants is variable and may determine milk yield (23). The average pH of milk is lower than that of plasma. Morriss et al. (24) have shown that the average pH of milk changes with time also; the pH is 7.45 in colostrum and 7.0–7.1 for transitional and mature milk. The pH gradually increases during lactation until it reaches 7.4 at 10 months. Milk composition varies throughout the day. There is diurnal variation in fat content, with the highest fat levels found in the morning (25–27). Infants will generally feed 10–15 minutes on each breast, and milk composition is variable in that time. The hindmilk contains more fat than foremilk (26). The lipid content of mature milk also increases with time (28).

The differences between milk from premature deliveries and term deliveries have been summarized by Anderson (29). Mother's milk from early lactation in preterm deliveries is higher in fat and protein, lower in lactose, and more varied in its composition than milk from mothers with full-term babies. Many of the differences between preterm and term milk, however, become less marked as the mother continues to nurse.

Drugs ingested by nursing mothers are not known to affect maturation of milk or the pH of milk. They may, however, affect the quantity of milk produced, or its composition. Bromocriptine, metoclopramide, and oral contraceptives represent a few examples of such drugs. The implications of the use of these medications are discussed later in this chapter.

DRUG EXCRETION INTO BREAST MILK

Determinants of Infant Exposure

Drugs taken by lactating women may be present in their infants through the consumption of breast milk. The extent of this exposure will depend on the pharmacokinetic properties of the drug in the child and mother (30). Breast physiology, milk composition, and infant suckling pattern also determine the extent of drug exposure in the infant.

Infant Drug Handling

There are differences between infants and adults in each of the following factors: drug absorption, drug distribution, drug metabolism, and drug excretion. In a review of these factors, Besunder et al. (31) concluded that neonatal gastric acid secretion and gastric emptying time are both decreased compared to adults; total body water of a newborn is higher than adult values; fat content is lower than adults; there is decreased protein binding in neonatal plasma; and there is decreased oxidative metabolism of drugs at birth. The capacity of this metabolizing pathway, however, increases in the first few weeks of life and soon exceeds proportionally adult capacity.

The infant's capacity for drug conjugation and glucuronidation of drugs is lower at birth. Sulfation, however, is relatively well developed in the newborn (32). Kidney blood flow, glomerular filtration, and tubular function are all reduced in the neonatal period. The infant's capacity does not reach adult levels until approximately 6 months (31). The decreased clearance rate in neonates has been used to provide a summary of drugs incompatible with breastfeeding based on likely infant plasma levels achieved during maternal therapy (33).

The susceptibility of an infant to adverse effects from drugs also depends on the pharmacokinetic characteristics of the drug and the sensitivity of the infant. Adverse reactions can be divided into two groups: dose-related reactions that reflect the pharmacological actions of the drug, and idiosyncratic reactions. Many of the adverse reactions reported in breastfed infants consuming drugs via milk are dose-related: that is, relatively large doses of the drug have been delivered to the infant via breast milk. The remainder of reports reflect an exaggerated response to the agent by the infant. Idiosyncratic reactions are not dose-related, and it is often difficult to quantify the risk of such a reaction occurring. Fortunately, idiosyncratic responses are not common in breastfed infants.

Summary of the Literature Regarding Drug Excretion in Breast Milk and the Milk-to-Plasma (M/P) Ratio

Drugs must pass from maternal mammary capillaries to the alveolar cells before they can be transferred into milk. During this process, drugs must cross a series of membrane barriers (11). Drug molecules may pass through membranes in two ways: passive diffusion and active transport. Lipid-soluble drugs may dissolve in the lipid phase of the membrane and diffuse through. Water-soluble drugs may diffuse through water-filled pores. Carrier proteins may also transport drugs across membranes (34). The rate of drug passage depends on degree of ionization of the drug, lipid solubility, size, and concentration gradient (34).

A drug transferred into milk may exist in association with the various milk components (35) such as the aqueous layer, the proteins, or fat. The protein-bound portion of a drug is not available for transfer into milk. Thus, a drug that is highly bound to maternal plasma protein may not appear in breast milk to as great an extent as a drug that is not protein-bound. Propranolol and warfarin are examples of highly protein-bound drugs that do not cross into breast milk in appreciable amounts.

The milk-to-plasma ratio (M/P ratio), which compares the concentration of a drug achieved in milk to maternal plasma, serves as an estimate of the dose of a drug delivered in milk as a function of the amount in maternal plasma. Different models have been described to explain and predict how drugs are transferred into breastmilk (36); however, a two-compartment model is usually sufficient to describe drug transfer in milk. This model assumes a central compartment and a peripheral compartment, which includes milk. There is a time dependency of the M/P ratio as a function of distribution characteristics. A method of deriving other mammary models has been described (37).

Drug diffusion between plasma and milk is a dynamic and reversible process. Thus, most drugs are not permanently "trapped" in milk. This implies that nursing mothers need not "pump and dump" milk in an attempt to promote drug elimination. This practice may be better suited for other purposes, such as alleviating the pain from engorged breasts or maintaining an adequate milk flow.

Numerous clinical trials have measured the M/P ratio of different drugs. The values from these trials have provided health professionals with some measurements as a basis for assessing the safety of drug usage while breastfeeding. However, some reported values have questionable validity because they were obtained from imperfectly designed studies. Namely, investigators have often failed to assure steady-state conditions, to measure metabolites, to account for infant suckling pattern, and to study an adequate number of patients. This topic has been reviewed by Wilson et al. (36), and a summary is provided.

Many trials report an M/P ratio obtained from only one simultaneously obtained milk and plasma drug level. Clearly, if the M/P ratio varies with time, this reading will not produce an accurate estimation of the amount of drug the infant may consume. The M/P ratio assumes that a constant ratio is maintained between the maternal plasma drug level and the milk drug level. For drugs in which the plasma and milk concentrations parallel each other over time, the M/P ratio is ideally calculated by taking the area under the curve (AUC) time course profile in milk and plasma and equating these values in a ratio. One of the basic assumptions for calculating an accurate M/P ratio is that the mother is at steady state. This is because drugs may accumulate in breast milk as a function of dosing. The M/P ratio calculated before steady state is achieved may underestimate the M/P ratio at steady state.

Another factor that often is overlooked in calculating the infant dose from drugs in breast milk is the contribution of metabolites with additional pharmacological activity (i.e., active metabolites). Metabolites may be formed in the maternal circulation or in breast tissue and transferred to the infant via breast milk. The M/P ratio of drug metabolites is not always measured. Case reports that measure metabolites offer valuable information to the overall transfer of a drug in breast milk. However, one of the drawbacks of many case reports lies in the sparseness of the details provided on the analytical methods used to achieve this.

The effect of infant suckling on the M/P ratio is not always known. Clinical trials often do not incorporate infant feeding between measurements. It is known that a long feeding time is associated with an increase in the percentage of lipid in the milk. Thus, for lipid-soluble drugs, the M/P ratio may increase throughout a feeding interval, and this variation may not be detected in the trial. The calculation of an M/P ratio may also vary depending on the type of milk sample obtained. Some trials analyze the first few drops of milk expressed, while others average the amount collected over an entire feeding interval. The M/P ratio may vary according to the maturity of the milk as well. Trials should report the exact stage of lactation at which drug analyses were made.

Finally, many of the trials involving measurement of drugs in breast milk use small sample sizes. This may be due to such factors as insufficient number of women taking medications while breastfeeding, difficulty in retrieving consent and meeting study criteria, unavailability of assay methods, and perhaps a perception that drug consumption by infants through breast milk is negligible. Results often show considerable variability within and between subjects. It is clear that conclusions made from such studies cannot be extrapolated to all lactating women with a measurable degree of certainty.

Estimating M/P Ratios

Studies of drug transfer into milk are not available for many agents, and the M/P ratio is not known for these drugs. Another method, however, can be employed to estimate a nursing infant's drug consumption. It involves calculating an M/P ratio from information known about the physiochemical properties of the drug. Much research has been done on drug transfer into milk in animal species. The principles of these findings are often used to estimate the M/P ratio of drugs if data are unavailable for humans.

Animal studies of drug transfer into milk have shown that the distribution of drugs between maternal plasma and milk can partially be explained using pH partition theory (38–41). Drug transfer occurs by passive diffusion of the un-ionized species, the degree of ionization at plasma pH determining the amount available for diffusion into milk. This can be determined using the pH partition theory (42) and the pK_a of the drug:

$$\text{Acidic drugs: } pK_a = pH + \log \frac{\text{un-ionized}}{\text{ionized}} \tag{1}$$

$$\text{Basic drugs: } pK_a = pH + \log \frac{\text{ionized}}{\text{un-ionized}}$$

Because the pH of milk is generally lower than that of plasma, the concentration that an electrolyte achieves in milk will depend on the pK_a of the drug. When the M/P ratio has not been measured, the milk-to-plasma ultrafiltrate ratio (M_u/P_u) (42) may be calculated instead using the Henderson-Hasselbach equation, a ratio that describes drug partitioning into ultrafiltrate fluids devoid of lipids or proteins.

$$\text{For acidic drugs: } M_u/P_u = \frac{1 + 10^{(pH_m - pK_a)}}{1 + 10^{(pH_p - pK_a)}} \tag{2}$$

$$\text{For basic drugs: } M_u/P_u = \frac{1 + 10^{(pK_a - pH_m)}}{1 + 10^{(pK_a - pH_p)}}$$

where pH_p is the pH of plasma and pH_m is the pH of milk.

Since most drugs are weak acids or weak bases, they will partition into breast milk according to their degree of ionization in the two media. Most acids are present in dissociated and undissociated forms in milk and plasma. Since only the undissociated form can pass from plasma to milk, an equilibrium is established across the mammary membrane, and the concentrations of the undissociated drug are equal in the ultrafiltrates. However, since the plasma pH is slightly higher, a larger portion of drug will be present in plasma than milk in the dissociated state. Thus $M_u/P_u < 1$. The situation is reversed for weak bases. Bases exist in dissociated and undissociated forms in plasma and milk. As a result of the lower pH in milk, a larger portion of drug will be ionized. Thus, the drug concentration in the milk ultrafiltrate will be higher than in the plasma. Thus, weak bases can achieve higher concentrations in the milk ultrafiltrate than in the plasma. This phenomenon is called "ion trapping." Un-ionized drugs will have M_u/P_u ratios of approximately 1.

The amount of drug available to cross into milk depends on protein binding. This is because only the unbound portion is able to diffuse into milk. Binding to milk proteins may also occur, and predictions of M/P ratios without considering protein binding may mislead conclusions (43). The Henderson-Hasselbach equation can be modified to allow for correction of protein binding of drugs in plasma and milk. The calculated milk-to-plasma ratio then reflects the ratio of drugs in skim milk to plasma (M_{skim}/P) (44). In this case, the milk is devoid of lipid constituents:

$$M_{skim}/P = \frac{M_u \times \text{plasma} f_u}{P_u \times \text{milk} f_u} \qquad (3)$$

where $f_u = 1 - $ fraction protein-bound.

Milk also contains other constituents, such as lipids, which can alter drug concentration. Atkinson and Begg (45) have designed a detailed model that accounts for drug octanol/water partition coefficient (or lipophilicity) and plasma protein binding. This model thus estimates a ratio of whole milk to plasma (M/P) instead of M_u/P_u or M_{skim}/P. The specific model is as follows:

For basic drugs: $\ln M/P = 0.025 + 2.3 \ln (M_u/P_u) + 0.9 \ln (F_{up}) + 0.5 \ln K$

For acidic drugs: $\ln M/P = -0.405 + 9.4 \ln (M_u/P_u) - 0.7 \ln (F_{up}) - 1.5 \ln K$

where $K = (0.955/f_{um}) \times (0.045 + \text{milk/lipid } P_{app})$, $f_{up} = $ fraction of drug unbound in plasma $(1 - $ plasma protein binding), $f_{um} = $ fraction unbound in milk, and $P_{app} = $ apparent partition coefficient at pH 7.2. An explanation of the derivation and use of the model is found in the cited paper.

As mentioned, experimentally or theoretically derived M/P ratios are used to estimate the amount of drug excretion in milk. For example, the drug concentration in milk (C_m) can be calculated as follows:

$$C_m = M/P \times C_{ss} \qquad (4)$$

where $C_{ss} = $ the average maternal plasma level at steady state, which is usually obtained from reference texts. If it is not known, the C_{ss} can be estimated using the following well-known equation:

$$C_{ss} = \frac{R \times F}{Cl} \qquad (5)$$

where $R = $ dose rate, $F = $ bioavailability, and $Cl = $ clearance. These variables are also obtained from reference texts.

Once the C_m has been calculated, it can be used to estimate infant drug exposure. This is done by estimating the volume of milk (V_m) that is ingested by a breastfeeding infant per day. An average value of 150 mL/kg/d (35) is often used. The following equation can then be used to calculate the infant dosage (D_{inf}) per unit time (35):

$$D_{inf} = C_m \times V_m \tag{6}$$

In addition, one can compare the infant dose with the maternal dose or with the therapeutic dose of the drug in infants. The former option involves calculating the percentage of maternal dose on a mg/kg basis, or the fraction of the dose the infant receives (F_{inf}), which is obtained as follows:

$$F_{inf} = \frac{D_{inf} \times 100}{\text{maternal dose}} \tag{7}$$

These calculations have been used by many investigators to estimate the drug consumption of nursing infants. It should be noted, however, that they are simply estimates of infant exposure to drugs through breast milk. The values obtained by these equations are not sufficient in estimating risk to the infant. Other variables will affect the risk/benefit analysis for drug exposure during breastfeeding. These include the pharmacology of the drug, the presence of active metabolites, the dose and length of therapy, the disposition of the drug in infants, infant age and clinical status, quantity of milk consumed, utilization of the drug in pediatric medicine, and possible effects of the drug on lactation. Most important, the probability of developing adverse reactions needs to be considered when risk is assessed.

Breastfeeding mothers should not be encouraged to take medications unless it is necessary. When drug therapy is required during lactation, the safest drug in a therapeutic class should be chosen, and the lowest dose that will achieve the therapeutic goal should be used. If the milk-plasma drug profile has been clearly defined, mothers can also tailor their dose times to avoid peak milk levels during infant feedings.

Information Sources on Drugs and Lactation

There are many reviews on the topic of drug excretion in breast milk. The most extensive review is from the World Health Organization (WHO) Working Group. In *Drugs and Human Lactation* (46), the WHO Working Group reviews breast physiology, mechanisms of drug excretion in milk, and clinical trials and case reports involving drugs and breast milk. The book also makes recommendations on the safety of the drugs reviewed. Another source of information is *Drugs in Pregnancy and Lactation* (47), which summarizes some of the findings from clinical trials and case reports. The recommendations of the American Academy of Pediatrics (AAP) Committee on Drugs are also given; the AAP publishes a summary of drugs considered to be compatible with breastfeeding (48).

Guidelines for studies on drug passage into milk have also been developed by the WHO Working Group (49). They address such factors as sample size of study, drug assay methods, and general study design. Clinical trials of drug excretion in milk are difficult to conduct, and the case report makes up much of the information that is available in this area. A brief discussion of the clinical usefulness of case reports is therefore warranted.

Obviously, case reports often provide information that is otherwise unavailable. Case reports identify possible adverse effects of drugs from exposure through breast milk. For example, acetaminophen is generally regarded as safe during lactation. However Matheson et al. (50) reported a 2-month-old infant who developed a rash after maternal ingestion of acetaminophen. Upon rechallenge at a later date, a similar type of rash developed. The milk concentrations found were similar to those reported earlier. Accordingly, it is apparent from this case report that recognizing potential drug-related reactions is important during breastfeeding.

Case reports can also verify that some drugs whose safety is suspect may indeed cause side effects in the breastfeeding neonate. For example, Atkinson et al. (33) recommended that atenolol be avoided in nursing mothers with infants less than 44 weeks postconceptual age. This recommendation was based on the estimated infant concentrations that would be achieved. Countering this concern, atenolol has been studied in puerperium lactating women without adverse effects. In a case report, however, Schmimmel et al. (51) reported a neonate who suffered from signs of β-adrenergic blockade while her mother was taking atenolol. This was the first report of toxic effects caused by atenolol through breastfeeding, and it lends credibility to the models that predicted it could occur.

Case reports are often simpler to produce than a clinical trial; sometimes only one patient is involved, and the time commitment may be proportionately smaller. Results are also rapidly available to the scientific community because the analysis of one patient is shorter than for a group. Case reports may also be useful in introducing analytical methods that can be used by others to analyze drugs in breast milk.

The potential disadvantage of case reports is that the events they describe may be interpreted by health professionals as common. It must be remembered that a single case report does not reflect the risk or safety following drug exposure for all nursing infants. In addition, it does not always prove a causal relationship between drug exposure and clinical effect. The information should be extrapolated to other settings with extreme caution. Whenever possible, it is best to incorporate the case report into an overall risk assessment together with other clinical data available, including the results of investigating other possible treatment modalities, considering infant age and clinical status, and observing the baby's breastfeeding pattern.

The appendix shows a table that summarizes the excretion of selected drugs in milk and includes data obtained from clinical trials and case reports. The legend appears before the table. Recommendations on the safety of selected drugs during nursing follow.

THERAPEUTIC IMPLICATIONS OF DRUG EXCRETION IN BREAST MILK

Assessing the Risk of Drug Exposure in Breast Milk

The dose of a drug ingested by an infant through breast milk provides an estimate of the risk to the infant. For most drugs that have been studied, the infant dose ingested through breast milk is less than 5% of the maternal dose on a weight-adjusted basis (F_{inf}). Because the therapeutic dose is similar in both adults and children on a milligram-for-kilogram basis, the dose ingested by the infant will not be sufficient to exert a pharmacological effect. Occasionally, however, the F_{inf} may approach the recognized infant therapeutic dose. In such cases, the clinician assumes that the risk for side effects is not negligible and may be similar to the risk of side effects for a drug directly given to the infant.

Drugs can be ranked and categorized according to the proportion of the maternal dose for the convenience of risk assessment (52). However, care should be exercised when these data are used in clinical settings. First, the risk to the infant is not entirely proportional to the F_{inf}. Even if the infant dose should happen to be a small fraction of a maternal dose, potent pharmacological actions or potential for severe side effects may make the drug incompatible with breastfeeding. In contrast, a drug that causes no known adverse effects may be compatible with breastfeeding even if the infant ingests close to a therapeutic dose via milk.

Assessing potential risks is a crucial step when counseling a mother about whether to breastfeed or formula-feed while taking medication. The potential risks of developing adverse reactions in the breastfed infants exposed to drugs in milk should be weighed against the risks associated with formula-feeding. Bottle feeding is associated with higher mortality rates for infants than breastfeeding. In industrialized countries, bottle feeding is associated with mortality rates of 1–5 per 1000 live births. In developing countries, the mortality rate is 300 per 1000 live births (9). Furthermore, recent studies have shown associations between premature infant exposure to cow's milk (which most infant formulas are based on) and immune system disorders such as insulin-dependent diabetes mellitus (53) and Crohn's disease (54). While there appears to be a real risk associated with formulas based on cow's milk, virtually nothing has been learned about the probability of developing adverse reactions in infants of breastfeeding mothers on medications.

When one assesses the risk associated with breastfeeding during maternal medications, any case report of adverse reactions in breastfed infants should be considered. One should also bear in mind that the incidence of such events may well be extremely low.

General guidelines have been proposed by Berlin (11) based on consistent findings from studies that have evaluated drug excretion in breast milk:

1. Most drugs (and environmental chemicals) are capable of crossing from plasma to milk.
2. The concentrations of drugs in milk parallel the levels achieved in plasma over a similar time course, and milk-to-plasma concentration ratios vary from 50 to 100%.
3. Following a single maternal dose of a drug, the observed half-lives are similar for plasma and milk.
4. The total amount of drug available for infant absorption is usually less than one percent of the maternal dose.
5. There are few studies or reports based on steady-state maternal dosing.
6. For most drugs, the risk of side effects in the infant can be assessed to be small or negligible.

In the Motherisk Program in Toronto, we have been prospectively collecting infant outcome data in a cohort of breastfed infants whose mothers were on medications. Women initially contacted Motherisk seeking advice on the safety of drug consumption during breastfeeding. They had not yet started drug therapy. Mothers were subsequently contacted for a follow-up interview (about 6 weeks after the initial consultation). The mothers who had ingested drugs while breastfeeding were asked whether the children had experienced any adverse reactions during drug therapy. This study included 838 mother–infant pairs and took place between 1985 and 1991. No major adverse events (defined as requiring medical attention) were identified. Overall, 11% of the mothers reported symptoms in the infants during their drug therapy. These symptoms did not require medical attention. Table 1 shows a partial list of the minor adverse effects on the breastfed infants exposed to drugs commonly inquired about in our program.

Long-term effects in infants from drug consumption in breast milk are not available. Studies of this nature are difficult to conduct. Large cohorts are necessary, and patients must be followed for long periods of time. Thus far, information is limited to long-term effects of oral contraceptives and social drugs (see Table 2 and related text).

REVIEW OF SELECTED DRUG CLASSES

We now list recommendations for the use of selected drugs (mostly taken from the table in the appendix) and breastfeeding. Infant monitoring guidelines are also recommended.

Table 1   Main Maternal Drug Exposures and Associated Minor Adverse Reactions in the Breastfed Infants (Data From Motherisk Cohort)

Drug	No. of mother–infant pairs	Number of infants with reactions			
		Diarrhea	Drowsiness	Irritability	Others
Antibiotics					
Amoxicillin	25	3	0	0	0
Erythromycin	17	2	0	2	0
Sulfamethoxazole + trimethoprim	12	0	0	0	2[a]
Cloxacillin	10	2	0	0	0
Cephalexin	7	2	0	0	0
Nitrofurantoin	6	2	0	0	1[a]
Ampicillin	5	1	0	0	0
Cefaclor	5	1	0	0	0
Analgesics/narcotics					
Acetaminophen	43	0	0	0	0
Acetaminophen + codeine + caffeine	26	0	5	1	2
Ibuprofen	21	0	0	0	0
Naproxen	20	0	2	0	1
Aspirin	15	0	0	0	0
Antihistamines					
Terfenadine	25	0	0	3	0
Diphenhydramine	12	0	1	0	0
Astemizole	10	0	0	2	0
Dimenhydrinate	7	0	0	1	0
Chlorpheniramine	5	0	0	0	0
Sedatives/antidepressants/ antiepileptics					
Carbamazepine	6	0	0	0	0
Alprazolam	5	0	1	0	0
Miscellaneous					
Oral contraceptive	16	0	1	2	4[a]
Pseudoephedrine	10	0	0	2	0
5-Aminosalicylic acid	8	1	0	0	0
Prednisone (-lone)	6	0	0	0	0
Levothyroxine	5	0	0	0	0
Permethrin	5	0	0	0	0
Warfarin	5	0	0	0	0

[a]Other reactions included poor feeding (2 cases with sulfamethoxazole/trimethoprim), decreased milk volume (1 with nitrofurantoin and 3 with oral contraceptives), constipation (2 with acetaminophen + codeine, 1 with oral contraceptives), and vomiting (1 with naproxen).

Analgesics

Acetaminophen is excreted into milk in small amounts. Narcotic analgesics such as codeine and morphine have also been detected in milk in small amounts. Therapeutic doses of codeine are generally considered to be safe to use. One recent case report found morphine plasma concentrations in the analgesic range in a 3-week-old infant whose mother was being tapered off high doses of morphine (see appendix table). No adverse effects were reported in this infant. Nursing infants, however, may be sensitive to the effects of narcotics and should be observed for signs of sedation or unexplained episodes of cyanosis and apnea during maternal therapy (264).

Anti-infectives

Penicillin and cephalosporin antibiotics are considered to be safe to use while breastfeeding. Infants should be observed for allergic reactions. Infants with glucose 6-phosphate dehydrogenase deficiency should avoid exposure to sulfonamides, nalidixic acid, nitrofurantoin, and other agents capable of causing hemolysis. Sulfonamides should be avoided if newborn infants have jaundice, because of theoretical risks of displacement of bilirubin from binding sites and kernicterus.

The use of metronidazole during lactation is controversial. Experimental studies have revealed that it has carcinogenic and mutagenic properties (265). However, human data have not substantiated the carcinogenic risk (266). Breastfeeding may be continued during metronidazole therapy. Close supervision of the nursing infant is warranted, however, since significant amounts may be present in milk and the infant may be at risk for adverse effects such as diarrhea. If a single dose of metronidazole has been prescribed, breastfeeding may be temporarily withheld for 12–24 hours while the drug is being excreted by the body. During this period, the breasts can be manually emptied to alleviate engorgement and to maintain milk flow.

Ciprofloxacin and ofloxacin have been measured in milk in small amounts. According to the drug monograph, norfloxacin was not detected in the milk of lactating women after a single dose of 200 mg (267). The use of quinolones during breastfeeding, however, has not gained wide acceptance in the medical community. The quinolones were shown to cause cartilage damage in juvenile animals (268) and were subsequently not recommended for use in children, pregnant women, and nursing women. Many pediatric patients, however, have received quinolone antibiotics. The current published data on more than 1000 pediatric patients treated with quinolones revealed no documentation of unequivocal quinolone-induced arthropathy (269,270). Even though the risk for quinolone-induced arthropathy in the nursing infant is unknown, it is probably very low. Nevertheless, quinolones are not first-line therapy for most infections nursing women may encounter, and other antibiotics are generally preferred. If maternal therapy with a quinolone such as ciprofloxacin is warranted, the data suggest that the baby may continue to nurse. As a precaution, the infants should be monitored closely for signs of arthropathy (e.g., limping, tenderness, stiffness).

Infant exposure to acyclovir through breast milk is small. Topical use of acyclovir is compatible with breastfeeding. Oral administration is unlikely to expose the infant to significant plasma levels because bioavailability is low.

Chloramphenicol should be used with caution because of risks of idiosyncratic reactions in the newborn, such as bone marrow suppression. The use of tetracycline during breastfeeding has not been documented to cause problems. However, there is some controversy regarding its use. Even though tetracycline crosses into breast milk in low amounts, and its bioavailability in nursing infants may be low as a result of complexation with calcium or magnesium ions in milk, the potential risk for tooth mottling in the breastfeeding infant is unknown. The AAP has commended tetracycline as safe to use during lactation (48). In most cases, however, safer antimicrobials can be substituted for both chloramphenicol and tetracycline.

One case report showed that isoniazid is excreted in large amounts in breast milk. Its use during lactation has not been recommended because there are concerns for infant liver toxicity.

Anti-inflammatory Agents

Salicyclic acid has been shown to cross into breast milk in small amounts following maternal acetylsalicylic acid (ASA) ingestion. Occasional use of ASA is not likely to harm the infant. Chronic high dose ASA therapy, however, has not been adequately studied. Inevitably, more salicylate will be present in milk and the infant may be at risk for salicylate toxicity (271).

Nonsteroidal anti-inflammatory drugs (NASIDs) such as diclofenac, ibuprofen, naproxen, flurbiprofen, ketoprofen, ketorolac, and mefenamic acid have been shown to be present in small amounts and are considered to be safe to use.

Antihypertensive Drugs

The special need for antihypertensive therapy in postpartum women has promoted the study of this class of drugs.

The transfer of different β-adrenergic blockers into breast milk has been well studied. The primary determinant of passage into breast milk for this drug class is protein binding (272). Drugs that are less lipophilic and less protein-bound, such as atenolol or sotalol, are present in higher quantities.

Any infant's exposure to these drugs will be further increased by poor elimination processes. For example, drug half-lives may be doubled or tripled for drugs excreted renally (273) in the postnatal period. Another consideration is that β-adrenergic blockers used throughout pregnancy may cause hypotension, bradycardia, and respiratory difficulties in newborns. Since a newborn's heart rate is lowest in the first few days postpartum, the added use of β-adrenergic blockers may be worrisome, especially if the newborn is premature (273).

Other antihypertensive agents, such as methyldopa, captopril, enalapril, nifedipine, diltiazem, and verapamil, have been measured in breast milk in small amounts. Adverse effects have not been reported, and the use of these drugs is considered to be compatible with breastfeeding.

Anticonvulsants

The anticonvulsants carbamazepine, valproic acid, and phenytoin are excreted into breast milk in low amounts. Breastfeeding may be continued during their use.

Phenobarbital, primidone, and ethosuximide, on the other hand, are excreted in much higher amounts, and infants may be exposed to *nearly* therapeutic doses. Phenobarbital is usually contraindicated during nursing (see Table 2). Infants exposed to these medications via milk should be closely supervised because they may be at risk for adverse effects such as lethargy, sedation, and poor feeding. Infant anticonvulsant plasma concentration monitoring is also advisable.

Antihistamines

Antihistamines are present in many over-the-counter medications, and ingestion of this class of drugs should not stop the nursing mother from breastfeeding. Although quantitative data on the excretion of most antihistamines in milk are lacking, their use is generally considered to be safe during nursing. Specific data on drug excretion in milk are present for loratadine, terfenadine, and triprolidine, all of which have been measured in milk in small amounts. There is one case report in the literature of sedation and irritability in an infant following maternal ingestion of clemastine (274). The Motherisk cohort data include 59 mother–infant pairs with 7 (12%) mothers reporting minor adverse effects in their children (Table 1). Antihistamines may be used during lactation; however, infants should be monitored for potential adverse effects.

Cardiovascular Drugs

Infant consumption of digoxin, flecainide, procainamide, or mexiletine from breast milk is small. Amiodarone and disopyramide, however, are present in larger amounts, which may affect the infant. Whenever possible, drug levels in breast milk and/or infant's plasma should be monitored during maternal therapy. During amiodarone therapy, infant thyroid function tests should be monitored as well, since amiodarone can cause hyper- or hypothyroidism.

Diuretics

Diuretics have been found in breast milk in low amounts. The theoretical concern that they may suppress lactation has been raised. However, lactogenesis itself has not been shown to be influenced by fluid intake (275), and the impact of taking diuretics is unknown.

Drugs Acting on the Central Nervous System (CNS)

Many puerperial women may require CNS medications to alleviate symptoms of depression, anxiety, or other psychiatric conditions. Most of the information available for these drugs, however, is in the form of case reports. Generalizations regarding "risk" are difficult to make.

Case reports of tricyclic antidepressants measured in breast milk show that infant exposure is consistently low for drugs of this class. Breastfeeding may be continued during their use, keeping in mind that the effects of long-term exposure of these drugs on the developing central nervous system is not known. Similarly, excretion of some neuroleptics into breast milk has been studied. Only small amounts have been found, but potential long-term behavioral effects are unknown.

Lithium therapy during breastfeeding warrants concern because the drug freely passes into breast milk and significant plasma levels have been detected in nursing infants (appendix table). For this reason, many health professionals advise against the use of lithium during lactation (see Table 2). If a woman chooses to nurse during lithium therapy, however, infant plasma lithium levels should be monitored.

Benzodiazepines should be used with caution in breastfeeding women. Metabolizing capacity of these drugs may be limited in the neonatal period, and accumulation may occur. If benzodiazepine therapy is necessary, short-term treatment with a short-acting agent devoid of pharmacologically active metabolites, such as lorazepam or alprazolam, is preferrable (276).

Thyroid and Antithyroid Drugs

Levothyroxine is compatible with breastfeeding. Thyroid hormones cross into breast milk in low amounts. Their presence is not likely to affect the infant's thyroid (277–280).

Propylthiouracil crosses into breast milk in small amounts and is the antithyroid drug of choice during breastfeeding. Infants have been safely breastfed on maternal doses of 50–300 mg/d (281). The infant should be tested regularly for thyroid function to monitor for toxicity (282,283), however, if clinically warranted.

Gastrointestinal Drugs and Laxatives

H_2 receptor blockers such as cimetidine and ranitidine should be used with caution in breastfeeding mothers. To date, adverse effects have not been reported in nursing infants, but the potential exists for inhibition of gastric acid secretion and enzyme metabolizing capability. Aluminum and magnesium salts are considered to be safe to use (284,285). Sucralfate is poorly absorbed from the gastrointestinal tract and is not likely to cause adverse effects in the nursing infant (285).

Metoclopramide and domperidone are excreted into milk in small amounts. Both increase prolactin levels (286–288), and metoclopramide has increased milk production in women with faltering milk production (287–289).

Several investigators studied the clinical effects on nursing infants after maternal ingestion of laxatives. Phenolphthalein (290), mineral oil, magnesia, and senna glycosides (291,292) have all been associated with normal infant bowel patterns after short-term maternal therapy. No harmful effects from docusate have been observed (293). Nonetheless, lactating women are generally advised to use drugs that are poorly absorbed from the gastrointestinal tract, such as psyllium or other bulk-forming agents.

Miscellaneous

5-Aminosalicyclic acid and sulfasalazine can be used by the lactating mother. The infant should be monitored for adverse reactions, such as diarrhea.

Chloroquine and hydroxychloroquine are both excreted in breast milk. Adverse effects have not been reported with their use. Weekly dosing of chloroquine for malaria is unlikely to expose the nursing infant to toxic amounts. There are no reports on the safety of daily chloroquine, administered for arthritis. Since the milk half-life of chloroquine is approximately one week (appendix table), daily administration would inevitably lead to accumulation of the drug in milk.

Prednisone and prednisolone have been detected in milk in small amounts. Breastfeeding need not be interrupted. Because systemic absorption following topical and inhalational steroids usually is not substantial, these drugs are also safe to use during lactation.

Theophylline is excreted in milk. Since clearance of theophylline is low in the neonatal period, close monitoring of the infant is necessary to detect adverse effects.

Warfarin is highly protein-bound. Levels in milk have been consistently below detection limits, and no adverse effects have been reported in nursing infants. Heparin therapy is also compatible with breastfeeding. Heparin does not pass into milk (294).

Topical Agents

The excretion of topically applied drugs into breast milk has not been widely studied. This fact does not, however, rule out their use in nursing women. For example, the excretion of inhalational β-adrenergic agonists (e.g., salbutamol) in breast milk has not been studied, but bioavailability of these agents is low. Breastfeeding during their use is considered to be safe. Similarly, ipratropium and sodium cromoglycate are unlikely to cause adverse effects.

Many other topical agents (eye drops, creams, ointments, etc.) with low bioavailability and a low order of toxicity may be used during the lactation period as well. Examples of these agents are lidocaine ointment, nystatin cream, and clotrimazole cream.

DRUGS USUALLY CONTRAINDICATED DURING BREASTFEEDING

Table 2 lists drugs commonly avoided during lactation. The sections that follow review the reasons for not using these drugs. Some drugs that fall into this category were discussed above (see "Review of Selected Drug Classes").

Antineoplastics

The use of antineoplastic drugs is generally contraindicated during lactation. Even if the absolute dose to which the infant is exposed is small, the

Table 2 Drugs Usually Contraindicated During Breastfeeding

Antineoplastics
Bromocriptine[a]
Ergotamine
Gold
Iodine-containing substances
Lithium
Oral contraceptives[a]
Phenobarbital
Radiopharmaceuticals
Social drugs and drugs of abuse

[a]May decrease milk supply.

possibility for immediate or long-term toxicity precludes breastfeeding during the use of these medications. Of these medications, azathioprine and methotrexate are two of the more commonly used antineoplastic agents in ambulatory care patients. Both have been measured in breast milk. The peak milk concentration of 6-mercaptopurine, the active metabolite of azathioprine, was 18 ng/mL in a woman taking 25 mg of azathioprine daily and 4.5 ng/mL in a woman taking 75 mg daily (295). There are three cases of infants breastfed during maternal azathioprine therapy without adverse effects (295,296). Methotrexate secretion in milk was measured in a patient receiving 22.5 mg daily. The peak milk methotrexate level was only 2.6 ng/mL. The highest M/P ratio was 0.08 (297). Based on these data, some have argued that methotrexate may be safe to use in rheumatic diseases (298), where it is administered only once a week. Further study seems warranted. Lactating mothers requiring these medications should be well informed of the risks to the baby. If antineoplastics are used during lactation, the following should be strictly monitored: milk drug levels, infant plasma drug levels, and infant hematological parameters.

Radiopharmaceuticals

The use of radiopharmaceuticals usually requires temporary cessation of breastfeeding to avoid infant exposure to excessive radioactivity. The time necessary before most radioactivity is excreted varies with the radioisotope used; reference texts or departments of nuclear medicine can be consulted for this information. While awaiting clearance of the isotope, breast pumping may be employed to preserve nursing function. Since most diagnostic testing is planned in advance, mothers may express milk (and keep it frozen) before the procedure. This milk will be given to the baby during the time that nursing has been suspended.

Ergot Alkaloids

Bromocriptine, an ergot alkaloid, is contraindicated during breastfeeding. It possesses prolactin-suppressing activity and is used to prevent lactation (299,300). Ergotamine is avoided because it entails risks of milk suppression (301) and ergotism in the infant (302). Methylergonovine, however, is used to assist uterine involution. Short-term therapy with methylergonovine is not associated with adverse effects.

Social Drugs and Drugs of Abuse

Social drugs such as alcohol are not recommended for use during lactation. Ethanol freely distributes into milk, and levels in milk are similar to those in plasma. Elimination from milk is also similar to elimination from blood (303,304). Occasional alcohol consumption exposes the nursing infant to small amounts of ethanol and is not considered to be harmful, but the infant may be at risk for sedation with higher doses (305). At higher doses, ethanol presents a risk to successful lactation also, since oxytocin release is blocked (306). Infant motor development is affected by maternal alcohol ingestion in a dose-dependent fashion (307). Interestingly, both alcoholic and non-alcoholic beer have been shown to increase prolactin secretion (308). In summary then, alcohol use should be limited during lactation.

Smoking during lactation is also not recommended. A nursing mother should be encouraged to stop smoking because there are well-documented health risks to herself and her nursing infant. Nicotine has been measured in milk (309). Cotinine, the major metabolite of nicotine, has also been measured in milk (310,311). In fact, infant urine cotinine levels have been correlated with maternal breast milk cotinine levels (312).

Maternal smoking has been linked to a higher incidence of respiratory tract infections in infants (312). Smoking has also been shown to have a negative effect on breast milk production (313). Smoking may be a contributing factor to infant colic (314). In addition, infants may also be exposed to other chemicals from cigarette smoking, such as carcinogens. As such, passive smoking by the infant (315,316) may lead to long-term adverse effects.

The use of "street drugs" by lactating women is contraindicated. The first concern should be that it may be difficult for nursing women to properly care for their infants if they are experiencing an altered state of mind when using these drugs. Also, there exists the potential for drug exposure through breast milk (or passive smoking) and therefore, adverse effects on the infant. These drugs are typically very potent, and smaller doses can have pharmacological effects. In a case report, intranasal use of cocaine resulted in the presence of the drug and its metabolite in the mother's milk and in the urine of her infant, who exhibited signs of cocaine toxicity (317). Phencyclidine has been detected in breast milk (318). Δ-9-Tetrahydrocannabinol (THC), considered to be the main psychoactive component of marijuana, is also excreted into breast milk (319). In a study of infant development after marijuana exposure during pregnancy and lactation, maternal use of marijuana in the first month postpartum was associated with lower motor development scores at one year of age in exposed infants compared to unexposed infants (320). Marijuana has also been shown to decrease plasma prolactin levels in women (321).

Gold

The use of gold therapy during breastfeeding is controversial. Variable milk levels have been reported, and the extent of absorption by the infant is unknown. In one report, the mean milk level of aurothioglucose was 41 μg/L in a nursing woman receiving weekly injections of 50 mg. The ratio of milk to serum was 0.01. The drug was not present in the infant's serum or urine (limit of detection 5 × 10⁻⁷ mg/L) (322). In another report, sodium auro-thiomalate given weekly at a dose of 25 mg produced maximum milk levels of 40 μg/L, and the infant's urine contained 0.4 μg/L. The infant experienced transient facial edema that could not be explained (323). The highest milk level reported in a woman receiving 10 mg of sodium aurothiomalate monthly was 93 μg/L. The ratio of milk to serum varied from 0.02 to 0.03. The infant plasma level was 51 μg/L; no adverse reactions were observed (324). Gold has a long half-life (approximately one week in serum), and long after a dose has been given to a nursing mother, her infant may continue to have exposure (322). Gold has also been shown to be excreted in increasing concentrations over time in milk (322,324). Infants who are nursing during maternal gold therapy should be monitored very closely for adverse effects.

Iodine

Drugs containing iodine (e.g., potassium iodide, povidone-iodine) are not recommended during breastfeeding. Iodine is transported into breast milk and can result in iodine-induced goiter and hypothyroidism in the infant (325). Extensive topical administration and vaginal use of povidone-iodine by breastfeeding mothers has led to transient congenital hypothyroidism (326,327) and grossly elevated serum iodine levels in their infants (328).

Oral Contraceptives

Much controversy has surrounded the use of oral contraceptives during lactation. The topic has been extensively reviewed by Koetsawang (329), who concluded that combination estrogen and progestogen oral contraceptives, even in low doses, can decrease milk yield. Progestogen-only contraceptives are associated with fewer changes. The World Health Organization (330) recently studied the effects of different types of contraception on milk and in nursing infants. They found that combined oral contraceptives caused slight changes in milk composition as well as a decrease in milk yield. Hormonal contraceptives, however, were not associated with any significant difference in infant weight, fat fold, or rate of discontinuation of breastfeeding by the mothers compared to a control group.

Oral contraceptives are not recommended for use in early lactation or in nutritionally deficient mothers because the potential adverse effects on milk supply may be clinically significant in these women. Overall, progestogen-only contraceptives may be preferrable. Initiation of oral contraceptives during nursing should be delayed. However, there is no consensus as to how long (331). Nursing prolongs amenorrhea in postpartum women, and oral contraceptives need not be started right away. Oral contraceptives probably should not begin until breastfeeding is fully established (approximately 6 weeks) or even later.

CONCLUSIONS

Most drugs taken by breastfeeding women are excreted into breast milk, and a determination of the risk to the infant must be made. For most drugs, risk assessment is made by considering the dose delivered to the infant from nursing. Other factors in risk assessment include the toxicity profile of the drug.

The amount of drug consumed by the infant during nursing is usually less than 5% of the maternal dose (mg/kg). This small amount is tolerable by most infants without toxicity. Common sense dictates that even though many drugs may be taken safely during nursing, mothers should not be exposed to them unnecessarily.

If maternal drug therapy is required, the specific agents used should be chosen with the intent of minimizing any risks to the infant. In this way, interruption of breastfeeding is rarely required. The following principles should be applied: the drug used should be appropriate for treating the mother's condition, it should be unlikely to cause adverse effects in the infant, and finally, the infant should be monitored for potential adverse effects.

APPENDIX

Table A1 is a review of the findings of clinical trials of drugs taken during lactation. It is inevitable that some of the details sought by the reader will be missing. Readers are encouraged to review the individual research papers cited and other resources for additional information.

Study Design

All drugs were taken orally unless otherwise specified. Where data were unavailable, a question mark (?) or blank space appears.

Ref. = reference.
No. = number of subjects (taken from the number of women donating milk samples for drug analysis, or from the number of women whose data appear in the paper)
MD = multiple dose
SD = single dose

Lactation Stage

The period of lactation is specified. Whether the infant was nursing during maternal drug therapy is noted in the column headed "BF" (breastfed). The mothers donating milk samples for study analysis were not always the same mothers who nursed their infants during drug therapy.

Dosage to Infant

The dosage to infant F_{inf} was calculated as a proportion of the maternal dose, in milligrams per kilogram. The following formula was used:

$$F_{inf} = \frac{C_m \times V_m \times 100}{D}$$

where C_m = milk concentration of drug, and V_m = volume of milk ingested by infant (150 mL/kg/d for MD studies and 30 mL/kg/dose for SD studies) (52); it is assumed that an infant nurses five times daily during MD therapy, and once during an SD study.

D is the maternal dose (mg/kg). A maternal weight of 60 kg was used to calculate infant exposure if maternal weight was not provided by the paper. The bioavailability of the drug was assumed to be 100%.

Mean F_{inf} = mean % maternal dose obtained through milk. This value was calculated using the average milk concentration reported, or the arithmetic average calculated from data shown; arithmetic means were calculated using milk levels reported in the first 8–16 hours after dosing, if appropriate.

Max F_{inf} = maximum % maternal dose obtained through milk. This value was calculated using the highest milk level observed in one subject or the average maximum concentration achieved.

Standard Adult Dose

The standard adult dose, taken from standard reference books (262,263), is provided so that an infant's dose (mg) may be estimated using the relationship:

$$D_{inf} = F_{inf} \times \text{standard adult dose}$$

Other Findings

M/P = milk-to-plasma ratio
M/S = milk-to-serum ratio
M/B = milk-to-blood ratio
$t_{\frac{1}{2}}$ = drug half-life in milk
t_{max} = time to maximum drug concentration in milk

The ratios above were derived from investigators in different ways (e.g., arithmetic mean, area under the curve).

Comments

Other findings of the study are noted.

Table A1 Summary of Data Obtained from Studies of Drugs in Breast Milk

Drug	Ref. No.	Dose	Lactation stage	Mean F_{inf}	Max F_{inf}	Standard adult dose	M/P	M/S	$t_{1/2}$ (h)	t_{max} (h)	BF	Comments
Analgesics												
Acetaminophen	55	11	SD	2-22 mo	0.91	4.15	325-650 mg q4-6h			2.3	1-2	Yes	No adverse reaction in infants Acetaminophen and metabolite not detected in urine of infants (limit of detection 0.5 µg/mL)
	50	1	SD	2 mo	1.02	1.28						Yes	Case report of infant rash on two occasions
	56	4	SD	2-8 mo	1.1	1.85		1.24				No	No metabolites detected in milk (limit of detection 100 ng/mL)
Codeine	57	3	SD	?	0.40 (0.45)	1.58		0.76		2.7	2	No	
	58	1	SD	7 wk		1.29 (1.35)	10-60 mg q4-6h	2.16		2.5	1	No	M/P morphine = 2.46 ( ) = including active metabolite morphine
	58	1	SD	13 wk	0.59 (0.61)	1.47 (1.5)						Yes	( ) = including active metabolite morphine

Drug	No.	n		Duration		Dose			Comments
Meperidine	59	2	MD	8-72 h	0.61 (1.27)	50-150 mg q3-4h	1.17	?	( ) = including active metabolite normeperidine
	60	5	MD	1 d	1.57 (2.2)			Yes	Intravenous infusion. Neurobehavioral depression observed in neonates during 3rd day of maternal therapy. ( ) = including active metabolite normeperidine
Morphine	61	5	SD	>1 mo	6.0	5-30 mg q4h PO	2.45	?	Epidural/intramuscular/intravenous injection
	60	5	MD	1 d	0.65 (0.89)			Yes	Intravenous infusion. No adverse effects in neonates. ( ) = including metabolite morphine-3-glucuronide
	62	1	MD	3 wk	2.25			Yes	No adverse reaction in neonate. Neonatal plasma level 4 ng/mL

(continued)

Table A1 (Continued)

Drug	Ref.	No.	Dose	Lactation stage	Mean F_{inf}	Max F_{inf}	Standard adult dose	M/P	M/S	$t_{1/2}$ (h)	t_{max} (h)	BF	Comments
Oxycodone	63	6	MD	Post cesarean		10.17	5 mg q6h	3.4				?	Maternal dose unspecified; calculation based on 5 mg q6h Peak milk level 226 ng/mL
Anti-infectives													
Acyclovir	64	1	MD	4 mo	0.77	1.17	200 mg t.i.d.-200 mg 5×/d	0.6-4.1				Yes	One infant urine sample contained 1.08 µg/mL
Amoxicillin	65	1	MD	1 y	0.94	1.28			3.24	2.8		?	
	66	6	SD	3 d	0.08	0.23	250-500 mg q8h		0.013-0.043		4-5	?	
Ampicillin	67	10	MD	?		0.75	250-500 mg q6h		0.23			Yes	No difference in monitored parameters in infants compared with control group
	68	2-3	SD	5-7 d	0.05	0.072						?	
	69	6	MD	1-8 d	0.19	1.17						5 of 6	Administered as pivampicillin
Cephalexin	66	6	SD	3 d	0.06	0.15	250-1000 mg q6h		0.008-0.14		4-5	?	
	68	2-3	SD	5-7 d	0.13	0.29						?	

Drug												
Cefadroxil	66	6	SD	3 d	0.16	0.43	500-1000 mg b.i.d.	0.009-0.019		6-7	?	
Chloramphenicol	68	2-3	SD	5-7 d		0.18					?	
	70	5	MD	First week	1.88	5.23	50 mg/kg/d divided q6h				?	Chemical method of analysis used measures of antimicrobially effective fraction along with ineffective metabolites
	70	5	MD	Puerperium	1.94	3.63					?	
	71	4	SD	4 d	0.56	1.49		0.6	1.8		?	
	71	5	MD	1 wk	0.71	2.28		0.47-0.59		1.4	?	
Ciprofloxacin	68	2-3	SD	5-7 d	1.38	1.51	250-750 mg q12h				?	
	72	1	SD	17 d		1.08					No	
	73	1	MD	3 mo	1.76						Yes	One milk level reported Infant serum level below detection limit (0.03 μg/mL)
Clindamycin	74	10	MD	?	0.91	2.27	150-450 mg q6h	1.6-2.14		2	?	
	75	5	MD	1-2 wk		6.2					No	

(continued)

Table A1 (Continued)

Drug	Ref.	No.	Dose	Lacta-tion stage	Mean F_{inf}	Max F_{inf}	Standard adult dose	M/P	M/S	$t_{1/2}$ (h)	t_{max} (h)	BF	Comments
Clindamycin (continued)	76	2	MD	?	0.93	1.35						?	
	68	2-3	SD	5-7 d	0.81	1.44						?	
	77	1	MD	1-5 d								Yes	Intravenous therapy No milk levels obtained Report of neonatal bloody stools, but neonate previously treated with gentamicin and ampicillin
Cloxacillin	68	2-3	SD	5-7 d	0.072	0.144	250-500 mg q6h					?	Intramuscular injection
Erythromycin	68	2-3	SD	5-7 d	0.4	0.504	250 mg q.i.d.					?	
Isoniazid	78	1	SD	?	10.0 (12.2)		5-10 mg/kg/d			5.9	3	No	Peak acetylisoniazid milk level 5 h postdose; milk half-life 13.5 h ( ) = including metabolite acetyl-isoniazid

| Metronidazole | 79 | 12 | MD | 1 wk | 9.0 (13.2) | 11.64 (15.9) | 250 mg b.i.d.-750 mg t.i.d. | 0.91 | Yes | Neonatal stool changes and *Candida* isolated in more cases than controls; no serious adverse reactions in neonates Neonatal plasma levels 1.27-2.41 μg/mL; metabolite levels 1.1-2.41 μg/mL (in 7 neonates) M/P metabolite = 0.77 ( ) = including active hydroxy-metabolite |
| | 80 | 11 | MD | First mo | 8.55 (11.7) | 18.3 (24) | | 1 | Yes | No adverse reactions in neonates Neonatal plasma metronidazole level 0.3-1.4 μg/mL; metabolite level 0.1-0.8 μg/mL M/P hydroxymetabolite = 1.2 ( ) = including active hydroxy-metabolite |

(continued)

Table A1 (Continued)

Drug	Ref.	No.	Dose	Lactation stage	Mean F_{inf}	Max F_{inf}	Standard adult dose	M/P	M/S	$t_{1/2}$ (h)	t_{max} (h)	BF	Comments
Metronidazole (continued)	80	4	MD	First mo	10.8 (13.4)	13.5 (18.2)		1				Yes	No adverse reactions in neonates Neonatal plasma metronidazole level 0.6-4.9 µg/mL; metabolite level 0.4-2.3 µg/mL M/P hydroxy-metabolite = 1.2 ( ) = including active hydroxy-metabolite
	81	3	SD	6-14 wk	2.78	5.04						No	
	82	13	SD	3-8 d	0.04	0.12						No	
Nalidixic acid	83	1	MD	2 wk			1000 mg q.i.d.		0.061		2-4	Yes	Case report of hemolytic anemia in neonate negative for G6PD deficiency
Nitrofurantoin	84	9	MD	?		1.13	50-100 mg q.i.d.		0.27-0.31			No	
	85	?	MD	1-4 d								No	None detected in 20 milk samples (detection limit 2 µg/mL)
	86	3	MD	2-5 d		4.2		2.2				No	
	86	3	MD	2-5 d		6.54		2.3				No	

Drug											
Ofloxacin	74	10	MD	?	1.46	2.71	200-400 mg q12h	0.98-1.66		2	?
Penicillin	87	7	SD	2-5 d		0.054	1-10 million units/d divided q4-6h			?	Intramuscular injection
Penicillin V	88	18	SD	?	0.04	0.21	125-500 mg q6-8h		1-8	2-8	14 infants	0.52 mg/L detected in urine of one infant; undetectable in another infant tested 3 infants with looser stools
Sulfamethoxazole	89	50	MD	First 10 d	2.0-2.5		400-1000 mg q12h	0.1			Yes
Sulfisoxazole	90	6	MD	?			1000 mg q.i.d.	0.06	7.2		1 of 6	A mean of 0.45% of the 24-h maternal dose was recovered in milk over a 48-h period (including metabolite) Detected in urine of the breast-feeding infant M/S N-acetyl-sulfisoxazole = 0.22; milk half-life 8.9 h

(continued)

165

Table A1 (Continued)

Drug	Ref.	No.	Dose	Lactation stage	Mean F_{inf}	Max F_{inf}	Standard adult dose	M/P	M/S	$t_{1/2}$ (h)	t_{max} (h)	BF	Comments
Tetracycline	91	5	MD	?	0.51	1.16	250-500 mg q6h					Yes	No adverse reactions in infants Infants' serum < 0.07 mg/L
Trimethoprim	68	2-3	SD	5-7 d	0.88	1.44						?	
	89	50	MD	First 10 d	3.75-5.51		80-160 mg q12h	1.25				Yes	
Vancomycin	92	1	MD	Puerperium	5.7		125-500 mg q6-8h PO					?	Intravenous therapy Single milk level obtained 4 h postdose
Anticonvulsants													
Carbamazepine	93	1	MD	2-30 d	3.0 (4.3)	3.32 (5.27)	10-20 mg/kg/d					Yes	No adverse reaction in infant Infant serum level 1.1-1.8 mg/L Mother also taking phenytoin ( ) = including active metabolite 10,11-epoxide
	94	4	MD	3-28 d	2.44 (2.97)	4.5 (5.0)			0.39			Yes	Steady-state serum level in neonates 1.0 μg/mL

Ref	N	Route	Age		M/P		Comments
95	19	MD	2-35 d	2.72 (4.35)	3.83 (6.4)	0.36	and hyperexcitability noted M/S 10,11-epoxide = 0.49 ( ) = including 10,11-epoxide
						?	No abnormalities noted in breast-fed infants Neonatal serum levels < 1.5 μg/mL in 3 tested neonates M/P 10,11-epoxide = 0.53 ( ) = including 10,11-epoxide
96	1	MD	5 wk	2.07		Yes	One milk level obtained No adverse reaction in infant Mother also taking primidone
97	3	MD	2 days-5 wk	3.78 (5.48)	4.66 (7.41)	0.6	Yes	No adverse reaction in infants Infant plasma level 0-1.8 μg/mL M/P 10,11-epoxide = 1.05 ( ) = including 10,11-epoxide

(continued)

Table A1 (Continued)

Drug	Ref.	No.	Dose	Lactation stage	Mean F_{inf}	Max F_{inf}	Standard adult dose	M/P	M/S	$t_{1/2}$ (h)	t_{max} (h)	BF	Comments
Carbamazepine (continued)	98	?	MD	3-32 d					0.39			?	Mean milk level 1.9 µg/mL (0.8-3.8 µg/mL)
	99	?	MD						0.41			?	Mean milk level 1.8 µg/mL (0.5-3.8 µg/mL)
	100	1	MD	3 wk								Yes	Neonatal cholestatic hepatitis after exposure throughout pregnancy and lactation
Ethosuximide	101	1	MD	3-5 d	48.9	53.8	1000-1500 mg/d		0.94			No	
	98	?	MD	3-32 d					0.79			?	Mean milk level 21.3 µg/mL (18-24 µg/mL)
	102	1	MD	3 d-5 mo	68.6	99		0.8				Yes	No adverse reaction in infant Peak infant plasma level 29.5 mg/L
	103	5	MD	3-28 d	51.2	81.3			0.86			Yes	4 of 6 breastfeeding neonates hyperexcitable or sedated; 5 of these mothers

Drug							Dose			Effect	Comments
Phenobarbital	99	?	MD	?	43.2	297	30-100 mg/d	0.36	?		taking additional antiepileptics Neonatal serum levels 15-40 µg/mL in 5 breast-fed neonates
	98	?	MD	3-32 d				0.46	?		Maternal dose unspecified; calculation based on 100 mg/d Mean milk level 4.8 µg/mL (0-33 µg/mL) Mean milk level 10.4 µg/mL (0.5-33 µg/mL)
Phenytoin	104	6	MD	1-3 mo	4.8	8.8 (9.84)	100 mg t.i.d.	0.13	Yes		No adverse reactions in infants 2 of 6 infants with measurable levels of 0.12 and 0.18 µg/mL ( ) = including conjugated and unconjugated 4-OH phenytoin
	98	?	MD	3-32 d				0.18	?		Mean milk level 0.8 µg/mL (0.5-1.4 µg/mL)

(continued)

Table A1 (Continued)

Drug	Ref.	No.	Dose	Lactation stage	Mean F_{inf}	Max F_{inf}	Standard adult dose	M/P	M/S	$t_{1/2}$ (h)	t_{max} (h)	BF	Comments
Phenytoin	99	?	MD	?					0.19			?	Mean milk level 0.7 µg/mL (0-2.2 µg/mL)
	105	1	MD	1 wk	0.58	0.68		0.45				Yes	5 infants breast-fed; nursing did not affect the elimination of phenytoin from exposure in utero
	106	2	MD	1-33 d	4.8	7.8						Yes	No adverse reactions in infants
Primidone	98	?	MD	3-32 d			250 mg t.i.d.-q.i.d.		0.81			?	Mean milk level 2.3 µg/mL (0.5-6.7 µg/mL)
	99	?	MD	?		7.47-9.96			0.71			?	Maternal dose unspecified; calculation based on standard adult dose
	107	?	MD	First mo					0.72			Yes	Mean milk level 2.1 µg/mL (0-8.3 µg/mL) Withdrawal reaction in 1 of 6 infants breastfed

| 108 | 4 | MD | 4-27 d | 8.49 (18.3) | 21.1 (37.8) | 0.72 | Yes | Peak neonatal serum level in 2 neonates tested; primidone, phenobarbital, (PEMA) level; 2.5 µg/mL; 13 µg/mL, 1.4 µg/mL, respectively M/S metabolite phenobarbital = 0.36 M/S metabolite PEMA = 0.64 | 2 of 5 breastfed neonates with poor feeding for first 5 days of life Serum levels of 1 neonate; primidone, phenobarbital, PEMA; 0.8-1 µg/mL, 1.5-3 µg/mL, 0.5-0.6 µg/mL, respectively |

(continued)

Table A1 (Continued)

Drug	Ref.	No.	Dose	Lacta-tion stage	Mean F_{inf}	Max F_{inf}	Standard adult dose	M/P	M/S	$t_{1/2}$ (h)	t_{max} (h)	BF	Comments
Primidone (continued)													M/S phenobarbital = 0.41 M/S PEMA = 0.76 ( ) = including metabolites phenobarbital and PEMA
Valproic acid	109	1	MD	5-29 d	2.88	4.06	15-60 mg/kg/d divided t.i.d.					Yes	No adverse reaction in infant Undetected in infant serum at 1 month
	110	11	MD	3-6 d	1.22	3.8		0.05				?	
	111	1	MD	62-130 h	0.58	0.85		0.01-0.02				?	
	112	6	MD	3-82 d	1.12 (1.25)	6.98 (7.63)			0.027			Yes	M/S 3-keto metabolite = 0.074 ( ) = including 3-keto metabolite; other metabolites not detected (< 0.1 µg/mL)

Antidepressants

Drug	No.						Dose			Comments
Amitriptyline	113	1	MD	4-6 mo	1.06 (1.89)	1.2 (2.1)	50-150 mg/d		Yes	No adverse reaction in infant; Infant serum amitriptyline < 5 ng/mL; nortriptyline < 15 ng/mL; ( ) = including active metabolite nortriptyline
	114	1	MD	6-8 wk	1.29 (1.79)	1.36 (1.89)			Yes	Infant plasma levels below limit of detection 10 ng/mL; ( ) = including active metabolite nortriptyline
Clomipramine	115	1	MD	4-35 d	2.4	3.75	75-150 mg/d	0.76-1.62	Yes	No adverse reaction in infant
Desipramine	116	1	MD	10 wk	0.84 (1.74)	1.38 (3.0)	75-150 mg/d		Yes	No adverse reaction in infant; Infant plasma desipramine < 1 ng/mL; hydroxydesipramine < 5 ng/mL; ( ) = including metabolite 2-hydroxydesipramine

(continued)

173

Table A1 (Continued)

Drug	Ref. No.	Dose	Lactation stage	Mean F_{inf}	Max F_{inf}	Standard adult dose	M/P	M/S	$t_{1/2}$ (h)	t_{max} (h)	BF	Comments
Doxepin	117	1 MD	1-4 mo	0.38 (1.09)		75-150 mg/d	1.08-1.66				Yes	No adverse reaction in infant Infant plasma doxepin <5 µg/L; N-desmethyl-doxepin 15 µg/L M/P N-desmethyl-doxepin = 1.02-1.53 ( ) = including metabolite N-desmethyldoxepin
	118	1 MD	8 wk	0.19 (0.29)	0.31 (0.43)						Yes	Case report of infant sleepiness Infant serum doxepin 3 mg/L; N-desmethyldoxepin 58 and 66 µg/L on 2 occasions ( ) = including metabolite N-desmethyldoxepin
Fluoxetine	119	1 MD	5 mo	1.3 (3.17)		20 mg/d					Yes	One milk level reported ( ) = including active metabolite norfluoxetine

No.	Drug	n	MD/SD	Time	Value 1	Value 2	Dose	Ratio	Adverse	Comments
120		1	MD	17 wk	1.89 (3.35)	3.02 (5.36)			Yes	No adverse reaction in infant ( ) = including active metabolite norfluoxetine
121	Fluvoxamine	1	MD	14 wk	0.65		100–200 mg/d		Yes	No adverse reaction in infant One milk level reported
122	Imipramine	1	MD	6 wk	0.07 (0.19)	0.13 (0.29)	75–150 mg/d		Yes	No adverse reaction in infant ( ) = including active metabolite desipramine
123		2	MD	1 mo		1.64 (4.97)		0.91	Yes	M/P desipramine = 0.91 ( ) = including active metabolite desipramine
124	Nortriptyline	1	MD	6–7 d	1.3	2.9	30–100 mg/d	0.87–3.71	Yes	No adverse reaction in infant; normal motor development at 4 months
125	Trazodone	6	SD	3–8 mo	0.27	0.43	150–400 mg/d	0.142	No	2
126	Zopiclone	3	SD	?	0.5	1.27	7.5 mg PRN	0.6	?	

(continued)

175

Table A1 (Continued)

Drug	Ref.	No.	Dose	Lactation stage	Mean F_{inf}	Max F_{inf}	Standard adult dose	M/P	M/S	$t_{1/2}$ (h)	t_{max} (h)	BF	Comments
Antihistamines													
Loratadine	127	6	SD	1-12 mo		0.18 (0.34)	10 mg/d	1.2			2	No	Peak metabolite level 5.3 h post-dose M/P metabolite = 0.8 ( ) = including active metabolite descarboethoxyl-oratadine
Terfenadine	128	4	MD	?	0.31		60 mg q12h	0.21		14.2	4.3	?	Terfenadine carboxylic acid metabolite measured
Triprolidine	129	3	SD	14 wk-18 mo	0.5	0.84	2.5 mg q4-6h	0.5-0.56				?	
Antihypertensives													
Acebutolol	130	3	MD	3-9 d	1.55 (5.31)	3.09 (8.07)	400-800 mg/d	1.9-9.2				?	Hypotension, bradycardia in one neonate M/P diacetolol = 2.3-24.7 ( ) = including active metabolite diacetolol

Drug	Ref	n		Time								Comments
Atenolol	131	1	MD	1-6 wk	19	25	50-200 mg/d	2.9		8	Yes	No adverse reaction in infant Infant plasma level below detection 10 ng/mL
	132	7	MD	Puerperium	9.44	15.43			4.5		?	Serum level 0.07 mg/L in 1 neonate; no adverse reaction
	133	4	MD	4-12 d	9.8	25		1.1-3.1		2-6	Yes	Infant plasma level < 3 µg/L
	134	11	MD	?	6.39						Yes	No adverse reactions in infants Detected in urine of 3 tested infants
	135	5	MD	Puerperium	5.67	9.36					Yes	No adverse reactions in infants
	51	1	MD	1 wk	4.22						Yes	One milk level reported Neonatal bradycardia, cyanosis Neonatal serum level 2010 ng/mL on one occasion
Captopril	136	11	MD	?	0.009	0.014	12.5-25 mg t.i.d.			3.8	No	Several mothers nursed their infants during therapy with no adverse reports in infants

(continued)

Table A1 (Continued)

Drug	Ref.	No.	Dose	Lacta-tion stage	Mean $\tilde{}_{inf}$	Max F_{inf}	Standard adult dose	M/P	M/S	$t_{1/2}$ (h)	t_{max} (h)	BF	Comments
Captopril (continued)													M/B AUC = 0.031
Clonidine	137	9	MD	1-5 d	4.14		0.2-1.2 mg/d divided q.i.d.					Yes	Mean neonatal serum level 0.65 ng/mL (mean maternal dose = 392 μg/d)
	137	9	MD	10-14 d	7.85							Yes	Mean neonatal serum level 0.5 ng/mL (mean maternal dose = 309 μg/d)
	137	9	MD	45-60 d	6.70							Yes	Mean infant serum level 0.25 ng/mL (mean maternal dose = 242 μg/d)
Diltiazem	138	1	MD	18 d	0.69	0.83	30-60 mg q6-8h					No	
Enalapril	139	3	SD	3-45 d			2.5-40 mg/d					?	Enalapril not measured; enala-prilat milk level < 0.2 ng/mL Normal angioten-sin-converting enzyme activity in milk

	Drug	No.	SD/MD	Time			Dose			Comments
140		5	SD	Puerperium	0.016 (0.03)	0.05 (0.07)		0.005-0.043	No	M/S enalaprilat = 0.021-0.031 ( ) = including active metabolite enalaprilat
141	Hydralazine	1	MD	8 wk		0.8	10-50 mg q.i.d.		Yes	
142	Labetolol	25	MD	3 d	0.10	0.45	200-600 mg b.i.d.		24 of 25	No adverse reactions in neonates
143		3	MD	6-9 d	0.30	0.59		0.8-2.6	Yes 2-3	Neonatal plasma level above detection (21 µg/L) in 1 of 2 neonates tested
144	Methyldopa	1	MD	17 d	1.22	1.75	250 mg b.i.d.-500 mg q.i.d.		Yes	No adverse reaction in neonate Neonatal serum level < 0.2 µg/mL
145		4	MD	30-60 h		0.09 (0.72)			?	( ) = including conjugated (and free) methyldopa
146		3	MD	1-8 wk		1.19 (3.2)		0.19-0.34	Yes	No adverse reactions in infants 1 of 3 infants with detectable plasma level of 0.09 µg/mL (detection limit 0.05 mg/mL) ( ) = including conjugated (and free) methyldopa

(continued)

Table A1 (Continued)

Drug	Ref.	No.	Dose	Lactation stage	Mean F_{inf}	Max F_{inf}	Standard adult dose	M/P	M/S	$t_{1/2}$ (h)	t_{max} (h)	BF	Comments
Methyldopa (continued)	147	8	MD	?	0.2 (0.51)			0.46				Yes	Maternal dose unspecified; calculation based on 750 mg/d ( ) = including conjugated (and free) methyldopa
Metoprolol	148	9	MD	?	1.0	3.6	50-100 mg b.i.d.	3.7				Yes	
	149	8	MD	3-5 d	0.75-1.5	2.95-5.9		2.8				Yes	Peak neonatal plasma level 0.5-45 μg/L
	132	3	MD	4-6 mo		3.0						No	
	133	3	MD	4-60 d	1.26	2.2		2-3.1	3.6			Yes	Infant plasma level < 3 μg/L
Minoxidil	150	1	MD	2 mo	1.34 (1.54)	5.0 (5.41)	10-40 mg/d					Yes	No adverse reaction in infant ( ) = including glucuronide metabolite
Nadolol	151	12	MD	>1 mo	4.1	5.0	80-240 mg/d		4.6	21.8	6	No	
Nifedipine	152	1	MD	?		0.53	10-20 mg q8h			3.3	1	No	
	153	1	MD	10 d		1.04 (1.53)					1	Yes	( ) = including pyridine metabolite

Drug	Ref	n	Route	Time			Dose				Adverse reaction	Comments
Nitrendipine	154	2	MD	> 3 mo	0.1 (0.26)	0.25 (0.54)	10-40 mg/d (155)	0.2-0.4		3-4	No	( ) = including inactive pyridine metabolite
Oxprenolol			MD	3-6 d	0.45	1.5	60-320 mg/d divided t.i.d.	0.45			?	
	157	12	MD	< 4 - > 8 d	0.72	2.1		0.29			?	
Propranolol	158	3	MD	First wk	0.3 (1.0)	1.0 (2.0)	20 mg b.i.d.-160 mg/d divided b.i.d.-t.i.d.	0.33-1.65	6.5		?	M/P naphthoxy-lactic acid 0.19-0.42; milk half-life 4.2 h
												( ) = including propranolol glucuronide and naphthoxylactic acid
	159	1	MD	2-3 mo	0.19	0.24				3	Yes	No adverse reaction in infant
	160	1	MD	3-6 d	0.26	0.45					Yes	No adverse reaction in neonate
	135	5	MD	Puerperium	0.30	0.41					Yes	No adverse reaction in neonates
Sotalol	161	5	MD	First wk	21.8	41.95	80-160 mg b.i.d.	5.4			Yes	No adverse reactions in neonates
	162	1	MD	5, 105 d	23.6				2.4-5.6		Yes	No adverse reaction in neonates
	163	1	MD	5-7 d	21.8	28.1		2.75-3.57			No	No adverse reaction in infant

(continued)

Table A1 (Continued)

Drug	Ref. No.	Dose	Lactation stage	Mean F_{inf}	Max F_{inf}	Standard adult dose	M/P	M/S	$t_{1/2}$ (h)	t_{max} (h)	BF	Comments
Timolol	157	11	MD	<4->8 d	1.1	3.3	5-10 mg b.i.d.	0.8				?	
Verapamil	164	1	MD	3-5 d	0.09	0.14	80 mg t.i.d.-q.i.d.		0.23			Yes	No adverse reaction in neonate Neonatal plasma level 2.1 ng/mL
	165	1	MD	8 wk	0.38 (0.51)	0.51 (0.68)		0.64				Yes	No adverse reaction in infant Infant plasma verapamil and norverapamil < 1 µg/L () = including metabolite norverapamil
	166	1	MD	13 d	0.55	0.91					2	No	Infant plasma verapamil and norverapamil < 1 µg/L
	167	1	MD	3 mo	0.10 (0.13)	0.30 (0.38)		0.6		4.29	1	Yes	Norverapamil peak milk level 2 h postdose; milk half-life 1.34 h; M/P = 0.16

Anti-inflammatory drugs

Acetylsalicyclic acid										
58	1	SD	7 wk	0.45	0.55	325-650 mg q4h antipyretic dose	0.05		No	
58	1	SD	13 wk		0.74		0.03-0.34		Yes	
168	1	MD	6 mo	1.8-2.6	3.2-4.7	2.6-3.9 g/d in divided doses (anti-inflammatory dose)	0.04-0.08	3	Yes	Maternal dose unspecified; calculation based on standard adult dose; Peak milk level 1 mg/dL
169	1	MD	9 wk						Yes	No milk levels obtained; No adverse reaction in infant; infant serum level 0.47 mmol/L (infant 50% breastfed)
170	1	MD	2 wk						Yes	No milk levels obtained; Neonatal metabolic acidosis; serum salicylate level 24 mg/dL

(continued)

Table A1 (Continued)

Drug	Ref.	No.	Dose	Lactation stage	Mean F_{inf}	Max F_{inf}	Standard adult dose	M/P	M/S	$t_{1/2}$ (h)	t_{max} (h)	BF	Comments
Diclofenac	171	6	SD	?			25-50 mg t.i.d.					?	Intramuscular injection No drug detected in milk
Flurbiprofen	172	12	MD	3-5 d		0.29	50 mg q6h	0.019				No	
	173	10	SD	>1 mo		0.17					3	No	
Ibuprofen	174	1	MD	Mature milk			400-800 mg q4-6h					Yes	Ibuprofen and major metabolites not detected in milk (limit of ibuprofen detection 0.5 µg/mL)
	175	12	MD	3-5 d								?	No ibuprofen detected in milk (limit of detection 1 µg/mL)
Indomethacin	176	16	MD	<10 d, 10 mo		1.21	25 mg b.i.d.-200 mg/d	0.37				Yes	Rectal administration No adverse reactions in neonates; plasma levels in 6 of 7 neonates tested < 20 µg/L; level 47 µg/L in 1 neonate

	177	1	MD	4-6 d						Yes	Neonatal seizures No milk or neonatal serum levels obtained
Ketorolac	178	10	MD	2-6 d		0.18	10 mg q.i.d.	0.015-0.037		No	
Mefenamic acid	179	10	MD	2-4 d	0.2 (1.2)	0.79 (2.4)	250 mg q6h			Yes	Mean infant level 0.08 μg/mL one hour after nursing; ( ) = including metabolites
Naproxen	180	1	MD	5 mo	1.79	2.21	250 mg b.i.d.-q.i.d.		4	Yes	
	180	1	MD	6 mo	2.45	2.80				Yes	0.47 mg of naproxen and conjugated naproxen excreted by infant over 12 h after maternal dose of 375 mg (0.26% of cumulative maternal value)
Piroxicam	181	1	MD	13 mo	3.6	7.65	20 mg/d			Yes	Not detected in infant serum
	181	1	MD	8 mo	3.6	4.95				No	
	182	4	MD	3-4.5 mo	3.51	6.35		0.01-0.03		Yes	No adverse reaction in infants

(continued)

Table A1 (Continued)

Drug	Ref.	No.	Dose	Lactation stage	Mean F_{inf}	Max F_{inf}	Standard adult dose	M/P	M/S	$t_{1/2}$ (h)	t_{max} (h)	BF	Comments
Piroxicam (continued)													Piroxicam and conjugate not detected in one infant's urine
Antipsychotic drugs													
Chlorpromazine	183	4	MD	?		0.44-2.94	10-50 mg t.i.d.-q.i.d.					2 of 4	Maternal dose unspecified; calculation based on standard adult dose Milk levels 7-98 ng/mL 1 of 2 breastfed infants was drowsy and lethargic
Haloperidol	184	1	MD	6 wk	0.15		0.5-2 mg b.i.d.-t.i.d.					No	No adverse reaction in infant; developmental milestones achieved at 6 mo and 1 y 1.5 µg/L detected in infant's urine
	185	1	MD	3-4 wk	1.87	2.1						Yes	

Perphenazine	1	MD	1 mo	0.12	0.17	2-8 mg t.i.d.	0.7-1.1	Yes	No adverse reaction in infant
Lithium	1	MD	5 d	16.6-33.3		900 mg-1.2 g/d divided b.i.d.-q.i.d. (as carbonate)		Yes	Neonatal cyanosis, lethargy 0.6 mEq/L detected in infant plasma and in milk sample Infant exposed to lithium in utero
	4	MD	1-4 wk					Yes	Milk level range 0.16-0.56 mmol/L Infant serum level range 0.1-0.3 mmol/L
	1	MD	0-10 wk	27.02				Yes	No adverse reaction in infant Infant serum level < 0.2 mmol/L throughout breastfeeding
	1	MD	70 d	4.0				Yes	One milk level obtained No adverse reaction in infant; lithium level 0.04 mEq/L

(continued)

Table A1 (Continued)

Drug	Ref.	No.	Dose	Lactation stage	Mean F_{inf}	Max F_{inf}	Standard adult dose	M/P	M/S	$t_{1/2}$ (h)	t_{max} (h)	BF	Comments
Antithyroid drugs													
Methimazole	191	1	MD	2-6 mo	2.1	4.5	5-15 mg/d	0.3-0.7				Yes	Given as carbimazole
													No adverse effects in breastfeeding twins; methimazole plasma levels 0-156 ng/mL (peak level 2-4 h postdose)
	192	1	MD	?	7.17	11.52			1.16			?	
	193	5	SD	2-6 wk		1.34			0.98		1	?	Given as carbimazole
Propylthiouracil	194	9	SD	1-8 mo	0.32		50 mg b.i.d.-t.i.d.					?	1 infant breastfeeding while mother on long-term treatment showed no adverse effects
	195	1	SD	?								No	0.077% of a radioactive dose of propylthiouracil excreted in 500 mL of milk over 24 h

188

Anxiolytics

Drug											Comments
Alprazolam	196	1	MD	7 d			0.25 mg b.i.d.-t.i.d.			Yes	No levels obtained; Neonatal restlessness and irritability; neonatal exposure in utero also
Clonazepam	197	1	MD	2-4 d	1.89	2.41	8-10 mg/d divided t.i.d.		4	Yes	Mother also taking phenytoin
	198	1	MD	3-14 d				0.3		Yes	Milk level range 11-13 ng/mL; Infant neurodevelopmental exam normal at 5 months
Diazepam	199	1	MD	1 y	4.2 (7.36)	4.7 (8.6)	2 mg b.i.d.-10 mg q.i.d.	0.2		Yes	No adverse reaction in infant; low levels of metabolites detected in infant plasma; M/P desmethyldiazepam = 0.13; M/P oxazepam = 0.10; M/P temazepam = 0.14

(continued)

Table A1 (Continued)

Drug	Ref. No.	Dose	Lactation stage	Mean F_{inf}	Max F_{inf}	Standard adult dose	M/P	M/S	$t_{1/2}$ (h)	t_{max} (h)	BF	Comments
Diazepam (continued)												( ) = including active metabolites n-desmethyldiazepam, oxazepam, temazepam
	200	1	MD	1 wk–3 mo	2.76–4.6 (6.07–10.12)	7.8–13.0 (14.8–24.6)						Yes	Normal infant development; infant sedation if feeding occurred within 8 h of maternal dose Infant diazepam level 0.7 ng/mL and n-desmethyldiazepam level 46 ng/mL at 32 days of age ( ) = including n-desmethyldiazepam
	201	4	MD	3–9 d	2.1 (5.4)	3.87 (11.5)		0.16				Yes	M/P n-desmethyldiazepam = 0.27; oxazepam not in milk ( ) = including n-desmethyldiazepam

190

Drug	No.	n		Duration	Level (SD)	Dose	Compatible	Comments
	202	1	MD	8 d			Yes	Neonatal lethargy and weight loss; urine positive for oxazepam
	203	3	MD	6 d	2.34 (3.9)		Yes	No adverse reactions in infants Mean infant level on 2 occasions for diazepam 74 and 172 ng/mL; 31 and 243 ng/mL for n-desmethyldiazepam Oxazepam not detected in any sample ( ) = including n-desmethyl-diazepam
Lorazepam	204	1	MD	5 d	2.16 (6.1)	2-3 mg/d divided b.i.d.-q.i.d.	Yes	One milk level obtained No adverse reaction in neonate ( ) = including conjugated and free lorazepam
Midazolam	205	12	MD	2-7 d		15 mg PRN	Yes	Morning milk level after evening dose < 3 µg/L

(continued)

Table A1 (Continued)

Drug	Ref.	No.	Dose	Lacta-tion stage	Mean F_{inf}	Max F_{inf}	Standard adult dose	M/P	M/S	$t_{1/2}$ (h)	t_{max} (h)	BF	Comments
Midazolam (continued)	205	2	SD	2-3 mo	0.06 (0.10)	0.11 (0.15)		0.15				?	( ) = including hydroxymida-zolam
Nitrazepam	205	10	MD	2-7 d	2.52	3.60	5-10 mg PRN	0.27				Yes	Plasma level < 3 µg/L in 1 infant tested
Oxazepam	206	1	MD	> 7 mo	0.68	0.75	10-15 mg t.i.d.-q.i.d.					?	
Temazepam	207	10	MD	< 15 d	1.31		30 mg h.s.	<0.2				Yes	No adverse reactions in neonates; plasma levels of temazepam and oxazepam below detection in 2 neonates that were tested. Milk oxazepam levels < 5 µg/L for all patients
Cardiovascular drugs													
Amiodarone	208	1	MD	6-9 wk	36.9 (51.5)		200-600 mg/d					Yes	Infant amiodar-one and desethyl-

209	1	MD	2-3 d	8.1 (11.7)		No	amiodarone plasma level at 9 weeks 0.4 mg/L and 0.15 mg/L, respectively; ( ) = including metabolite desethylamiodarone
210	1	MD	First mo	5.67 (7.7) / 8.21 (11.0)		Yes	( ) = including metabolite desethylamiodarone; No adverse reaction in infant; Infant serum amiodarone level < 0.1 mg/L; desethylamiodarone < 0.05 mg/L; ( ) = including metabolite desethylamiodarone
211	3	MD	0-6 wk	10.35 (15.3) / 13.7 (21.8)	7.8	Yes	One infant stopped breastfeeding owing to hypothyroidism; Desethylamiodarone M/P = 1.9; ( ) = including metabolite desethylamiodarone

(continued)

Table A1 (Continued)

Drug	Ref. No.	Dose	Lactation stage	Mean F_{inf}	Max F_{inf}	Standard adult dose	M/P	M/S	$t_{1/2}$ (h)	t_{max} (h)	BF	Comments
Bretylium	212	1	MD	First 4 mo			100 mg t.i.d.-600 mg q6h					Yes	No milk levels obtained No adverse events in infants
Digoxin	213	2	MD	14 d	2.14	3.5	0.125-0.25 mg/d	0.8-0.9			4-6	Yes	No adverse reaction in neonates; neonatal plasma levels < 0.1 ng/mL
	214	11	MD	3-7 d	2.3			0.59				No	
	215	1	MD	7 d	2.28			0.9				Yes	One milk level obtained Neonatal serum level 0.2 ng/mL
	216	11	SD	?					0.62			No	Intravenous injection
Disopyramide	217	1	MD	4 d-1 mo	5.85 (10.7)	8.55 (15.8)	100-200 mg q.i.d.	0.9				Yes	No adverse reaction in infant; infant plasma level 0.5 mg/L at 28 days M/P n-monodesalkyl metabolite = 5.6 ( ) = including n-monodesalkyl metabolite

Drug	Ref	N		Duration			Dose				Compatible	Comments
	218	1	MD	2-16 d	2.75	3.05			0.4		Yes	No adverse reaction in neonate; neonatal plasma level < 0.5 mg/L
	219	1	MD	2 mo	1.75	2.21		0.46-0.53			Yes	Infant disopyramide level 0.1-0.14 mg/L
Flecainide	163	1	MD	5-7 d	3.70	4.92	100-150 mg q12h	1.57-2.18			No	
	220	11	MD	1-6 d	3.7	7.0		2.6-3.7	14.7	3-6	No	
Mexiletine	221	1	MD	2 d, 6 wk	1.1	1.2	200-300 mg q8h	1.14-2			Yes	No adverse reaction in infant; infant serum level < 0.05 mg/L
Procainamide	222	1	MD	2-5 d	1.04	1.58		1.45			Yes	
	223	1	MD	2 d	2.43 (4.0)	4.59 (6.84)	50 mg/kg/d divided q3h-q6h	4.3			Yes	M/P NAPA = 3.8 ( ) = including active metabolite NAPA
Propafenone	224	1	MD	3 d	0.03 (0.08)		150 mg q8h				No	( ) = including metabolite 5-OH-propafenone
Quinidine	225	1	MD	4-5 d	5.58	6.27	300-600 mg q8-12h (as sulfate)	0.71			No	Administered as quinidine sulfate

(continued)

Table A1 (Continued)

Drug	Ref.	No.	Dose	Lactation stage	Mean F_{inf}	Max F_{inf}	Standard adult dose	M/P	M/S	$t_{1/2}$ (h)	t_{max} (h)	BF	Comments
Diuretics													
Acetazolamide	226	1	MD	10-11 d	1.53	1.89	250 mg daily -250 mg q.i.d.					Yes	No adverse reaction in neonate; neonatal plasma level 0.2-0.6 $\mu g/mL$
Chlorothiazide	227	11	SD	> 3 mo		<0.36	500-2000 mg/d					No	Milk levels < 1 mg/L; calculation assumes milk level of 1 mg/L
Chlorthalidone	228	7	MD	3 d	6.66	15.5	25-100 mg/d					?	M/B = 0.06
Furosemide	229	120	MD	First wk			20-40 mg b.i.d.					No	Furosemide and fluid restriction successfully suppressed lactation
Hydrochlorothiazide	230	1	MD	28 d	1.94	2.92	50-100 mg/d					Yes	No adverse reaction in neonate; neonatal blood level < 20 ng/mL
Spironolactone	231	1	MD	17 d	0.84	1.15	25-200 mg/d					Yes	No adverse reaction in neonate

Gastrointestinal drugs

Drug										
Cimetidine	232	1	MD	6 mo	4.42	4.77	800-1200 mg/d		No	Canrenone levels measured; spironolactone levels not measured M/S canrenone = 0.51-0.72
	232	1	SD	6 mo	0.92	1.67			No	
Cisapride	233	10	MD	1-5 d	0.08	0.26	5-10 mg t.i.d.-q.i.d.	0.045	No	
Domperidone	234	2	MD	3-6 d	0.08		10 mg t.i.d.-q.i.d.		No	
Famotidine	235	10	SD	2-8 d	0.006	0.01			No	
	235	4	MD	1-3 mo	0.07				?	
	236	8	SD	?		0.32	20-40 mg/d	0.41-1.78	No	
Loperamide	237	6	MD	First 3 d	0.024	0.07 (0.09)	2 mg PRN		No	( ) = including loperamide and loperamide oxide
Metoclopramide	238	5	MD	1-3 wk	3.3	4.7	5-10 mg t.i.d.-q.i.d.		Yes	Metoclopramide detected in plasma from 1 of 5 neonates tested; peak level 20.9 ng/mL
	238	18	MD	9-14 wk	1.44	3.75			Yes	
	239	10	SD	7-10 d	2.26				?	

(continued)

Table A1 (Continued)

Drug	Ref. No.	Dose	Lactation stage	Mean F_{inf}	Max F_{inf}	Standard adult dose	M/P	M/S	$t_{1/2}$ (h)	t_{max} (h)	BF	Comments
Nizatidine	240	3	MD	3-8 mo	1.47	3.6	150 mg/d-150 mg b.i.d.			<2		?	
Ranitidine	241	6	SD	6-10 d	1.4	4.4	150 mg/d-150 mg b.i.d.	1.92-6.7				?	
	242	1	MD	54 d	4.86	8.6		6.8-23.8			5.5	No	
Miscellaneous												
5-Aminosalicyclic acid	243	1	MD	6 wk			800 mg-4000 mg/d					Yes	Rectal administration Milk levels not reported Case report of watery diarrhea in infant
	244	1	MD	?	0.07 (7.5)			0.27				Yes	One milk level reported M/P acetyl-5-ASA = 5.1 ( ) = including metabolite acetyl 5-ASA
Chloroquine	245	3	SD	2-5 d			500 mg/wk for malaria (as phosphate)	1.96-4.26				No	Mean amount excreted in milk over 9 days was 0.19% of maternal dose

											Comments
	246	11	SD	?	6.6/d[a]	11.25/d[a]		6.6	8.8 d	14.4	Yes	M/P metabolite desethylchloroquine = 0.54–3.89 [a]Dose calculation based on infant consumption on a daily basis owing to chloroquine's long milk half-life 4 infants of 4 tested had positive urine samples for chloroquine and desethylchloroquine M/P desethylchloroquine = 1.5
	247	5	SD	2–2.5 mo	4.71/d[a]	11.91/d[a]			5.5 d	3	No	
Hydroxychloroquine	248	1	MD	9 mo	2.81	3.67	200–600 mg/d arthritis (as sulfate)	5.5			Yes	
Methylergometrine	249	1	MD	8 wk	<0.05						No	
	250	8	MD	5 d	2.4	3.38	0.2–0.4 mg q6-12h				?	

(continued)

Table A1 (Continued)

Drug	Ref.	No.	Dose	Lactation stage	Mean F_{inf}	Max F_{inf}	Standard adult dose	M/P	M/S	$t_{1/2}$ (h)	t_{max} (h)	BF	Comments
Prednisolone	251	6	MD	3-152 d		4.51	5-60 mg/d (prednisone)	0.1-0.2			1	?	One milk level reported
	252	1	SD	?	0.51							Yes	Prednisolone and prednisone measured
	253	7	SD	?								No	Mean total recovery per 1 L of milk during 48 h from radiolabeled prednisolone was 0.14%
Pseudo-ephedrine	129	3	SD	14 wk-18 mo	1.6	2.6	60 mg q.i.d. PRN	2.2-2.8			4.2-7	1-1.5	?
Sulfasalazine	254	12	MD	5-6 wk		0.9 (11.1)	2-4 g/d divided q.i.d.					Yes	Sulfasalazine milk level < 1 µg/mL in 26 of 31 samples M/S sulfapyridine = 0.4 ( ) = including metabolite sulfapyridine

| 255 | 1 | MD | 4.5-6.5 mo | (2.25) | (5.85) | Yes | No sulfasalazine, 5-ASA, acetyl-5-ASA detected in milk No adverse reaction in infant; infant sulfapyridine and metabolites urine levels 3-4.1 µg/mL M/P sulfapyridine = 0.6-0.63 ( ) = including sulfapyridine and metabolites |
| 256 | 8 | MD | 2-24 wk | 1.42 (11.7) | | Yes | Sulfasalazine undetected in 6 of 7 milk samples and 6 of 8 infants (< 1 mg/L); peak infant plasma sulfapyridine level 4.8 mg/L M/S sulfapyridine = 0.48 ( ) = including sulfasalazine and sulfapyridine |

(continued)

Table A1 (Continued)

Drug	Ref. No.	Dose	Lactation stage	Mean F_{inf}	Max F_{inf}	Standard adult dose	M/P	M/S	$t_{1/2}$ (h)	t_{max} (h)	BF	Comments
Sulfasalazine (continued)	257	1	MD	2 mo								Yes	Bloody diarrhea in infant; infant blood sulfapyridine level 5.3 μg/mL Mother found to be a poor acetylator
Theophylline	258	3	SD	?		8.14–13.48	400-900 mg/d PO divided b.i.d.	0.67				No	Intravenous injection
	259	1	SD	9 mo		2.82			0.7		1-3	Yes	Agitation in infant; 5 other nursing infants with no adverse effects
Warfarin	260	13	MD	3-10 d			2-10 mg/d					7-Yes	No adverse reactions in neonates Milk and neonatal plasma levels below limit of detection 25 ng/mL
	261	2	MD	?								Yes	No adverse reactions in infants No warfarin detected in milk

^aSee Comments column for chloroquine.

Answer

Tell the woman that large amounts of amiodarone are excreted into milk, and the drug is generally considered to be incompatible with breastfeeding. Although the baby appears normal, amiodarone could cause fetal/neonatal hypothyroidism. If the woman chooses to breastfeed, the baby's plasma amiodarone levels and thyroid function tests should be regularly monitored. Breastfeeding should be discontinued if there are any clinical or laboratory signs of toxicity.

REFERENCES

1. Forman MR. Review of research on the factors associated with choice and duration of infant feeding in less-developed countries. Pediatrics 1984; 74(suppl): 667–694.
2. Simopoulos AP, Grave GD. Factors associated with the choice and duration of infant-feeding practice. Pediatrics 1984; 74(suppl):603–614.
3. Matheson I. Drugs taken by mothers in the puerperium. Br Med J 1985; 290: 1588–1589.
4. Passmore CM, McElnay JC, D'Arcy PF. Drugs taken by mothers in the puerperium: Inpatient survey in Northern Ireland. Br Med J 1984; 289:1593–1596.
5. Martinez GA, Krieger FW. 1984 Milk-feeding patterns in the United States. Pediatrics 1985; 76:1004–1008.
6. McNally E, Hendricks S, Horowitz I. A look at breast-feeding trends in Canada (1963–1982). Can J Public Health 1985; 76:101–107.
7. Ryan AS, Rush D, Krieger FW, et al. Recent declines in breast-feeding in the United States, 1984 through 1989. Pediatrics 1991; 88:719–727.
8. Kovar MG, Serdula MK, Marks JS, et al. Review of the epidemiologic evidence for an association between infant feeding and infant health. pediatrics 1984; 74(suppl):615–638.
9. Cunningham AS, Jelliffe DB, Jelliffe EFP. Breast-feeding and health in the 1980s: A global epidemiologic review. J Pediatr 1991; 118:659–666.
10. Anderson JE, Marks JS, Park T-K. Breast-feeding, birth interval, and infant health. Pediatrics 1984; 74(suppl):695–701.
11. Berlin CM. The excretion of drugs and chemicals in human milk. In Pediatric Pharmacology: Therapeutic Principles in Practice (Yaffe SJ, ed.). Grune & Stratton, New York, 1980, pp 137–147.
12. Kirksey A, Groziak SM. Maternal drug use: Evaluation of risks to breast-fed infants. World Rev Nutr Diet 1984; 43:60–79.
13. Catz CS, Giacoia GP. Drugs and breast milk. Pediatr Clin North Am 1972; 19:151–166.
14. Noel GL, Suh HK, Frantz AG. Prolactin release during nursing and breast stimulation in postpartum and nonpostpartum subjects. J Clin Endocrinol Metab 1974; 38:413–423.
15. Vorherr H. The Breast: Morphology, Physiology and Lactation. Academic Press, New York, 1974, p 73.
16. Jenness R. The composition of human milk. Semin Perinatol 1979; 3:225–239.

17. Casey CE, Hambidge KM. Nutritional aspects of human lactation. In Lactation Physiology, Nutrition, and Breast-Feeding (Neville MC, Neifert MR, eds). Plenum Press, New York, 1983, pp 199–248.
18. Jenness R. The composition of human milk. Semin Perinatol 1979; 3:225–239.
19. Hartmann PE, Prosser CG. Physiological basis of longitudinal changes in human milk yield and composition. Fed Proc 1984; 43:2448–2453.
20. Lonnerdal B. Effects of maternal dietary intake on human milk composition. J Nutr 1986; 116:499–513.
21. Pickles VR. Blood-flow estimations as indices of mammary activity. J Obstet Gynaec Br Emp 1953; 60:301–311.
22. Neville MC, Keller R, Seacat J, et al. Studies in human lactation: Milk volumes in lactating women during the onset of lactation and full lactation. Am J Clin Nutr 1988; 48:1375–1386.
23. Dewey KG, Heinig MJ, Nommsen LA, et al. Maternal versus infant factors related to breast milk intake and residual milk volume: The Darling study. Pediatrics 1991; 87:829–837.
24. Morriss FH, Brewer ED, Spedale SB, et al. Relationship of human milk pH during course of lactation to concentrations of citrate and fatty acids. Pediatrics 1986; 78:458–464.
25. Prentice A, Prentice AM, Whitehead RG. Breast-milk fat concentrations of rural African women. 1. Short-term variations within individuals. Br J Nutr 1981; 45:483–494.
26. Hytten FE. Clinical and chemical studies in human lactation. Br Med J 1954; 1:175–182.
27. Lammi-Keefe CJ, Ferris AM, Jensen RG. Changes in human milk at 0600, 1000, 1400, 1800, and 2200 h. J Pediatr Gastroenterol Nutr 1990; 11:83–88.
28. Changes with time in the lipids of human milk. Nutr Rev 1984; 42:12–13.
29. Anderson GH. The effect of prematurity on milk composition and its physiological basis. Fed Proc 1984; 43:2438–2442.
30. WHO Working Group. Determinants of drug excretion in breast milk. In Drugs and Human Lactation (Bennett PN, Matheson I, Dukes NMG, et al., eds). Elsevier, Amsterdam, 1988, pp 27–48.
31. Besunder JB. Reed MD, Blumer JL. Principles of drug biodisposition in the neonate. A critical evaluation of the pharmacokinetic-pharmacodynamic interface (part 1). Clin Pharmacokinet 1988; 14:189–216.
32. Dutton GJ. Developmental aspects of drug conjugation, with special reference to glucuronidation. Annu Rev Pharmacol Toxicol 1978; 18:17–35.
33. Atkinson HC, Begg EJ, Darlow BA. Drugs in human milk: Clinical pharmacokinetic considerations. Clin Pharmacokinet 1988; 14:217–240.
34. Schanker LS. Passage of drugs across body membranes. Pharmacol Rev 1962; 14:501–530.
35. Wilson JT. Determinants and consequences of drug excretion in breast milk. Drug Metab Rev 1983; 14:619–652.
36. Wilson JT, Brown RD, Hinson JL, et al. Pharmacokinetic pitfalls in the estimation of the breast milk/plasma ratio for drugs. Annu Rev Pharmacol Toxicol 1985; 25:667–689.

37. Benet LZ. General treatment of linear mammillary models with elimination from any compartment as used in pharmacokinetics. J Pharm Sci 1972; 61: 536–541.
38. Miller GE, Banerjee NC, Stowe CM. Diffusion of certain weak organic acids and bases across the bovine mammary gland membrane after systemic administration. J Pharmacol Exp Ther 1967; 157:245–253.
39. Rasmussen F. Mammary excretion of sulphonamides. Acta Pharmacol (Kbh) 1958; 15:139–148.
40. Rasmussen F. Mammary excretion of benzylpenicillin, erythromycin and penethamate hydroiodide. Acta Pharmacol (Kbh) 1959; 16:194–200.
41. Sisodia CS, Stowe CM. The mechanism of drug secretion into bovine milk. Ann NY Acad Sci 1964; 111:650–661.
42. Wilson JT, Brown RD, Cherek DR, et al. Drug excretion in human breast milk: Principles, pharmacokinetics and projected consequences. Clin Pharmacokinet 1980; 5:1–66.
43. Fleishaker JC, Desai N, McNamara PJ. Factors affecting the milk-to-plasma drug concentration ratio in lactating women: Physical interactions with protein and fat. J Pharm Sci 1987; 76:189–193.
44. Atkinson HC, Begg EJ. Prediction of drug concentrations in human milk from plasma protein binding and acid-base characteristics. Br J Clin Pharmacol 1988; 25:495–503.
45. Atkinson HC, Begg EJ. Prediction of drug distribution into human milk from physiochemical characteristics. Clin Pharmacokinet 1990; 18:151–167.
46. Bennett PN, Matheson I, Dukes NMG, et al. eds. Drugs and Human Lactation. Elsevier, Amsterdam, 1988.
47. Briggs GG, Freeman RK, Yaffe SJ, comps. Drugs in Pregnancy and Lactation, 3rd ed. Williams & Wilkins, Baltimore, 1990.
48. Roberts RJ, Blumer JL, Gorman RL, et al. American Academy of Pediatrics Committee on Drugs. Transfer of drugs and other chemicals into human milk. Pediatrics 1989; 84:924–936.
49. WHO Working Group. Guidelines for studies on the passage of drugs into breast milk. In Drugs and Human Lactation (Bennett PN, Matheson I, Dukes NMG, et al., eds). Elsevier, Amsterdam, 1988, pp 59–64.
50. Matheson I, Lunde PKM, Notarianni L. Infant rash caused by paracetamol in breast milk? Pediatrics 1985; 76:651–652.
51. Schmimmel MS, Eidelman AJ, Wilschanski MA, et al. Toxic effects of atenolol consumed during breast feeding. J Pediatr 1989; 114:476–478.
52. WHO Working Group. Use of the monographs on drugs. In Drugs and Human Lactation (Bennett PN, Matheson I, Dukes NMG, et al, eds). Elsevier, Amsterdam, 1988, pp 65–75.
53. Karjalainen J, Martin JM, Knip M, et al. A bovine albumin peptide as a possible trigger of insulin-dependent diabetes mellitus. N Engl J Med 1992; 327:302–307.
54. Koletzko S, Sherman P, Corey M, et al. Role of infant feeding practices in development of Crohn's disease in childhood. Br Med J 1989; 298:1617–1618.
55. Berlin CM, Yaffe SJ, Ragni M. Disposition of acetaminophen in milk, saliva, and plasma of lactating women. Pediatr Pharmacol (New York) 1980; 1:135–141.

56. Notarianni LJ, Oldham HG, Bennett PN. Passage of paracetamol into breast-milk and its subsequent metabolism by the neonate. Br J Clin Pharmacol 1987; 24:63–67.
57. Bitzen P-O, Gustafsson B, Jostell KG, et al. Excretion of paracetamol in human breast milk. Eur J Clin Pharmacol 1981; 20:123–125.
58. Findlay JWA, DeAngelis RL, Kearney MF, et al. Analgesic drugs in breast milk and plasma. Clin Pharmacol Ther 1981; 29:625–633.
59. Quinn PG, Kuhnert BR, Kaine CJ, et al. Measurement of meperidine and nor-meperidine in human breast milk by selected ion monitoring. Biomed Environ Mass Spectrom 1986; 13:133–135.
60. Wittels B, Scott DT, Sinatra RS. Exogenous opioids in human breast milk and acute neonatal neurobehavior: A preliminary study. Anesthesiology 1990; 73: 864–869.
61. Feilberg VL, Rosenborg D, Christensen CB, et al. Excretion of morphine in human breast milk. Acta Anaesthesiol Scand 1989; 33:426–428.
62. Robieux I, Koren G, Vandenbergh H, et al. Morphine excretion in breast milk and resultant exposure of a nursing infant. Clin Toxicol 1990; 28:365–370.
63. Marx CM, Pucino F, Carlson JD, et al. Oxycodone excretion in human milk in the puerpium. DICP. 1986; 20:474.
64. Lau RJ, Emergy MG, Galinsky RE. Unexpected accumulation of acyclovir in breast milk with estimation of infant exposure. Obstet Gynecol 1987; 69:468–471.
65. Meyer LJ, de Miranda P, Sheth N, et al. Acyclovir in human breast milk. Am J Obstet Gynecol 1988; 158:586–588.
66. Kafetzis DA, Siafas CA, Georgakopoulos PA, et al. Passage of cephalosporins and amoxicillin into the breast milk. Acta Paediatr Scand 1981; 70:285–288.
67. Campbell AC, McElnay JC, Passmore CM. The excretion of ampicillin in breast milk and its effect on the suckling infant. Br J Clin Pharmacol 1991; 31:230P.
68. Matsuda S. Transfer of antibiotics into maternal milk. Biol Res Pregnancy Perinatol 1984; 5:57–60.
69. Matheson I, Samseth M, Sande HA. Ampicillin in breast milk during puerperal infections. Eur J Clin Pharmacol 1988; 34:657–659.
70. Havelka J, Hejzlar M, Popov V, et al. Excretion of chloramphenicol in human milk. Chemotherapy 1968; 13:204–211.
71. Plomp TA, Thiery M, Maes RAA. The passage of thiamphenicol and chloramphenicol into human milk after single and repeated oral administration. Vet Hum Toxicol 1983; 25:167–172.
72. Cover DL, Mueller BA. Ciprofloxacin penetration into human breast milk: A case report. DICP. 1990; 24:703–704.
73. Gardner DK, Gabbe SG, Harter C. Simultaneous concentrations of ciprofloxacin in breast milk and in serum in mother and breast-fed infant. Clin Pharm 1992; 11:352–354.
74. Giamarellou H, Kolokythas E, Petrikkos G, et al. Pharmacokinetics of three newer quinolones in pregnant and lactating women. Am J Med 1989; 87:49S–51S.
75. Steen B, Rane A. Clindamycin passage into human milk. Br J Clin Pharmacol 1982; 13:661–664.

76. Smith JA, Morgan JR, Rachlis AR, et al. Clindamycin in human breast milk. Can Med Assoc J 1975; 112:806.
77. Mann CF. Clindamycin and breast-feeding. Pediatrics 1980; 66:1030.
78. Berlin CM, Lee C. Isoniazid and acetylisoniazid disposition in human milk, saliva and plasma. Fed Proc 1979; 38:426.
79. Passmore CM, McElnay JC, Rainey EA, et al. Metronidazole excretion in human milk and its effect on the suckling neonate. Br J Clin Pharmacol 1988; 26: 45-51.
80. Heisterberg L, Branebjerg PE. Blood and milk concentrations of metronidazole in mothers and infants. J Perinat Med 1983; 11:114-120.
81. Erickson SH, Oppenheim GL, Smith GH. Metronidazole in breast milk. Obstet Gynecol 1981; 57:48-50.
82. Traeger A, Peiker G. Excretion of nalidixic acid via mother's milk. Arch Toxicol 1980; 4(suppl):388-390.
83. Belton EM, Jones RV. Haemolytic anaemia due to nalidixic acid. Lancet 1965; 2:691.
84. Varsano I, Fischl J, Shochet SB. The excretion of orally ingested nitrofurantoin in human milk. J Pediatr 1973; 82:886-887.
85. Hosbach RE, Foster RB. Absence of nitrofurantoin from human milk. JAMA 1967; 202:145.
86. Pons G, Rey E, Richard M-O, et al. Nitrofurantoin excretion in human milk. Dev Pharmacol Ther 1990; 14:148-152.
87. Greene HJ, Burkhart B, Hobby GL, et al. Excretion of penicillin in human milk following parturition. Am J Obstet Gynecol 1946; 51:732-733.
88. Matheson I, Samseth M, Loberg R, et al. Milk transfer of phenoxymethylpenicillin during puerperal mastitis. Br J Clin Pharmacol 1988; 25:33-40.
89. Miller RD, Salter AJ. The passage of trimethoprim/sulphamethoxazole into breast milk and its significance. In Progress in Chemotherapy. Vol 1. Antibacterial Chemotherapy (Daikos CK, ed). Hellenic Society for Chemotherapy, Athens, 1974, pp 687-691.
90. Kauffman RE, O'Brien C, Gilford P. Sulfisoxazole secretion into human milk. J Pediatr 1980; 97:839-841.
91. Posner AC, Prigot A, Konicoff NG. Further observations on the use of tetracycline hydrochloride in prophylaxis and treatment of obstetric infections. In Antibiotics Annual 1954-1955. Medical Encyclopedia, New York, 1954-1955, pp 594-598.
92. Reyes MP, Ostrea EM, Cabinian AE, et al. Vancomycin during pregnancy: Does it cause hearing loss or nephrotoxicity in the infant? Am J Obstet Gynecol 1989; 161:977-981.
93. Pynnonen S, Sillanpaa M. Carbamazepine and mother's milk. Lancet 1975; 2:563.
94. Kuhnz W, Jager-Roman E, Rating D, et al. Carbamazepine and carbamazepine-10,11-epoxide during pregnancy and postnatal period in epileptic mothers and their nursed infants: Pharmacokinetics and clinical effects. Pediatr Pharmacol (New York) 1983; 3:199-208.
95. Froescher W, Eichelbaum M, Niesen M, et al. Carbamazepine levels in breast milk. Ther Drug Monit 1984; 6:266-271.
96. Niebyl JR, Blake DA, Freeman JM, et al. Carbamazepine levels in pregnancy and lactation. Obstet Gynecol 1970; 53:139-140.

97. Pynnonen S, Kanto J, Sillanpaa M, et al. Carbamazepine: Placental transport, tissue concentrations in foetus and newborn, and level in milk. Acta Pharmacol Toxicol (Kbh) 1977; 41:244-253.
98. Kaneko S, Sato T, Suzuki K. The levels of anticonvulsants in breast milk. Br J Clin Pharmacol 1979; 7:624-627.
99. Kaneko S, Suzuki K, Sato T, et al. The problems of antiepileptic medication in the neonatal period: Is breastfeeding advisable? In Epilepsy, Pregnancy, and the Child (Janz D, Bossi L, Dam M, et al, eds). Raven Press, New York, 1982, pp 343-348.
100. Frey B, Schubiger G, Musy JP. Transient cholestatic hepatitis in a neonate associated with carbamazepine exposure during pregnancy and breast-feeding. Eur J Pediatr 1990; 150:136-138.
101. Koup JR, Rose JQ, Cohen ME. Ethosuximide pharmacokinetics in a pregnant patient and her newborn. Epilepsia 1978; 19:535-539.
102. Rane A, Tunell R. Ethosuximide in human milk and in plasma of a mother and her nursed infant. Br J Clin Pharmacol 1981; 12:855-858.
103. Kuhnz W, Koch S, Jakob S, et al. Ethosuximide in epileptic women during pregnancy and lactation period. Placental transfer, serum concentrations in nursed infants and clinical status. Br J Clin Pharmacol 1984; 18:671-677.
104. Steen B, Rane A, Lonnerholm G, et al. Phenytoin excretion in human breast milk and plasma levels in nursed infants. Ther Drug Monit 1982; 4:331-334.
105. Rane A, Garle M, Borga O, et al. Plasma disappearance of transplacentally transferred diphenylhydantoin in the newborn studied by mass fragmentography. Clin Pharmacol Ther 1974; 15:39-45.
106. Mirkin BL, Diphenylhydantoin: Placental transport, fetal localization, neonatal metabolism, and possible teratogenic effects. J Pediatr 1971; 78:329-337.
107. Kuhnz W, Koch S, Helge H, et al. Primidone and phencbarbital during lactation period in epileptic women: Total and free drug serum levels in the nursed infants and their effects on neonatal behavior. Dev Pharmacol Ther 1988; 11: 147-154.
108. Nau H, Rating D, Hauser I, et al. Placental transfer and pharmacokinetics of primidone and its metabolites phenobarbital, PEMA and hydroxyphenobarbital in neonates and infants of epileptic mothers. Eur J Clin Pharmacol 1980; 18:31-42.
109. Alexander FW. Sodium valproate and pregnancy. Arch Dis Child 1979; 54: 240.
110. von Unruh GE, Froescher W, Hoffmann F, et al. Valproic acid in breast milk: How much is really there? Ther Drug Monit 1984; 6:272-276.
111. Dickinson RG, Harland RC, Lynn RK, et al. Transmission of valproic acid (Depakene) across the placenta: Half-life of the drug in mother and baby. J Pediatr 1979; 94:832-835.
112. Nau H, Rating D, Koch S, et al. Valproic acid and its metabolites: Placental transfer, neonatal pharmacokinetics, transfer via mother's milk and clinical status in neonates of epileptic mothers. J Pharmacol Exp Ther 1981; 219:768-777.
113. Brixen-Rasmussen L, Halgrener J. Jorgensen A. Amitriptyline and nortriptyline excretion in human breast milk. Psychopharmacology 1982; 76:94-95.

114. Bader TF, Newman K. Amitriptyline in human breast milk and the nursing infant's serum. Am J Psychiatry 1980; 137:855–856.
115. Schimmel MS, Katz EZ, Shaag Y, et al. Toxic neonatal effects following maternal clomipramine therapy. J Toxicol Clin Toxicol 1991; 29:479–484.
116. Stancer HC, Reed KL. Desipramine and 2-hydroxydesipramine in human breast milk and the nursing infant's serum. Am J Psychiatry 1986; 143:1597–1600.
117. Kemp J, Ilett KF, Booth J, et al. Excretion of doxepin and *n*-desmethyldoxepin in human milk. Br J Clin Pharmacol 1985; 20:497–499.
118. Matheson I, Pande H, Alertsen AR. Respiratory depression caused by *n*-desmethyldoxepin in breastmilk. Lancet 1985; 2:1124.
119. Isenberg KE. Excretion of fluoxetine in human breast milk. J Clin Psychiatry 1990; 51:169.
120. Burch KJ, Wells BG. Fluoxetine/norfluoxetine concentrations in human milk. Pediatrics 1992; 89:676–677.
121. Wright S, Dawling S, Ashford JJ. Excretion of fluvoxamine in breast milk. Br J Clin Pharmacol 1991; 31:209.
122. Sovner R, Orsulak PJ. Excretion of imipramine and desipramine in human breast milk. Am J Psychiatry 1979; 136:4A:451–452.
123. Ware MR, DeVane CL. Imipramine treatment of panic disorder during pregnancy. J Clin Psychiatry 1990; 51:482–484.
124. Matheson I, Skjaeraasen J. Milk concentrations of flupenthixol, nortriptyline and zuclopenthixol and between-breast differences in two patients. Eur J Clin Pharmacol 1988; 35:217–220.
125. Verbeeck RK, Ross SG, McKenna EA. Excretion of trazodone in breast milk. Br J Clin Pharmacol 1986; 22:367–370.
126. Gaillot J, Heusse D, Houghton GW, et al. Pharmacokinetics and metabolism of zopiclone. Pharmacology 1983; 27(suppl):76–91.
127. Hilbert J, Radwanski E, Affrime MB, et al. Excretion of loratadine in human breast milk. J Clin Pharmacol 1988; 28:234–239.
128. Lucas BD, Purdy CY, Scarim SK, et al. Terfenadine breast milk excretion and pharmacokinetics in lactating women. Pharmacotherapy 1992; 12:506.
129. Findlay JWA, Butz RF, Sailstad JM, et al. Pseudoephedrine and triprolidine in plasma and breast milk of nursing mothers. Br J Clin Pharmacol 1984; 18:901–906.
130. Boutroy MJ, Bianchetti G, Dubruc C, et al. To nurse when receiving acebutolol: Is it dangerous for the neonate? Eur J Clin Pharmacol 1986; 30:737–739.
131. White WB, Andreoli JW, Wong SH, et al. Atenolol in human plasma and breast milk. Obstet Gynecol 1984; 63:42S–44S.
132. Liedholm H, Melander A, Bitzen P-O, et al. Accumulation of atenolol and metoprolol in human breast milk. Eur J Clin Pharmacol 1981; 20:229–231.
133. Kulas J, Lunell N-O, Rosing U, et al. Atenolol and metoprolol. A comparison of their excretion into human breast milk. Acta Obstet Gynecol Scand Suppl 1984; 118:65–69.
134. Thorley KJ. Pharmacokinetics of atenolol in pregnancy and lactation. Drugs 1983; 25(suppl 2):215–218.

135. Thorley KJ, McAinsh J. Levels of the beta-blockers atenolol and propranolol in the breast milk of women treated for hypertension in pregnancy. Biopharm Drug Dispos 1983; 4:299–301.
136. Devlin RG, Fleiss PM. Captopril in human blood and breast milk. J Clin Pharmacol 1981; 21:110–113.
137. Hartikainen-Sorri A-L, Heikkinen JE, Koivisto M. Pharmacokinetics of clonidine during pregnancy and nursing. Obstet Gynecol 1987; 69:598–600.
138. Okada M, Inoue H, Nakamura Y, et al. Excretion of diltiazem in human milk. N Engl J Med 1985; 312:992–993.
139. Huttunen K, Gronhagen-Riska C, Fyhrquist F. Enalapril treatment of a nursing mother with slightly impaired renal function. Clin Nephrol 1989; 31:278.
140. Redman CWG, Kelly JG, Cooper WD. The excretion of enalapril and enalaprilat in human breast milk. Eur J Clin Pharmacol 1990; 38:99.
141. Liedholm H, Wahlin-Boll E, Hanson A, et al. Transplacental passage and breast milk concentrations of hydralazine. Eur J Clin Pharmacol 1982; 21: 417–419.
142. Michael CA. Use of labetalol in the treatment of severe hypertension during pregnancy. Br J Clin Pharmacol 1979; 8:211S–215S.
143. Lunell NO, Kulas J, Rane A. Transfer of labetalol into amniotic fluid and breast milk in lactating women. Eur J Clin Pharmacol 1985; 28:597–599.
144. Hauser GJ, Almog S, Tirosh M, et al. Effect of α-methyldopa excreted in human milk on the breast-fed infant. Helv Paediatr Acta ;1985; 40:83–86.
145. Jones HMR, Cummings AJ. A study of the transfer of α-methyldopa to the human foetus and newborn infant. Br J Clin Pharmacol 1978; 6:432–434.
146. White WB, Andreoli JW, Cohn RD. Alpha-methyldopa disposition in mothers with hypertension and in their breast-fed infants. Clin Pharmacol Ther 1985; 37:387–390.
147. Hoskins JA, Holliday SB. Determination of α-methyldopa and methyldopate in human breast milk and plasma by ion-exchange chromatography using electrochemical detection. J Chromatogr 1982; 230:162–167.
148. Sandstrom B, Regardh C-G. Metoprolol excretion into breast milk. Br J Clin Pharmacol 1980; 9:518–519.
149. Lindeberg S, Sandstrom B, Lundborg P, et al. Disposition of the adrenergic blocker metoprolol in the late-pregnant woman, the amniotic fluid, the cord blood and the neonate. Acta Obstet Gynecol Scand Suppl 1984; 118:61–64.
150. Valdivieso A, Valdes G, Spiro TE, et al. Minoxidil in breast milk. Ann Intern Med 1985; 102:135.
151. Devlin RG, Duchin KL, Fleiss PM. Nadolol in human serum and breast milk. Br J Clin Pharmacol 1981; 12:393–396.
152. Ehrenkranz RA, Ackerman BA, Hulse JD. Nifedipine transfer into human milk. J Pediatr 1989; 114:478–480.
153. Penny WJ, Lewis MJ. Nifedipine is excreted in human milk. Eur J Clin Pharmacol 1980; 36:427–428.
154. White WB, Yeh SC, Krol GJ. Nitrendipine in human plasma and breast milk. Eur J Clin Pharmacol 1989; 36:531–534.
155. Santiago TM, Lopez LM. Nitrendipine: A new dihydropyridine calcium-channel antagonist for the treatment of hypertension. DICP. 1990; 24:167–175.

156. Sioufi A, Hillion D, Lumbroso P, et al. Oxprenolol placental transfer, plasma concentrations in newborns and passage into breast milk. Br J Clin Pharmacol 1984; 18:453–456.

157. Fidler J, Smith V, DeSwiet M. Excretion of oxprenolol and timolol in breast milk. Br J Obstet Gynaecol 1983; 90:961–965.

158. Smith MT, Livingstone I, Hooper WD, et al. Propranolol, propranolol glucuronide, and naphthoxylactic acid in breast milk and plasma. Ther Drug Monit 1983; 5:87–93.

159. Bauer JH, Pape B, Zajicek J, et al. Propranolol in human plasma and breast milk. Am J Cardiol 1979; 43:860–862.

160. Taylor EA, Turner P. Anti-hypertensive therapy with propranolol during pregnancy and lactation. Postgrad Med J 1981; 57:427–430.

161. O'Hare MF, Murnaghan GA, Russell CJ, et al. Sotalol as a hypotensive agent in pregnancy. Br J Obstet Gynaecol 1980; 87:814–820.

162. Hackett LP, Wojnar-Horton RE, Dusci LJ, et al. Excretion of sotalol in breast milk. Br J Clin Pharmacol 1990; 29:277.

163. Wagner X, Jouglard J, Moulin M, et al. Coadministration of flecainide acetate and sotalol during pregnancy: Lack of teratogenic effects, passage across the placenta, and excretion in human breast milk. Am Heart J 1990; 119:700–702.

164. Anderson HJ. Excretion of verapamil in human milk. Eur J Clin Pharmacol 1983; 25:279–280.

165. Miller MR, Withers R, Bhamra R, et al. Verapamil and breast-feeding. Eur J Clin Pharmacol 1986; 30:125–126.

166. Inoue H, Unno N, Ou M-C, et al. Level of verapamil in human milk. Eur J Clin Pharmacol 1984; 26:657–658.

167. Anderson P, Bondesson U, Mattiasson I, et al. Verapamil and norverapamil in plasma and breast milk during breast feeding. Eur J Clin Pharmacol 1987; 31:625–627.

168. Bailey DN, Weibert RT, Naylor AJ, et al. A study of salicylate and caffeine excretion in the breast milk of two nursing mothers. J Anal Toxicol 1982; 6: 64–68.

169. Unsworth J, d'Assis-Fonseca A, Beswick DT, et al. Serum salicylate levels in a breast fed infant. Ann Rheum Dis 1987; 46:638–639.

170. Clark JH, Wilson WG. A 16-day-old breast-fed infant with metabolic acidosis caused by salicylate. Clin Pediatr 1981; 20:53–54.

171. Fowler PD. Voltarol: Diclofenac sodium. Clin Rheum Dis 1979; 5:427–464.

172. Smith IJ, Hinson JL, Johnson VA, et al. Flurbiprofen in post-partum women: Plasma and breast milk disposition. J Clin Pharmacol 1989; 29:174–184.

173. Cox SR, Forbes KK. Excretion of flurbiprofen into breast milk. Pharmacotherapy 1987; 7:211–215.

174. Weibert RT, Townsend RJ, Kaiser DG, et al. Lack of ibuprofen secretion into human milk. Clin Pharm 1982; 1:457–458.

175. Townsend RJ, Benedetti TJ, Erickson SH, et al. Excretion of ibuprofen into breast milk. Am J Obstet Gynecol 1984; 149:184–186.

176. Lebedevs TH, Wojnar-Horton RE, Yapp P, et al. Excretion of indomethacin in breast milk. Br J Clin Pharmacol 1991; 32:751–754.

177. Eeg-Olofsson O, Malmros I, Elwin C-E, et al. Convulsions in a breast-fed infant after maternal indomethacin. Lancet 1978; 2:215.

178. Wischnik A, Manth SM, Lloyd J, et al. The excretion of ketorolac tromethamine into breast milk after multiple oral dosing. Eur J Clin Pharmacol 1989; 36:521-524.

179. Buchanan RA, Eaton CJ, Koeff ST, et al. The breast milk excretion of mefenamic acid. Curr Ther Res 1968; 10:592-596.

180. Jamali F, Stevens DRS. Naproxen excretion in milk and its uptake by the infant. DICP. 1983; 17:910-911.

181. Ostensen M. Piroxicam in human breast milk. Eur J Clin Pharmacol 1983; 25: 829-830.

182. Ostensen M, Matheson I, Laufen H. Piroxicam in breast milk after long-term treatment. Eur J Clin Pharmacol 1988; 35:567-569.

183. Wiles DH, Orr MW, Kolakowska T. Chlorpromazine levels in plasma and milk of nursing mothers. Br J Clin Pharmacol 1978; 5:272-273.

184. Stewart RB, Karas B, Springer PK. Haloperidol excretion in human milk. Am J Psychiatry 1980; 137:849-850.

185. Whalley LJ, Blain PG, Prime JK. Haloperidol secreted in breast milk. Br Med J 1981; 282:1746-1747.

186. Olesen OV, Bartels U, Poulsen JH. Perphenazine in breast milk and serum. Am J Psychiatry 1990; 147:1378-1379.

187. Tunnessen WW, Hertz CG. Toxic effects of lithium in newborn infants: A commentary. J Pediatr 1972; 81:804-807.

188. Schou M, Amdisen A. Lithium and pregnancy—III. Lithium ingestion   ' children breast-fed by women on lithium treatment. Br Med J 1973; 2:138.,.

189. Sykes PA, Quarrie J, Alexander FW. Lithium carbonate and breast-feeding. Br Med J 1976; 4:1299.

190. Weinstein MR, Goldfield M. Lithium carbonate treatment during pregnancy; report of a case. Dis Nerv Syst 1969; 30:828-832.

191. Rylance GW, Woods CG, Donnelly MC, et al. Carbimazole and breastfeeding. Lancet 1987; 1:928.

192. Tegler L, Lindstrom B. Antithyroid drugs in milk. Lancet 1980; 2:591.

193. Johansen K. Anderson AN, Kampmann JP, et al. Excretion of methimazole in human milk. Eur J Clin Pharmacol 1982; 23:339-341.

194. Kampmann JP, Johansen K, Hansen JM, et al. Propylthiouracil in human milk. Revision of a dogma. Lancet 1980; 1:736-737.

195. Low LCK, Lang J, Alexander WD. Excretion of carbimazole and propylthiouracil in breast milk. Lancet 1979; 2:1011.

196. Anderson PO, McGuire GG. Neonatal alprazolam withdrawal-possible effects of breast feeding. DICP. 1989; 23:614.

197. Soderman P, Matheson I. Clonazepam in breast milk. Eur J Pediatr 1988; 147:212-213.

198. Fisher JB, Edgren BE, Mammel MC, et al. Neonatal apnea associated with maternal clonazepam therapy: A case report. Obstet Gynecol 1985; 66:34S-35S.

199. Dusci LJ, Good SM, Hall RW, et al. Excretion of diazepam and its metabolites in human milk during withdrawal from combination high dose diazepam and oxazepam. Br J Clin Pharmacol 1990; 29:123–126.
200. Wesson DR, Camber S, Harkey M, et al. Diazepam and desmethyldiazepam in breastmilk. J Psychoactive Drugs 1985; 17:55–56.
201. Brandt R. Passage of diazepam and desmethyldiazepam into breast milk. Arzneimittelforschung 1976; 26:454–457.
202. Patrick MJ, Tilstone WJ, Reavey P. Diazepam and breast-feeding. Lancet 1972; 1:542–543.
203. Erkkola R, Kanto J. Diazepam and breast-feeding. Lancet 1972; 1:1235–1236.
204. Whitelaw AGL, Cummings AJ, McFadyen IR. Effect of maternal lorazepam on the neonate. Br Med J 1981; 282:1106–1108.
205. Matheson I, Lunde PKM, Bredesen JE. Midazolam and nitrazepam in the maternity ward: Milk concentrations and clinical effects. Br J Clin Pharmacol 1990; 30:787–793.
206. Wretlind M. Excretion of oxazepam in breast milk. Eur J Clin Pharmacol 1987; 33:209–210.
207. Lebedevs TH, Wojnar-Horton RE, Yapp P, et al. Excretion of temazepam in breast milk. Br J Clin Pharmacol 1992; 33:204–206.
208. McKenna WJ, Harris L, Rowland E, et al. Amiodarone therapy during pregnancy. Am J Cardiol 1983; 51:1231–1233.
209. Pitcher D, Leather HM, Storey GCA, et al. Amiodarone in pregnancy. Lancet 1983; 1:597–598.
210. Strunge P, Frandsen J, Andreasen F. Amiodarone during pregnancy. Eur Heart J 1988; 9:106–109.
211. Plomp TA, Vulsma T, de Vijlder JJM. Use of amiodarone during pregnancy. Eur J Obstet Gynecol Reprod Biol 1992; 43:201–207.
212. Gutgesell M, Overholt E, Boyle R. Oral bretylium tosylate use during pregnancy and subsequent breastfeeding: A case report. Am J Perinatol 1990; 7: 144–145.
213. Loughnan PM. Digoxin excretion in human breast milk. J Pediatr 1978; 92: 1019–1020.
214. Chan V, Tse TF, Wong V. Transfer of digoxin across the placenta and into breast milk. Br J Obstet Gynaecol 1978; 85:605–609.
215. Finley JP, Waxman MB, Wong PY, et al. Digoxin excretion in human milk. J Pediatr 1979; 94:339–340.
216. Reinhardt D, Richter O, Genz T, et al. Kinetics of the translactal passage of digoxin from breast feeding mothers to their infants. Eur J Pediatr 1982; 138: 49–52.
217. Barnett DB, Hudson SA, McBurney A. Disopyramide and its *n*-monodesalkyl metabolite in breast milk. Br J Clin Pharmacol 1982; 14:310–312.
218. MacIntosh O, Buchanan N. Excretion of disopyramide in human breast milk. Br J Clin Pharmacol 1985; 19:856–857.
219. Hoppu K, Neuvonen PJ, Korte T. Disopyramide and breast feeding. Br J Clin Pharmacol 1986; 21:553.

220. McQuinn RL, Pisani A, Wafa S, et al. Flecainide excretion in human breast milk. Clin Pharmacol Ther 1990; 48:262–267.
221. Timmis AD, Jackson G, Holt DW. Mexiletine for control of ventricular dysrhythmias in pregnancy. Lancet 1980; 2:647–648.
222. Lewis AM, Johnston A, Patel L, et al. Mexiletine in human blood and breast milk. Postgrad Med J 1981; 57:546–547.
223. Pittard WB, Glazier H. Procainamide excretion in human milk. J Pediatr 1983; 102:631–633.
224. Libardoni M, Piovan D, Busato E, et al. Transfer of propafenone and 5-OH-propafenone to foetal plasma and maternal milk. Br J Clin Pharmacol 1991; 32:527–528.
225. Hill LM, Malkasian GD. The use of quinidine sulfate throughout pregnancy. Obstet Gynecol 1979; 54:366–368.
226. Soderman P, Hartvig P, Fagerlund C. Acetazolamide excretion into human breast milk. Br J Clin Pharmacol 1984; 17:599–600.
227. Werthmann MW, Krees SV. Excretion of chlorothiazide in human breast milk. J Pediatr 1972; 81:781–783.
228. Mulley BA, Parr GD, Pau WK, et al. Placental transfer of chlorthalidone and its elimination in maternal milk. Eur J Clin Pharmacol 1978; 13:129–131.
229. Cominos DC, Van der Walt A, Van Rooyen AJL. Suppression of postpartum lactation with furosemide. S Afr Med J 1976; 50:251–252.
230. Miller ME, Cohn RD, Burghart PH. Hydrochlorothiazide disposition in a mother and her breast-fed infant. J Pediatr 1982; 101:789–791.
231. Phelps DL, Karim A. Spironolactone: Relationship between concentrations of dethioacetylated metabolite in human serum and milk. J Pharm Sci 1977; 66:1203.
232. Somogyi A, Gugler R. Cimetidine excretion into breast milk. Br J Clin Pharmacol 1979; 7:627–629.
233. Hofmeyr GJ, Sonnendecker EWW. Secretion of the gastrokinetic agent cisapride in human milk. Eur J Clin Pharmacol 1986; 30:735–736.
234. Hofmeyr GJ, van Iddekinge B. Domperidone and lactation. Lancet 1983; 1:647.
235. Hofmeyr GJ, van Iddekinge B, Blott JA. Domperidone: Secretion in breast milk and effect on puerperal prolactin levels. Br J Obstet Gynaecol 1985; 92:141–144.
236. Courtney TP, Shaw RW, Cedar E, et al. Excretion of famotidine in breast milk. Br J Clin Pharmacol 1988; 26:639P.
237. Nikodem VC, Hofmeyr GJ. Secretion of the antidiarrhoeal agent loperamide oxide in breast milk. Eur J Clin Pharmacol 1992; 42:695–696.
238. Kauppila A, Arvela P, Koivisto M, et al. Metoclopramide and breast-feeding: Transfer into milk and the newborn. Eur J Clin Pharmacol 1983; 25:819–823.
239. Lewis PJ, Devenish C, Kahn C. Controlled trial of metoclopramide in the initiation of breast feeding. Br J Clin Pharmacol 1980; 9:217–219.
240. Obermeyer BD, Bergstrom RF, Callaghan JT, et al. Secretion of nizatidine into human breast milk after single and multiple doses. Clin Pharmacol Ther 1990; 47:724–730.

241. Riley AJ, Crowley P, Harrison C. Transfer of ranitidine to biological fluids: Milk and semen. In The Clinical Use of Ranitidine (Misiewicz JJ, Wormsley KG, eds). Medicine Publishing Foundation, Oxford, 1981, pp 78-81.

242. Kearns GL, McConnell RF, Trang JM, et al. Appearance of ranitidine in breast milk following multiple dosing. Clin Pharm 1985; 4:322-324.

243. Nelis GF. Diarrhea due to 5-aminosalicylic acid in breast milk. Lancet 1989; 1:383.

244. Jenss H, Weber P, Hartmann F. 5-Aminosalicyclic acid and its metabolite in breast milk during lactation. Am J Gastroenterol 1990; 85:331.

245. Edstein MD, Veenendaal JR, Newman K, et al. Excretion of chloroquine, dapsone and pyrimethamine in human milk. Br J Clin Pharmacol 1986; 22: 733-735.

246. Ogunbona FA, Onyeji CO, Bolaji OO, et al. Excretion of chloroquine and desethylchloroquine in human milk. Br J Clin Pharmacol 1987; 23:473-476.

247. Ette EI, Essien EE, Ogonor JI, et al. Chloroquine in human milk. J Clin Pharmacol 1987; 27:499-502.

248. Nation RL, Hackett LP, Dusci LJ, et al. Excretion of hydroxychloroquine in human milk. Br J Clin Pharmacol 1984; 17:368-369.

249. Ostensen M, Brown ND, Chiang PK, et al. Hydroxychloroquine in human breast milk. Eur J Clin Pharmacol 1985; 28:357.

250. Erkkola R, Kanto J, Allonen H, et al. Excretion of methylergometrine (methylergonovine) into the human breast milk. Int J Clin Pharmacol Biopharm 1978; 16:579-580.

251. Ost L, Wettrell G, Bjorkhem I, et al. Prednisolone excretion in human milk. J Pediatr 1985; 106:1008-1011.

252. Katz FH, Duncan BR. Entry of prednisone into human milk. N Engl J Med 1975; 293:1154.

253. McKenzie SA, Selley JA, Agnew JE. Secretion of prednisolone into breast milk. Arch Dis Child 1975; 50:894-896.

254. Jarnerot G, Into-Malmberg M-B. Sulphasalazine treatment during breast feeding. Scand J Gastroenterol 1979; 14:869-871.

255. Berlin CM, Yaffe SJ. Disposition of salicylazosulfapyridine (azulfidine) and metabolites in human breast milk. Dev Pharmacol Ther 1980; 1:31-39.

256. Esbjorner E, Jarnerot G, Wranne L. Sulphasalazine and sulphapyridine serum levels in children to mothers treated with sulphasalazine during pregnancy and lactation. Acta Paediatr Scand 1987; 76:137-142.

257. Branski D, Kerem E, Gross-Kieselstein E, et al. Bloody diarrhea—A possible complication of sulfasalazine transferred through human breast milk. J Pediatr Gastroenterol Nutr 1986; 5:316-317.

258. Stec GP, Greenberger P, Ruo TI, et al. Kinetics of theophylline transfer to breast milk. Clin Pharmacol Ther 1980; 28:404-408.

259. Yurchak AM, Jusko WJ. Theophylline secretion into breast milk. Pediatrics 1976; 57:518-520.

260. Orme M L'E, Lewis PJ, de Swiet M, et al. May mothers given warfarin breastfeed their infants? Br Med J 1977; 1:1564-1565.

261. McKenna R, Cole ER, Vasan U. Is warfarin sodium contraindicated in the lactating mother? J Pediatr 1983; 103:325–327.

262. Krogh CME, ed. Compendium of Pharmaceuticals and Specialties, 27th ed. Canadian Pharmaceutical Association, Ottawa, 1992.

263. McElvoy GK, Litvak K, Welsh OH, et al, eds. American Hospital Formulary Service Drug Information. American Society of Hospital Pharmacists, Bethesda, MD, 1992.

264. Naumburg EG, Meny RG. Breast milk opioids and neonatal apnea. Am J Dis Child 1988; 142:11–12.

265. Rhône-Poulenc. Flagyl. In Compendium of Pharmaceuticals and Specialties, 24th ed (Krogh CME, ed). Canadian Pharmaceutical Association, Ottawa, 1989, pp 409–410.

266. Beard CM, Noller KL, O'Fallon WM, et al. Lack of evidence for cancer due to use of metronidazole. N Engl J Med 1979; 301:519–522.

267. Stoukides CA. The galactopharmacopedia: Quinolone antibiotics and breast-feeding. J Hum Lact 1991; 7:143–144.

268. Schluter G. Toxicology of ciprofloxaxin. In First International Ciprofloxacin Workshop (Neu HC, Weuta H, eds). Excerpta Medica, Leverkusen, 1985, pp 61–67.

269. Chysky V, Kapila K, Hullmann R, et al. Safety of ciprofloxacin in children: Worldwide clinical experience based on compassionate use. Emphasis on joint evaluation. Infection 1991; 19:289–296.

270. Schaad UB, Stoupis C, Wedgwood J, et al. Clinical, radiologic and magnetic resonance monitoring for skeletal toxicity in pediatric patients with cystic fibrosis receiving a three-month course of ciprofloxacin. Pediatr Infect Dis J 1991; 10:723–729.

271. Needs CJ, Brooks PM. Antirheumatic medication during lactation. Br J Rheumatol 1985; 24:291–297.

272. Riant P, Urien S, Albengres E, et al. High plasma protein binding as a parameter in the selection of betablockers for lactating women. Biochem Pharmacol 1986; 35:4579–4581.

273. Boutroy MJ. Fetal and neonatal effects of the beta-adrenoceptor blocking agents. Dev Pharmacol Ther 1987; 10:224–231.

274. Kok THHG, Taitz LS, Bennett MJ, et al. Drowsiness due to clemastine transmitted in breast milk. Lancet 1982; 1:914–915.

275. Duckman S, Hubbard JF. The role of fluids in relieving breast engorgement without the use of hormones. Am J Obstet Gynecol 1950; 60:200–204.

276. Kanto JH. Use of benzodiazepines during pregnancy, labour and lactation, with particular reference to pharmacokinetic considerations. Drugs 1982; 23: 354–380.

277. Mallol J, Obregon MJ, Morreale de Escobar G. Analytical artifacts in radioimmunoassay of L-thyroxin in human milk. Clin Chem 1982; 28:1277–1282.

278. Moller B, Bjorkhem I, Falk O, et al. Identification of thyroxine in human breast milk by gas chromatography-mass spectrometry. J Clin Endocrinol Metab 1983; 56:30–34.

279. Jansson L, Ivarsson S, Larsson I, et al. Tri-iodothyronine and thyroxine in human milk. Acta Paediatr Scand 1983; 73:703–705.
280. Mizuta H, Amino N, Ichihara K, et al. Thyroid hormones in human milk and their influence on thyroid function of breast-fed babies. Pediatr Res 1983; 17: 468–471.
281. Momotani N, Yamashita R, Yoshimoto M, et al. Recovery from foetal hypothyroidism: Evidence for the safety of breast-feeding while taking propylthiouracil. Clin Endocrinol 1989; 31:591–595.
282. Cooper DS. Antithyroid drugs: To breast-feed or not to breast-feed. Am J Obstet Gynecol 1987; 157:234–235.
283. Cooper DS. Antithyroid drugs. N Engl J Med 1984; 311:1353–1362.
284. McGuire TM, Mitchell IB, Wright AH, et al. Update on excretion of drugs in breast milk – Part 2. Aust J Hosp Pharm 1988; 18:150–164.
285. Lewis JH, Weingold AB, Committee on FDA-Related Matters, American College of Gastroenterology. The use of gastrointestinal drugs during pregnancy and lactation. Am J Gastroenterol 1985; 80:912–923.
286. Camanni F, Genazzani AR, Massara F, et al. Prolactin-releasing effect of domperidone in normoprolactinemic and hyperprolactinemic subjects. Neuroendocrinology 1980; 30:2–6.
287. Kauppila A, Anunti P, Kivinen S, et al. Metoclopramide and breast feeding: Efficacy and anterior pituitary responses of the mother and the child. Eur J Obstet Gynecol Reprod Biol 1985; 19:19–22.
288. Ehrenkranz RA, Ackerman BA. Metoclopramide effect on faltering milk production by mothers of premature infants. Pediatrics 1986; 78:614–620.
289. Sousa PLR. Metoclopramide and breast-feeding. Br Med J 1975; 1:513.
290. Fantus B, Dyniewicz JM. Phenolphthalein administration to nursing women. Am J Digest Dis Nutr 1936; 3:184–185.
291. Baldwin WF. Clinical study of senna administration to nursing mothers: Assessment of effects on infant bowel habits. Can Med Assoc J 1963; 89:566–568.
292. Werthmann MW, Krees SV. Quantitative excretion of senokot in human breast milk. Med Ann DC. 1973; 42:4–5.
293. White GJ, White M. Breastfeeding and drugs in human milk. Vet Hum Toxicol 1984; 26(suppl 1).
294. O'Reilly RA. Anticoagulant, antithrombotic, and thrombolytic drugs. In Goodman and Gilman's The Pharmacological Basis of Therapeutics, 7th ed (Gilman AG, Goodman LS, Rall TW, et al, eds). Collier MacMillan Canada, Toronto, 1985, pp 1338–1359.
295. Coulam CB, Moyer TP, Jiang N-S, et al. Breast-feeding after renal transplantation. Transplant Proc 1982; 13:605–609.
296. Grekas DM, Vasiliou SS, Lazarides AN. Immunosuppressive therapy and breast-feeding after renal transplantation. Nephron 1984; 37:68.
297. Johns DG, Rutherford LD, Leighton PC, et al. Secretion of methotrexate into human milk. Am J Obstet Gynecol 1972; 112:978–980.
298. Brooks PM, Needs CJ. The use of antirheumatic medication during pregnancy and in the puerperium. Rheum Dis Clin North Am 1989; 15:789–806.

299. Peters F, Del Pozo E, Conti A, et al. Inhibition of lactation by a long-acting bromocriptine. Obstet Gynecol 1986; 67:82–85.
300. Scapin F, Buonaccorsi S, Tronconi G, et al. Metergoline versus bromocriptine in the prevention of puerperal lactation: A double-blind clinical trial. Eur J Clin Pharmacol 1982; 22:181–183.
301. Varga L, Lutterbeck PM, Pryor JS, et al. Suppression of puerperal lactation with an ergot alkaloid: A double-blind study. Br Med J 1972; 2:743–744.
302. Illingworth RS. Abnormal substances excreted in human milk. Practitioner 1953; 171:533–538.
303. Kesaniemi YA. Ethanol and acetaldehyde in the milk and peripheral blood of lactating women after ethanol administration. J Obstet Gynaecol Br Commonw 1974; 81:84–86.
304. Lawton ME. Alcohol in breast milk. Aust N Z J Obstet Gynaecol 1985; 25: 71–73.
305. Wyckerheld Bisdom CJ. Alcohol and nicotine poisoning in nurslings. JAMA 1937; 109:178.
306. Cobo E. Effect of different doses of ethanol on the milk-ejecting reflex in lactating women. Am J Obstet Gynecol 1973; 115:817–821.
307. Little RE, Anderson KW, Ervin CH, et al. Maternal alcohol use during breast-feeding and infant mental and motor development at one year. N Engl J Med 1989; 321:425–430.
308. Carlson HE, Wasser HL, Reidelberger RD. Beer-induced prolactin secretion: A clinical and laboratory study of the role of salsolinol. J Clin Endocrinol Metab 1985; 60:673–677.
309. Ferguson BB, Wilson DJ, Schaffner W. Determination of nicotine concentrations in human milk. Am J Dis Child 1976; 130:837–839.
310. Labrecque M, Marcoux S, Weber J-P, et al. Feeding and urine cotinine values in babies whose mothers smoke. Pediatrics 1989; 83:93–97.
311. Schwartz-Bickenbach D, Schulte-Hobein B, Abt S, et al. Smoking and passive smoking during pregnancy and early infancy: Effects on birth weight, lactation period, and cotinine concentrations in mother's milk and infant's urine. Toxicol Lett 1987; 35:73–81.
312. Schulte-Hobein B, Schwartz-Bickenbach D, Abt S, et al. Cigarette smoke exposure and development of infants throughout the first year of life: Influence of passive smoking and nursing on cotinine levels in breast milk and infants' urine. Acta Paediatr 1992; 81:550–557.
313. Vio F, Salazar G, Infante C. Smoking during pregnancy and lactation and its effects on breast-milk volume. Am J Clin Nutr 1991; 54:1011–1016.
314. Said G, Patois E, Lellouch J. Infantile colic and parental smoking. Br Med J 1984; 289:660.
315. Greenberg RA, Haley NJ, Etzel RA, et al. Measuring the exposure of infants to tobacco smoke: Nicotine and cotinine in urine and saliva. N Engl J Med 1984; 310:1075–1078.
316. Luck W, Nau H. Nicotine and cotinine concentrations in serum and urine of infants exposed via passive smoking or milk from smoking mothers. J Pediatr 1985; 107:816–820.

317. Chasnoff IJ, Lewis DE, Squires L. Cocaine intoxication in a breast-fed infant. Pediatrics 1987; 80:836–838.
318. Kaufman KR, Petrucha RA, Pitts FN, et al. PCP in amniotic fluid and breast milk: Case report. J Clin Psychiatry 1983; 44:269–270.
319. Perez-Reyes M, Wall ME. Presence of Δ9-tetrahydrocannabinol in human milk. N Engl J Med 1982; 307:819–820.
320. Astley SJ, Little RE. Maternal marijuana use during lactation and infant development at one year. Neurotoxicol Teratol 1990; 12:161–168.
321. Mendelson JH, Mello NK, Ellingboe J. Acute effects of marihuana smoking on prolactin levels in human females. J Pharmacol Exp Ther 1985; 232:220–222.
322. Rooney TW, Lorber A, Veng-Pedersen P, et al. Gold pharmacokinetics in breast milk and serum of a lactating woman. J Rheumatol 1987; 14:1120–1122.
323. Bell RAF, Dale IM. Gold secretion in maternal milk. Arthritis Rheum 1976; 19:1374.
324. Bennett PN, Humphries SJ, Osborne JP, et al. Use of sodium aurothiomalate during lactation. Br J Clin Pharmacol 1990; 29:777–779.
325. Braverman LE. Iodine induced thyroid disease. Acta Med Austriaca 1990; 17:29–33.
326. Delange F, Chanoine JP, Abrassart C, et al. Topical iodine, breastfeeding, and neonatal hypothyroidism. Arch Dis Child 1988; 63:106–107.
327. Danziger Y, Pertzelan A, Mimouni M. Transient congenital hypothyroidism after topical iodine in pregnancy and lactation. Arch Dis Child 1987; 62:295–296.
328. Postellon DC, Aronow R. Iodine in mother's milk. JAMA 1982; 247:463.
329. Koetsawang S. The effects of contraceptive methods on the quality and quantity of breast milk. Int J Gynaecol Obstet 1987; 25(suppl):115–127.
330. World Health Organization (WHO) Task Force on Oral Contraceptives, Special Programme of Research, Development, and Research Training in Human Reproduction. Effects of hormonal contraceptives on breast milk composition and infant growth. Stud Fam Plann 1988; 19:361–369.
331. Laukaran VH. The effects of contraceptive use on the initiation and duration of lactation. Int J Gynaecol Obstet 1987; 25(suppl):129–142.

Part II

Poisoning and Radiation in Pregnancy

11

Poisoning in Pregnancy

Milton Tenenbein
University of Manitoba, Winnipeg, Manitoba, Canada

Clinical Case

You attend a 16-year-old pregnant (12 weeks gestation) woman who had tried to commit suicide by taking 60 caplets of Tylenol (325 mg each). The patient, who weighs 50 kg, did not tell anyone about her action for 24 hours, but then became frightened by her continued vomiting. Her boyfriend did not suspect anything because "she had morning sickness anyway."

INTRODUCTION

Exposure to drugs and chemicals can have an adverse effect on the outcome of a pregnancy. We generally consider low level exposures (doses insufficient to harm the expectant mother), which we evaluate by the criteria of reproductive wastage and production of dysmorphic offspring. Very little attention has been addressed to the issue of acute poisoning during pregnancy. In such situations there is potential risk for the mother as well as the fetus.

The fetal and maternal risks are not necessarily equal. Extent of toxin exposure may be different on both sides of the placenta. Although most agents that are absorbed across the gastrointestinal epithelium freely traverse the placenta, some, such as iron, have specialized transplacental absorptive mechanisms (1,2). In a massive overdose situation, this mechanism may become a rate-limiting step, thus resulting in a relatively smaller fetal exposure. Conversely, some agents, such as salicylates, are present in higher concentrations in the fetus (3,4). Fetal metabolic pathways are often immature. While this may seem to put the fetus at greater risk, it can also be protective when, for example, toxicity is due to an intracellularly generated metabolite, not the ingestant itself. Acetaminophen is an example of such an agent.

Because the mother is at risk, she often requires treatment. Does the presence of a conceptus demand modified therapy? Do poisoning-managing interventions such as syrup of ipecac, hemodialysis, or specific antidotes present a risk to the fetus? In some cases, a unique decision in the management of the acutely poisoned patient may be required: Should a potentially viable fetus be delivered on an emergency basis to prevent damage or death?

This chapter reviews the management of the poisoned expectant mother. Adverse effects to the neonate from drugs administered in therapeutic doses to the mother are discussed elsewhere in this book, as are teratogenesis and the fetal and neonatal effects of substance abuse. First, the epidemiology of acute poisonings during pregnancy is reviewed. Then we discuss the general management of the overdosed expectant mother and the management of various specific poisonings.

EPIDEMIOLOGY OF POISONING DURING PREGNANCY

Most poisonings during pregnancy are suicidal gestures. However, in one large series of hospitalized poisoned pregnant patients, 14% were accidental (5). In this series of 162 patients, there were two maternal and four fetal deaths. This cohort, which was gleaned from a specialized unit for the treatment of intoxications, consisted of relatively serious cases. The occurrence of only four fetal deaths, a 2.5% rate, would seem to indicate a relative resistance to an acute toxic insult. If indeed this is so, it may help to explain the limited number of published cases of overdoses during pregnancy, since most patients do well.

Pregnant women may threaten suicide to strengthen their case for a therapeutic abortion (6). Conversely, pregnancy provides a unique motivation for drug overdose (i.e., an attempt to induce an abortion). In Czeizel's series, 8% overdosed for the expressed purpose of inducing an abortion, and 23% subsequently had a therapeutic abortion (5). Some agents are commonly considered as abortifacients. If overdose of quinine during pregnancy is encountered, one should strongly consider the possibility that an attempt was made to induce abortion (7). Historically, lead was often ingested to induce abortions (8), and from time to time various herbal remedies have been utilized for this purpose (9). Whitlock and Edwards, who reviewed pregnancy and attempted suicide (10), felt that the indicence of suicidal gestures by pregnant women was at least equal to that of nonpregnant women. These authors reported that 7% of all women making suicidal gestures are likely to be pregnant. Although pregnant women are less likely to kill themselves, suicide does account for 1% of all deaths during pregnancy, and pregnancy is an associated factor in 5% of all female suicides (10).

Rayburn et al. reviewed drug overdose during pregnancy in an ambulatory population (11). Their cohort was gleaned from the case records of a poison control center. In a 4-year period, 0.07% of all telephone consultations involved overdoses by pregnant women. Although the ingestants were similar to those of the general population, one notable difference was an increased frequency of ingestion of vitamins and iron, which constituted the second most common group of ingestants. This should not be surprising, since pregnant women are routinely placed on these supplements. However, it is worrisome because the management of iron overdose is complex enough without the presence of a fetus.

Czeizel studied drug overdose and pregnancy from another perspective (12). He wondered whether the prior occurrence of an overdose adversely affects subsequent reproductive function. Happily he found that a severe overdose does not lead to decreased fertility, increased pregnancy wastage, or subsequent dysmorphology (12).

APPROACH TO THE POISONED PREGNANT PATIENT

The general management of the pregnant patient who has taken an acute overdose should not differ from that of the nonpregnant individual. The proper approach is well described elsewhere (13), and it includes acute stabilization (airway, breathing, circulation), history, physical examination, supportive care, nonspecific antipoison therapy (prevention of absorption, enhancement of elimination), and specific antipoison therapy (administration of an antidote). In addition to such routine management, fetal well-being must be monitored.

Recently, the approach to preventing the absorption of ingested poisons has undergone reappraisal and modification. The time-honored interventions of ipecac-induced emesis and orogastric lavage have been questioned, and activated charcoal administration has become the primary gastrointestinal decontamination procedure (14–16). In addition to this change in the approach to the prevention of absorption of poisons, an additional procedure, whole-bowel irrigation with polyethylene glycol-electrolyte lavage solution has been introduced as a new intervention (17). Its use in a pregnant patient has been reported (18). From the perspective of the management of the overdosed pregnant patient, the trend away from syrup of ipecac circumvents potential concerns regarding the teratogenic potential and safety of this drug during pregnancy. Unlike ipecac, activated charcoal is not absorbed; thus adverse effects on the fetus would not be expected.

The risk to the fetus from the administration of most antidotes is unknown. The scant available information is discussed below in connection with the poison in question. These risks may manifest as teratogenesis or as acute fetal toxicity if the antidote has agonistic properties. An example of the latter situation is the administration of atropine for organophosphate pesticide poisoning. Since the transplacental delivery of the poison and the antidote may not be similar, although the mother's atropine dose may be optimal, the fetus is at risk to receive a relative underdose or overdose of this antidote. The latter situation has been documented (19). Despite these potential fetal risks, the needs of the mother are paramount. If the indication for an antidote exists, the presence of a gravid uterus must not be considered to contraindicate its administration. A tragic case of a maternal death associated with the withholding of an antidote because of teratogenic fears has been published (20,21).

Although there is very limited literature on most forms of therapy for poisoning during pregnancy, some experiences with hemodialysis have been published. There are at least three reports of the use of acute hemodialysis during pregnancy to treat acute drug overdose (22–24), as well as reviews of pregnancy in hemodialysis patients (25–27). Acute hemodialysis does not seem to have an adverse effect on the fetus. Although women on chronic hemodialysis have increased reproductive wastage, premature labors, and growth-retarded newborns, these are more likely a consequence of their underlying renal disease.

ACETAMINOPHEN

Published Experience

After nutritional supplements, acetaminophen is the commonest drug taken by pregnant women (28). It has been documented as the drug most frequently overdosed on during pregnancy (11), and the published experience of overdoses during pregnancy is greatest for this agent (Table 1) (29–38). Since it crosses the placenta (40), the fetus is at potential risk.

The first case was published in 1978 but was poorly documented. The overdose occurred during the first half of pregnancy and was not treated with specific antidote; the mother suffered severe hepatotoxicity: serum aspartate transaminase (AST) of 9550 IU/L. The fetus survived only to be therapeutically aborted 2 weeks later. Since there was no description of a pathological examination of the abortus, it is not known whether there was any fetal toxicity.

Between 1982 and 1986, eight case reports were found. Byer et al. (30) described a 26-year-old, 36-week-pregnant woman who ingested 32.5 g of acetaminophen. Four and one-half hours after the ingestion, her serum concentration was just barely into the potential toxicity section of the nomogram,

Table 1 Acetaminophen Overdose During Pregnancy

Case	Gestation (weeks)	Potential maternal toxicity	Full course of antidote	Maternal toxicity	Timing of delivery after overdose	Fetal outcome	Ref.
1	20	Yes	No	Yes	na	Survival; subsequent thera-peutic abortion	29
2	36	Yes	Yes	No	6 weeks	Normal	30
3	29	Yes	No	Yes	16 h	Survival; no hepatotoxicity	31
4	38	Yes	Yes	No	17 h	Survival; no hepatotoxicity	32
5	18	Yes	Yes, but late	Yes	23 weeks	Normal	33
6	36	No	Yes	No	7 h	Survival; no hepatotoxicity	34
7	28	Yes	No	Yes	na	Stillborn	35
8	16	Yes	Yes	No	24 weeks	Normal	36
9	16	Yes	Yes, but late	Yes	16 weeks	Normal	37
10	33	Yes	Yes	Yes	na	Stillborn	38

Note: na, not available.

and she was treated with a full course of the antidote *N*-acetylcysteine. No hepatotoxicity ensued, and the patient delivered a normal neonate 6 weeks later. The following year, Lederman et al. (31) reported a 22-year-old woman in her 29th week of pregnancy who had ingested 32.5 g of acetaminophen. Her serum concentration of 160 mg/L at 10 h after the overdose was toxic by nomogram. She did not receive a course of antidotal therapy and went on to develop severe hepatotoxicity (AST of 4300 IU/L), from which she fully recovered. Sixteen hours after this overdose she spontaneously delivered a 1.22 kg female who developed hyaline membrane disease and required assisted ventilation. Cord blood acetaminophen concentration was 76 mg/L, which falls into the toxic range of the adult nomogram. Neonatal therapy included four exchange transfusions, but no specific antidote. No hepatotoxicity occurred, and the child survived.

Four cases were published in 1984. Ruthnum and Goel (32) described a 22-year-old, 38-week-pregnant woman who ingested 26 g of acetaminophen. At 4 h her serum concentration was in the toxic range of the nomogram. Labor was induced, and she delivered a 3.1 kg male 17 h after the overdose. Cord blood acetaminophen concentration was nontoxic on the adult nomogram and the infant did not develop hepatotoxicity. Stokes (33) described a 17-year-old, 18-week-pregnant girl who ingested 10 and 15 g of acetaminophen at 18 and 8 h prior to admission. Her plasma concentration was toxic by nomogram and she was treated with intravenous *N*-acetylcysteine. She developed severe hepatotoxicity from which she fully recovered. She subsequently delivered a full-term male with some mild perinatal difficulties unassociated with the acetaminophen overdose.

The third 1984 case, described by Roberts et al. (34), was a 25-year-old, 36-week-pregnant woman who ingested 20 g of acetaminophen 4 h prior to presentation. Although her serum concentration was just barely toxic by nomogram, the half-life was not prolonged, indicating probable nontoxicity. The baby, a male, was delivered by cesarean section 7 h after the overdose and the mother was then treated with *N*-acetylcysteine. The baby's cord plasma acetaminophen concentration was toxic by nomogram, and treatment with an exchange transfusion was initiated. Neither the neonate nor the mother developed hepatotoxicity. Haibach et al. (35) described a case that is unique in that although the mother recovered, the fetus died. The mother was 27 years old and in her 27th to 28th week of pregnancy when she consumed 29.5 g of acetaminophen over a 24 h period. Fetal death was confirmed by ultrasound examination at presentation, 16 hours later. Treatment with oral *N*-acetylcysteine was not tolerated, and the mother went on to develop severe hepatotoxicity from which she recovered. At autopsy, a high concentration of acetaminophen was found in the fetal liver, indicating that the baby had been alive at the time of the overdose. Although the death occurred earlier than expected (16–24 h after overdose), the hepatic microscopy supported acetaminophen toxicity. Thus, toxicity must be considered to be the probable cause for the fetal death.

Two cases were described in 1986. Robertson et al. (36) described a 21-year-old, 16-week-pregnant woman who ingested 36 g of acetaminophen. Her serum concentration was well into the toxic range of the nomogram. Because oral *N*-acetylcysteine was not tolerated, this antidote was administered intravenously. There was no maternal hepatotoxicity, and a normal newborn was delivered at term. The second patient, described by Ludmir et al. (37), was 16 weeks pregnant and had ingested 64 g of acetaminophen. Her serum concentrations were also well into the toxic range, and *N*-acetylcysteine therapy was begun at 20 h after the overdose, a time unlikely to alter the course. This patient developed severe hepatotoxicity from which she fully recovered. A premature labor and delivery resulted in a normal 32-week newborn that subsequently thrived.

The largest experience of acetaminophen overdose during pregnancy was published in 1989 (38). In this multicenter study, complete data were available in 60 of 113 cases, and one of these is of particular interest: a stillborn fetus at 33 weeks gestation, with death having occurred 2 days after maternal overdose. The mother's serum acetaminophen concentration was toxic by nomogram and she received a full oral course of *N*-acetylcysteine beginning at 12 hours after acetaminophen ingestion. Significant hepatotoxicity occurred in the mother, who survived. The fetal serum acetominophen concentration was grossly elevated, and at autopsy the fetus was found to have massive hepatonecrosis. This case is very similar to that of Haibach et al. (35), strengthening the hypothesis that the fetus is at greatest risk if the acetaminophen overdose occurs during the third trimester. Riggs et al. (38) also attributed a first trimester fetal loss to an acetaminophen overdose. However, the mother was also very seriously affected and she died. It was not determined whether the fetal loss was secondary to the mother's critical condition or primary to fetal hepatotoxicity.

Another large series describing 48 cases was published in 1990 (39). Details of individual cases are sketchy, making commentary difficult. Of interest, though, was the observation of no birth defects associated with first-trimester *N*-acetylcysteine therapy.

Of the 10 cases summarized in Table 1, case 6 is of little interest because of negligible potential for toxicity. Cases 1, 3, 5, 7, 9, and 10 all exhibited maternal hepatotoxicity. The two intrauterine deaths, cases 7 and 10, were third-trimester overdoses. The other four fetuses did well. Of these, only one was in the third trimester (case 3), and this baby was delivered 6 hours after the overdose. Thus, it would seem that maternal hepatotoxicity in the third trimester is a marker for potential fetal demise. However, the clinical usefulness of this association (if it exists at all) is quite limited, since both fetuses died prior to or during the early development of maternal toxicity.

Pharmacology and Toxicology

Estimation of the fetal risk from a maternal acetaminophen overdose requires an understanding of the metabolism of this drug by the mature organism and the differences that may exist in the fetus. We discuss only briefly the metabolism of this drug, since it is well reviewed elsewhere (41). In therapeutic amounts, acetaminophen is largely excreted as urinary sulfates or glucuronides. A small amount is oxidized by the cytochrome P-450 mixed function oxidase system. This produces a highly reactive metabolite that binds to hepatocellular macromolecules, producing hepatotoxicity. This effect can be prevented by complexation with hepatic glutathione. In overdose situations, sulfation and glucuronidation become saturated, thus presenting an increased load to the cytochrome P-450 pathway. Hepatotoxicity ensues after glutathione has been depleted. Thus it is an intracellularly generated metabolite, not the parent acetaminophen, that produces toxicity. Administration of N-acetylcysteine is protective because it acts as a glutathione precursor (42).

Therefore, for hepatotoxicity to occur, the fetal hepatocyte must have an active cytochrome P-450 system. Absent or decreased capacity for sulfation, glucuronidation, and glutathione generation would increase the risk of fetal liver damage. In general, cytochrome P-450, sulfation, and glutathione are present in human fetal livers but glucuronidation is not (43,44). Not surprisingly, the extent of the activities of these processes is poorly documented. It varies among xenobiotics and with gestational age.

However, acetaminophen is one of the few drugs that has undergone human fetal metabolic studies (45). Hepatocytes were harvested from fetuses at 18 to 23 week gestation. Cytochrome P-450 activity, glutathione generation, and sulfation were demonstrated along with an absence of glucuronidation. Mean cytochrome P-450 activity was only 10% of adult values, with a linear increase occurring over the gestational period under study. Thus, degree of fetal risk from maternal acetaminophen ingestion would seem to correlate with gestational age. This suggestion is supported by the observation that the two fetal deaths (35,38) were third-trimester gestations.

Treatment of Acetaminophen Overdose During Pregnancy

The management of the pregnant woman with an acetaminophen overdose should not differ from that of the nonpregnant individual, that is, stabilization, supportive care, appropriate gastrointestinal decontamination, and specific therapy (N-acetylcysteine administration), ideally based on serum acetaminophen concentration determination. The safety of this antidote for the fetus has not been established, but preliminary information is encouraging (38). In any event, *N*-acetylcysteine should not be withheld if the mother is at risk. However, it has been shown to have negligible transplacental passage in sheep (46). Since oral administration in humans produces significantly lower plasma concentrations (46), the intravenous route in the mother seems to be the logical choice for protection of her fetus. Also, the fetal delivery of *N*-acetylcysteine may be compromised after maternal oral administration because of first-pass hepatic uptake, particularly if the maternal liver is in a relatively glutathione-depleted state owing to the acetaminophen overdose. Furthermore, the oral route is often poorly tolerated because of vomiting (47).

Nevertheless, the findings of Selden et al. (46) point to a poor fetal prognosis in significant third-trimester acetaminophen overdose. The limited data available support immediate delivery of a mature fetus, for direct extrauterine *N*-acetylcysteine therapy if the maternal serum acetaminophen concentration is well into the toxic range by nomogram. If the risk for delivery is too great because of fetal immaturity, direct intrauterine cannulation of the umbilical vasculature for *N*-acetylcysteine administration could be considered. However, neither of these options is likely to be practical because of the duration of time required for their organization and implementation.

SALICYLATES

Published Experience

Five reports of in utero salicylate intoxication in pregnant women were found. Three were due to an acute ingestion (48–50), whereas the other two were the result of subacute or chronic toxicity (51,52). There were two deaths, both in the acute group (48,50). Jackson (48), in 1948, described a woman in her eighth month of pregnancy who delivered a 2.7 kg stillborn 17 hours after an overdose of 200 g of acetylsalicylic acid. Although at autopsy tentorial tears and cerebral hemorrhage were found, there was "a high concentration of salicylate" in the cord blood, indicating at least that the fetus was alive prior to the overdose. Nevertheless, the contribution of salicylate toxicity to the fetal demise is unclear. Also, given the mother's benign course, it is unlikely that she actually ingested 200 g of acetylsalicylic acid.

In 1961 Earle (49) described a 3.5 kg neonate whose mother had ingested 15–18 g of acetylsalicylic acid 27 hours prior to delivery. At 20 h of age, the baby was acidemic with a salicylate concentration of 350 mg/L. One hour earlier, the mother's concentration had been 220 mg/L; it had been 380 mg/L 20 h prior to delivery. An exchange transfusion resulted in removal of an estimated 135 mg of salicylate. Since this represents only 40 mg/kg, and is equivalent to two-fifths of a tablet, it is difficult to ascribe benefit to this intervention. Mother and baby did well.

Rejent and Baik described a woman in her eighth month of pregnancy who ingested 36.5 g of acetylsalicylic acid (50). She was manifesting salicylism, but the fetus was not felt to be in distress. However, 20 hours later, the baby was dead. The postmortem fetal serum salicylate concentration was 243 mg/L, with a brain concentration of 200 μg/g. Since the latter amount is similar to fatal brain concentrations in mice (53), it is likely that the fetal death was due to intrauterine salicylate toxicity.

Lynd et al. (51) described a case of chronic intrauterine salicylism in a 2.6 kg male neonate who was irritable and feeding poorly at 36 h of age. It was learned that his mother had self-medicated with undetermined amounts of salicylates throughout her ninth month. The baby was hyperpneic and hypertonic, and he appeared malnourished. His serum salicylate level was 310 mg/L at 36 h. A concentration of 383 mg/L was found upon analysis of the cord blood. The baby was treated with induced diuresis and his condition improved. His irritability, hypertonia, poor feeding, and intrauterine malnutrition may have been due to the salicylism, but other causes such as maternal drug abuse were not conclusively ruled out.

Ahlfors et al. (52) described a 3 kg, 37-week female neonate delivered by cesarean section for fetal distress. Her mother had consumed 3 g of acetylsalicylic acid daily for several days prior to delivery for a flulike illness. Shortly after birth, tachypnea, a compensated metabolic acidosis, and a cord blood concentration of 473 mg/L were documented. An exchange transfusion at 21 h had a negligible effect on the serum salicylate concentration, but the neonate gradually recovered. An interesting observation was that the salicylate displaced bilirubin from its albumin binding sites, thus necessitating interventions to lower bilirubin concentrations to prevent kernicterus.

Pharmacology and Toxicology

The toxic effects of salicylates on the mother are well described elsewhere (54). Because lungs do not function in the fetus, stimulation of respiration is of no concern. However, the ability of salicylates to uncouple oxidative phosphorylation makes them a general cellular poison, with the brain in particular being a target organ because of its inability to compensate with anaerobic energy production. Hill's work with mice supports central nervous system toxicity as the mechanism of death in salicylism (53).

Unlike acetaminophen, the parent compound rather than the metabolite produces the toxicity of salicylate overdose, thus placing the fetus at risk. Several factors would seem to support the hypothesis that there may be a greater fetal than maternal risk. Salicylate traverses the placenta and is found in higher concentrations in the fetus (3,4). The fetus has a lower arterial pH than the adult, making the blood-to-intracellular pH gradient less. Since the drug is a weak acid, this lower gradient favors a relatively greater proportion of the fetal salicylate load entering the central nervous system. In addition, the fetus has less capacity to buffer the acidemic stress imposed by the salicylate and, relative to the mother, a reduced capacity to metabolize and excrete this toxin. Indeed, in at least three cases paired newborn-maternal sera demonstrated salicylate persistence in the neonate (49-51).

Treatment of Salicylate Overdose During Pregnancy

The treatment of salicylate poisoning is supportive care (54). This includes patient stabilization, appropriate gastrointestinal decontamination, administration of fluid, electrolyte and glucose, and, when indicated, an extracorporeal removal intervention. In pregnancy, it is hoped that the positive effects of these maneuvers will be reflected transplacentally. However, several of the previously described fetal factors (higher serum concentrations, larger proportion of salicylate in the brain, lower buffering capacity, and decreased salicylate metabolism) would somewhat negate such benefits. Therefore, when the fetus is potentially viable ex utero, consideration should be given to prompt delivery. This provides the opportunity for direct provision of care to the newborn.

IRON

Published Experience

Prenatal vitamins and iron have been documented as the second most common overdosed drug group during pregnancy (11). A series of 49 cases from the United Kingdom has been published (55). However, the vast majority were either nontoxic or negligibly toxic overdoses, and the retrospective nature of the review makes analysis difficult. We have managed five cases, and there are six other case reports in the literature (20,21,56-60). The most notable observation is that the fetus seems to fare better than the mother.

The literature reports one overdose in the first trimester (56), two in the second (20,21,57), and three during the third (58-60). One case was nontoxic by serum iron concentration and deferoxamine challenge criteria (57). The only fetal death occurred as a spontaneous abortion in a 17-year-old girl who was seriously ill and subsequently died of the overdose (20,21). The other five babies did well, although two maternal deaths (59,60) occurred shortly after the delivery of neonates who showed no signs of iron toxicity. Three mothers were treated with deferoxamine (one second trimester and two third trimester), and these babies were normal. Two other cases occurred prior to deferoxamine availability and were treated with other chelators no longer used in iron poisonin g (56,59). Both these babies did well. Three pregnancies were delivered within 36 h of overdose, and the cord blood or early postpartum serum iron concentrations were in the normal range (58–60). The fetus that died and its placenta were examined histologically for evidence of iron toxicity and for the presence of increased iron. Neither was found (20,21). This is also true for the only other placenta that was examined (58).

Pharmacology and Toxicology

The pathophysiology of acute iron poisoning is well reviewed elsewhere (61, 62). This can be a difficult poisoning to treat, and several aspects of its therapy are controversial (61). Major features of iron poisoning include gastrointestinal hemorrhage, shock, acidosis, hepatic failure, and coagulopathy. Death is usually the result of cardiovascular collapse or hepatic failure. Although the introduction of the specific iron chelator deferoxamine improved the prognosis, optimal use of this antidote has not been established. The well-being of a fetus presents an additional challenge to the management of an already complex problem.

The passage of iron across cellular membranes and its transport throughout the body involve complex processes. Iron, in physiological conditions, exists in its oxidized (ferric) state. Since ferric iron is insoluble, the plasma protein transferrin is required for its transport. Iron traverses membranes by receptor-mediated endocytosis, which is an active, rapid, unidirectional process able to function against a concentration gradient. Transferrin is bound by its specific receptor and is then internalized by endocytosis. The iron is cleaved from the transferrin and retained, whereas the former is returned as apotransferrin. This has been documented as the iron transport system across the human placenta (1,2).

Therefore, only transferrin-bound iron would be eligible for transplacental passage. This is further supported by studies in pregnant ewes (Fig. 1). Despite massive induced hyperferremia, only a negligible amount of iron was passed to the fetus (63). Thus, unlike other poisons discussed in this chapter, the placenta acts as a barrier to iron. This would explain why the fetus seems to do better than the mother. This "placental block" is supported by lack of neonatal hyperferremia (58–60), lack of histological iron toxicity (20,21,58), and two maternal deaths despite survival of the offspring (59,60). Thus, it would seem that the risk to the fetus is not from the iron itself but is secondary to the induced pathophysiological derangements in the mother.

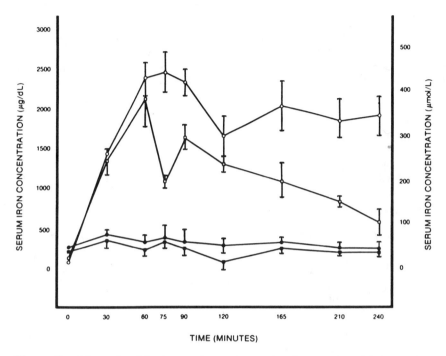

Figure 1 Maternal and fetal serum iron concentrations in control- and deferoxamine-treated animals. Plotted values are mean + / − standard error. Ewes in both groups received 2 mg iron per kg maternal body weight IV over the first 60 minutes. Ewes in the deferoxamine group then received 50 mg deferoxamine mesylate per kg maternal body weight IV over 15 minutes. Open circles = control ewes, solid circles = control fetuses, open squares = deferoxamine ewes, solid squares = deferoxamine fetuses. (By permission, Steven C. Curry, M.D.)

The use of the specific iron chelator deferoxamine during pregnancy is of concern because the product monograph cites it as a proved animal teratogen. These studies have not been published but have been referred to as personal communications in two case reports (57,64). They were briefly described as the prolonged administration of very high doses to pregnant nonhyperferremic mice and rabbits during early gestation. This resulted in skeletal anomalies and decreased ossification in the offspring.

Because deferoxamine is negligibly absorbed across the gastrointestinal tract and is a charged and relatively large molecule, it would not be expected to cross the placenta. Therefore, the adverse effects observed in the rodents would most likely be due to chelation of essential nutrients required for skeletal maturation. This would occur over periods of time more prolonged than would typify the treatment of an iron overdose. In addition, chelation of other nutrients would be less likely in a hyperferremic state.

These speculations are supported by three case reports of deferoxamine therapy during pregnancy (64–66). In two of these, deferoxamine was administered for the first 16 and 19 weeks of pregnancy in thalassemic women (64,65). In the third case, a woman received two intramuscular injections during her tenth week. In no cases was there evidence of teratogenesis. In the three published cases of iron overdose in pregnant women treated with deferoxamine, all the babies did well (57,58,60). However, these were second- and third-trimester pregnancies.

Treatment of Iron Overdose During Pregnancy

Management principles should follow those of the nonpregnant patient (61, 62). The teratogenic risk of deferoxamine is probably overstated. Nevertheless, as in all situations, maternal well-being takes precedence over fetal concerns. The death of an iron-poisoned mother associated with the withholding of deferoxamine because of concern over teratogenesis was especially tragic (20,21).

ORGANOPHOSPHORUS PESTICIDES

Published Experience

At least five cases of organophosphate pesticide poisoning during pregnancy have been described (19,67–69), but two are of limited interest. One of the latter provides only the results of postmortem analysis of various maternal and fetal tissues from a 19-year-old girl who, in her fifth month of pregnancy, committed suicide by ingesting mecarbam (67). The authors demonstrated that this pesticide crosses the placenta and at least in this maternal-fetal pair, was found in higher concentrations in the conceptus. The other is a 24-year-old woman in her third month of pregnancy whose malathion overdose was successfully treated with atropine, obidoxime, and assisted ventilation (68). She underwent a therapeutic abortion 2 months later, and there was no description of the products of conception. Thus, all that can be concluded is that appropriate treatment of organophosphorus poisoning during early pregnancy can result in full recovery of the mother and maintenance of her pregnancy.

Two others, a 22-year-old woman in her 36th week who overdosed with methamidophos, and a 25-year-old in her 16th week poisoned with fenthion, were both appropriately managed with atropine, pralidoxime, and respiratory support (69). No abnormalities of pregnancy were described, and both women delivered normal babies at term. Thus, it is possible to successfully manage organophosphate poisoning in the second and third trimesters.

Perhaps the most interesting is the case report of Weis et al. (19). Although this 21-year-old female in her 34th to 35th week of pregnancy never admitted to ingesting a pesticide, the rapid onset of a severe cholinergic syndrome, the absence of plasma and erythrocyte cholinesterase activity, and the dramatic response to large doses of atropine preclude any other diagnosis. However, the stress of spontaneous onset of labor early on, along with the atropine therapy, resulted in fetal heart rate of 200 beats/min. An emergency cesarean section was done, resulting in the delivery of a small, floppy, depressed neonate. As in the mother, assisted ventilation and atropine infusions were required. Curiously, the mother seemed to have been more severely affected, since she had a longer requirement for assisted ventilation and atropine, her cholinesterases took longer to return to normal, and her therapeuric atropine dose was a toxic dose for the fetus in utero.

Pharmacology and Toxicology

The pathophysiology of acute organophosphorus pesticide is well described elsewhere (70). Of interest is the occurrence of two delayed paralytic syndromes. The better known is a peripheral neuropathy involving the distal extremities (71). Onset is a few weeks after the acute phase and is separated from it by a period of recovery. Respiratory failure is not a feature, and at worse its occurrence could complicate subsequent labor and delivery.

The second paralytic syndrome was described in 1987 as the "intermediate syndrome" (72). It consists of proximal muscle weakness, multiple cranial nerve palsies, and respiratory failure beginning within 24–96 h after ingestion. There may not be an apparent period of recovery between onset and the acute phase. The occurrence of this syndrome along with its required therapeutic interventions represent a more serious risk to pregnancy. Interestingly, this intermediate syndrome occurred in three of the cases above (68,69).

Not surprisingly, little is known regarding the human transplacental passage of the many organophosphate pesticides. However, if maternal toxicity follows ingestion, transgastrointestinal epithelial passage has occurred, making fetal entry a result to be expected. This was confirmed for mecarbam (67). The amount passed on to the fetus relative to the maternal body burden would likely differ from compound to compound. Although mecarbam was found in higher concentration in the fetus (67), the more severe maternal course in the case of Weis et al. (19) suggests a relatively smaller fetal burden in that situation.

Of additional concern is the possibility of innate differences in the sensitivity to organophosphates by maternal and fetal cholinesterase systems.

Decreased activities of neonatal plasma and red cell cholinesterase ranging from 50 to 70% of adult values have been consistently documented (73–75). Therefore, increased fetal sensitivity to cholinesterase-inhibiting pesticides would be expected.

These issues of relative placental passage and potentially differing fetal and maternal sensitivities are important because the chief antidote, atropine, has potent agonistic properties. Therefore, there is the potential for a therapeutic maternal atropine dose being either subtherapeutic or toxic for the fetus.

Treatment of Organophosphorus Insecticide Poisoning During Pregnancy

The basic management in a pregnant woman should not differ from the non-pregnant patient. It includes appropriate life support and gastrointestinal decontamination, meticulous respiratory care, and the administration of atropine and pralidoxime (70). The fetus should be closely monitored. If the maternal condition is satisfactory but distress is documented in a potentially viable fetus, consideration should be given to immediate delivery to permit the initiation of therapy ex utero.

DIGITALIS

Published Experience

With the advent of specific antidotal therapy for digitalis poisoning (76), it is important to discuss poisoning in pregnancy with this drug. However, only one case could be located (77): a 26-year-old woman who during her seventh month of pregnancy ingested 8.9 mg of digitoxin, demonstrating clinical and electrocardiographic evidence of digitalis toxicity. Although the patient was quite ill, she did well with supportive care. On presentation, fetal heart tones were irregular, with a rate of 68 beats/min. They became inaudible for 5 h and were then noted to be 150 beats/min and regular. Spontaneous labor on the fourth day produced a female weighing 2160 g, in poor condition, who died three days postpartum. An electrocardiogram at 15 minutes of age supported a digitalis effect on the neonate. Autopsy findings were consistent with prolonged intrauterine anoxia.

Because this report goes back to 1960, documentation does not meet current standards. Notably absent are serum drug concentrations and sophisticated fetal monitoring data. Nevertheless, there is a strong case for intrauterine digitalis toxicity.

Pharmacology and Toxicology

Acute digitalis poisoning and its treatment with Fab antibody fragments is well described elsewhere (78). Therefore, our discussion is limited to issues pertinent to this problem in pregnancy (the transplacental passage of these cardiac glycosides and of the Fab antidigoxin antibody fragments). Radioactive tracer studies have demonstrated transplacental passage of both digoxin (79) and digitoxin (80) in humans during the first half of pregnancy. This result is further supported by the practice of treating fetal tacharrhythmias with maternal digitalization. Nagashima et al. report three such cases (81). They demonstrated arrhythmia conversion and similar cord and maternal serum digoxin concentrations. They also cite several other similar case reports. Therefore, the fetus is at risk for cardiovascular dysfunction due to maternal cardiac glycoside overdose. Indeed, Sherman and Locke documented fetal bradycardia (77).

Data on the transplacental passage of Fab antibody fragments are lacking. If this antidote does not cross the placenta, its administration to the mother would be of no direct benefit to the fetus. However, transplacental passage is likely, since these fragments are freely excreted in the urine. Nevertheless, a brief case report exploring the use of this agent in eclampsia suggests otherwise (82). This conclusion is questionable, however, since the fetal presence of the fragments was only indirectly inferred from measurements of an endogenous digitalis-like factor, and the maternal, and newborn samples were not simultaneous.

Treatment of Digitalis Poisoning During Pregnancy

The management of the pregnant woman with an acute digitalis overdose should be based on the same principles advised for nonpregnant individuals (78), namely initial stabilization, appropriate gastrointestinal decontamination, measurement of serum electrolyte and digoxin concentrations, cardiac monitoring, and supportive care. In addition, fetal cardiac rhythm should be monitored [with fetal echocardiography (81) if available]. If there is maternal indication (hyperkalemia or life-threatening rhythm disturbances) for the administration of antidigoxin antibody fragment, this should be done even though its safety and efficacy for the fetus is unknown. Hopefully, coexistent fetal cardiac arrhythmias would be simultaneously corrected. If not, a second maternal dose should be considered. If still unsuccessful, a viable fetus could be delivered and the antidote directly administered. In the case of a previable fetus, intrauterine cannulation of the fetal vasculature for direct antidote administration and for possible fetal blood sampling could be considered. Another possibility, albeit seemingly unlikely, would be the occurrence of a fetal indication for antidotal therapy in a healthy mother. If this were to occur, the same approach would seem to be appropriate.

CAMPHOR

Published Experience

Camphor ingestions have become a relative rarity, likely owing to concerted efforts to dissuade the use of this substance. However, since at least four poisonings during pregnancy have been described (83–86), the topic is reviewed for historical interest.

Weiss and Catalano (83) described a 26-year-old woman at term who ingested 60 mL of camphorated oil instead of castor oil. She had two seizures but delivered a normal baby, who had the obvious odor of camphor. Camphor was qualitatively demonstrated in the newborn's blood. Riggs et al. (84) described a 40-year-old woman at term who also ingested 60 mL of camphorated oil instead of castor oil. She too had a seizure. Thirty-six hours later, she delivered a daughter in very poor condition, who died in 30 minutes. Since the course was complicated by preeclampsia, abruptio placentae with hemorrhage, and breech presentation, the contribution of camphor to the fetal demise is uncertain. Camphor was qualitatively demonstrated in the maternal blood, cord blood, and amniotic fluid and in the infant's brain, liver, and kidneys. Blackmon and Curry (85) described a hospitalized 32-year-old women in her third month of pregnancy with a threatened abortion who was given 45 mL of camphorated oil in error. Although the patient had four seizures, she carried to term, delivering a normal baby. Jacobziner and Raybin (86) mentioned in passing a 17-year-old pregnant girl who drank 60 mL of camphorated oil to induce an abortion. Although she recovered and her conceptus remained vital, further details were not given.

Pharmacology, Toxicology, and Treatment

Camphor is both a gastrointestinal irritant and a central nervous system stimulant. Acute symptoms include nausea, vomiting, abdominal pain, tremors, convulsions, and coma. In two of the cases above, placental passage was demonstrated (83,84). The extent of this phenomenon was not quantified. No adverse effects on the conceptus were detected in three of the four cases, and the contribution of camphor to the one postpartum newborn death is uncertain. There is no specific therapy for camphor poisoning.

LEAD

Published Experience

Aspects to be considered in the discussion of lead exposure during pregnancy include spontaneous abortion, teratogenesis, symptoms and signs of toxicity in the mother or infant, and neurodevelopmental sequelae in the offspring. In keeping with the mandate of this chapter, we discuss only maternal and fetal toxicity. Five such case reports were located (87–92). In two of these, only the mothers demonstrated clinical toxicity (87–89), whereas in three others toxicity developed only in the offspring during early infancy (90–92). Two other cases of significantly increased maternal and fetal lead burdens are reviewed even though the mother-child pairs had no evidence of clinical toxicity (93,94).

In 1964 Angle and McIntyre described a woman in her eighth month of pregnancy who complained of fatigue and abdominal pain (87). She had been exposed to the fumes of burning battery casings for the preceding 2 months, and her blood lead concentration was 240 μg/dL. The patient was treated with parenteral calcium disodium edetate (EDTA) for 1 week. Four weeks later she delivered a normal male. Cord blood lead concentration was reported as less than 60 μg/dL. However, the polarographic methodology used in this assay is questionable because of its low sensitivity. The other example of maternal toxicity is a 17-year-old girl who presented in her eighth month of pregnancy with abdominal pain, paresthesias in her feet, calf pain, gingival lead lines, and moderate anemia. She had been eating plaster chips from her apartment walls during her pregnancy. Blood lead and amniotic fluid lead concentrations were 86 and 90 μg/dL, respectively. The patient was treated with a 3-day course of EDTA. At delivery 8 days later, her blood lead had fallen to a near normal of 26 μg/dL, while the cord and amniotic fluid remained elevated at 79 and 86 μg/dL, respectively. There was no evidence of clinical toxicity in the neonate; however, skeletal radiographs demonstrated lead lines in the long bones. The baby was treated with a course of EDTA at 2 weeks and at 5 months of age, and her developmental evaluation was normal at 18 months.

Three cases of fetal lead exposure presenting as toxicity in early infancy were located (90–92). The mothers were asymptomatic. Palmisano et al. (90) described a 2.5-month-old female infant with failure to thrive, hypertonic legs, spontaneous tremors, and hyperactive deep tendon reflexes; she had been born at term with a weight of 1900 g. The mother frequently drank illicit whiskey, which in this region was known to be contaminated by lead. No other sources of lead were found. Although there were no blood lead concentrations, increased lead burdens were documented in both mother and child by urinary excretion criteria. The infant received a 3-day course of EDTA. This baby's intrauterine grown retardation, failure to thrive, and neurological abnormalities cannot solely be attributed to her fetal experience with lead because of the concomitant intrauterine alcohol exposure. However, the following two cases offer more convincing evidence that intrauterine lead acquisition produces toxicity during early infancy.

Sensirivantana et al. (91) described a 2-month-old girl whose symptoms were seizures, anemia, basophilic stippling of red blood cells, skeletal lead lines, and brown nails. There had been a significant exposure to lead fumes during the seventh month of pregnancy because the mother had burned several electric motor rotors in a metal-salvaging operation. Pregnancy, labor, delivery, and neonatal course were otherwise unremarkable. Lead concentration in the maternal hair was markedly elevated, as was the baby's blood concentration (113 μg/dL). Extremely high values were also found in the baby's hair and nails (brown nails). The elevated hair (maternal and child) and nail values as well as the presence of skeletal lead lines support an intrauterine lead acquisition. The infant was treated with dimercaprol, EDTA, and *d*-penicillamine.

The second case, described by Ghafour et al. (92), was a 36-h-old neonate with seizures, opisthotonic posturing, and frequent spasms. Her blood lead concentrations were subsequently found to be elevated at 66 and 81 μg/dL at 12 and 17 days of age, with a maternal value of 76. The mother used lead-glazed cooking utensils and a lead-based eye cosmetic, both known to cause lead poisoning. She had a history of two miscarriages and two other children with neonatal seizures. This baby was treated with both dimercaprol and EDTA.

In the other two reports of fetal lead exposure, both the mother and the baby were asymptomatic. Singh et al. (93) described a 20-year-old woman who sustained an acute lead exposure in the third trimester as a result of removing paint in her home. A blood lead concentration of 61 μg/dL was found, which declined to 39 at delivery with cord blood of 50. Ryu et al. (94) described a normal female neonate whose mother had worked for the past 3 years in a battery manufacturing plant. The mother's blood lead concentration varied from a high of 57 μg/dL to 33 at delivery. Elevated concentrations were also documented in the cord blood and at 3 and 6 days of age.

Pharmacology, Toxicology, and Treatment

Lead serves no useful purpose in the body. It produces chronic rather than acute toxicity, and most individuals with increased body burdens are asymptomatic. Lead is a well-known reproductive toxin, producing spontaneous abortions, decreased fertility, and possible teratogenesis. Exposure to lead during infancy can result in adverse neurodevelopmental sequelae, and it is speculated that the developing fetal nervous system may have an increased sensitivity.

Maternal cord blood screening studies (95–97) as well as several of the case reports above demonstrate that lead freely crosses the placenta. However, it is unlikely that EDTA, the most commonly used lead chelator, enters the fetus. There has been only one well-documented case of EDTA therapy during pregnancy (88,89). Although the mother's blood lead level declined from 86 to 26 μg/dL, the cord blood concentration remained elevated at 79, suggesting nonpassage of this chelator. Furthermore, human studies have demonstrated negligible penetration through the gastrointestinal epithelium, red blood cell membranes, and the blood-brain barrier (98), making transplacental passage unlikely. There are no similar data for dimercaprol, but because it penetrates the central nervous system, fetal penetration would seem more likely. However, its use in adults is seldom indicated. Since dimercaprol must be given intramuscularly and is associated with several adverse effects, it is a poor candidate for maternal administration for fetal benefit.

Dimercaptosuccinic acid (99), a new lead chelator that is structurally similar to dimercaprol and is given orally, seems to be the best choice. However, there is no reported experience with this drug during pregnancy.

Even with a chelator exhibiting good fetal penetration, transplacental chelation would be difficult. Although chelators efficiently clear the blood, this compartment is refilled from tissue stores during the first few days after administration. Thus, prolonged courses would be required; this practice could deny the fetus essential trace elements.

Thus, maternal indications would seem to be the only valid reason for the administration of lead chelators during pregnancy.

MISCELLANEOUS POISONINGS DURING PREGNANCY

The following toxicants are discussed together because of limited experience with women who have ingested them during pregnancy.

Arsenic

Historically, organic arsenicals were used as antisyphilitics and antiparasitics. Iatrogenic toxicities were not uncommon, and Kantor and Levin described one such case during pregnancy and cited others (100). Since other therapeutic agents have long since replaced these compounds, they are not discussed further.

Two cases of acute inorganic arsenic poisonings during pregnancy were found (101,102). A 17-year-old girl in her seventh month of pregnancy ingested a rat poison containing arsenic trioxide (101). She received one dose of dimercaprol 24 h after the ingestion. Three days later, the patient spontaneously delivered an 1100 g female who died of hyaline membrane disease. High concentrations of arsenic were found in the infant's liver, kidneys, and brain. The mother survived, although she required hemodialysis for renal failure in the postpartum period.

A 30-year-old woman in her 28th week of pregnancy was poisoned with arsenic trioxide (102). She survived despite multiple organ failure and adult respiratory distress syndrome. Intrauterine death occurred during the fourth or fifth day after ingestion. Toxic concentrations of arsenic were found in the fetal liver, kidneys, stomach, and spleen.

Both the foregoing cases show that inorganic arsenic freely crosses the placenta, and mother and fetus alike are at risk. Ideally, supportive and specific therapy should be effective for both patients.

The management of arsenic poisoning is well reviewed elsewhere (103). The experience of Lugo et al. (101) regarding the safety of dimercaprol during pregnancy is not helpful, since only one dose was given during the third trimester and the baby died of hyaline membrane disease. Kantor and Levin (100) administered a course of dimercaprol to a woman in her 26th week of pregnancy (iatrogenic organic arsenic toxicity) and concluded that "it probably had no deleterious effect on the pregnancy." However, dimercaptosuccinic acid, an orally effective analog of dimercaprol, is now available for the treatment of lead poisoning (99). It has been widely used elsewhere for arsenic poisoning and seems to be a better choice (104). However, there is no reported experience with this drug during pregnancy.

Paraquat

Overdoses of the herbicide paraquat is associated with a very high mortality. Hemoperfusion, its touted intervention, is at best of questionable efficacy. The few described cases of paraquat poisoning during pregnancy reflect this dismal prognosis (105–107). Because of decreased substrate for free oxygen radical generation, there is at least theoretical advantage for the fetus in the relative hypoxic intrauterine milieu. And since hemoperfusion is of questionable value and technically difficult in the neonate, the argument for nonintervention of a potentially viable pregnancy is tenable unless fetal distress is present.

Nutmeg

The common spice nutmeg has anticholinergic properties, and being an hallucinogen, is abused from time to time. A 29-year-old woman in her 30th week of pregnancy ingested a large amount of nutmeg secondary to a cooking error (108). She experienced mild to moderate anticholinergic syndrome. Fetal tachycardia (170 beats/min) was documented, suggesting transplacental passage. The mother did well with supportive care and delivered a normal baby at term.

Quinine

When quinine overdose occurs during pregnancy, the desire to induce an abortion should be suspected. Dannenberg et al. (7) described 4 such cases and reviewed 66 others. The maternal death rate was 16% and the abortion rate without maternal death was only 4%. In addition, at least 59% of the offspring had congenital anomalies. Therefore, quinine is of dubious efficacy as an abortifacient, has significant associations with maternal morbidity and mortality, and may be teratogenic.

In overdose, quinine produces tinnitus, deafness, nausea. vomiting, vasodilation, visual impairment, and cardiac arrhythmias (109,110). Permanent visual disturbances and blindness are potential sequelae. Fatalities usually are due to cardiac toxicity. Treatment is nonspecific (general supportive measures and gastrointestinal decontamination as needed). From a theoretical perspective, acid diuresis would hasten the renal elimination of quinine and is often touted in the management of this poisoning. However, this intervention as well as dialysis and hemoperfusion have been shown to be ineffective (109). Since these are far from benign interventions, they should be avoided.

Naphthalene

Naphthalene poisoning during pregnancy has been twice reported (111,112). In both instances, the mothers were chronic mothball ingestors who presented at term with a hemolytic anemia. Hemolytic anemia and jaundice were found in both babies in the immediate postpartum period. Management of this problem should include the discontinuation of the ingestion of naphthalene and transfusion therapy of both mother and newborn as indicated. The latter should be monitored for hyperbilirubinemia and managed accordingly. It is conceivable that fetal anemia may be identified prior to term. In such instances, intrauterine transfusion should be considered.

Ciguatera

Ciguatera is a fishborne food poisoning characterized by gastrointestinal and neurological symptoms occurring within a few hours of ingestion (113). Two cases of ciguatera poisoning during pregnancy have been reported (114,115).

One patient was in the early part of her second trimester (114). She had typical symptoms soon after ingestion, including increased fetal movements that persisted for a few hours. Her baby was normal at term and for the 10 months that he was followed thereafter. There were no neurological or muscular abnormalities. The other case involved a woman at term (115). She also developed typical symptoms soon after ingestion of the bad fish, and she experienced "bizarre," "tumultuous" fetal movements for 24 hours. An elective cesarean section 2 days later produced a term male with left-sided facial palsy and possible myotonia of the hands. The liquor was meconium stained, and a mild meconium aspiration syndrome was managed without assisted ventilation. In both instances assays of specimens from the fish confirmed ciguatera poisoning. The differences in the two newborns are probably a consequence of the timing of the fetal exposures. The treatment of this poisoning is symptomatic and supportive (114).

Amanita phalloides

Poisoning during pregnancy with *Amanita phalloides*, a very toxic wild mushroom, has been briefly documented in a 21-year-old woman in her eighth month of pregnancy (116). Early in her course, both blood and amniotic fluid were sampled for the toxin. The former was positive and the latter was negative. Two months later, a healthy baby without biochemical evidence of hepatotoxicity was born. Belliardo et al. (116) suggest that their negative amniotic fluid assay and the neonate's lack of hepatotoxicity support nonpassage of the toxin across the placenta. More data are needed to support this claim.

Poisonous Snake Bites

Dunnihoo et al. (117) reviewed the literature on poisoning by members of the Crotalidae family (rattlesnakes, cottonmouths, and copperheads) during pregnancy. The venom of these reptiles has procoagulant activity. The authors described 30 cases in limited detail. The maternal mortality rate was 10%, and fetal wastage (intrauterine deaths plus spontaneous abortions) was 43%.

There was no mention of antivenin therapy. Significant transplacental passage of this antidote would seem unlikely because of its high molecular weight. This, along with an apparent increase in risk for the fetus, prompts consideration of emergency delivery of a mature fetus in cases of severe maternal envenomation. However, this decision must be balanced against the risk this procedure presents to a mother with compromised coagulation.

Answer

This young woman has ingested acetaminophen in a toxic dose, where fatalities are not uncommon. She postponed treatment, thus substantially further increasing her risk for severe, or even fatal liver damage. Recent research suggests that N-acetylcysteine (NAC) therapy may have some efficacy even at this late stage. Her general status and especially liver function should be closely followed. In some institutions she may receive NAC even at this stage. Although the drug has been implicated in interrupting collagen formation in some babies, there is no clear-cut established causation. Available literature, although scarce, suggests that the fetus has an increased risk of liver damage and stillbirth.

REFERENCES

1. Aisen P, Brown EB. The iron binding function of transferrin in iron metabolism. Semin Hemat 1977; 14:31–53.
2. Huebers HA, Finch CA. Transferrin. Physiologic behavior and clinical implications. Blood 1984; 64:763–767.
3. Garrettson LK, Procknal JA, Levy G. Fetal acquisition and neonatal elimination of a large amount of salicylate. Clin Pharmacol Ther 1975; 17:98–103.
4. Levy G, Procknal JA, Garrettson LK. Distribution of salicylate between neonatal and maternal serum at diffusion equilibrium. Clin Pharmacol Ther 1975; 18:210–214.
5. Czeizel A, Szentesi I, Szekeres J, Glauber A, Bucski P, Molnar C. Pregnancy outcome and health conditions of offspring of self-poisoned women. Acta Pediatr Hung 1984; 25:209–236.
6. Sim M. Abortion and the psychiatrist. Br Med J 1963; 2:145–148.
7. Dannenberg AL, Dorfman SF, Johnson J. Use of quinine for self-induced abortion. South Med J 1983; 76:846–849.
8. Hall A. The increasing use of lead as an abortifacient. Br Med J 1905; 1:584–587.
9. Gold J, Cates W Jr. Herbal abortifacients. JAMA 1980; 243:1365–1366.
10. Whitlock FA, Edwards JE. Pregnancy and attempted suicide. Comp Psychiatry 1968; 9:1–12.
11. Rayburn W, Aronow R, Delancy B, Hogan MJ. Drug overdose during pregnancy. An overview from a metropolitan poison control center. Obstet Gynecol 1984; 64:611–614.
12. Czeizel A, Szentesi I, Molnar G. Lack of effect of self-poisoning on subsequent reproductive outcome. Mutat Res 1984; 127:175–182.
13. Kulig K. Initial management of ingestions of toxic substances. N Engl J Med 1992; 326:1677–1681.

14. Kulig K, Bar-Or D, Cantrill SV, Rosen P, Rumack BH. Management of acutely poisoned patients without gastric emptying. Ann Emerg Med 1985; 14:562–567.
15. Albertson TE, Derlet RW, Foulke GE, Minguillon MC, Tharratt SR. Superiority of activated charcoal alone compared with ipecac and activated charcoal in the treatment of acute toxic ingestions. Ann Emerg Med 1989; 18:56–59.
16. Merigian KS, Woodard M, Hedges J Jr, Roberts J Jr, Stuebing R, Rashkin MC. Prospective evaluation of gastric emptying in the self-poisoning patient. Am J Emerg Med 1990; 8:479–483.
17. Tenenbein M. Whole bowel irrigation as a gastrointestinal decontamination procedure after acute poisoning. Med Toxicol 1988; 3:77–84.
18. Van Ameyde KJ, Tenenbein M. Whole bowel irrigation during pregnancy. Am J Obstet Gynecol 1989; 160:646–647.
19. Weis OF, Muller FO, Lyell H, Badenhorst CH, van Niekerk P. Materno-fetal cholinesterase inhibitor poisoning. Anesth Analg 1983; 62:233–235.
20. Strom RL, Schiller P, Seeds AF, ten Bensel R. Fatal iron poisoning in a pregnant female. Minn Med 1976; 59:483–489.
21. Manoguerra AS. Iron poisoning. Report of a fatal case in an adult. Am J Hosp Pharm 1976; 33:1088–1090.
22. Theil GB, Richter RW, Powell MR, Doolan PD. Acute Dilantin poisoning. Neurology 1961; 11:138–142.
23. Kurtz GG, Michael UF, Morosi HJ, Vaamonde CA. Hemodialysis during pregnancy. Report of a case of glutethimide poisoning complicated by acute renal failure. Arch Intern Med 1966; 118:30–32.
24. Vaziri ND, Kumar KP, Mirahmadi K, Rosen SM. Hemodialysis in treatment of acute chloral hydrate poisoning. South Med J 1977; 70:377–378.
25. Trebbin WM. Hemodialysis in pregnancy. JAMA 1979; 241:1811–1812.
26. Wing AJ, Brunner FP, Brynger H, Chantler C, Donckerwoicke RA, Gurland HJ, Jacobs C, Mansell MA. Successful pregnancies in women treated by dialysis and kidney transplantation. Br J Obstet Gynecol 1980; 87:839–845.
27. Hou S. Pregnancy in women requiring dialysis for renal failure. Am J Kidney Dis 1987; 368–373.
28. Rayburn W, Wible-Kant J, Bledsoe P. Changing trends in drug use during pregnancy. J Reprod Med 1982; 27:569–575.
29. Silverman JJ, Carithers RL Jr. Acetaminophen overdose. Am J Psychiatry 1978; 135:114–115.
30. Byer AJ, Trayler TR, Semmer JR. Acetaminophen overdose in the third trimester of pregnancy. JAMA 1982; 247:3114–3115.
31. Lederman S, Fysh WJ, Tredger M, Gamsu HR. Neonatal paracetamol poisoning. Treatment by exchange transfusion. Arch Dis Child 1983; 58:631–633.
32. Ruthnum P, Goel KM. ABC of poisoning: Paracetamol. Br Med J 1984; 289:1538–1539.
33. Stokes IM. Paracetamol overdose in the second trimester of pregnancy. Br J Obstet Gynaecol 1984; 91:286–288.
34. Roberts I, Robinson MJ, Mughal MZ, Ratcliffe JG, Prescott LF. Paracetamol metabolites in the neonate following maternal overdose. Br J Clin Pharmacol 1984; 18:201–206.

35. Haibach H, Akhter JE, Muscato MS, Cary PL, Hoffman MF. Acetaminophen overdose with fetal demise. Am J Clin Pathol 1984; 82:240–242.
36. Robertson RG, Van Cleave BL, Collins JJ Jr. Acetaminophen overdose in the second trimester of pregnancy. J Fam Pract 1986; 23:267–268.
37. Ludmir J, Main DM, Landon MB, Gabbe SG. Maternal acetaminophen overdose at 15 weeks of gestation. Obstet Gynecol 1986; 67:750–751.
38. Riggs BS, Bronstein AC, Kulig K, Archer PG, Rumack BH. Acute acetaminophen overdose during pregnancy. Obstet Gynecol 1989; 74:247–253.
39. McElhatton PT, Sullivan GM, Volans GN, Fitzpatrick R. Paracetamol overdose during pregnancy: An analysis of the outcomes of cases referred to the Teratology Information Service of the National Poison Information Service. Hum Exp Toxicol 1990; 9:147–153.
40. Levy G, Garrettson LK, Soda DM. Evidence of placental transfer of acetaminophen. Pediatrics 1975; 55:895.
41. Jackson CH, MacDonald NC, Cornett JWD. Acetaminophen. A practical pharmacologic review. Can Med Assoc J 1984; 131:25–37.
42. Lauterberg BH, Corcoran GB, Mitchell JR. Mechanism of action of N-acetylcysteine in the protection against hepatotoxicity of acetaminophen in rats in vivo. J Clin Invest 1983; 71:980–991.
43. Rane A, Tomson G. Prenatal and neonatal drug metabolism in man. Eur J Clin Pharmacol 1980; 18:9–15.
44. Perucca E. Drug metabolism in pregnancy, infancy and childhood. Pharmacol Ther 1987; 34:129–143.
45. Rollins DE, von Bahr C, Glaumann H, Moldeus P, Rane A. Acetaminophen. Potentially toxic metabolite formed by human fetal and adult liver microsomes and isolated fetal liver cells. Science 1979; 205:1414–1416.
46. Selden BS, Curry SC, Clark RF, Johnson BC, Meinhart R, Pizziconi VB. Transplacental transport of N-acetylcysteins in an ovine model. Ann Emerg Med 1991; 20:1069–1072.
47. Prescott LF. Treatment of severe acetaminophen poisoning with intravenous acetylcysteine. Arch Intern Med 1981; 141:386–389.
48. Jackson AV. Toxic effects of salicylate on the fetus and mother. J Pathol Bacteriol 1948; 60:587–593.
49. Earle R Jr. Congenital salicylate intoxication — Report of a case. N Engl J Med 1961; 265:1003–1004.
50. Rejent TA, Baik S. Fatal in utero salicylism. J Forensic Sci 1985; 30:942–944.
51. Lynd PA, Andreasen AC, Wyatt RJ. Intrauterine salicylate intoxication in a newborn. Clin Pediatr (Phil) 1976; 15:912–913.
52. Ahlfors CE, Shwer ML, Ford KW. Bilirubin-albumin binding in neonatal salicylate intoxication. Dev Pharmacol Ther 1982; 4:47–60.
53. Hill JB. Salicylate intoxication. N Engl J Med 1973; 288:1110–1113.
54. Temple AR. Acute and chronic effects of aspirin toxicity and their treatment. Arch Intern Med Med 1981; 141:364–369.
55. McElhatton PR, Roberts JC, Sullivan FM. The consequences of iron overdose and its treatment with desferrioxamine in pregnancy. Hum Exp Toxicol 1991; 10:251–259.

56. Dugdale AE, Powel LW. Acute iron poisoning. Its effects and treatment. Med J Aust 1965; 2:990–992.
57. Blanc P, Hryhorczuk D, Danel I. Deferoxamine treatment of acute iron intoxication in pregnancy. Obstet Gynecol 1984; 64:12S–14S.
58. Rayburn WF, Donn SM, Wulf ME. Iron overdose during pregnancy. Successful therapy with deferoxamine. Am J Obstet Gynecol 1983; 147:717–718.
59. Richards R, Brooks SEH. Ferrous sulphate poisoning in pregnancy with afibrinogenaemia as a complication. West Indian Med J 1966; 15:134–140.
60. Olenmark M, Biber B, Dottori O, Rybo G. Fatal iron intoxication in late pregnancy. J Toxicol Clin Toxicol 1987; 25:347–359.
61. Banner W Jr, Tong TG. Iron poisoning. Pediatr Clin North Am 1986; 33:393–409.
62. Proudfoot AT, Simpson D, Dyson EH. Management of acute iron poisoning. Med Toxicol 1986; 1:83–100.
63. Curry SC, Bond GR, Raschke R, Tellez D, Wiggins D. An ovine model of maternal iron poisoning in pregnancy. Ann Emerg Med 1990; 19:632–638.
64. Thomas RM, Skalicka AE. Successful pregnancy in transfusion-dependent thalassemia. Arch Dis Child 1980; 55:572–574.
65. Martin K. Successful pregnancy in β-thalassemia major. Aust Paediatr J 1983; 19:182–183.
66. Christiaens GCML, Rijksen G, Marx J, Hofsteded P, Staal GEJ. Desferrioxamine in pregnancy. Arch Gynecol 1985; 237(suppl):80.
67. Papadopoulou-Tsoukali H, Njau S. Mother-fetus postmortem toxicologic analysis in a fatal overdose with mecarbam. Forensic Sci Int 1987; 35:249–152.
68. Gadoth N, Fisher A. Late onset of neuromuscular block in organophosphorus poisoning. Ann Intern Med 1978; 88:654–655.
69. Karalliedde L, Senanayake N, Ariaratam A. Acute organophosphorus insecticide poisoning during pregnancy. Hum Toxicol 1988; 7:363–364.
70. Tafuri J, Roberts J. Organophosphate poisoning. Ann Emerg Med 1987; 16:193–202.
71. Sananayake N, Johnson MK. Acute polyneuropathy after poisoning by a new organophosphate insecticide. N Engl J Med 1982; 306:155–157.
72. Sananayazke N, Karalliedde L. Neurotoxic effects of organophosphorus insecticides. An intermediate syndrome. N Engl J Med 1987; 316:761–763.
73. Jones PEH, McCance RA. Enzyme activities in the blood of infants and adults. Biochem J 1949; 45:464–467.
74. Zsigmond EK, Downs JR. Plasma cholinesterase activity in newborns and infants. Can Anaesth Soc J 1971; 18:278–285.
75. Karlsen RL, Sterri S, Lyngaas S, Fonnum F. Reference values for erythrocyte acetylcholinesterase and plasma cholinesterase activities in children, implications for organophosphate intoxication. Scand J Clin Lab Invest 1981; 41:301–302.
76. Smith TW, Butler VP Jr, Haber F, Fozzard H, Marcus FI, Bremner WF, Schulman IC, Phillips A. Treatment of life-threatening digitalis intoxication with digoxin-specific Fab antibody fragments. Experience in 26 cases. N Engl J Med 1982; 307:1357–1362.

77. Sherman JL Jr, Locke RV. Transplacental neonate digitalis intoxication. Am J Cardiol 1960; 6:834–837.
78. Ellenhorn MJ, Barceloux DG. Digitalis. In Medical Toxicology. Diagnosis and Treatment of Human Poisoning, Elsevier, New York, 1988, pp 200–207.
79. Saarikoski S. Placental transfer and fetal uptake of H-digoxin in humans. Br J Obstet Gynaecol 1976; 83:879–884.
80. Okita GT, Plotz EJ, Dans ME. Placental transfer of radioactive digitoxin in pregnant women and its fetal distribution. Circ Res 1956; 4:376–380.
81. Nagashima M, Asai T, Suzuki C, Matsushima M, Ogawa A. Intrauterine supraventricular tacharrhythmias and transplacental digitalization. Arch Dis Child 1986; 61:996–1000.
82. Goodlin RC. Antidigoxin antibodies in eclampsia. N Engl J Med 1988; 318: 518–519.
83. Weiss J, Catalano P. Camphorated oil intoxication during pregnancy. Pediatrics 1973; 52:713–714.
84. Riggs J, Hamilton R, Hamel S, McCabe J. Camphorated oil intoxication in pregnancy. Obstet Gynecol 1965; 25:255–258.
85. Blackmon WP, Curry HB. Camphor poisoning. Report of case occurring during pregnancy. J Fla Med Assoc 1957; 43:999–1000.
86. Jacobziner H, Raybin HW. Camphor poisoning. Arch Pediatr 1962; 79:28–30.
87. Angle CR, McIntire MS. Lead poisoning during pregnancy. Am J Dis Child 1964; 108:436–439.
88. Pearl M, Boxt LM. Radiographic findings in congenital lead poisoning. Radiology 1980; 136:83–84.
89. Timpo AE, Amin JS, Casalino MB, Yuceoglu AM. Congenital lead intoxication. J Pediatr 1979; 94:765–767.
90. Palmisano PA, Sneed RC, Cassady G. Untaxed whiskey and fetal lead exposure. J Pediatr 1969; 75:869–872.
91. Sensirivantana R, Supachadhiwong O, Phancharoen S, Mitrakul C. Neonatal lead poisoning. Clin Pediatr (Phil) 1983; 22:582–584.
92. Ghafour SY, Khuffash FA, Ibrahim HS, Reavey PC. Congenital lead intoxication with seizures due to prenatal exposure. Clin Pediatr (Phil) 1984; 23:282–283.
93. Singh N, Donovan CM, Hanshaw JB. Neonatal lead intoxication in a prenatally exposed infant. J Pediatr 1978; 93:1019–1021.
94. Ryu JE, Ziegler EE, Fomon SJ. Maternal lead exposure and blood lead concentration in infancy. J Pediatr 1978; 93:476–478.
95. Gershanik JJ, Brooks GG, Little JA. Blood lead values in pregnant women and their offspring. Am J Obstet Gynecol 1974; 119:508–511.
96. Zetterlund B, Winberg J, Lundgren G, Johansson G. Lead in umbilical cord blood correlated with the blood lead of the mother in areas of low, medium or high atmospheric pollution. Acta Paediatr Scand 1977; 66:169–175.
97. Angell NF, Lavery JP. The relationship of blood lead levels to obstetric outcome. Am J Obstet Gynecol 1982; 142:40–45.
98. Foreman H, Trujillo TT. The metabolism of C-14 labeled ethylenediaminetetraacetic acid in human beings. J Lab Clin Med 1954; 43:566–571.

99. Graziano JH, Siris ES, Loiancono N, Silverberg SJ, Turgeon L. 2,3-Dimer-captosuccinic acid as an antidote for lead intoxication. Clin Pharmacol Ther 1985; 37:431–438.

100. Kantor HI, Levin PM. Arsenical encephalopathy in pregnancy with recovery. Am J Obstet Gynecol 1948; 56:370–374.

101. Lugo G, Cassady G, Palmisano P. Acute maternal arsenic intoxication with neonatal death. Am J Dis Child 1969; 117:328–330.

102. Bolliger CT, van Zijl P, Louw JA. Multiple organ failure with the adult respiratory distress syndrome in homicidal arsenic poisoning. Respiration 1992; 59:57–61.

103. Ellenhorn MJ, Barceloux DG. Arsenic. In Medical Toxicology. Diagnosis and Treatment of Human Poisonings, Elsevier, New York, 1988, pp 1012–1016.

104. Aposhian HV. DMSA and DMPS — Water-soluble antidotes for heavy metal poisoning. Annu Rev Pharmacol Toxicol 1983; 23:193–215.

105. Talbot AR, Fu CC. Paraquat intoxication during pregnancy. A report of 9 cases. Vet Hum Toxicol 1988; 30:12–17.

106. Fennelly JJ, Gallagher JT, Carroll RJ. Paraquat poisoning in a pregnant woman. Br Med J 1968; 3:722–725.

107. Musson FA, Porter CA. Effect of ingestion of paraquat on a 20-week gestation fetus. Postgrad Med J 1982; 58:731–732.

108. Lavy G. Nutmeg intoxication in pregnancy. J Reprod Med 1987; 32:63–64.

109. Batemman DN, Blin PG, Woodhouse KW, Rawlins MD, Dyson H, Heyworth R, Prescott LF, Proudfoot AT. Pharmacokinetics and clinical toxicity of quinine overdose. Lack of efficacy of techniques intended to enhance elimination. Q J Med 1985; 54:125–131.

110. Dyson EH, Proudfoot AT, Prescott LF, Heyworth R. Death and blindness due to overdose of quinine. Br Med J 1985; 291:31–33.

111. Anziulewicz JA, Dick HJ, Chiarulli EE. Transplacental naphthalene poisoning. Am J Obstet Gynecol 1959; 78:519–521.

112. Zinkham WH, Childs B. A defect of glutathione metabolism in erythrocytes from patients with a naphthalene-induced hemolytic anemia. Pediatrics 1958; 22:461–471.

113. Gillespie NC, Lewis RJ, Pearn JH, Bourke ATC, Holmes MJ, Bourke JB, Shields WJ. Ciguatera in Australia. Occurrence, clinical features, pathophysiology and management. Med J Aust 1986; 145:584–590.

114. Senecal PE, Osterloh JD. Normal fetal outcome after maternal ciguateric toxin exposure in the second trimester. J Toxicol Clin Toxicol 1991; 29:473–478.

115. Pearn J, Harvey P, DeAmbrosis W, Lewis R, McKay R. Ciguatera and pregnancy. Med J Aust 1982; 1:57–58.

116. Belliardo F, Massano G, Accomo S. Amatoxins do not cross the placental barrier. Lancet 1983; 1:1381.

117. Dunnihoo DR, Rush BM, Wise RB, Brooks GG, Otterson WN. Snake bite poisoning in pregnancy. A review of the literature. J Reprod Med 1992; 37: 653–658.

12

A Multicenter, Prospective Study of Fetal Outcome Following Accidental Carbon Monoxide Poisoning in Pregnancy

Gideon Koren, Teresa Sharav, and Anne Pastuszak
The Hospital for Sick Children, Toronto, Ontario, Canada

Lorne K. Garrettson
Emory University, Atlanta, Georgia

R. Kelly Hill, Jr.
Our Lady of the Lake Regional Medical Center, Baton Rouge, Louisiana

Ivan Samson
Community Group Health Centre, St. Catherines, Ontario, Canada

Mark Rorem
Geisinger Medical Center, Danville, Pennsylvania

Arlene King
Fairview Health Complex, Fairview, Alberta, Canada

Jill E. Dolgin
Children's Hospital of Buffalo, Buffalo, New York

Clinical Case

At 16 weeks of gestation a woman was poisoned by carbon monoxide from a leak in the family's furnace. She got up in the morning with dizziness, severe headache, and palpitations. The family's dog had died. The patient's carboxyhemoglobin level 2 hours after leaving the house, before any treatment, was 25%. The fetus appears to be doing well clinically and by ultrasound examination, but the patient wants to know the risks to the baby.

Reprinted with permission of Pergamon Press, from Reproductive Toxicology 1991; 5:397–403.

INTRODUCTION

Carbon monoxide (CO) poisoning accounts for many fatalities in North America and Europe. This odorless, colorless gas binds to hemoglobin 250 times more avidly than oxygen does and reduces the capacity of the blood to transport oxygen. In addition, CO poisons a variety of intracellular enzymes, including cytochrome oxidase and cytochrome P-450, further impairing cellular respiration.

Carbon monoxide readily crosses the placenta and, although it takes several hours for fetal carboxyhemoglobin to equilibrate with maternal levels, final fetal concentrations are higher because fetal hemoglobin has greater affinity for the gas (1). Equally important, the elimination half-life of CO from the fetal circulation is longer than from the maternal circulation (1).

While the hypoxic damage of CO to the fetus is biologically predictable, available experience is sketchy, retrospective, and uncontrolled.

Most reported cases in the literature involved severe poisoning, often with loss of maternal consciousness; in many of these, stillbirths and anoxic fetal brain damage were noted (2–32). However, as documented by the National Data Collection System of the American Association of Poison Control Centers, most cases of CO poisoning are not severe (33). While the adult or pediatric patient can be expected to recover completely from less severe poisoning, no study has addressed fetal safety following exposure at lower grades of CO poisoning, especially when the pregnant woman does not exhibit changes in state of consciousness.

In the past, there have been no data to permit the construction of a dose-response relationship of CO toxicity on the human fetus; consequently it has been impossible to counsel the pregnant woman and her family on the likelihood of the unborn baby suffering permanent anoxic damage. While available case reports partially address the risk of severe cases (2–32), the lack of a denominator (i.e., total number of exposed cases in pregnancy) precludes an accurate risk assessment. More important, available reports have not dealt with the more commonly occurring mild or moderate maternal poisoning.

The Motherisk Program in Toronto is an antenatal counseling clinic for women exposed to drugs, chemicals, radiation, and infections in pregnancy and lactation (34). Lack of data to help counsel women with mild-to-moderate carbon monoxide poisoning in pregnancy led us to conduct this prospective, multicenter study.

PATIENTS AND METHODS

In October 1985, letters explaining the purpose of the study were sent to all the listed poison control centers in North America, to various hyperbaric treatment units, and to teratogen information programs. In addition, the study was advertised at the annual meetings of the American Academy of Clinical Toxicology, the American Board of Medical Toxicology, the American Association of Poison Control Centers, and the Canadian Association of Poison Control Centres, and in the official journals of these organizations (35). Referrals were, in most instances, by telephone to the Motherisk Program or, less frequently, by mail. When a referral was made by a physician, the study questionnaire was sent to him or her to complete, in addition to the information obtained by the telephone. When the contact was made by the pregnant woman, she was interviewed according to the same protocol and referred to her physician. Women living within a reasonable distance of Toronto were offered the opportunity of counseling at the Motherisk Clinic.

The questionnaire explored the type and duration of CO exposure, nature and severity of symptoms, time elapsed before treatment (if any), carboxyhemoglobin (COHb) levels, and measurements of the CO in the ambient air. In six cases we estimated COHb levels from the known ambient CO concentrations (38). The type, timing, and duration of treatment (e.g., hyperbaric or high flow oxygen) were recorded. A general medical and obstetric history was obtained, including cigarette smoking, alcohol consumption, and nonmedical drug/chemical use in pregnancy. The clinical severity of the CO exposure was graded according to the system used by the New York Hyperbaric Group (Table 1) (36).

A second telephone contact was made a few weeks after the expected day of confinement to record the final course of pregnancy and birth. Infant follow-up was repeated annually by telephone and included items concerning health and physical growth. A developmental questionnaire derived from the Denver Developmental Screening Test (37) was used. Detailed, structured

Table 1 Severity of CO Exposure

Grade 1	Alert, oriented
	Symptoms: headache, dizziness, nausea
Grade 1 +	As above but a relative was unconscious
Grade 2	Alert, alterations of mental state
	Symptoms: more pronounced than above
Grade 3	Not alert, disorientation, loss of recent memory, muscle weakness or incoordination
Grade 4	Disoriented, depressed sensorium, response to simple commands limited and inappropriate
Grade 5	Comatose, responding only to pain or not responding to any stimulus

Source: Ref. 36.

questions were asked of the mother by a developmental pediatrician to determine milestones in the areas of gross motor, adaptive, language, and personal social development. In addition, an attempt was made to obtain qualitative information of the child's development, including not only milestones but whether the child was floppy or hypertonic or showed inappropriate lateralization. Structured questions were asked about the child's temperament and behavior, the mother's own assessment of the child, and any anxieties she might have concerning his or her health or development.

DATA ANALYSIS

We recorded fetal outcome and correlated it with the severity of maternal exposure by stratifying the exposures to mild stages (grades 1–2) versus severe stages (grades 3–5).

STATISTICAL ANALYSIS

Means of values among subgroups (birth weight by trimester of CO exposure) were compared by analysis of variance. Differences in proportions of adverse pregnancy outcome in relation to grade of clinical severity (grades 1–2 vs. 3–5) were compared by the Fisher's exact test.

RESULTS

Between December 1985 and March 1989, a total of 40 cases of CO poisoning during pregnancy were collected. Their geographical locations are presented in Table 2. All pregnant women were in good health prior to the CO poisoning and had not suffered from a known chronic illness. The 40 pregnancies included three twin births, one termination of pregnancy at 16 weeks gestation, and four pending births. Analyses are based on a total of 38 babies. The CO poisoning was secondary to malfunctioning furnaces in 23 cases; also implicated were malfunctioning water heaters ($n = 7$), car fumes ($n = 6$), methylene chloride ($n = 3$), and yacht engine fumes ($n = 1$). The exposure occurred during the first trimester in 12 pregnancies, second trimester in 14, and third trimester in 14. The clinical grade of poisoning was based on clinical symptoms and signs in all cases. Table 3 summarizes cases for which COHb levels were available or could be estimated from the known ambient CO concentrations.

The trimester at the time of CO exposure did not affect mean birth weight. Mean birth weight of the infants was 3.4 ± 0.5 kg, excluding the three twin pregnancies, whose mean birth weight was 2.1 ± 0.9 kg, two infants of moth-

Table 2 Geographic Distribution of CO Poisoning in Pregnancy

Province or state	Number
Ontario (Canada)	18[a]
Wisconsin	5
Pennsylvania	3
Alberta (Canada)	2
Georgia	2
Louisiana	2
Minnesota	2
Connecticut	2
Illinois	1
Nebraska	1
New York	1
Ohio	1
	40

[a]Of this number, eight were from Toronto.

ers who smoked more than 20 cigarettes a day during pregnancy (birth weights 3.4 and 3.9 kg), and an infant exposed at term.

Table 4 presents stratification of clinical severity of CO outcomes (grades 1–2 vs. 4–5) by proportion of adverse pregnancy outcome. Adverse fetal outcome occurred only after grade 4 or 5 poisoning. There were two cases with grade 5 symptoms. The first case, a stillbirth at 29 weeks of gestation with COHb level of 26%, was treated with high flow oxygen. The second case for which COHb levels were available resulted in fetal death at term, followed by maternal demise. In both cases fetal death was temporally related to the poisoning.

Of the three cases with grade 4 severity, two pregnancies resulted in normal fetal outcome and one infant was diagnosed as having cerebral palsy at the age of 8 months. The two women who had grade 4 poisoning and had normal outcome were exposed to CO at 27 and 28 weeks gestation, had COHb levels of 39 and 21%, respectively, an hour after the end of exposure, and were treated with hyperbaric oxygen. Both infants were developing well at one year of age. The women with grade 4 symptoms and adverse outcome was poisoned by CO at 23 weeks of gestation and had a COHb of 25%, measured 2 hours after the exposure. She was treated with high flow 100% oxygen for 2 hours. The remainder of the pregnancy was uneventful, and a baby girl was born at term after an uneventful delivery, with birth weight of 4 kg. The infant had an apneic spell immediately after birth, but there was no

Table 3 Relationship Between Measured or Calculated COHb, Clinical Scoring, and Fetal Outcome

COHb (%)	Time of exam (h) after exposure[a]	Grade	Treatment[b]	Length treatment (h)	Outcome
40–50	2	5	HfO_2	2	Elective termination
39	2	4	$HybO_2$	2	Normal
26	1	4	HfO_2	3	Stillborn
25	2	4	HfO_2	2	Cerebral palsy
21	2	4	$HybO_2$	2	Normal
18	nk	1	HfO_2	12	Normal
14	nk	1	nil		Normal
13.8	1	2	HfO_2	7	
			$+ HybO_2$	2	Normal
6.2	1.5	1	nil		Normal
2.4	nk	1	nil		Normal
0.8	2	1	nil		Normal
2	nk	1	nil		Normal
Indirect measures of exposure (converted from ambient ppm)					
32[c]	2	1+	HfO_2	12	Normal DQ
32		1+	nil		Fetal bradycardia
32		1	nil		Normal
14		1	nil		Normal
14		1	nil		36 weeks gestation
5		1	nil		Normal

[a]nk, not known.
[b]$HybO_2$, hyperbaric oxygen; HfO_2, high flow oxygen.
[c]COHb measurement of affected son.

Table 4 Outcome of Pregnancy as Related to Severity of CO Poisoning and Treatment

Outcome	Grades 1 and 2	Grades 4 and 5[a] Hyperbaric O_2	High flow O_2
Normal	31	2	0
Adverse	0	0	3

[a]Grades 4 and 5 were associated with significantly worse outcome compared with grades 1 and 2 ($p < 0.0001$, Fisher's exact test).

recurrence. At 8 months she was examined by a neurologist because head control was poor and developmental delay had been noted. A CAT scan showed enlargement of the ventricles, bilateral calcification in the basal ganglia, and altered white matter density. The changes were judged to be compatible with postanoxic encephalopathy.

There were two cases with grade 2 severity. One woman was exposed at 20 weeks gestation and the baby, born at 25 weeks, had respiratory distress syndrome and jaundice. Follow-up at 3 months of age showed the infant to be developing appropriately. The second grade 2 poisoning occurred at 30 weeks gestation; maternal COHb was 13.8% at the time of exposure, and the patient was treated initially with high flow oxygen for 7 hours followed by 2 hours of hyperbaric oxygen. The rest of this pregnancy was uneventful and resulted in delivery of a 3.2 kg infant who was developing normally at 3 weeks.

All infants born to mothers with grade 1 symptoms had a normal outcome. Some of these women were treated with high flow oxygen ($n = 10$), but most of them were untreated after cessation of CO exposure ($n = 19$).

To date, follow-up has been completed at 3 years in six children, 2 years in six children, 1 year in twelve children, up to 6 months in six infants, and up to 1 month in five infants. Apart from the single infant with cerebral palsy described above, the development of the children has been normal (Table 5). All physical growth parameters were within age-appropriate growth percentiles. The mean age of sitting without support was 6.5 ± 1.4 months; mean age of walking independently was 12 ± 1.4 months and kicking a ball

Table 5 Developmental Milestones of Babies Exposed In Utero to CO Poisoning[a]

First instance of	Mean age range (months, ± SD)	Normal range (months)
Smile	1.4 ± 0.5	0–2
Sitting without support	6.5 ± 1.4	4.8–7.8
Object constancy	8 ± 0.5	
Pincer grasp	8.6 ± 1.5	9.4–14.7
Waving goodbye	10.8 ± 2.4	9 months
Walking independently	12 ± 1.4	11.3–14.3
Building a tower of two cubes	16.2 ± 1.8	12.5–20
Independent use of spoon	16.3 ± 2.9	
First word	11.4 ± 2.1	8.5–13.5
Combination of two words	15.6 ± 1.2	14–26

[a]Excluded 1 child with cerebral palsy (see text).

22 ± 1.5 months. Object constancy was observed at 8 ± 0.5 months, a pincer grasp at 8.6 ± 1.5 months, building a tower of two cubes at 16.2 ± 1.8 months, and independent use of a spoon at 16.3 ± 2.9 months. The first smile was noted at 1.4 ± 0.5 months and waving goodbye at 10.8 ± 2.4 months. The first word was at 11.4 ± 2.1 months, and combining two words was reported at 15.6 ± 1.2 months. All the children above 3 years of age were integrating socially and were reported to have normal developmental milestones. All the mothers reported satisfaction with the development of their children.

DISCUSSION

Acute CO poisoning became a common part of life after the introduction of coal heating. Incomplete combustion of carbonaceous compounds may be associated with faulty furnaces and stoves, malfunctioning gas and kerosene space heaters, improperly vented charcoal or sterno fires, and engine fumes. Inhaled methylene chloride is metabolized in the body to CO and may cause various degrees of CO poisoning and even death (39). Smoking is by far the most common source of chronic exposure to CO, and smokers of 20 cigarettes per day may maintain COHb levels up to 10% (normal value for nonsmokers is 0.85%) (1,38,40).

After crossing the placenta and binding to fetal hemoglobin, CO decreases the amount of oxygen reaching the developing organism, thus creating a state of hypoxia. Initial animal studies documented that at CO levels causing severe maternal toxicity, fetuses are invariably affected, with permanent damage to the developing brain being the most consistent finding (41). Recent studies have documented that chronic exposure of pregnant animals to CO levels not associated with measurable maternal toxicity may be related to developmental delay and permanent damage to the central nervous system (CNS) (1,41).

Recent human studies suggest that offspring of heavy smokers may have lower scores in developmental tests (42) or may have lower scholastic achievement in high school (43). These studies have attempted to correct for a variety of maternal socioeconomic and environmental variables before identifying heavy smoking as the culprit.

The available 51 case reports of accidental CO poisoning in pregnancy (Tables 6 and 7) are consistent with controlled animal studies, showing stillbirth and permanent fetal brain damage consistent with hypoxia. However, very few of these cases dealt with mild-to-moderate CO exposures (grades 1–3), which are much more common than the more severe accidents (33). The literature suggests that of the 22 cases of grade 5 exposures, 17 resulted in stillbirth and 5 in fetal brain damage. None of the grade 5 cases were judged to be healthy, although most reports do not specify their diagnostic criteria

Table 6 Maternal CO Toxicity Grade in Relation to Fetal Outcome

Maternal grade of toxicity	Number of cases	Fetal outcome		
		Normal	CNS damage	Stillbirth
1	3	3		
1 +	1	1		
2				
3	1	1[a]		
4				
5	22		5	17
Unknown	24	9	12	3
Total	51	14	17	20

[a]Patient received 100% O_2 at 2.4 atm for 90 minutes.
Source: All cases published to date (see ref. list).

or length of follow-up. Because of poor documentation, the clinical grade of severity could not be determined in half of these cases, of which 9 babies were normal, 12 were reported to have CNS damage, and 3 were stillborn (Table 6).

Methodologically, any assessment of fetal outcome following maternal CO poisoning is seriously hampered. The accidental exposure is never a "controlled" event, and the exposure may have been much longer than initially assumed. Second, upon suspecting CO poisoning, the pregnant woman is often evacuated from the contaminated area and treated before COHb levels can be established. Similarly, the source of CO (e.g., furnace, engine) is usually stopped and proper ventilation of the area restored, thus making interpretation of ambient CO levels impossible or inaccurate. In addition, there is a poor correlation between COHb levels and clinical toxicity (36,44); clinical symptoms and signs may better correlate with the degree of CO toxicity (36,38,43).

As with any adverse event in pregnancy, it is crucial to rule out other risk factors that may cause adverse fetal outcome before incriminating CO as a potential fetotoxin. These factors include drug and alcohol consumption, genetic background, and maternal general health and obstetric history.

Assessment of fetal outcome imposes additional methodological problems. Because our series was collected prospectively from all over North America, the evaluation of pregnancy outcome had to be based on maternal reports. Without an appropriate control group, these reports may not identify subtle CNS damage that would be unmasked by elaborate developmental tests.

Table 7 Reported Cases of Fetal/Infant Neurological Disorders Resulting from Maternal Carbon Monoxide Poisoning

Reference (No.)	Neurological disorders
1. Maresch, 1929 (2)	Softening in the basal ganglia
2. Neubuerger, 1935 (3)	Hydrocephalis internus
3. Brander, 1940 (4)	Microcephalis and tetraplegia
4. Zourbas, 1947 (5)	Retardation of psychomotor development
5. Hallervorden, 1949 (6)	Extensive damage to the globus pallidus, striatum, red zone of substantia nigra, and lateral nucleus of the thalamus areas of the cortex; manifested a diffuse loss of neurons; polymicrogyria affected the frontal and anterior central regions
6. Desclaux et al., 1951 (7)	Mental retardation
7. Beau et al., 1956 (8)	Injury to putamen and globus pallidus; injury to cerebral cortex
8. Beau et al., 1956 (8)	Convulsions and behavior indicative of brain toxicity
9. Beau et al., 1956 (8)	Slight retardation in development; strabismus
10. Beau et al., 1956 (8)	Cyanotic, no reflexes
11. Solcher, 1957 (9)	Bilateral status marmoratus of the putamen; medial globus pallidus and subthalamic nucleus suffered neural loss
12. Schwedenberg, 1959 (10)	Injury to putamen and globus pallidus; injury to cerebral cortex extensive; damage to centrum semiovale
13. Csermely, 1962 (11)	Multicystic cavitary degeneration of the white matter; cortex and basal ganglia showed a total loss of nerve cells
14. Colmant and Wever, 1963 (12)	Injury to putamen and globus pallidus; injury to cerebral cortex; extensive damage to centrum semiovale
15. Bankl and Jellinger, 1967 (13)	Symmetrical temporal microgyria was present, along with massive hemispheral destruction
16. Lombard, cited by Longo, 1977 (15)	Mental retardation, strabismus
17. Lombard, cited by Longo, 1977 (15)	Mental retardation, athetosis, spasticity

Bearing in mind these limitations, this prospective study was designed to record data available a few hours after the initial contact. The grading of clinical toxicity was based on a widely accepted system (36); and follow-up of fetal outcome was performed by a developmental pediatrician. In Toronto, several children had a more complete assessment with the Bayley Scales. The child with cerebral palsy had additional tests.

The data represent the first multicenter prospective collection and evaluation of CO poisoning in pregnancy. The proportion of numbers between mild-to-moderate and severe poisoning closely reflects that of CO poisoning in the general population (33), thus ruling out a reporting bias toward milder cases.

Pregnancy outcome following grades 4 and 5 in our patients closely resembles that described in case reports (Tables 6 and 7). Two of our patients were treated with hyperbaric oxygen and had normal outcome, whereas the three treated with high flow oxygen masks had adverse fetal outcome. Although these numbers are too small to permit one to draw definite conclusions, they agree with recent case reports (29) documenting good outcome after hyperbaric oxygen treatment. Equally important, in none of these cases could we detect adverse maternal or fetal effects caused by this mode of treatment.

The elimination half-life of COHb in the body is 5 hours in room air, 1 hour in high-flow oxygen, and 23 minutes with hyperbaric oxygen (HBO) (45). While HBO is efficacious in treating adults and children with severe CO poisoning, it may be even more important for fetal therapy. After equilibration, fetal COHb levels are higher and have a longer half-life than the maternal COHb (1). Because the potential for developing irreversible CNS damage depends on the severity of anoxia, it makes biological sense to try to remove fetal CO as quickly as possible. It is generally recommended that maternal oxygen therapy continue five times longer than was needed for maternal COHb to return to normal (1).

The mother with grade 4 severity who gave birth to a child with cerebral palsy was treated with high-flow oxygen for 2 hours only. Based on a COHb elimination half-life of 1 hour, this therapy would have not reduced her COHb level (25%) to normal; the fetal COHb levels would be pathological for a longer period.

Pregnancy outcome following grade 1 and 2 accidental exposures to CO was normal in all cases. Excluding the three sets of twins, which tend to be small for their gestational age, the other babies, including two preterm infants, did not appear to suffer from intrauterine growth retardation. It is conceivable that short, albeit substantial, hypoxia does not impair the growth potential when pregnancy continues normally.

Of special concern to the pregnant woman, her family, and the health professionals who counsel her about fetal risk is the potential long-term CNS damage that may be caused by mild CO poisoning of the fetus. Within the limitations of the follow-up that could be performed in the present study, we could not document adverse developmental effects in these babies (Table 5). Because of the rarity of CO poisoning in pregnancy, it is very unlikely that more sensitive, controlled tests can be performed. It is, therefore, theoretically possible that our analysis missed more subtle CNS damage.

In summary, this prospective study confirmed the substantial fetal risks following grades 4 and 5 CO poisoning in pregnancy. It is possible that hyperbaric oxygen therapy improves fetal outcome.

In the case of mild poisoning (grades 1 and 2), the present study did not detect increased fetal risk: the outcome measurements were compatible with normal infant neurobehavioral development.

Answer

According to the only prospective study available today, this patient's symptomatology puts her in a low-risk category. We did not conduct cognitive tests, but at her level of exposure the baby is expected to develop normally according to the milestones of the Denver Developmental Screening Test.

REFERENCES

1. Longo LD. The biological effects of carbon monoxide on the pregnant woman, fetus, and newborn infant. Am J Obstet Gynecol 1977; 129:69–102.
2. Maresch R. Über einen Fall von Kohlenoxydgasschadigung des Kindes in der Gebarmutter. Wien Med Wochenschr 1929; 79:454–456.
3. Neubuerger F. Fall einer intrauterinen Hirnschadigung nach Leuchtgasvergiftung der Mutter. Beitr Gerichtl Med 1935; 13:85–95.
4. Brander T. Microcephalus und Tetraplegie bei einem Kinde nach Kohlenoxydvergiftung der Mutter wahrend der Schwangerschaft. Acta Paediatr Scand 1940; suppl 1, 28:123–132.
5. Zourbas J. Encephalopathie congenitale avec troubles du tonus neuromusculaire vraisemblablement consécutive à une intoxication par l'oxyde de carbone. Arch Fr Pediatr 1947; 4:513–515.
6. Hallervorden J. Über eine Kohlenoxydvergiftung im Fetalleben mit Entwicklungsstorung der Hirnrinde. Allg Z Psychiat 1949; 124:289–298.
7. Desclaux P, Soulairae A, Morlon C. Intoxication oxycarbonée au cours d'une gestation (5me mois), mentale consécutive. Arch Fr Pediatr 1951; 8:316–318.
8. Beau A, Neimann N, Pierson M. Du role de l'intoxication oxycarbonée gravidique dans la génèse des encephalopaties néonatales. Arch Fr Pediatr 1956; 13:130–143.

9. Solcher H. Über einen Fall von überstandener fötaler Kohlenoxydvergiftung. Z Hirnforsch 1957; 3:49–55.
10. Schwedenberg TH. Leukoencephalopathy following carbon monoxide asphyxia. J Neuropathol Exp Neurol 1959; 18:597–608.
11. Csermely H. Über die Pathogenese des Cerebrum polycysticum. In IV Internationaler Kongress für Neuropathologie, Munich (Jacob H, ed). Thieme, Stuttgart, 1962, pp 44–48.
12. Colmant HJ, Wever H. Pranatale Kohlenoxydvergiftung mit "Organtod" des Zentrainervensystems. Arch Psychiatr Nervenkr 1963; 204:271–287.
13. Bankl H, Jellinger K. Zentrainervose Schaden nach foetaler Kohlenoxydvergiftung. Beitr Pathol 1967; 135:350–376.
14. Beaudoing A, Gachon L, Butin L-P, et al. Les conséquences foetales de l'intoxication oxycarbonée de la mère. Pediatre 1969; 24:539–553.
15. Longo LD. Carbon monoxide in the pregnant mother and fetus and its exchange across the placenta. Ann NY Acad Sci 1970; 174:313–341.
16. Balthazard V, Nicloux M. Intoxication mortelle oxycarbonée chez une femme enceinte de 8 mois: Dosage de l'oxyde de carbone dans le sang maternel et dans le sang foetal. Arch Mens Obstet Gynec 1913; 3:161–165.
17. Breslau F. Intoxication zweier Schwangeren mit Holzleuchtgas: Tod und vorzeitige Geburt eines Kindes. Monatsschr Geburtsk Frauenkrankh 1859; 13:449–456.
18. Derobert L, Le Breton R, Bardon J. De la perméabilité placentaire à l'oxyde de carbone. Ann Med Leg 1949; 29:336–339.
19. Freund MB. Ein Fall von Absterben der Frucht in Siebenten Schwangerschaftsmonate in Folge von nur massiger Intoxication der Mutter durch Kohlenoxydgas. Monatsschr Geburtsk Frauenkrankh 1859; 14:31–33.
20. Helpern M, Strassman G. Differentiation of fetal and adult human hemoglobin. Arch Pathol 1943; 35:776–782.
21. Martland HS, Martland HS Jr. Placental barrier in carbon monoxide, barbiturate and radium poisoning. Am J Surg 1950; 80:270–279.
22. Phillips P. Carbon monoxide poisoning during pregnancy. Br M J 1924; 1:14–15.
23. Seifert P. Kohlenoxydvergiftung und Schwangerschaft. Zentralbl Gynaekol 1952; 23:895–900.
24. Tissier P. Asphyxie par le gaz d'éclairage d'une femme au terme de sa grossesse: Mort foetale, survie de la mère. Obstetrique 1909; 14:911–914.
25. Copel J, Bowen F, Bolognese RJ. Carbon monoxide intoxication in early pregnancy. Obstet Gynecol 1982; 59:26S–28S.
26. Caravati EM, Adams CJ, Joyce SM, Schaler NC. Fetal toxicity associated with maternal carbon monoxide poisoning. Ann Emerg Med 1988; 17:714–717.
27. Lombard J. Du role de l'intoxication oxycarbonée au cours de la grossesse comme facteur de malformations. Thesis, Université de Nancy (France), 1950.
28. Cramer CR. Fetal death due to accidental maternal carbon monoxide poisoning. J Toxicol Clin Toxicol 1982; 19:297–301.
29. Van Hoesen KB, Camporesi EM, Moon RE, Hage MK, Piantadosi CA. Should hyperbaric oxygen be used to treat the pregnant patient for acute carbon monoxide poisoning? JAMA 1989; 261:1039–1043.

30. Curtis GW, Algeri EJ, McBay AJ, Ford R. The transplacental diffusion of carbon monoxide. A review and experimental study. Arch Pathol 1955; 59:677–690.
31. Ginsberg MD, Myers RE. Fetal brain injury after maternal carbon monoxide intoxication: Clinical and neuropathologic aspects. Neurology 1976; 26:15–23.
32. Muller GL, Graham S. Intrauterine death of the fetus due to accidental carbon monoxide poisoning. N Engl J Med 1955; 252:1075–1078.
33. Litovitz TL, Schmitz BF, Matyunas N, Martin TG. 1987 annual report of the American Association of Poison Control Centers National Data Collection System. Am J Emerg Med 1988; 6:479–515.
34. Bologa-Campeanu M, Koren G, Rieder M, McGuigan M. Drugs and chemicals most commonly concerning pregnant women; A review of reproductive hazards. Med Toxicol 1988; 3:307–323.
35. Mac R. Motherisk Program. Vet Hum Toxicol 1988; 30:603.
36. Peirce EC, Kaufmann H, Bensky WH, et al. A registry for carbon monoxide poisoning in New York City. Clin Toxicol 1988; 26:419–441.
37. Frankenburg WK, Dobbs JB. The Denver Developmental Screening Test. J Pediatr 1967; 71:181–191.
38. Tintinalli JE, Rominger M, Kittleson K. Carbon monoxide. In Poisoning and Drug Overdose (Haddad LM, Winehester JF, eds). Saunders, Philadelphia, 1983, pp 748–753.
39. Langehermig PL, Seeler RA, Berman E. Paint removers and carboxyhemoglobin. N Engl J Med 1976; 295:1137.
40. Schardain J. Chemically Induced Birth Defects. Marcel Dekker, New York, 1985, pp 754–756.
41. Singh J. Early behavioral alterations in mice following prenatal carbon monoxide exposure. Neurotoxicology 1986; 7:475–482.
42. Sexton MJ, Fox NL, Heber JR. The effect of maternal smoking on the cognitive development of three-year-old children. Teratology 1986; 33:31c–32c.
43. Fogelman KR, Manor O. Smoking in pregnancy and development into early adulthood. Br Med J 1988; 297:1233–1236.
44. Goldbaum LG, Orellando T, Dergal E. Mechanism of toxic action of carbon monoxide. Ann Clin Lab Sci 1976; 6:372–376.
45. Goldfrank L. Toxic emergencies, 2nd ed. Appleton-Century Crofts, New York, 1982, pp 223–230.

13

Direct Drug Toxicity to the Fetus

Monica Bologa
The Hospital for Sick Children and The Upjohn Company of Canada,
Toronto, Ontario, Canada

Izhar ul Qamar, Warif Laila, and Gideon Koren
The Hospital for Sick Children, Toronto, Ontario, Canada

Clinical Case

One of your patients, a hypertensive woman, is well controlled on captopril. In fact, after stormy years with β-adrenergic blockers she is for the first time doing well. Upon learning that she is pregnant, the patient says that she would like very much to stay on captopril.

Counseling pregnant women who have been exposed to drugs during pregnancy commonly entails the need to define teratogenic risk. However, many agents may exert toxic rather than teratogenic effects, which may have a major impact on the health and prognosis of the neonate, and it is most appropriate to define these risks, as well (1–3).

In most cases data on direct toxicity of drugs that significantly cross the placenta stem from clinical and laboratory findings in newborn infants. As clearly documented in Table 1, in most instances the toxic effects can be predicted from the known pharmacological and toxicological effects in older children and adults (3–5).

We have attempted, in addition to describing reported cases and series of fetal toxicity, to define the rate of occurrence of a given finding. This figure, which is of course lacking in some instances, is crucial for risk assessment. Because the use of any drug in pregnancy must be subjected to a risk-benefit analysis, the lack of such data for many agents often makes it impossible to decide whether a certain drug should be used. Whenever known toxic effects are based on case reports, it is impossible to derive risk rates, because the denominator (total number of exposed cases) is not known.

Table 1 Direct Drug Toxicity to the Fetus

No.	Drugs	Toxic fetal effects	Reported rate of occurrence	Comments/recommendations	Ref.
1.	Acebutolol	IUGR (BW < 2500 g)	12.5% (7/56)	More frequent than after pindolol, less frequent than after atenolol	9
		β-Adrenergic blockade: hypotension, bradycardia, transient hypoglycemia	40% (4/10)	Observe newborn (first 24–48 h) for symptoms of β-adrenergic blockade	10
2.	Acetazolamide	Metabolic acidosis	C/R	Resolved spontaneously	11
		Hypocalcemia, hypomagnesemia		Resolved with treatment	
3.	Acetohexamide	Hypoglycemia	C/R	Does not provide good control of diabetes during pregnancy, therefore not recommended in pregnancy	12
4.	Albuterol	Respiratory distress syndrome	2.9% (1/35)	From exposure during labor	13
5.	Alphaprodine	Respiratory depression with severe anoxia	3.5% (7/199)	Concomitant use of levallorphan	14
			6.7% (13/192)		
6.	Aminoglutethimide	Virilization	C/R	From intake throughout pregnancy	15
7.	Amiodarone	Bradycardia, hypothyroidism	C/R	Half-life of weeks	16
				Should follow neonatal thyroid function	
8.	Ammonium chloride	Acidosis	100%	Induced in a dose-related manner near term in 100% of cases	17
				No clinical symptoms or long-term effects	
9.	Amphetamine	Neonatal withdrawal	C/R	After heavy IV use	18
				Contraindicated during pregnancy except for absolute indication for narcolepsy	

			C/R		
10.	Aspirin	Congenital salicylate intoxication	C/R		19
		IUGR (mean BW significantly reduced in 144 exposed newborns as compared to matched controls)			20
		Depressed platelet aggregation laboratory tests	100% (7/7)		21
		Partial suppression of thromboxane B production	100% (10/10)		22
			100% (17/17)	No hemorrhagic complications in the fetus	23
		Hemorrhages	21.4% (3/14)	Due to hemorrhages	24
		Stillbirths and neonatal deaths	3.6% (5/138)		25
		Increased incidence of intraventricular hemorrhage (IVH) in premature or low birth weight infants	70.5% (12/17) vs. 45% (41/90) in controls	May be due to prematurity itself	26
		Premature closure of the ductus arteriosus and death	C/R	Due to prostaglandin-inhibiting activity; avoid as much as possible chronic use of aspirin during pregnancy and especially near term	27
11.	Atenolol	IUGR (BW < 2500 g)	32.3% (10/31)	More frequent than after acebutolol or pindolol	9
		Respiratory distress	5.8% (3/52)	Transient, not requiring ventilation	28
		Apgar score < 7 at 1 min	7.6% (4/52)	Improved at 5 min in all except one	
12.	Azathioprine	Immunosuppression	C/R	Concomitant exposure to prednisone	29
		Prematurity	43% (40/93)	Analysis of reports on 238 pregnancies in renal transplant patients, 1980–1989, comparing immunosuppression with azathioprine to cyclosporin A	
		Small for gestational age	19% (18/93)		30

(continued)

Table 1 (Continued)

No.	Drugs	Toxic fetal effects	Reported rate of occurrence	Comments/recommendations	Ref.
13.	Benztropine	Paralytic ileus	C/R		31
14.	Betamethasone	Hypoglycemia < 40 mg/dL	37.7% (55/146)		32
		< 30 mg/dL	24.7% (36/146)		
15.	Bretylium	Leukocytosis	C/R		33
		Hypotension	50% (numbers not available)		34
16.	Bromides	IUGR, with subsequent retarded growth	C/R		35
		Neonatal bromism: hypotonia, poor suck response, diminished reflexes	C/R		36
17.	Butalbital	Neonatal withdrawal	C/R	Concomitant exposure to caffeine	37
18.	Caffeine	IUGR (< 2500 g at term)	7.5% (177/2357) vs. 4.7% (47/998) in unexposed controls	Heavy maternal coffee intake; incidence of IUGR increased to 9.9% (34/343) in neonates of mothers who also smoked regularly during pregnancy	38
19.	Camphor	Neonatal respiratory failure	C/R	From accidental ingestion	39
20.	Captopril	Acute renal failure reversible fatal anuria	C/R 28.6% (2/7)	Concomitant exposure to furosemide	40
		IUGR with prematurity	C/R	Concomitant intake of acebutolol for nephrotic syndrome with hypertension	41
		Oligohydramnios	14.5% (11/76)	Analysis of results of use of either captopril or enalapril in 76 patients with hypertension during pregnancy	42

No.	Drug	Adverse effect	Incidence/Type	Comments	Ref.
21.	Carbamazepine	Anuria	5% (2/44)	Those patients were described in 25 various publications up to 1990	43
		Cholestatic hepatitis	C/R	Hepatitis resolved upon cessation of breastfeeding	44
22.	Chloramphenicol	Cardiovascular collapse (gray syndrome)	C/R	From exposure near term; contra-indicated near term	45
23.	Chlordiazepoxide	Neonatal withdrawal: irritability, tremors	C/R		46
		Hypotonia, hypothermia, unresponsiveness, poor feeding	C/R		
24.	Chlorothiazide	Hypoglycemia	0.1% (14/13725) vs. 0.02% in controls	From exposure within hours of delivery	47
		Thrombocytopenia	0.85% (2/234)	From exposure near term due to transfer of antiplatelet antibodies from mother	48
		Hemolytic anemia	C/R		49
		Electrolyte imbalance			50
		Hyponatremia with hypotonia	C/R		51
		Hypokalemia with bradycardia	C/R		51
		Fatal acute hemorrhagic pancreatitis	C/R	From exposure after first trimester	53
25.	Chlorpropamide	Hypoglycemia	C/R	Does not provide good control of diabetes during pregnancy; therefore not recommended during pregnancy	54

(continued)

Table 1 (Continued)

No.	Drugs	Toxic fetal effects	Reported rate of occurrence	Comments/recommendations	Ref.
26.	Chlorpromazine	Hypotension	C/R		55
		Extrapyramidal syndrome: tremors, hypertonia, spasticity, hyperreflexia	C/R		56
		Hypotonia, lethargy, hypo-reflexia, jaundice	C/R		57
		Paralytic ileus	C/R		58
27.	Cimetidine	Transient liver impairment	C/R	From exposure near term	59
28.	Clomipramine	Lethargy, hypotonia, hypothermia, jitteriness, irregular breathing	C/R		60
29.	Clonazepam	Apnea, cyanosis, lethargy, hypotonia	C/R		61
30.	Cocaine	Microcephaly	17% (6/35)	Compared with a group of mothers on heroin during pregnancy	62
		IUGR	26% (9/35)		
		Changes in sleep pattern (irritability/sleepiness)	26% (9/35) 6% (2/35)		
31.	Codeine and dihydro-codeine bitartrate	Neonatal withdrawal	C/R		63
		Respiratory depression	2.6% (3/115)	Less pronounced than after meperidine	64
32.	Coumarin derivatives	Hemorrhage	3% (of normal newborns)	Numbers not available from review	3
		Stillbirth/neonatal death	8%		
		Prematurity	46.5% (14/30)	Vs. 10.5% (2/19) in controls	65
		Low birth weight	50% (15/30)	Vs. 10.5% (2/19) in control newborns of mothers with prosthetic heart valves not on anticoagulants	

#	Drug	Effect	Incidence	Comment	Ref
33.	Cyclosporin A	Prematurity	66% (21/32)	Analysis of reports of 238 pregnancies in patients with renal transplants, 1980–1989, comparing immunosuppression with cyclosporin A to azathioprine	30
		Small for gestational age	56% (18/32)		
34.	Danazol	Virilization of female infant	66% (10/15)	Mostly mild	66
35.	Desipramine	Neonatal withdrawal: tachycardia, diaphoresis, weight loss	C/R	From exposure throughout pregnancy	67
36.	Dexamethasone	Leukocytosis	C/R		68
37.	Diazepam	Floppy infant syndrome: hypotonia, lethargy, poor feeding	71.4% (10/14)		69
		Neonatal withdrawal: irritability, tremors, hypertonicity, diarrhea, vomiting	C/R		70
		Hypothermia (mean body temperature significantly lower in 12 exposed newborns vs. 13 controls)		Avoid chronic intake, especially near term	71
38.	Diazoxide	Transient bradycardia	8.3% (1/12)		72
		Hyperglycemia	100% (4/4)		73
		Tachycardia	50% (2/4)	Cautious use in small dosages, if absolute indication (after other therapies have failed)	
39.	Diethylstilbesterol	Benign lesions of the cervix (in adolescents):	8.3% (10/121)		74
		Carcinoma in situ	1/121		
		Polyp	3/121		
		Abnormal smear	6/121		

(continued)

273

Table 1 (Continued)

No.	Drugs	Toxic fetal effects	Reported rate of occurrence	Comments/recommendations	Ref.
39.	Diethylstilbesterol (continued)	Carcinoma of the vagina	C/R		75
		Masculinization of the female infant: hirsutism	72% (23/32)		76
		Testicular tumor: seminoma	C/R		77
		Cervical cytological abnormalities	14% (45/321)		
		Cervical neoplasia	6.2% (20/321)		
		Changes in psychosexual behavior (in male offspring)	15% (39/259)		79
40.	Digitalis	Neonatal death	C/R	From maternal overdose	80
		Prematurity (mean GA at delivery = 1 week less in 22 exposed patients vs. 64 controls)			81
41.	Diphenhydramine	Neonatal withdrawal: tremors, diarrhea	C/R		82
42.	Docusate Na	Electrolyte imbalance: hypomagnesemia	C/R		83
43.	Doxepin	Paralytic ileus	C/R	Concomitant exposure to chlorpromazine	84
44.	Enalapril	Reversible acute renal failure	C/R	From exposure 2 weeks prior to cesarean section at 35 weeks	85
		Oligohydramnios	14.5% (11/76)	Analysis of results of use of either enalapril or captopril in 76 patients with hypertension during pregnancy described in various publications up to 1990	42
		Anuria	41% (7/17)		

	Drug	Effect	Incidence	Comment	Ref.
45.	Esmolol	Decreased fetal heart rate	C/R	Improved on termination of esmolol infusion	86
46.	Ethchlorvynol	Hypotonia, hyporeflexia, hypoactivity	C/R		87
47.	Ethosuximide	Hemorrhage	C/R		88
48.	Fentanyl	Respiratory depression	C/R	From peridural administration during labor	89
49.	Fluorouracil	Cyanosis, jerking extremities	C/R		90
50.	Fluphenazine	Extrapyramidal syndrome	C/R		91
51.	Haloperidol	Withdrawal emergent syndrome with tongue thrusting, tremors of all extremities, abnormal hand posturing	C/R	Most symptoms resolved spontaneously within several days	92
52.	Heroin	Neonatal withdrawal: hyperactivity, respiratory distress, convulsions, sweating and excessive mucus secretion, diarrhea	55-75%	Related to dosage and length of exposure	93
			91% (42/45)	Withdrawal more frequent but less severe as compared to methadone-exposed newborns	94
		Intrauterine death from meconium aspiration	C/R		95
		Growth retardation		Comparable to methadone-exposed	96
		IUGR	45% (10/22)		97
		Fetal distress	65% (14/22)		
		Withdrawal syndrome	66% (15/22)		
		Prematurity	9% (2/22)		
53.	Hexamethonium	Paralytic ileus	C/R		98
54.	Hydralazine	Thrombocytopenia	C/R	May be related to maternal disease rather than the drug	99

(continued)

Table 1 (Continued)

No.	Drugs	Toxic fetal effects	Reported rate of occurrence	Comments/recommendations	Ref.
54.	Hydralazine (continued)	Arrhythmia due to premature atrial contraction	C/R		100
		Fetal distress	71% (5/7)	Associated with rapid uncontrolled decline in maternal blood pressure when given intravenously to the mother for hypertension	101
		Lupuslike syndrome	C/R	Pericardial effusion, cardiac tamponade, death	102
				103	
55.	Hydroxyprogesterone	Masculinization of female infant	C/R		
56.	Ibuprofen	Oligohydramnios	27% (8/30)	Vs. 70% (26/37) with indomethacin, possibly due to impaired renal function in fetus; oligohydramnios resolved on discontinuation of treatment	104
57.	Imipramine	Neonatal withdrawal: irritability, rapid breathing, cyanosis, colic	C/R		105
58.	Indomethacin	Stillbirth	C/R	Most likely due to premature closure of the ductus arteriosus	106
		Hydrops fetalis, renal insufficiency, ileal perforation	C/R		107
		Renal functional impairment	9 preterm neonates	Usually transient change	108
		Periventricular leukomalacia	34% (26/76)		109
		Oligohydramnios	70% (27/37)		104
59.	Insulin	Hypoglycemia Hyperbilirubinemia Hypocalcemia Polycythemia	65% (169/260)	Difficult to separate the effects of exogenous insulin from maternal diabetes	110

#	Drug	Adverse effect	Incidence	Comments	Ref
		Macrosomia	47% (21/46)	Due to transplacental transfer of biologically active insulin as insulin and insulin antibody complex, more with animal than human insulin	111
60.	Iodides				
	Potassium iodide	Hypothyroidism with goiter, cardiomegaly	28.6% (14/49) 8.2% (4/49)	Goiter may be large enough to cause tracheal compression and death	112
	Radioactive iodides	Hypothyroidism with goiter, tracheal hypoplasia with stridor	C/R		113
61.	Isoniazid	Hemorrhages	C/R		114
62.	Isoxsuprine	Hypotension	63% (27/43)		115
		Hypocalcemia	59% (23/39)		
		Paralytic ileus	40% (17/43)		
		Death	16% (7/43)		
		Myocardial ischemia	67% (6/9)	Transient ischemic ECG changes	116
63.	Kanamycin	Ototoxicity	2.3% (9/351)	From exposure near term	117
64.	Labetolol	β-adrenergic blockade	C/R	Inhibition of compensatory response due to β-adrenergic blockade	118
		Decreased tolerance to hypoxia	C/R		119
65.	Lithium	Hypotonia	C/R	Self-limited (return to normal within 2 weeks)	3
		Cyanosis			
		Bradycardia			
		Hyperthyroidism		Review of case reports	
		Atrial flutter			
		T-wave inversion on ECG			
		Cardiomegaly			
		Hepatomegaly			
		Gastrointestinal bleeding			
		Diabetes insipidus			
		Shock			

(continued)

Table 1 (Continued)

No.	Drugs	Toxic fetal effects	Reported rate of occurrence	Comments/recommendations	Ref.
65.	Lithium (continued)	Neonatal jaundice	C/R	Transient unconjugated bilirubinemia	120
66.	Magnesium sulfate	Stillbirth	C/R		121
		IUGR, low Apgar scores; toxicity: hypotonia, hyporeflexia	75.7% (28/37)		122
		CNS depression with no spontaneous breathing, movements or reflexes	C/R		123
		Impaired muscular activities; sucking, cry response, ventral suspension (mean group scores in 36 exposed newborns significantly lower vs. 43 controls)		124	
67.	Medroxyprogesterone	Ambiguous genitalia	C/R		125
68.	Meperidine	CNS depression (Apgar scores ≤ 7)	38.6% (11/29)	Time and dose related with maximum incidence (100%) if drug administered > 3 h prior to delivery (5/5)	126
		Impaired behavioral response	87.9% (29/33) vs. 12.5% (1/8) in controls	Concomitant exposure to promethazine/phenobarbital prochlorperazine/morphine	127
		EEG changes	12.5% (1/8) in controls		
		Transient decrease in oxygenation	84.8% (28/33) vs. 100% (10/10)	Mean decline in TcP_{O_2} 11.7 torr mean duration 4.6 min after injection	

	Drug	Effect	Incidence	Comments	Ref.
69.	Mepivacaine	Bradycardia and acidosis	41% (7/17)	Clinical signs correlated with high levels of mepivacaine in fetal blood following paracervical block with mepivacaine in the mother	128
70.	Methadone	Withdrawal syndrome		Withdrawal is more severe than in heroin-exposed newborns	94
		With seizures	76% (34/46)		
		Irritability	10.9% (5/46)		
		Tremulousness	91.7% (66/72)		96
		Hypertonicity	75% (54/72)		
		IUGR (mean BW significantly lower in 72 newborns of addicted mothers vs. 72 controls)	40.3% (29/72)		96
		Hyperbilirubinemia	9.7% (7/72)		96
		Jaundice	13% (6/46)		94
		Thrombocytosis	100% (33/33)		129
		Hyaline membrane disease	4.3% (2/46)		92
		Stillbirth	6.4% (3/47)		130
		Neonatal death	8.5% (4/47)		
		Sudden infant death syndrome	2.8% (20/702)		131
71.	Methimazole	Hypothyroidism			
		Present at birth	C/R		132
		With goiter	C/R		133
		Becoming evident later in infancy (2 mo)	C/R		134
72.	Methyldopa	Neonatal nasal obstruction with respiratory distress	C/R	Due to edema of nasopharyngeal mucosa requiring topical vasoconstrictors, resolved within 2 days	135

(continued)

Table 1 (Continued)

No.	Drugs	Toxic fetal effects	Reported rate of occurrence	Comments/recommendations	Ref.
72.	Methyldopa (continued)	Low birth weight in 25 newborns vs. 20 control newborns		Greater decrease in birth weight in newborns of mothers on high dose (1.25–2.0 g/day) vs. low dose (1.0 g/day)	136
73.	Methylene Blue	Hemolytic anemia, hyperbilirubinemia, jaundice	C/R	From diagnostic intraamniotic injection of 30–50 mg of the dye	137
		Intestinal obstruction, jejunal atresia	9.5% (17/178)	Possible cause, spasm of mesenteric artery after fetal oral ingestion	138
74.	Metoprolol	Increased immunoglobin E levels	45% (13/29)	Vs. 15% (3/23) in placebo group, β-adrenoceptor blocking agents possibly stimulate IgE antibody formation and promote allergy	139
75.	Morphine	Congenital "morphinism" with neonatal withdrawal	91% (20/22)		140
76.	Minoxidil	Hypertrichosis	C/R		141
77.	Nadolol	IUGR; tachypnea, mild hypoglycemia	C/R		142
78.	Naloxone	Fatal respiratory depression	C/R		143
		Seizures	C/R	Due to neonatal opioid withdrawal in infant of opioid abuser mother	144
79.	Naproxen	Primary pulmonary hypertension with severe hypoxemia, increased blood clotting, times, hyperbilirubinemia, impaired renal function	C/R	Exposure at 30 weeks for 2–6 days, attributed to prostaglandin-inhibiting action	145
80.	Nifedipine	Hyperbilirubinemia	8.7% (2/23)	Vs. 31.6% (6/19) in newborns of mothers who had tocolysis with ritodrine	146

No.	Drug	Effect	Incidence/Type	Comment	Ref.
81.	Norethindrone	Masculinization of the female fetus	0.3%–18.3% (15/82)		147
82.	Norethynodrel	Masculinization of the female fetus	25% (1/4)		148
83.	Nortryptyline	Urinary retention	C/R		149
84.	Opium	Narcotic withdrawal	C/R		150
85.	Oral contraceptives	Hyperbilirubinemia ± kernicterus	C/R	Symptoms begin 48 h after birth	151
		Mean bilirubin levels were significantly higher in 16 newborns exposed to progestogens in utero vs. 73 newborns exposed to oral contraceptives and 83 unexposed newborns; significantly higher in 40 bottle-fed newborns exposed to oral contraceptives vs. 33 breastfed exposed newborns and 83 unexposed		Risk for toxic effects of constituent hormones (progestogens and estrogens)	152
86.	Pentazocine	Choreoathetosis	C/R	Resolved spontaneously	153
		Neonatal withdrawal: trembling, jitteriness, hyperirritability, hyperactivity, hypertonia, diaphoresis, diarrhea, vomiting, high-pitched cry, opisthotonic posturing	C/R	After chronic maternal ingestion; Symptoms disappear within 24 h of birth	154
		Prematurity	37.5% (9/24)		155
		IUGR	8.3% (2/24)		
		Metabolic acidosis			156

(continued)

Table 1 (Continued)

No.	Drugs	Toxic fetal effects	Reported rate of occurrence	Comments/recommendations	Ref.
87.	Phencyclidine	Irritability, jitteriness, hypertonicity, poor feeding	C/R		157
		IUGR	32% (12/37)		158
88.	Phenobarbital	Hemorrhagic disease	C/R	Early onset (first 24 h after birth), probably due to induction of liver microsomal enzymes that deplete vitamin K	159
		Barbiturate withdrawal	C/R	Onset within 6 days	160
89.	Phenytoin	Hemorrhagic disease of the newborn	C/R	Early onset (first 24 h after birth), probably due to induction of liver microsomal enzymes that deplete vitamin K	161
90.	Pindolol	IUGR (BW < 2500 g)	7.9% (3/38)	Less frequent than after atenolol, acebutolol	9
91.	Prednisone	Immunosuppression	C/R	Concomitant exposure to azathioprine throughout pregnancy	29
		Stillbirth	23.5% (8/34) vs. 3% (1/34) in controls (with same diagnosis)	Attributed to failure of placental function	162
92.	Primidone	Overactivity, tremors, jitteriness	C/R	Malformed newborn, died at 3 weeks	163
		Hemorrhagic disease	C/R	Due to suppression of vitamin-K-dependent clotting factors	164
93.	Promazine	Hyperbilirubinemia (mean bilirubin levels significantly higher in 317 exposed patients vs. 272 controls)		From exposure during labor	165

	Effect	Incidence	Comments	Ref.
94. Promethazine	Transient behavioral and EEG changes	100% (28/28)	27/28: concomitant exposure to meperidine or phenobarbitol persisted for ≤ 3 days	166
95. Propoxyphene	Impaired platelet aggregation tests	88.9% (16/18)		167
	Neonatal withdrawal: irritability, tremors, hyperactivity, hypertonicity, high-pitched cry, fever, diaphoresis, ± seizures	C/R		168
96. Propranolol	Bradycardia (transient)	20% (2/10)	Exposure during labor	169
	Bradycardia	7%	From analysis of 23 reports involving 167 liveborn infants exposed chronically to the drug in utero	3
	IUGR	14%		
	Hypoglycemia	10%		
	Respiratory depression	4%		
	Hyperbilirubinemia	4%		
	Polycythemia	1%		
	Thrombocytopenia	0.6%		
	Respiratory depression	80% (4/5)	Drug given prior to cesarean section	170
	Prematurity	33% (3/9)		171
97. Propylthiouracil	Hypothyroidism with goiter	12% (28/240)	From exposure close to term; self-limited, resolving within a few days. Goiter usually smaller than iodine-induced goiter	172
	Clinically evident at birth with subsequent retardation in mental and physical development	C/R	50% of cases concomitant exposure to high doses of iodide	173
	Neonatal hepatitis	C/R	Possible hypersensitivity mechanism with spontaneous remission	174

(continued)

Table 1 (Continued)

No.	Drugs	Toxic fetal effects	Reported rate of occurrence	Comments/recommendations	Ref.
98.	Pyridoxine	Convulsions	C/R	High doses early in pregnancy presumably altered pyridoxine metabolism in two successive pregnaices	175
				"Dependency-induced" convulsions in offsprings of three successive pregnancies	176
				Additional 50 cases reported; some fatalities	3
99.	Quinidine	Thrombocytopenia	0.9% (2/234)		177
100.	Quinine	Auditory and optic nerve damage			
		Hearing loss	1% (2/200)		178
		Hypoplasia of optic nerve	C/R		179
		Thrombocytopenic purpura	C/R		180
		Hemolysis in G6PD-deficient infants	C/R		181
101.	Reserpine	Jitteriness	C/R	Due to quinine withdrawal	182
		Nasal discharge + cyanosis; lethargy + poor feeding	100% (12/12) 25% (3/12) 41.7% (5/12)	From exposure near term	183
102.	Rifampicin	Hemorrhagic disease of the newborn	C/R	Due to hypoprothrombinemia	184

No.	Drug	Effect	Incidence	Comments	Ref.
103.	Ritodrine	Tachycardia (increased mean heart rate in 20 exposed cases vs. 20 controls); transient hypoglycemia (less significant, in same 20 cases)			185
		Stillbirth	C/R		186
		Cardiac ischemia	29% (6/21)	ECG changes lasting several weeks	116
		Hyperbilirubinemia	31.6% (6/19)	Vs. 8.7% (2/23) in newborns of mothers who had tocolysis with nifedipine	146
104.	Scopolamine	Acute toxicity: tachycardia, fever, lethargy	C/R		187
105.	Streptomycin	Ototoxicity: cochlear and vestibular	C/R	From exposure in the last month of gestation	188
106.	Sulfonamides	Hyperbiliburinemia, jaundice	7.7% (1/13)	From exposure near term; premature infants especially susceptible	189
		Severe hemolytic anemia with hydrops fetalis and stillbirth	C/R	Neonates with G6PD deficiency more prone	190
107.	Terbutaline	Hypoglycemia	C/R	Secondary to maternal insulin production in response to hyperglycemia that has not been determined prior to delivery	191
		Bradycardia			
		Cardiovascular decompensation	75%, three infants of a quadruplet pregnancy	Down-regulation of fetal β-adrenergic receptors leading to decreased myocardial function and cardiac output	192

(continued)

Table 1 (Continued)

No.	Drugs	Toxic fetal effects	Reported rate of occurrence	Comments/recommendations	Ref.
107.	Terbutaline (continued)	Metabolic acidosis			
		Decreased urine output			
		Myocardial necrosis	C/R		193
108.	Tetracycline	Yellow discoloration of deciduous teeth	13.8% (13/94)–77.8% (7/9)	From exposure > 16–25 weeks of gestation	194
				Due to chelating ability of the drug with calcium orthophosphate	195
		Stillbirths and prematurity	C/R	Due to maternal hepatotoxicity (fatty degeneration) after IV tetracycline, usually occurring after 35 weeks of gestation	196
109.	Theophylline	Transient tachycardia, irritability, vomiting	C/R	With maternal serum concentrations in the high therapeutic range	197

110. Thioridazine	Neonatal withdrawal: apneic spells	C/R	From chronic exposure throughout pregnancy. Resolved with theophylline treatment	198
	Extrapyramidal syndrome	C/R	Concomitant exposure to chlorpromazine, trifluoperazine effect considered most likely due to chlorpromazine	56
111. Tolbutamide	Thrombocytopenia	C/R	Persisted for 2 weeks	199
112. Trifluoperazine	Extrapyramidal syndrome	C/R	Concomitant exposure to chlorpromazine, thioridazine effect considered most likely due to chlorpromazine	56
113. Vancomycin	Fetal bradycardia	C/R	1 g given IV prior to delivery	200
	Anemia	19% (6/31)		
114. Zidovudine	IUGR	4% (2/45)		201

BW, birth weight; CNS, central nervous system; C/R, case report(s); ECG, electrocardiogram; EEG, electroencephalogram; GA, gestational age; IUGR, intrauterine growth retardation; SIDS, sudden infant death syndrome.

287

For each toxic effect caused by a drug, a representative reference is given; for obvious reasons we could not include the thousands of references available. This chapter mentions only some substances of abuse, other than medications, which are detailed in Chapters 14 and 15. Clearly, agents such as cigarettes and ethanol (6–8) may have significant toxic effects on the fetus, which will have to be included in the assessment of risks caused by medications.

Answer

Captopril and other drugs that inhibit the angiotensin converting enzyme have been shown to seriously affect renal function in the fetus, causing neonatal anuria and even death. The drug should not be used in pregnancy unless other options have been exhausted.

REFERENCES

1. Ellenhorn MJ, Barceloux DG. Toxic exposure during pregnancy. In Medical Toxicology. Diagnosis and Treatment of Human Poisoning. Elsevier, New York, 1988; pp131–152.
2. Riley EP, Vorhees CV. Handbook of Behavioral Teratology. Plenum, New York, 1986.
3. Briggs GG, Freeman RK, Yaffe SJ. Drugs in Pregnancy and Lactation, 2nd ed. Williams & Wilkins, Baltimore, 1986.
4. Hill LM, Kleinberg F. Effects of drugs and chemicals on the fetus and newborn. First part. Mayo Clin Proc 1984; 59:707–716.
5. Schenkel B, Vorherr H. Nonprescription drugs during pregnancy: Potential teratogenic and toxic effects upon embryo and fetus. J Reprod Med 1974; 12:27–45.
6. Rosett H, Weiner L. Alcohol and the Fetus. A Clinical Perspective. Oxford University Press, New York, 1984.
7. Coles CD, Smith IE, Fernhoff PM, Falek A. Neonatal ethanol withdrawal: Characteristics in clinically normal nondysmorphic neonates. J. Pediatr 1984; 105:445–451.
8. Ioffe S, Childiaeva R, Chernick V. Prolonged effects of maternal alcohol ingestion on the neonatal electroencephalogram. Pediatrics 1984; 74:330–335.
9. Dubois D, Petitcolas J, Temperville B, Klepper A, Catherine P. Treatment of hypertension in pregnancy with β-adrenoceptor antagonists. Br J Clin Pharmacol 1982; 13(suppl):375S–378S.
10. Dumez Y, Tchobroutsky C, Hornych H, Amiel-Tison C. Neonatal effects of maternal administration of acebutolol. Br Med J 1981; 283:1077–1079.
11. Merlob P, Litwin A, Mor N. Possible association between acetazolamide administration during pregnancy and metabolic disorders in the newborn. Eur J Obstet Gynecol Reprod Biol 1990; 35:85–88.

12. Kemball ML, McIver C, Milnar RDG, Nourse CH, Schiff D, Tiernan JR. Neonatal hypoglycaemia in infants of diabetic mothers given sulphonylurea drugs in pregnancy. Arch Dis Child 1970; 45:696-701.
13. Hastwell G. Salbutamol aerosol in premature labour. Lancet 1975; 2: 1212-1213.
14. Roberts H, Kuck MAC. Use of alphaprodine and levallorphan during labour. Can Med Assoc J 1960; 83:1088-1093.
15. Marek J, Horky K. Aminoglutethimide administration in pregnancy. Lancet 1970; 2:1312-1313.
16. McKenna WJ, Harris L, Rowland E, Whitelaw A, Storey G, Holt D. Amiodarone therapy during pregnancy. Am J Cardiol 1983; 51:1231-1233.
17. Goodlin RC, Kaiser IH. The effect of ammonium chloride induced maternal acidosis on the human fetus at term. I. pH, hemoglobin, blood gases. Am J Med Sci 1957; 233:666-674.
18. Ramer CM. The case of an infant born to an amphetamine addicted mother. Clin Pediatr (Phil) 1974; 13:596-597.
19. Earle R Jr. Congenital salicylate intoxication—Report of a case. N Engl J Med 1961; 265:1003-1004.
20. Turner G, Collins E. Fetal effects of regular salicylate ingestion in pregnancy. Lancet 1975; 2:338-339.
21. Corby DG, Schulman I. The effects of antenatal drug administration on aggregation of platelets of newborn infants. J Pediatr 1971; 79:307-313.
22. Casteels-Van Daele M, Eggermont E, de Gaetano G, Vermijlen J. More on the effects of antenatally administered aspirin on aggregation of platelets of neonates. J Pediatr 1972; 80:685-686.
23. Benigni A, Gregorini G, Frusca T, Chiabrando C, Ballerini S, Valcamonico, Orisio S, Piccinelli A, Pincirolo V, Fanelli R, Gastaldi A, Remuzzi G. Effect of low-dose aspirin on fetal and maternal generation of thromboxane by platelets in women at high risk for pregnancy-induced hypertension. N Engl J Med 1989; 321:357-362.
24. Bleyer WA, Breckenridge RJ. Studies on the detection of adverse drug reactions in the newborn. II. The effects of prenatal aspirin on newborn hemostasis. JAMA 1970; 213:2049-2053.
25. Collins E, Turner G. Maternal effects of regular salicylate ingestion in pregnancy. Lancet 1975; 2:335-337.
26. Rumack CM, Guggenheim MA, Rumack BH, Peterson RG, Johnson ML, Braithwaite WR. Neonatal intracranial hemorrhage and maternal use of aspirin. Obstet Gynecol 1981; 58(suppl):52S-56S.
27. Shapiro S, Monson RR, Kaufman DW, Siskind V, Heinonen OP, Slone D. Perinatal mortality and birth-weight in relation to aspirin taken during pregnancy. Lancet 1976; 1:1375-1376.
28. Fabregues G, Alvarez L, Varas Juri P, Drisaldi C, Cerrato C, Moschettoni C, Pituelo D, Baglivo HP, Esper RJ. Effectiveness of atenolol in the treatment of hypertension during pregnancy. Hypertension 1992; 19(suppl II):II 129-131.

29. Cote CJ, Meuwissen HJ, Pickering RJ. Effects on the neonate of prednisone and azathioprine administered to the mother during pregnancy. J Pediatr 1974; 85:324–328.
30. Pabelick C, Kemmer F, Koletzko B. Befunde bei neugeborenen nierentransplantierter Mutter. Monatsschr Kinderheilkd 1991; 139:136–140.
31. Falterman CG, Richardson CJ. Small left colon syndrome associated with maternal ingestion of psychotropic drugs. J Pediatr 1980; 97:308–310.
32. Papageorgiou AN, Desgranges MF, Masson M. Colle E, Shatz R, Gelfand MM. The antenatal use of betamethasone in the prevention of respiratory distress syndrome: A controlled double-blind study. Pediatrics 1979; 63:73–79.
33. Bielawski D, Hiatt IM, Hegyi T. Betamethasone-induced leukaemoid reaction in preterm infant. Lancet 1978; 1:218–219.
34. Product information. Bretylol. American Critical Care, 1985.
35. Opitz JM, Grosse RF, Haneberg B. Congenital effects of bromism? Lancet 1972; 1:91.
36. Pleasure JR, Blackburn MG. Neonatal bromide intoxication: Prenatal ingestion of a large quantity of bromides with transplacental accumulation in the fetus. Pediatrics 1975; 55:503–506.
37. Ostrea EM. Neonatal withdrawal from intrauterine exposure to butalbital. Am J Obstet Gynecol 1982; 143:597–599.
38. Mau G, Netter P. Kafee- und alkoholkonsum-risikofaktoren in der Schwangerschaft? Geburtshilfe Frauenheilkd 1974; 34:1018–1022.
39. Blackman WB, Curry HB. Camphor poisoning: Report of case occurring during pregnancy. J Fla Med Assoc 1957; 43:99–101.
40. Plouin PF, Tchobroutsky C. Inhibition of angiotensin converting enzyme in human pregnancy. 15 case-reports (in French). Presse Med 1985; 14:2175–2178.
41. Boutroy MJ, Vert P, Hurault de Ligny B, Miton A. Captopril administration in pregnancy impairs fetal angiotensin converting enzyme activity and neonatal adaptation. Lancet 1984; 2:935–936.
42. Hanssens M, Keirse MJNC, Vankelecom F, Van Assche FA. Fetal and neonatal effects of treatment with angiotensin-converting enzyme inhibitors in pregnancy. Obstet Gynecol 1992; 78:128–35.
43. Frey B, Schuigr G, Musy JP. Transient cholestatic hepatitis in a neonate associated with carbamazepine exposure during pregnancy and breast feeding. Eur J Pediatr 1990; 150:136–138.
44. Oberheuser F. Praktische Erfahrungen mit Medikamenten in der Schwangerschaft. Therapiewoche 1971; 31:2200. As reported in Manten A. Antibiotic drugs. In Meyler's Side Effects of Drugs, Vol VIII (Dukes MNG, ed). New York, 1975; pp 604–613.
45. Athinarayanan P, Pierog SH, Nigam SK, Glass L. Chlordiazepoxide withdrawal in the neonate. Am J Obstet Gynecol 1976; 124:212–213.
46. Stirrat GM, Edington PT, Berry DJ. Transplacental passage of chlordiazepoxide. Br Med J 1974; 2:729–732.
47. Senior B, Slone D, Shapiro S, Mitchell AA, Heinonen OP. Benzothiadiazides and neonatal hypoglycaemia. Lancet 1976; 2:377.

48. Karpatkin S, Strick N, Karpatkin MB, Siskind GW. Cumulative experience in the detection of antiplatelet antibody in 234 patients with idiopathic thrombocytopenic purpura, systemic lupus erythematosus and other clinical disorders. Am J Med 1972; 52:776–785.
49. Harley JD, Robin H, Robertson SEJ. Thiazide-induced neonatal haemolysis? Br Med J 1964; 1:696–697.
50. Pritchard JA, Walley PJ. Severe hypokalemia due to prolonged administration of chlorothiazide during pregnancy. Am J Obstet Gynecol 1961; 81:1241–1244.
51. Alstatt LB. Transplacental hyponatremia in the newborn infant. J Pediatr 1965; 66:985–988.
52. Anderson GG, Hanson TM. Chronic fetal bradycardia: Possible association with hypokalemia. Obstet Gynecol 1974; 44:896–898.
53. Minkowitz S, Soloway HB, Hall JE, Yermakov V. Fatal hemorrhagic pancreatitis following chlorothiazide administration in pregnancy. Obstet Gynecol 1964; 24:337–342.
54. Zucker P, Simon G. Prolonged symptomatic neonatal hypoglycemia associated with maternal chlorpropamide therapy. Pediatrics 1968; 42:824–825.
55. Bryans C Jr, Mulherin CM. The use of chlorpromazine in obstetrical analgesia. Ann J Obstet Gynecol 1959; 77:406–411.
56. Hill RM, Desmond MM, Kay JL. Extrapyramidal dysfunction in an infant of a schizophrenic mother. J Pediatr 1966; 69:589–595.
57. Tamer A, McKay R, Arias D, Worley L, Fogel BJ. Phenothiazine-induced extrapyramidal dysfunction in the neonate. J Pediatr 1969; 75:479–480.
58. Falterman CG, Richardson J. Small left colon syndrome associated with maternal ingestion of psychotropic drugs. J Pediatr 1980; 97:308–310.
59. Glade G, Saccar CL, Pereira GR. Cimetidine in pregnancy: Apparent transient liver impairment in the newborn. Am J Dis Child 1980; 134:87–88.
60. Ben Muza A, Smith CS. Neonatal effects of maternal clomipramine therapy. Arch Dis Child 1979; 54:405–409.
61. Fisher JB, Edgren BE, Mammel MC, Coleman JM. Neonatal apnea associated with maternal clonazepam therapy: A case report. Obstet Gynecol 1985; 66(suppl):34S–35S.
62. Fulroth R, Phillips B, Durand DJ. Perinatal outcome of infants exposed to cocaine and/or heroin in utero. Am J Dis Child 1989; 143:905–910.
63. Van Leeuwen G, Guthrie R, Strange F. Narcotic withdrawal reaction in a newborn infant due to codeine. Pediatrics 1965; 36:635–636.
64. Ruch WA, Ruch RM. A preliminary report on dihydrocodeine-scopolamine in obstetrics. Am J Obstet Gynecol 1957; 74:1125–1127.
65. Born D, Martinez EE, Almeida PA, Santos DV, Carvalho AC, Moron AF, Miyasaki CH, Moraes SD, Ambrose JA. Pregnancy in patients with prosthetic heart valves: The effects of anticoagulation on mother, fetus, and neonate. Am Heart J 1992; 124:413–417.
66. Brunskill PJ. The effects of fetal exposure to danazol. Br J Obstet Gynaecol 1992; 99:212–215.
67. Webster PA. Withdrawal symptoms in neonates associated with maternal antidepressant therapy. Lancet 1973; 2:318–319.

68. Otero L, Conlon C, Reynolds P, Duval-Armould B, Golden SM. Neonatal leukocytosis associated with prenatal administration of dexamethasone. Pediatrics 1981; 68:778–780.

69. McAllister CB. Placental transfer and neonatal effects of diazepam when administered to women just before delivery. Br J Anaesth 1980; 52:423–427.

70. Backes CR, Cordero L. Withdrawal symptoms in the neonate from presumptive intrauterine exposure to diazepam: Report of case. J Am Osteopath Assoc 1980; 79:584–585.

71. Owen JR, Irani SF, Blair AW. Effect of diazepam administered to mothers during labour on temperature regulation of neonate. Arch Dis Child 1972; 47: 107–110.

72. Morris JA, Arce JJ, Hamilton CJ, et al. The management of severe preeclampsia and eclampsia with intravenous diazoxide. Obstet Gynecol 1977; 49:675–680.

73. Neuman J, Weiss B, Rabello Y, Cabal L, Freeman RK. Diazoxide for the acute control of severe hypertension complicating pregnancy: A pilot study. Obstet Gynecol 1979; 53(suppl):50S–55S.

74. Vessey MP, Fairweather DVI, Norman-Smith B, Buckley J. A randomized double-blind controlled trial of the value of stilboestrol therapy in pregnancy: Long-term follow-up of mothers and their offspring. Br J Obstet Gynaecol 1983; 90:1007–1017.

75. Kaufman RH, Korhonen MO, Strama T, Adam E, Kaplan A. Development of clear cell adenocarcinoma in DES-exposed offspring under observation. Obstet Gynecol 1982; 59(suppl):68S–72S.

76. Peress MR, Tsai CC, Mathur RS, Williamson HO. Hirsutism and menstrual patterns in women exposed to diethylstibestrol in utero. Am J Obstet Gynecol 1982; 144:135–140.

77. Conley GR, Sant GR, Ucci AA, Mitcheson HD. Seminoma and epididymal cysts in a young man with known diethylstilbestrol exposure in utero. JAMA 1983; 249:1325–1326.

78. Verheijen RH, Schijf CP, Van Dongen PW, Van der Zanden PH, Bakker EH. Refocusing on the gynecological and obstetrical consequences of intrauterine exposure to diethylstilbesterol (DES) (in Dutch). Ned Tijdschr Geneeskd 1991; 135:89–93.

79. Yalom ID, Green R, Fisk N. Prenatal exposure to female hormones. Effect on psychosexual development in boys. Arch Gen Psychiatry 1973; 28:554–561.

80. Sherman JL Jr, Locke RV. Transplacental neonatal digitalis intoxication. Am J Cardiol 1960; 6:834–837.

81. Weaver JB, Pearson JF. Influence of digitalis on time of onset and duration of labour in women with cardiac disease. Br Med J 1973; 3:519–520.

82. Parkin DE. Probable benadryl withdrawal manifestations in a newborn infant. J Pediatr 1974; 85:580–582.

83. Schindler AM. Isolated neonatal hypomagnesaemia associated with maternal overuse of stool softener. Lancet 1984; 2:822.

84. Falterman CG, Richardson CJ. Small left colon syndrome associated with maternal ingestion of psychotropic drugs. J Pediatr 1980; 97:308–310.

85. Schubiger G, Flury G, Nussberger J. Enalapril for pregnancy-induced hypertension: Acute renal failure in a neonate. Ann Intern Med 1988; 108:215–216.
86. Larson CP Jr, Shuer LM, Cohen SE. Maternally administered esmolol decreases fetal as well as maternal heart rate. J Clin Anesth 1990; 2:427–9.
87. Rumack BH, Walravens PA. Personal communication. Department of Pediatrics, University of Colorado Medical Center, 1981.
88. Speidel BD, Meadow SR. Epilepsy, anticonvulsants and congenital malformations. Drugs 1974; 8:354–365.
89. Carrie LES, O'Sullivan GM, Seegobin R. Epidural fentanyl in labour. Anaesthesia 1981; 36:965–969.
90. Stadler HE, Knowles J. Fluorouracil in pregnancy: Effect on the neonate. JAMA 1971; 217:214–215.
91. Cleary MF. Fluphenazine decanoate during pregnancy. Am J Psychiatry 1977; 134:815–316.
92. Sexon WR, Barak Y. Withdrawal emergent syndrome in an infant associated with maternal haloperidol therapy. J Perinatal 1989; 9:170–172.
93. Zelson C, Rubio E, Wasserman E. Neonatal narcotic addiction: 10 year observation. Pediatrics 1971; 48:178–189.
94. Zelson C, Lee SJ, Casalino M. Neonatal narcotic addiction. N Engl J Med 1973, 289:1216–1220.
95. Rementeria JL, Nunag NN. Narcotic withdrawal in pregnancy: Stillbirth incidence with a case report. Am J Obstet Gynecol 1973; 116:1152–1156.
96. Strauss ME, Andresko M, Styker JC, Wardell JN, Dunkel LD. Methadone maintenance during pregnancy: Pregnancy, birth and neonate characteristics. Am J Obstet Gynecol 1974; 120:895–900.
97. Ciraru Vigneron N, Rafowicz E, Nguyen Tan Lung R, Brunner C, Barrier J Drug addiction and pregnancy: Principal obstetrical and pediatric complications (in French). J Gynecol Obstet Biol Reprod Paris 1989; 18:637–648.
98. Hallum JL, Hatchuel WLF. Congenital paralytic ileus in a premature baby as a complication of hexamethonium bromide therapy for toxemia of pregnancy. Arch Dis Child 1954; 29:354–356.
99. Widerlov E, Karlman I, Storsater J. Hydralazine-induced neonatal thrombocytopenia. N Engl J Med 1980; 303:1235–1238.
100. Lodeiro JG, Feinstein SJ, Lodeiro SB. Fetal premature atrial contractions associated with hydralazine. Am J Obstet Gynecol 1989; 160:105–107.
101. Kirshon B, Wasserstrum N, Cotton DB. Should continuous hydralazine infusions be utilized in severe pregnancy-induced hypertension? Am J Perinatol 1991; 8:206–208.
102. Yemini M, Shoham Z. Lupus-like syndrome in a mother and a newborn following administration of hydralazine. Eur J Obstet Gynecol Reprod Biol 1989; 30:193–197.
103. Wilkins L. Masculinization of female fetus due to use of orally given progestins. JAMA 1960; 172:1028–1032.
104. Hendricks SK, Smith JR, Moore DE, Brown ZA. Oligohydramnios associated with prostaglandin synthetase inhibitors in preterm labour. Br J Obstet Gynaecol 1990; 97:312–316.

105. Shrand H. Agoraphobia and imipramine withdrawal? Pediatrics 1982; 70:825–828.
106. Itskovitz J, Abramovici H, Brandes JM. Oligohydramnion, meconium and perinatal death concurrent with indomethacin treatment in human pregnancy. J Reprod Med 1980; 24:137–140.
107. Vanhaesebrouk P, Thiery M, Leroy JG, Govert P, de Praeter C, Coppens M, Cuvelier, Dhont M. Oligohydramnios, renal insufficiency and ileal perforation in preterm infants after intrauterine exposure to indomethacin. J Pediatr 1988; 113(4):738–743.
108. Heijden AJ, Provost AP, Nauta J, Grose W, Oranje WA, Wolff ED, Sauer PJJ. Renal functional impairment in preterm neonates related to intrauterine indomethacin exposure. Pediatr Res 1988, 24:644–648.
109. Baerts W, Fetter WPF, Hop WCJ, Wallenburg HCS, Spritzer R, Sauer PJJ. Cerebral lesions in preterm infants after tocolytic indomethacin. Dev Med Child Neurol 1990, 32:910–918.
110. Gabbe SG, Mestman JH, Freeman RK, et al. Management and outcome of pregnancy in diabetes mellitus, classes B to R. Am J Obstet Gynecol 1977; 129:723–732.
111. Menon RK, Cohen RM, Sperling MA, Cutfield WS, Mimouni F, Khoury JC. Transplacental passage of insulin in pregnant women with insulin dependent diabetes mellitus: Its role in fetal macrosomia. N Engl J Med 1990; 323:309–315.
112. Mehta PS, Mehta SJ, Vorherr H. Congenital iodide goiter and hypothyroidism: A review. Obstet Gynecol Surv 1983; 38:237–247.
113. Wolff J. Iodide goiter and the pharmacologic effects of excess iodide. Am J Med 1969; 47:101–124.
114. Eggermont E, Logghe N, Van De Casseye W, Casteels-Van Daele M, Jaeken J, Cosemans J, Verstraete M, Renaer M. Haemorrhagic disease of the newborn in the offspring of rifampicin and isoniazid treated mothers. Acta Paediatr Belg 1976; 29:87–90.
115. Brazy JE, Pupkin MJ. Effects of maternal isoxuprine administration on preterm infants. J Pediatr 1979; 94:444–448.
116. Gemelli M, De Luca F, Manganaro R, Leonardi R, Rando F, Agnetti A, Mami C, Di Pasquale G. Transient electrocardiographic changes suggesting myocardial ischaemia in newborn infants following tocolysis with beta-sympathomimetics. Eur J Pediatr 1990; 149:730–733.
117. Nishimura H, Tanimura T. Clinical Aspects of Teratogenicity of Drugs. Excerpta Medica, Amsterdam, 1976; pp 131–145.
118. Michael CA, Potter JM. A comparison of labetalol with other antihypertensive drugs in the treatment of hypertensive disease of pregnancy. In The Investigation of Labetalol in the Management of Hypertension in Pregnancy, (Riley A, Symonds EM, eds). Excerpta Medica, Amsterdam, 1982, pp 111–122.
119. Kjellmer I, Dagbjartsson A, Hrbek A, et al. Maternal beta-adrenoceptor blockade reduced fetal tolerance to asphyxia. Acta Obstet Gynecol Scand 1984 (suppl); 118:75–80.

120. Connoley G, Menahem S. A possible association between neonatal jaundice and long-term maternal lithium ingestion. Med J Aust 1990; 152:272-273.
121. Khandelwal SK, Sagar RS, Saxena S. Lithium in pregnancy and stillbirth: A case report. Br J Psychiatry 1989, 154:114-6.
122. Lipsitz PJ. The clinical and biochemical effects of excess magnesium in the newborn. Pediatrics 1971; 47:501-509.
123. Brady JP, Williams HC. Magnesium intoxication in a premature infant. Pediatrics 1967; 40:100-103.
124. Rasch DK, Huber PA, Richardson CJ, L'Hommedieu CS, Nelson TE, Reddi R. Neurobehavioral effects of neonatal hypermagnesemia. J Pediatr 1982; 100: 272-276.
125. Dayan E, Rosa FW. Fetal ambiguous genitalia associated with sex hormone use early in pregnancy. US Food and Drug Administration, Division of Drug Experience. ADR Highlights 1981:1-14.
126. Morrison JC, Wiser WL, Rosser SI, et al. Metabolites of meperidine related to fetal depression. Am J Obstet Gynecol 1973; 115:1132-1127.
127. Borgstedt AD, Rosen MG. Medication during labor correlated with behavior and EEG of the newborn. Am J Dis Child 1968; 115:21-25.
128. Baxi LV, Petrie RH, James LS. Human fetal oxygenation (TcPO$_2$), heart rate and uterine activity following maternal administration of meperidine. J Perinat Med 1988; 16:23-30.
129. Burstein Y, Giardina PJV, Rausen AR, Kandall SR, Siljestrom K, Peterson CM. Thrombocytosis and increased circulating platelet aggregates in newborn infants of polydrug users. J Pediatr 1979; 94:895-899.
130. Rementeria JL, Nunag NN. Narcotic withdrawal in pregnancy: Stillbirth Incidence with a case report. Am J Obstet Gynecol 1973; 116:1152-1156.
131. Chavez CJ, Ostrea EM, Stryker JC, Smialek Z. Sudden infant death syndrome among infants of drug-dependent mothers. J Pediatr 1979; 95:407-409.
132. Low L, Ratcliffe W, Alexander W. Intrauterine hypothyroidism due to anti-thyroid-drug therapy for thyrotoxicosis during pregnancy. Lancet 1978; 2: 370-371.
133. Refetoff S, Ochi Y, Selenkow HA, Rosenfield RL. Neonatal hypothyroidism and goiter in one infant of each of two sets of twins due to maternal therapy with antithyroid drugs. J Pediatr 1974; 85:240-244.
134. Hawe P, Francis HH. Pregnancy and thyrotoxicosis. Br Med J 1962; 2:817-822.
135. Le Gras MD, Seifert B, Casiro O. Neonatal nasal obstruction associated with methyldopa treatment during pregnancy [letter]. Am J Dis Child 1990; 144: 143-144.
136. Sulyok E, Bodis J, Hartman G, Ertl T. Neonatal effects of methyldopa therapy in pregnancy hypertension. Acta Pediatr Hung 1991; 31:53-65.
137. Crooks J. Haemolytic jaundice in a neonate after intra-amniotic injection of methylene blue. Arch Dis Child 1982; 57:872-873.
138. Van der Pol JG, Wolf H, Boer K, Treffers PE, Leschot NJ, Hey HA, Vos A. Jejunal atresia related to the use of methylene blue in genetic amniocentesis in twins. Br J Obstet Gynaecol 1992; 99:141 – 143.

296   *Bologa et al.*

139. Bjorksten B, Finnstrom O, Wichman K. Intrauterine exposure to the beta adrenergic receptor-blocking agent metoprolol and allergy. Int Arch Allergy Appl Immunol 1988; 87:59-62.
140. Cobrinik RW, Hodd RT Jr, Chusid E. The effect of maternal narcotic addiction on the newborn infant. Pediatrics 1959; 24:288-304.
141. Rosa FW, Idanpaan-Heikkila J, Asanti R. Fetal minoxidil exposure [letter]. Pediatrics 1987; 80:120.
142. Fox RE, Marx C, Stark AR. Neonatal effects of maternal nadolol therapy. Am J Obstet Gynecol 1985; 152:1045-1046.
143. Goodlin RC. Naloxone and its possible relationship to fetal endorphin levels and fetal distress. Am J Obstet Gynecol 1981; 139:16-19.
144. Gibbs J, Newson T, Williams J, Davidson DC. Naloxone hazard in infant of opioid abuser [letter]. Lancet 1989 2(8655):159-160.
145. Wilkinson AR, Aynsley-Green A, Mitchell MD. Persistent pulmonary hypertension and abnormal prostaglandin E levels in preterm infants after maternal treatment with naproxen. Arch Dis Child 1979; 54:942-945.
146. Bracero LA, Leikin E, Kirshenbaum N, Tejani N. Comparison of nifedipine and ritodrine for the treatment of preterm labor. Am J Perinatol 1991; 8:365-9.
147. Bongiovanni AM, McFadden AJ. Steroids during pregnancy and possible fetal consequences. Fertil Steril 1960; 11:181-184.
148. Jacobson BD. Hazards of norethindrone therapy during pregnancy. Am J Obstet Gynecol 1962; 84:962-968.
149. Hagler S, Schulz A, Hankin H, Kunstadter RN. Fetal effects of steroid therapy during pregnancy. Am J Dis Child 1963; 106:586-590.
150. Shearer WT, Schreiner RL, Marshall RE. Urinary retention in a neonate secondary to maternal ingestion of nortriptyline. J Pediatr 1972; 81:570-572.
151. Fisch GR, Henley WL. Symptoms of narcotic withdrawal in a newborn infant secondary to medical therapy of the mother. Pediatrics 1961; 28:852-853.
152. McConnell JB, Glasgow JF, McNair R. Effect on neonatal jaundice of oestrogens and progestogens taken before and after conception. Br Med J 1973; 3:605-607.
153. Profumo R, Toce S, Kotagal S. Neonatal choreoathetosis following prenatal exposure to oral contraceptives [letter]. Pediatrics 1990; 86:648-649.
154. Goetz RL, Bain RV. Neonatal withdrawal symptoms associated with maternal use of pentazocine. J Pediatr 1974; 84:887-888.
155. Dunn DW, Reynolds J. Neonatal withdrawal symptoms associated with T's and Blue's (pentazocine and tripelennamide). Am J Dis Child 1982; 136:644-645.
156. Wahab SA, Askalani AH, Amar RA, Ramadan ME, Neweigy SB, Saleh AA. Effects of some recent analgesics on labor pain and maternal and fetal blood gases and pH. Int J Gynaecol Obstet 1988; 26:75-80.
157. Strauss AA, Modanlou HD, Bosu SK. Neonatal manifestations of maternal phencyclidine (PCP) abuse. Pediatrics 1981; 68:550-552.
158. Tabor BL, Smith-Wallace T, Yonekura ML. Perinatal outcome associated with PCP versus cocaine use. Am J Drug Alcohol Abuse 1990; 16(3-4):337-348.

159. Lawrence A. Anti-epileptic drugs and the foetus. Br Med J 1963; 2:1267–1273.
160. Desmond MM, Schwanecke RP, Wilson GS, Yasunaga S, Burgdorff I. Maternal barbiturate utilization and neonatal withdrawal symptomatology. J Pediatr 1972; 80:190–197.
161. Allen RW Jr, Ogden B, Bentley FL, Jung AL. Fetal hydantoin syndrome, neuroblastoma and hemorrhagic disease in a neonate. JAMA 1980; 244:1464–1465.
162. Warrell DW, Taylor R. Outcome for the foetus of mothers receiving prednisolone during pregnancy. Lancet 1968; 1:117–118.
163. Rudd NL, Freedom RM. A possible primidone embryopathy. J Pediatr 1979; 94:835–837.
164. Bleyer WA, Skinner AL. Fatal neonatal hemorrhage after maternal anticonvulsant therapy. JAMA 1976; 235:626–627.
165. John E. Promazine and neonatal hyperbilirubinemia. Med J Aust 1975; 2:342–344.
166. Borgstedt AD, Rosen MG. Medication during labor correlated with behavior and EEG of the newborn. Am J Dis Child 1968; 115:21–24.
167. Corby DG, Shulman I. The effects of antenatal drug administration on aggregation of platelets of newborn infants. J Pediatr 1971; 79:307–313.
168. Quillan WW, Dunn CA. Neonatal drug withdrawal from propoxyphene. JAMA 1976; 235:2128.
169. Mitrani A, Oettinger M, Abinader EG, Sharf M, Klein A. Use of propranolol in dysfunctional labour. Br J Obstet Gynaecol 1975; 82:651–655.
170. Tunstall ME. The effect of propranolol on the onset of breathing at birth. Br J Anaesth 1969; 41:792–496.
171. Goodlin RC. Beta blocker in pregnancy-induced hypertension. Am J Obstet Gynecol 1982; 143:237–241.
172. Cheron RG, Kaplan MM, Larsen PR, Selenkow HA, Crigler JF Jr. Neonatal thyroid function after propylthiouracil therapy for maternal Graves' disease. N Engl J Med 1981; 304:525–528.
173. Man EB, Shaver BA Jr, Cooke RE. Studies of children born to women with thyroid disease. Am J Obstet Gynecol 1958; 75:728–741.
174. Hayashida CY, Duarte AJS, Sato AE, Yamashiro-Kanashiro EH. Neonatal hepatitis and lymphocyte sensitization by placental transfer of propylthiouracil. J Endocrinol Invest 1990; 13:937–941.
175. Hunt AD Jr, Stokes J Jr, McCrory WW, Stroud HH. Pyridoxine dependency: Report of a case of intractable convulsions in an infant controlled by pyridoxine. Pediatrics 154; 13:140–145.
176. Bejsovec MIR, Kulenda Z, Ponca E. Familial intrauterine convulsions in pyridoxine dependency. Arch Dis Child 1967; 42:201–207.
177. Domula VM, Weissach G, Lenk H. Über die auswirkung medikamentoser Behandlung in der Schwangerschaft auf das Gerennungspotential des Neugeborenen. Zentralbl Gynaekol 1977; 99:473–479.
178. Robinson GC, Brummitt JR, Miller JR. Hearing loss in infants and preschool children. II. Etiological considerations. Pediatrics 1963; 32:115–124.

179. McKinna AJ. Quinine induced hypoplasia of the optic nerve. Can J Ophthalmol 1966; 1:261–264.
180. Mauer MA, De Vaux W, Lahey ME. Neonatal and maternal thrombocytopenic purpura due to quinine. Pediatrics 1957; 19:84–87.
181. Glass L, Rajegowda BK, Bowne E, Evans HE. Exposure to quinine and jaundice in a G6PD-deficient newborn infant. Pediatrics 1973; 82:734–735.
182. Evans ANW, Brooke OG, West RJ. The ingestion by pregnant women of substances toxic to foetus. Practitioner 1980; 224:315.
183. Budnick IS, Leikin S, Hoeck LE. Effect in the newborn infant to reserpine administration ante partum. Am J Dis Child 1955; 90:286–289.
184. Eggermont E, Logghe N, Van De Casseye W, Casteels-Van Daele M, Jaeken J, Cosemans J, Verstaete M, Renaer M. Hemorrhagic disease of the newborn in the offspring of rifampicin and isoniazid treated mothers. Acta Paediatr Belg 1976; 29:87–90.
185. Leake RD, Hobel CJ, Oh W, Thiebeault DW, Okada DM, Williams PR. A controlled, prospective study of the effects of ritodrine hydrochloride for premature labor. Clin Res 1980; 28:90A (abstr).
186. Schilthius MS, Aarnaoudse JG. Fetal death associated with severe ritodrine induced ketoacidosis. Lancet 1980; 1:1145.
187. Evens RP, Leopold JC. Scopolamine toxicity in a newborn. Pediatrics 1980; 329–330.
188. Donald PR, Sellars SL. Streptomycin ototoxicity in the unborn child. South Afr Med J 1981; 60:316–318.
189. Kantor HI, Sutherland DA, Leonard JT, Kamholz FH, Fry ND, White WL. Effect on bilirubin metabolism in the newborn of sulfisoxazole administration to the mother. Obstet Gynecol 1961; 17:494–500.
190. Perkins RP. Hydrops fetalis and stillbirth in a male glucose-6-phosphate dehydrogenase-deficient fetus possible due to maternal ingestion of sulfisoxazole. Am J Obstet Gynecol 1971; 111:379–381.
191. Epstein MF, Nicholls RN, Stubblefield PG. Neonatal hypoglycemia after beta-sympathomimetic tocolytic therapy. J Pediatr 1979; 94:449–453.
192. Thorkelsson T, Loughead JL. Long-term subcutaneous terbutaline tocolysis: Report of possible neonatal toxicity. J Perinatol 1991; 11:235–8.
193. Fletcher SE, Fyfe DA, Case CL, Wiles HB, Upshur JK, Newman RB. Myocardial necrosis in a newborn after long-term maternal subcutaneous terbutaline infusion for suppression of preterm labor. Am J Obstet Gynecol 1991; 165 (5 pt 1):1401–1404.
194. Toaff R, Ravid R. Tetracyclines and the teeth. Lancet 1966; 2:281–282.
195. Kline AH, Blattner RJ, Lunin M. Transplacental effect of tetracyclines on teeth. JAMA 1964; 188:178–180.
196. Kaplan MM. Acute fatty liver of pregnancy. N Engl J Med 1985; 313:367–370.
197. Arwood LL, Dasta JF, Friedman C. Placental transfer of theophylline: Two case reports. Pediatrics 1979; 63:844–846.
198. Horowitz DA, Jablonski W, Mehta KA. Apnea associated with theophylline withdrawal in a term neonate. Am J Dis Child 1982; 136:73–74.

199. Schiff D, Aranda J, Stern L. Neonatal thrombocytopenia and congenital malformation associated with administration of tolbutamide to the mother. J Pediatr 1970; 77:457–458.
200. Hill LM. Fetal distress secondary to vancomycin-induced maternal hypotension. Am J Obstet Gynecol 1985; 153:74–75.
201. Sperling RS, Stratton P, O'Sullivan MJ, Boyer P, Watts DH, Lambert JS, Hammil H, Livinston EG, Gloeb DJ, Minkoff H, Fox HE. A survey of zidovudine use in pregnant women with human immunodeficiency virus infection. Am J Obstet Gynecol 1990; 163:728–732.

14

Nonmedical Drug and Chemical Use in Pregnancy

Joyce F. Schneiderman
The Addiction Research Foundation and The University of Toronto, Toronto, Ontario, Canada

Clinical Case

One of your pregnant patients admits having used narcotic opioids for several years. She wishes very much to discontinue this addiction pattern but does not know how.

INTRODUCTION

Nonmedical drug use can be defined as the taking of any psychoactive drug in the absence of a clearly defined medical indication (1). People ingest many chemicals to modify mood: as part of a social or recreational activity, as part of a lifestyle, or to self-medicate. Drugs are widely available in modern society. Alcohol, caffeine, and nicotine are so commonly used that they are not always considered to be drugs. Prescription drugs, like narcotics and benzodiazepines, may be obtained via a physician or via other sources. Illicit drugs, whose purity, dose, and sometimes even the substance itself are unknown include narcotics, stimulants, cannabinoids, and hallucinogens.

This chapter focuses on the management of women who use psychoactive drugs during pregnancy; it covers advice appropriate to the woman who plans to discontinue her drug use and discusses the care of the drug abuser who will require intensive treatment and support in a specialized setting. Neonatal withdrawal and drug use while breastfeeding are discussed in Chapters 10 and 15. Detailed discussion of drug abuse treatment and of the teratogenicity of psychoactive drugs is beyond the scope of this chapter.

Women of childbearing age have been increasing their nonmedical drug use over the last two decades (2–5). This increase and the thalidomide tragedy have fueled a concern for the effects of drugs on pregnancy. Recreational drug users and drug-dependent women may appear unconcerned about health risks to themselves, but they, too, usually wish to spare their unborn children from risks associated with drug use.

Our experience at the Motherisk Clinic in Toronto suggests that many women and their primary care physicians overestimate the risk of drugs to the fetus (6). Some women will consider therapeutic abortion, often on the recommendation of their doctor, fearing a major teratogenic effect. It is therefore extremely important to provide accurate information on the known risks of maternal drug-taking.

There is no evidence that the father's drug and alcohol consumption directly influences the outcome of pregnancy. His use may nonetheless be a marker for other factors contributing to increased risk. Concerns that previous drug use in either parent, particularly of hallucinogens and cannabinoids, may lead to an adverse outcome based on permanent chromosomal damage are unwarranted.

In the 1990s, it is rare to find a woman drug abuser who uses only one drug or even one drug class. The synergistic effects of drug interactions on the fetus remain largely unknown. An adverse outcome may be related to drug exposure at a critical period in gestation, to maximal drug level obtained, to cumulative exposure, or to a combination of these and other factors. The outcome of pregnancy in the alcohol- or drug-dependent woman depends on more than just her drug-taking behavior. The pharmacological effects are often compounded by lack of prenatal care, higher risk for other complications of pregnancy, cigarette smoking, and poor diet.

The outcome in women of the inner city drug subculture cannot be extrapolated to the woman who has used a substance one or several times socially, nor to the woman who has received a short course of parenteral narcotics in the treatment of an acute medical or surgical illness prior to knowledge of the pregnancy.

Neurobehavioral abnormalities have been reported in neonates of drug-using mothers (7); alcohol (8), marijuana (9), methadone (10), and cocaine (11) have been among the substances implicated. However, it is not possible to separate the contribution of prenatal drug exposure from the effects of persistent drug levels at birth, withdrawal symptoms, difficulties with mother-infant bonding, and continued drug exposure if the mother is breast-feeding. Data on long-term sequelae of prenatal drug use are limited, and results must be interpreted in light of the frequently suboptimal postnatal environment (Table 1).

Table 1 Risks Associated with Individual Drugs

Drug class	Alcohol	Narcotics	Cocaine	Marijuana	LSD, PCP	Solvents	Benzodiazapines	Barbiturates	Tobacco
Risk for withdrawal									
Mother	X							X	
Fetus	X	X							
Growth retardation	X	X	X	X		X			X
Neurobehavioral abnormalities	X	X	X	X	X	X			
Neonatal withdrawal syndrome	X	X	X				X	X	
Congenital malformation	X					X			

GENERAL GUIDELINES FOR CLINICAL MANAGEMENT

Because pregnancy is usually diagnosed at 6-8 weeks after the last menstrual period, it is important to consider the woman's usual drug-taking behavior. Confirmation of pregnancy may be further delayed in the drug abuser because the menstrual cycle is often irregular, and prolonged amenorrhea is common in this population. Early symptoms of pregnancy such as nausea, cramps, and fatigue, if they are attributed to drug withdrawal, may result in an increase in drug use.

For the woman presenting early in pregnancy and motivated to discontinue her drug use, a single counseling session addressing the adverse effects on pregnancy outcome if drug use is not curtailed may be sufficient. Even the problem user with some social stability can be managed by the primary care physician as an outpatient with a tailored detoxification regimen (see below) and a short course of weekly or biweekly counseling. If the patient is unsuccessful in following through on this plan after a 2-week trial, or if she is severely drug dependent and in crisis, referral for specialized alcohol and drug treatment services is indicated.

The initial approach to the woman with a significant alcohol or drug problem should include a complete medical and obstetrical assessment. The drug history is part of data collection and should be taken in a nonjudgmental manner. Alcohol, tobacco, caffeine, over-the-counter drugs, prescription medications, and illicit substance use should each be asked about specifically, including drug names, dose, route, timing in relation to conception, adverse reactions, and symptoms of overdose and withdrawal. Familiarity with street names and local availability of illicit drugs is helpful. A detailed psychosocial history provides the information on the patient's attitude about the pregnancy, the involvement of the baby's father, the condition of other children, and the current housing, financial, employment, and legal situations necessary to plan treatment.

The physical examination should screen for associated medical problems, such as trauma, hepatitis, abscesses, and sexually transmitted diseases. Urine toxicology for alcohol, benzodiazepines, barbiturates, cannabinoids, narcotics, and stimulants should be done at the first visit and repeated regularly throughout the pregnancy. An ultrasound examination is useful to establish gestational age and to assess fetal morphology. For women who are ambivalent about discontinuing drug use, this procedure may have therapeutic benefit (12). By making the pregnancy more "real," it may be possible to increase the commitment of such a woman to ensure the best possible outcome for her child.

Women with a long history of alcohol- and drug-related problems will usually require inpatient detoxification or methadone maintenance substitution. Prenatal care should be integrated with drug treatment. A multidisciplinary staff team comprising a physician, a nurse, a social worker, an addiction counselor, and a dietician is useful for case management. These patients can be difficult and time-consuming. A consistent approach by all team members is crucial so that the patient receives a clear message. The individual patient situation will dictate the need for a residential treatment program, or outpatient individual or group counseling. If a spouse or partner who also has a drug problem is involved, every attempt should be made to facilitate his treatment. Liaison with Alcoholics Anonymous, Narcotics Anonymous, and other voluntary self-help groups is valuable.

The ideal situation assumes a motivated patient presenting early in pregnancy and the availability of resources to provide intensive treatment if necessary. In many cases, prenatal care is sporadic at best, and crisis intervention (medical or psychosocial) may be the only treatment accepted. Each patient contact should be taken as an opportunity to engage her in ongoing care. At present, there is little to offer the woman who refuses treatment, but with sensitive handling she may ultimately comply voluntarily with a treatment plan. In Ontario, the Children's Aid Society will not intervene until after the birth of the child. This is also the case for child protection agencies in most other jurisdictions. If the woman presents before 12 weeks of gestation and wishes to consider a therapeutic abortion, this should be discussed if applicable laws permit, but this option should not be recommended as a standard practice.

The clinician's personal views on the use of illicit substances and alcohol should not be allowed to interfere with forming a therapeutic alliance with the patient. The pregnant substance-abusing patient is generally ambivalent about seeking treatment and responds best to a nonthreatening approach. She should be provided with specific objective information on the known effects of her drug use on the pregnancy, and she should be encouraged to stop all use in the context of ensuring the best possible fetal outcome. After the birth, mother and child should be closely followed. Postnatal care should include supportive counseling, contraception counseling, public health nurse visits, and training in parenting skills.

ILLICIT SUBSTANCES AND INTRAVENOUS DRUG ABUSE

The lifestyle of intravenous drug-using women plays a very important part in the formulation of the treatment plan. If they and their children remain in the drug-using community, they are not likely to abstain. Furthermore, pregnancy does not guarantee protection from the high incidence of physical violence these women experience (13). Exchange of sexual favors for drugs in addition to prostitution puts these women at high risk for sexually transmitted diseases. Sharing unsterilized needles puts them at risk both for hepatitis B and human immunodeficiency virus (HIV) infections. With prenatal screening and immunization as required, perinatal transmission of hepatitis B can now largely be prevented.

Women account for 7% of AIDS cases in the United States (14–16). More than half these women are intravenous drug users (17), and over 80% are of childbearing age. The incidence of perinatal transmission of AIDS is still uncertain. Friedland and Klein estimate a rate of roughly 40–50% based on information available in 1987 (16). Infants retain maternal antibody to a median age of 10 months (18) and must be monitored for the development of symptoms of AIDS. Prevention must be based on education and counseling of all intravenous drug users and their sexual partners. Routine screening for HIV in this population is controversial. Instead, serological testing should be offered to any high risk woman contemplating a pregnancy. Contraceptive counseling is mandatory in any woman known to be HIV positive.

Individual Drugs

Alcohol

Most women are aware that heavy drinking in pregnancy can harm the fetus. The fetal alcohol syndrome (FAS), first described by Smith and Jones in 1973, is now generally accepted to occur in the offspring of alcoholic women, that is, women who drink at least six standard drinks per day throughout the first trimester [one standard drink = 12 oz beer = 5 oz glass of wine = 1.5 oz liquor or approximately 15 g (0.5 oz) absolute alcohol]. The signs of

FAS are prenatal and postnatal growth retardation, central nervous system dysfunction (often including mental retardation), facial dysmorphology, and many other congenital abnormalities (19–24). A proposed minimum criterion for the diagnosis of FAS recommends that at least two of the following be present: microcephaly (head circumference less than the third percentile), microphthalmia and/or short palpebral fissures, poorly developed philtrum, thin upper lip, and flattening of the maxillary area, in addition to growth and neurological abnormalities (25).

The fetal alcohol syndrome has been estimated to occur in between one and two live births per 1000 in the general population and is a major preventable cause of mental retardation. An incidence of greater than 40% has been reported in alcoholic women. However, prospectively collected data suggest a true incidence closer to 2.5% (26).

On long-term follow-up, FAS children display lack of catch-up growth, attentional deficits, mental retardation, and dysmorphic features. With time, some improvement in all these areas occurs owing to biological maturation, but the children manifest poor school performance which is independent of environment (27).

Other adverse fetal outcomes in heavy drinkers include increased spontaneous abortions (26), premature placental separation, stillbirth, low birth weight (28), and congenital malformations (29). Drinking by the father in the month prior to conception has been associated with decreased birth weight (30), but as indicated above, this finding does not necessarily represent causality.

The data on women drinking less than six drinks per day are more difficult to interpret. Studies may rely on retrospective self-reports, use averaged amounts throughout the pregnancy, and employ varying definitions for moderate drinking. At drinking levels greater than two drinks per day, a partial FAS not meeting the minimum criteria, termed *fetal alcohol effects*, has been described. No such effects have been reported when consumption is less than two drinks per day (31). A prospective study examining first-trimester alcohol use evaluated congenital malformations by chart review, including 32,409 patients drinking two or fewer drinks per day. There was no significant increase in malformations between the group drinking up to two drinks and abstainers (32). Another study of more than 12,000 pregnancies showed an increase in abruptio placentae, but no other adverse outcome associated with an intake of less than two drinks per day (33).

There is no known safe lower limit for alcohol consumption in pregnancy, and many authorities recommend complete abstinence on this basis. Clearly, this is the most conservative approach. If all women of childbearing age were to abstain from alcohol, presumably FAS would disappear. The absence of risk is of course very difficult to demonstrate scientifically. Pregnancy should not be a time for undue restriction of lifestyle, and most women do drink. Even women who plan to abstain during pregnancy usually continue their customary drinking pattern until they confirm they are pregnant. The mother of an infant with an unrelated congenital abnormality should not have to bear the guilt of thinking that her minimal alcohol intake was responsible.

Rosett and Weiner conclude that there is no measurable risk from consuming less than 1 oz absolute alcohol (two standard drinks) per day (34). A Canadian committee has recommended abstinence, "or at least to limit consumption to less than 4 drinks per week" (35). Setting reasonable goals for moderation may enhance clinical credibility and compliance, while fairly emphasizing the hazards of heavy drinking.

Alcohol consumption in the month preceding recognition of pregnancy most accurately reflects early postconception drinking. Even among the heaviest drinkers, more than 50% of women spontaneously decrease their intake at the diagnosis of pregnancy (36). The social drinker also markedly decreases her drinking, often citing distaste, lack of appeal, or adverse physiological effects (37).

In the heavy social drinker or physically dependent woman, detoxification should occur as early as possible, and complete abstinence should be the only treatment goal considered. For a woman who is drinking greater than 80 g per day, a gradual reduction over 3-4 days is preferable (34). Intensive supportive counseling should be available during detoxification and throughout the pregnancy. If the woman uses other drugs, has a medical illness, or seems unlikely to be successful as an outpatient because of prior failure or current circumstances, inpatient admission should be arranged. We have successfully used a diazepam-loading regimen in women requiring hospitalization and pharmacological treatment of alcohol withdrawal (38). The long half-life of diazepam offers a "pharmacological taper," so that the patient usually does not require further drug after the first day of admission. This regimen is well tolerated by the pregnant woman, allowing early initiation of a global treatment plan instead of focusing on withdrawal symptomatology.

Disulfiram interferes with the intermediary metabolism of ethanol. The alcohol-disulfiram reaction is believed to be due to accumulation of acetaldehyde, and this pharmacological effect has been used as an adjunct in the treatment of alcohol dependence. Since the efficacy of disulfiram is unproven and the potential for a severe reaction and teratogenic effect must be considered, this drug is contraindicated in the woman who is pregnant or planning a pregnancy (39). The woman taking disulfiram who has an unplanned pregnancy should be counseled with respect to the reported associations of teratogenesis. One series of five cases reported one spontaneous abortion and two cases of clubfoot (40). Another group described two case reports of infants with limb reduction (41). Isolated case reports do not necessarily mean teratogenesis, and therefore therapeutic abortion should not routinely be recommended. A detailed ultrasound examination may be helpful.

Narcotics

Heroin use is associated with decreased birth weight and a higher incidence of medical, primarily infectious, and obstetrical complications. Narcotics do not appear to be teratogenic in humans (42). Infants of narcotic-dependent women are at risk for neonatal withdrawal (43) and sudden infant death syndrome (44). Although total abstinence seems preferable, this is often not realistically feasible. Pregnant women recently detoxified from narcotics have the same high rate of recidivism as nonpregnant addict (45,46). Rapid detoxification has been associated with fetal distress and death (47,48).

Methadone maintenance has been the treatment of choice for the heroin addict (49). Pharmacologically methadone suppresses withdrawal symptoms and in high enough doses will block opioid effects. It provides a constant drug level rather than the wide fluctuations that occur with illicit intravenous use, thus avoiding fetal risks from overdose or withdrawal. In addition to decreasing illicit use, methadone maintenance provides a framework for ongoing, often daily, contact with a treatment facility and institution of counseling and prenatal care.

With methadone maintenance, fetal outcome improves and birth weights increase albeit less than those in matched nondrug-using controls. Kandall et al. (50) report mean birth weights of 2490 g in heroin-abusing mothers, 2961 g in methadone-maintained mothers, and 3176 g in controls. Birth weight correlates to the methadone dose (50); however, it is likely that other factors are responsible. For example, there may be less illicit use in women receiving high doses. A good outcome also correlates with the number of prenatal visits.

A short initial hospitalization may provide the opportunity for prenatal assessment, treatment of concurrent medical problems, crisis intervention, introduction of the members of the multidisciplinary team, and stabilization on methadone (46). Ideally, the methadone dose should be carefully titrated to withdrawal symptoms with special attention to lower abdominal cramping, which may reflect uterine irritability, so that the woman is on the lowest possible dose. With a starting dose of 10–20 mg and additional doses every 6–8 hours, the maintenance dose can be arrived at within 24–48 hours. In some programs, this is not feasible and higher doses of 50–80 mg daily are chosen empirically. If a woman can be maintained on 20–25 mg daily, significant neonatal withdrawal usually does not occur (51,52).

Areas outside major urban centers often lack methadone maintenance clinics. In such areas, for the prescription abuser, or other highly motivated women with good community supports, a gradual outpatient detoxification with methadone or another narcotic can be undertaken over one to several weeks. This is most safely accomplished in the second trimester, when the risk of spontaneous abortion or precipitation of premature labor is lowest.

What are the long-term effects of prenatal methadone exposure? Longitudinal studies of infants to age 2 have found mental and physical development to be well within the normal range, although some differences from controls were noted. When evaluated at age 4 and 5, no differences were found from controls, but both groups had low scores, most likely an effect of low socioeconomic status (53,54). Accepting the difficulties in attempting to control for confounding variables, it appears that methadone in utero is one of the least important factors in the developmental outcome of these children.

Cocaine and Other Stimulants

The use of the stimulant cocaine increased rapidly in the past decade but now appears to have passed its peak. By 1986, nearly 40% of the U.S. population in the age range of 25–30 years had tried cocaine (55,56). Women of childbearing age are of particular concern because of the potential risk to the fetus.

The first report of cocaine effects on pregnancy outcome appeared in 1985 (11). Spontaneous abortions, prematurity, and intrauterine growth retardation are increased in cocaine-using mothers. Labor may be precipitated following a large intravenous bolus of cocaine, and there is a 10-fold increase in the incidence of abruptio placentae (57–60). Several infants have been reported with perinatal cerebral infarction (59). These adverse effects can be explained by the physiological alterations of acute cocaine intoxication.

A withdrawal syndrome and neurobehavioral abnormalities have been described in a small number of infants of cocaine-using mothers (11). There does not appear to be an increase in the rate of major congenital abnormalities. Because of the small sample size, difficulty in controlling for other drug use, and differing inclusion criteria in all the reports above, these findings must be considered to be preliminary.

Management of the mother depends on the extent of her drug use as well as concurrent medical and social problems. Many women can be managed as outpatients. Cocaine use often follows a cyclical pattern. Periods of abstinence of one to several weeks do not imply a less severe dependence, and counseling aimed at preventing relapse is crucial. Residential treatment should be made available to patients unable to abstain. Cocaine withdrawal consists of the "crash": several hours to days of depression, hypersomnolence, and hyperphagia, followed by a period of anergia and intense cocaine craving (56). No specific pharmacological therapy is required, since this syndrome does not appear to have any serious consequences to mother or fetus unless depression is severe enough to cause suicidal ideation.

Heavy cocaine users often take central nervous system depressants such as alcohol and benzodiazepines for symptom relief during the crash phase and may have significant cross-dependence on these agents. A complete drug and alcohol history should be obtained to identify patients at risk for depressant withdrawal, since this information is not always volunteered.

Amphetamines and other stimulants have a pharmacological profile similar to that of cocaine. Owing to restrictions on prescription use and limited illicit availability, the abuse of stimulants, with the exception of cocaine, is now a rarity. The Collaborative Perinatal Project found no evidence of teratogenesis with this class of drugs (61). Schardein, who reviewed the reports citing increased malformations, concluded that the evidence is generally negative (42). Clinically, the amphetamine-using mother presents in much the same way as the cocaine user and should be managed similarly (60,62).

Cannabinoids

The prevalence of marijuana use at the time of conception, which has been reported as 9–20% (9,63), varies with the population studied. More than half these women become abstainers during the first trimester. Although marijuana is not usually thought to be associated with a physical withdrawal syndrome, many regular users report irritability, sleep disturbance, and decreased appetite upon abrupt cessation (64). We have had a number of pregnant patients complain of severe nausea and vomiting on discontinuing marijuana smoking in the first trimester. This is consistent with the antiemetic effect of the cannabinoids.

Several studies have reported a decrease in birth weight and an increase in the prevalence of small-for-gestational-age babies and preterm infants in marijuana users (65,66). This has not been a consistent finding; it is likely related to a wide range of intake. Wu et al. reported a nearly fivefold greater increment in the blood carboxyhemoglobin level and a threefold increase of inhaled tar with smoking marijuana compared with tobacco cigarettes (67). Thus, effects similar to those in tobacco users would be expected in heavy marijuana users in addition to any effect from its active ingredient, Δ-9-tetrahydrocannabinol. Marijuana has not been associated with congenital abnormalities in humans. Fried found a dose-related association between marijuana smoking and alterations in visual responsiveness as well as increased tremors and startle reflexes in the newborn (9).

Hallucinogens, Phencyclidine, and Solvents

Prenatal exposure to lysergic acid diethylamide (LSD) has been implicated in an increased incidence of limb defects (68) and central nervous system and ocular abnormalities (42), but the evidence for teratogenic effects in humans is not convincing. With the widespread use of LSD in the 1970s, it is unlikely that a major teratogenic effect would have been missed. An early ultrasound examination is nonetheless recommended to rule out serious dysmorphogenesis.

Phencyclidine (PCP) was used by 0.8% of pregnant patients in one study; 7.3% gave a history of past use (69). A single case report describes an infant born with abnormal appearance and behavior who subsequently developed a spastic quadriparesis (70). Chasnoff et al. described seven infants with sudden outbursts of agitation and rapid changes in the level of consciousness at birth, but no congenital abnormalities (71).

Recreational solvent abusers choose toluene-containing products preferentially. Toluene can be obtained in relatively pure form in a variety of readily available and inexpensive products, such as lacquer thinner and contact cement cleaner. Acute solvent intoxication is similar to that of alcohol; there is no significant withdrawal syndrome (72). With chronic use, a persistent encephalopathy may develop, characterized by signs of cortical and cerebellar dysfunction. This is at least partially reversible with abstinence (73). The evidence for teratogenicity from occupational exposure is inconclusive. Hersh reported three cases whose mothers regularly inhaled a toluene product throughout pregnancy. All the infants had microcephaly, central nervous system dysfunction, attentional deficits, developmental delay, growth deficiency, and facial dysmorphology, a pattern quite similar to fetal alcohol syndrome (74). Users tend to have deprived backgrounds and limited social supports; inpatient treatment is usually indicated to initiate abstinence, but prognosis is generally poor.

Withdrawal from hallucinogens, PCP, and solvents can usually be managed supportively. When severe agitation in the intoxication phase is unresponsive to reassurance, benzodiazepines can be administered. The acutely psychotic patient may require a neuroleptic; haloperidol, a butyrophenone, is usually better tolerated than the phenothiazines.

Benzodiazepines

Benzodiazepines are in widespread use therapeutically and are frequently consumed by polydrug abusers. Although isolated abuse of high doses of benzodiazepines is rare, it is not uncommon to find women who have been maintained on chronic therapeutic doses for many years. In 1975 two groups reported an increase in risk of cleft lip and palate with first-trimester exposure to benzodiazepines (75,76). A subsequent case control study did not confirm this effect (77). The newer benzodiazepines have not been associated with specific abnormalities. Seven cases of a fetal benzodiazepine syndrome have been reported, but without adequate controls it is difficult to attribute a causative role (78). Given the high prevalence of benzodiazepine use, a human teratogenic effect is not likely to be large, if it exists at all (79).

A woman planning a pregnancy should be encouraged to discontinue her benzodiazepine use prior to conception (80). In counseling the woman with a history of first-trimester use, the clinician should provide a balanced summary of the reported effects. Although benzodiazepines are probably not teratogenic in humans, an ultrasound examination can be reassuring even if it does not guarantee the absence of abnormalities. A neonatal benzodiazepine abstinence syndrome has been reported (81), so detoxification should be advised regardless of the time in pregnancy that the woman presents.

Attempts at withdrawal are often unsuccessful when abrupt cessation leads to uncomfortable symptoms. In addition to anxiety and insomnia, these patients characteristically complain of sensory misperceptions and illusions, as well as depersonalization. A tapering regimen with diazepam obviates the fluctuations in drug levels that occur with the shorter-acting benzodiazepines. A rough guideline for converting to an equivalent dose of diazepam is to assume that the largest unit dose available is equipotent to 10 mg diazepam. The socially stable patient can generally be tapered by 5 mg diazepam per week with weekly outpatient supportive counseling (82). Abstinence can usually be achieved in 6–8 weeks. If outpatient detoxification is unsuccessful, a rapid diazepam taper may be tried in an inpatient unit. If abstinence cannot be achieved, the patient should be maintained on the lowest possible dose.

Barbiturates and Hypnosedatives

Owing to limited availability, the barbiturates and nonbarbiturate hypnosedatives (chloral hydrate, glutethimide, meprobamate, methaqualone) are no longer commonly abused substances. Butalbital, available only as a proprietary combination with aspirin and caffeine with or without codeine (Fiorinal-C), is the only barbiturate we see frequently (83). Heinonen et al., in the Boston Collaborative Study, found little evidence for a teratogenic effect in this group of drugs (61).

Because of the danger of a major withdrawal syndrome (tonic-clonic seizures and delirium) the pregnant woman ingesting more than 400 mg of barbiturate or equivalent daily should be admitted to the hospital for detoxification. Phenobarbital is the drug of choice, given either on a tapering schedule (84) or by an oral loading technique (85). A neonatal abstinence syndrome has been described.

Tobacco

Annual per capita cigarette consumption has decreased steadily in North America since 1973. However, the decrease has been much less in women than in men and the percentage of heavy smokers has increased, perhaps suggesting that many less severely dependent individuals have successfully quit (86). For married white women age 20 and over, the prevalence of smoking during pregnancy decreased from 40% to 25% between 1967 and 1980. This drop was greatest in women with high educational levels (87).

The smoker is 80% more likely than the nonsmoker to have a spontaneous abortion and is 100% more likely to have a low birth weight infant (< 2500 g). Cigarette smoking in pregnancy is associated with decreased birth weight, by an average of 200 g. This effect is dose dependent, is independent of other factors, and can be reversed by cessation of smoking in early pregnancy. Smoking during pregnancy leads to increased perinatal mortality, prematurity, placenta previa, and abruption (88,89). Although some studies have shown an increase in congenital malformations, most have not, and summing the data, we can say that tobacco smoking does not appear to cause human teratogenicity.

Sexton and Hebel performed a randomized controlled study of an intensive smoking cessation intervention during pregnancy. Prior to randomization both groups had decreased their mean number of cigarettes smoked by half and about 15% had quit. The reported quitting rate at 8 months gestation was 20% for the control group and 43% for the treatment group (91). Use of a self-help booklet has been shown to increase smoking cessation in public health maternity clinics (92). Education and support to decrease smoking can be effective in patients who do not spontaneously change their smoking behavior at the onset of pregnancy (93) and may result in improved fetal outcome. Nicotine chewing gum, although a useful adjunct to smoking cessation therapy, should not be used in pregnancy.

Caffeine

The average intake of caffeine in pregnancy is 144 mg/day, or about one cup of filtered coffee or two cups of tea (94). Several studies have demonstrated little or no fetal effect of caffeine (95,96). Animal studies using high doses and some human studies reporting adverse outcome have led most clinicians to recommend caution in beverage caffeine consumption. Since many of the adverse physiological effects of caffeine do not occur at doses below 400 mg/day (97), it is reasonable to limit consumption to this level.

SUMMARY

The mood-altering drugs have not been documented to be major teratogens with the exception of alcohol and possibly organic solvents. Most have been associated with intrauterine growth retardation, and a neonatal withdrawal syndrome at birth in infants of chronic, heavy users. In many women, a brief intervention consisting of education and support in the primary care setting can limit the morbidity of nonmedical drug use. A comprehensive prenatal program for drug-dependent women can help improve outcome in this high-risk population.

Answer

It is important to link this patient without delay with a program that specializes in addiction. Therapy should include all domains of life, since addiction cannot be effectively treated without accounting for its psychosocial aspects. Pharmacologically, most favorable experience comes from protocols using the long-acting opioid methadone.

FURTHER READING

Chasnoff IJ (ed). Drug Use in Pregnancy: Mother and Child, MTP Press, Norwell, MA, 1986.

Finnegan LP (ed). Drug Dependence in Pregnancy: Clinical Management of Mother and Child, National Institute on Drug Abuse, Washington, DC, 1979.

Jaffe JH. Drug addiction and drug abuse. In The Pharmacologic Basis of Therapeutics, 7th ed (Gilman AG, Goodman LS, Rall TW, Murad F, eds), Macmillan, 1985, New York, 532–851.

Rosett HL, Weiner L. Alcohol and the Fetus: A Clinical Perspective, Oxford University Press, New York, 1984.

REFERENCES

1. Jaffe JH. Drug addiction and drug abuse. In The Pharmacological Basis of Therapeutics, 7th ed (Gilman AG, Goodman LS, Rall TW, Murad F, eds), Macmillan, New York, 1985, pp 532–581.
2. Nicholi AM. The nontherapeutic use of psychoactive drugs. N Engl J Med 1983; 308:925–933.
3. Smart RG, Adlaf EM. Alcohol and other drug use among Ontario adults. Alcoholism and Drug Addiction Research Foundation, Toronto, Ont., Canada, 1987, pp 1–57.
4. Rayburn W, Wible-Kant J, Bledsoe P. Changing trends in drug use during pregnancy. J Reprod Med 1982; 27:569–575.
5. Freid PA, Watkinson B, Grant A, Knights RM. Changing patterns of soft drug use prior to and during pregnancy: A prospective study. Drug Alcohol Depend 1980; 6:323–343.
6. Koren G, Bologa-Campeanu M, Long D, et al. The perception of teratogenic risk by pregnant women exposed to drugs and chemicals during the first trimester. Am J Obstet Gynecol 1989; 160:1190–1194.
7. Chasnoff IJ, Schnoll SH, Burns WJ, Burns K. Maternal nonnarcotic substance abuse during pregnancy: Effects on infant development. Neurobehav Toxicol Teratol 1984; 6:277–280.

8. Landesman-Dwyer S, Keller S, Streissguth AP. Naturalistic observations of newborns: Effects of maternal alcohol intake. Alcoholism Clin Exp Res 1978; 2: 171–177.
9. Fried PA. Marijuana use by pregnant women: Neurobehavioral effects in neonates. Drug Alcohol Depend 1980; 6:415–424.
10. Rosen TS, Johnson HL. Methadone exposure: Effects on behavior in early infancy. Pediatr Pharmacol 1982; 2:192–196.
11. Chesnoff IJ, Burns WJ, Schnoll SH, Burns KA. Cocaine use in pregnancy. N Engl J Med 1985; 313:666–669.
12. Fletcher JC, Evans MI. Maternal bonding in early fetal ultrasound examinations. N Engl J Med 1983; 308:392–393.
13. Regan DO, Ehrlich SM, Finnegan LP. Infants of drugs addicts: At risk for child abuse, neglect, and placement in foster care. Neurotoxicol Teratol 1987; 9:315–319.
14. Scott GB, Fischl MA, Klimas N, et al. Mothers of infants with the acquired immunodeficiency syndrome: Evidence for both symptomatic and asymptomatic carriers. JAMA 1985; 253:363–366.
15. Thomas PA, Lubin K. Milberg J, et al. Cohort comparison study of children whose mothers have acquired immunodeficiency syndrome and children of well inner city mothers. Pediatr Infect Dis 1987; 6:247–251.
16. Friedland GH, Klein RS. Transmission of the human immunodeficiency virus. N Engl J Med 1987; 317:1125–1135.
17. Guinan ME, Hardy A. Epidemiology of AIDS in women in the United States 1981 through 1986. JAMA 1987; 257:2039–2042.
18. Mok JQ, Guaguinto C, De Rossi A, et al. Infants born to mothers seropositive for human immunodeficiency virus. Lancet 1987; 1:1164–1168.
19. Jones KL, Smith DW. Recognition of the fetal alcohol syndrome in early infancy. Lancet 1973; 2:999–1001.
20. Jones KL, Smith DW, Ulleland CN, et al. Pattern of malformation in offspring of chronic alcoholic mothers. Lancet 1973; 1:1267–1271.
21. Clarren SK, Smith DW. The fetal alcohol syndrome. N Engl J Med 1978; 298: 1063–1067.
22. Jones KL, Smith DW, Streissguth AP, Myrianthopoulos NC. Outcome in offspring of chronic alcoholic women. Lancet 1974; 1:1076–1078.
23. Hanson JW, Jones KL, Smith DW. Fetal alcohol syndrome: Experience with 41 patients. JAMA 1976; 235:1458–1460.
24. Streissguth AP, Herman CS, Smith DW. Intelligence, behavior, and dysmorphogenesis in the fetal alcohol syndrome: A report on 20 patients. J Pediatr 1978; 92:363–367.
25. Rosett HL. A clinical perspective of the fetal alcohol syndrome. Alcohol Clin Exp Res 1980; 4:119–122.
26. Sokol RJ, Miller SI. Reed G. Alcohol abuse during pregnancy: An epidemiologic study. Alcohol Clin Exp Res 1980; 4:135–145.
27. Spohr HL, Steinhausen HC. Follow-up studies of children with fetal alcohol syndrome. Neuropediatrics 1987; 18:13–17.

28. Kaminski M, Rumeau-Rouquette C, Schwartz D. Alcohol consumption in pregnant women and the outcome of pregnancy. Alcohol Clin Exp Res 1978; 2:155-163.
29. Ouellette EM, Rosett HL, Rosman NP, Weiner L. Adverse effects on offspring of maternal alcohol abuse during pregnancy. N Engl J Med 1977; 297:528-530.
30. Little RE, Sing CF. Association of father's drinking and infant's birth weight. N Engl J Med 1986; 314:1644-1645.
31. Hanson JW, Streissguth AP, Smith DW. The effects of moderate alcohol consumption during pregnancy on fetal growth and morphogenesis. J Pediatr 1978; 92:457-460.
32. Mills JL, Graubard BI. Is moderate drinking during pregnancy associated with an increased risk for malformations? Pediatrics 1987; 80:309-314.
33. Marbury MC, Linn S, Monson R, et al. The association of alcohol consumption with outcome of pregnancy. Am J Public Health 1983; 73:1165-1168.
34. Rosett HL, Weiner L. Alcohol and the fetus: A clinical perspective. Oxford University Press, New York, 1984.
35. The effects of alcohol on the outcome of pregnancy. Bull Soc Obstet Gynaecol Can 1984; 6:1-2.
36. Little RE, Streissguth AP. Drinking during pregnancy in alcoholic women. Alcohol Clin Exp Res 1978; 2:179-182.
37. Little RE, Schultz FA, Mandell W. Drinking during pregnancy. J Stud Alcohol 1976; 37:375-379.
38. Sellers EM, Naranjo CA, Harrison M, et al. Diazepam loading: Simplified treatment of alcohol withdrawal. Clin Pharmacol Ther 1983; 34:822-826.
39. Briggs GG, Freeman RK, Yaffe SJ. Drugs in Pregnancy and Lactation. Williams & Wilkins, Baltimore, 1986.
40. Favre-Tissot M, Delatour P. Psychopharmacologie et teratogṅѕe à propos du disulfirame: Essai experimental. Ann Med Psychol 1965; 123:735-740.
41. Nora AH, Nora JJ, Blu J. Limb-reduction anomalies in infants born to disulfiram-treated alcoholic mothers. Lancet 1977; 2:664.
42. Schardein JL. Chemically Induced Birth Defects. Marcel Dekker, New York, 1985.
43. Zelson C, Rubio E, Wasserman E. Neonatal narcotic addition: 10 year observation. Pediatrics 1971; 48:178-189.
44. Chavez CJ, Ostrea EM, Stryker JC, et al. Sudden infant death syndrome among infants of drug-dependent mothers. J Pediatr 1979; 95:407-409.
45. Blinick G, Wallach RC, Jerez E. Pregnancy in narcotics addicts treated by medical withdrawal. Am J Obstet Gynecol 1969; 105:997-1003.
46. Finnegan LP (ed). Drug Dependence in Pregnancy: Clinical Management of Mother and Child. National Institute on Drug Abuse, Washington, DC, 1979.
47. Zuspan FP, Gumpel JA, Mejia-Zelaya A, et al. Fetal stress from methadone withdrawal. Am J Obstet Gynecol 1975; 122:43-46.
48. Rementeria JL, Nunag NN. Narcotic withdrawal in pregnancy: Stillbirth incidence with a case report. Am J Obstet Gynecol 1973; 116:1152-1156.
49. Connaughton JF, Reeser D,f Schut J, Finnegan LP. Perinatal addiction: Outcome and management. Am J Obstet Gynecol 1977; 129:679-686.

50. Kandall SR, Albin S. Lowinson J, et al. Differential effects of maternal heroin and methadone use on birthweight. Pediatrics 1976; 58:681-685.
51. Ostrea EM, Chavez CJ, Strauss ME. A study of factors that influence the severity of neonatal narcotic withdrawal. J Pediatr 1976; 88:642-645.
52. Strauss ME, Andresko M, Stryker JC, Wardell JN. Relationship of neonatal withdrawal to maternal methadone dose. Am J Drug Alcohol Abuse 1976; 3: 339-345.
53. Kaltenbach K. Finnegan LP. Perinatal and developmental outcome of infants exposed to methadone in utero. Neurotoxicol Teratol 1987; 9:311-313.
54. Kaltenbach K. Finnegan LP. Developmental outcome of children born to methadone maintained women: A review of longitudinal studies. Neurobehav Toxicol Teratol 1984; 6:271-275.
55. Abelson HI, Miller JD. A decade of trends in cocaine use in the household population. Natl Inst Drug Abuse Res Monogr Ser 1985; 61:35-49.
56. Gawin FH, Ellinwood EH. Cocaine and other stimulants: Actions, abuse, and treatment. N Engl J Med 1988; 318:1173-1182.
57. Madden JD, Payne TF, Miller S. Maternal cocaine abuse and effect on the newborn. Pediatrics 1986; 77:209-211.
58. Bingol N, Fuchs M, Diaz V, et al. Teratogenicity of cocaine in humans. J Pediatr 1987; 110:93-96.
59. Chasnoff IJ, Bussey ME, Savich R, Stack CM. Perinatal cerebral infarction and maternal cocaine use. J Pediatr 1986; 108:456-459.
60. Oro AS, Dixon SD. Perinatal cocaine and methamphetamine exposure: Maternal and neonatal correlates. J Pediatr 1987; 111:571-578.
61. Heinonen OP, Slone D, Shapiro S. Birth defects and drugs in pregnancy. PSG Publishing, Littleton, CO, 1977.
62. Eriksson M, Larsson G, Winbladh B, Zetterstrom R. The influence of amphetamine addiction on pregnancy and the newborn infant. Acta Paediatr Scand 1978; 67:95-99.
63. Hatch EE, Bracken MB. Effect of marijuana use in pregnancy on fetal growth. Am J Epidemiol 1986; 124:986-993.
64. Hollister LE. Health aspects of cannabis. Pharmacol Rev 1985; 38:1-20.
65. Linn S, Schoenbaum SC, Monson RR, et al. The association of marijuana use with outcome of pregnancy. Am J Public Health 1983; 73:1161-1164.
66. Hingson R, Alpert JJ, Day N, et al. Effects of maternal drinking and marijuana use on fetal growth and development. Pediatrics 1982; 70:539-546.
67. Wu TC, Tashkin DP, Djahed B, Rose JE. Pulmonary hazards of smoking marijuana as compared with tobacco. N Engl J Med 1988; 318:347-351.
68. Long S. Does LSD induce chromosomal damage and malformations? A review of the literature. Teratology 1972; 6:75-90.
69. Golden NL, Kuhnert BR, Sokol RJ, et al. Phencyclidine use during pregnancy. Am J Obstet Gynecol 1984; 148:254-259.
70. Golden NL, Sokol RJ, Rubin IL. Angel dust: Possible effects on the fetus. Pediatrics 1980; 65:18-20.
71. Chasnoff IJ, Burns WJ, Hatcher RP, Burns KA. Phencyclidine: Effects on the fetus and neonate. Dev Pharmacol Ther 1983; 6:404-408.

72. Hayden JW, Comstock EG, Comstock BS. The clinical toxicology of solvent abuse. Clin Toxicol 1976; 9:169-184.
73. King MD. Day RE, Oliver JS, et al. Solvent encephalopathy. Br Med J 1981; 283:663-665.
74. Hersh JH, Podruch PE, Rogers G, Weisskopf B. Toluene embryopathy. J Pediatr 1985; 106:922-927.
75. Saxen I, Saxen L. Association between maternal intake of diazepam and oral clefts. Lancet 1975; 2:498.
76. Safra MJ, Oakley GP. Association between cleft lip with or without cleft palate and prenatal exposure to diazepam. Lancet 1975; 2:478-480.
77. Rosenberg L, Mitchell AA, Parsells JL, et al. Lack of relation of oral clefts to diazepam use during pregnancy. N Engl J Med 1983; 309:1282-1285.
78. Laegreid L, Olegard R, Wahlstrom J, Conradi N. Abnormalities in children exposed to benzodiazepines in utero. Lancet 1987; 1:108-109.
79. Weber LWD. Benzodiazepines in pregnancy—Academical debate or teratogenic risk? Biol Res Pregnancy 1985; 6:151-167.
80. Loudon JB. Psychotropic drugs. Br Med J 1987; 294:167-169.
81. Rementeria JL, Bhatt K. Withdrawal symptoms in neonates from intrauterine exposure to diazepam. Pediatr Pharmacol 1977; 90:123-126.
82. Busto U, Sellers EM, Naranjo CA, et al. Withdrawal reaction after long-term therapeutic use of benzodiazepines. N Engl J Med 1986; 315:854-859.
83. Devenyi P, Rideout J, Schneiderman J. Abuse of a commonly prescribed analgesic preparation. Can Med Assoc J 1985; 133:294-296.
84. Smith DE, Wesson DR. Phenobarbital technique for treatment of barbiturate dependence. Arch Gen Psychiatry 1971; 24:56-60.
85. Robinson GM, Sellers EM, Janecek E. Barbiturate and hypnosedative withdrawal by a multiple oral phenobarbital loading dose technique. Clin Pharmacol Ther 1981; 309:71-76.
86. Fielding JE. Smoking: Health effects and control. N Engl J Med 1985; 313: 491-498.
87. Kleinman JC, Kopstein A. Smoking during pregnancy, 1967-80. Am J Public Health 1987; 77:823-825.
88. Murphy JF, Mulcahy R. The effect of age, parity, and cigarette smoking on baby weight. Am J Obstet Gynecol 1971; 111:22-25.
89. Landesman-Dwyer S, Emanuel I. Smoking during pregnancy. Teratology 1979; 19:119-126.
90. Hebel JR, Nowicki P, Sexton M. The effect of antismoking intervention during pregnancy: An assessment of interactions with maternal characteristics. Am J Epidemiol 1985; 122:135-148.
91. Sexton M, Hebel JR. A clinical trial of change in maternal smoking and its effect on birth weight. JAMA 1984; 251:911-915.
92. Windsor RA, Cutter G, Morris J, et al. The effectiveness of smoking cessation methods for smokers in public health maternity clinics: A randomized trial. Am J Public Health 1985; 75:1389-1392.
93. Donovan JW. Randomised controlled trial of anti-smoking advice in pregnancy. Br J Prev Soc Med 1977; 31:6-12.

94. Morris MB, Weinstein L. Caffeine and the fetus—Is trouble brewing? Am J Obstet Gynecol 1981; 140:607–610.
95. Rosenberg L, Mitchell AA, Shapiro S, Slone D. Selected birth defects in relation to caffeine-containing beverages. JAMA 1982; 247:1429–1432.
96. Linn S, Schoenbaum SC, Monson RR, et al. No association between coffee consumption and adverse outcomes of pregnancy. N Engl J Med 1982; 306:141–145.
97. Curatolo PW, Robertson D. The health consequences of caffeine. Ann Intern Med 1983; 98:641–653.

15

Neonatal Drug Withdrawal Syndromes

James B. Besunder
Metro Health Medical Center and Case Western Reserve University School of Medicine, Cleveland, Ohio

Jeffrey L. Blumer
Rainbow Babies and Children's Hospital and Case Western Reserve University School of Medicine, Cleveland, Ohio

Clinical Case

You are consulted about a baby who is suspected of having an opioid withdrawal syndrome: restlessness, intractable crying, diarrhea, vomiting, sweating, tremor, and poor feeding. The mother claims that although she is a heroin user, she has not been able to get any drug for several days. Neonatal urine test is negative, and the house staff suspects that the neonatal presentation is something other than drug withdrawal.

INTRODUCTION

Drug abuse is a global problem within our society. As a result, the fetus, by passive addiction, has become an unfortunate victim of increasing maternal substance abuse. Although most pediatricians are acquainted with the neonatal narcotic withdrawal syndrome, substance withdrawal syndromes have now been described for many other classes of drugs, including sedative-hypnotics, stimulants, antidepressants, neuroleptics, antihistamines, and alcohol (1,2). The pediatrician, in particular, must be cognizant of the potential that signs or symptoms observed in a young infant may be the consequence of drug withdrawal. This chapter reviews drugs known to precipitate withdrawal syndromes in newborns, their clinical manifestations and therapy, and, when known, the mechanism for induction of the substance withdrawal syndrome.

OPIOIDS

Although addiction to heroin and methadone is encountered most frequently, the narcotic withdrawal syndrome has also been described with propoxyphene (3–5), codeine (6,7), and the opiate agonist/antagonist pentazocine (8–10). A great deal is known about the short-term clinical effects of maternal opiate addiction on the newborn; however, many confounding variables such as polydrug abuse, improper nutrition, and socioeconomic factors obscure a description of their potential long-term effects.

Mechanism of Opiate Withdrawal

Evidence exists that at least part of the clinical manifestation of narcotic withdrawal results from α_2-adrenergic supersensitivity in the locus ceruleus (LC) (11). Increased firing of neurons located in the LC of monkeys produces many of the central nervous system symptoms associated with narcotic withdrawal, including behavioral changes, increased wakefulness, and tremors (12,13). α_2-Adrenergic receptors (14) as well as opiate receptors (15–17) are located in the LC, and stimulation of these receptors by clonidine and morphine, respectively, inhibits activation of the LC in primates and rats (18, 19). Hamburg and Tallman (20) demonstrated an increased number of α_2-adrenergic receptors in rat brains following chronic morphine administration.

In 1978 Aghajanian (21) observed similar depressant effects on LC neuronal firing by morphine and clonidine in rats, although the two drugs appeared to act at independent receptors within the LC. Initially, the administration of morphine markedly depressed LC-neuronal activation. However, tolerance developed rapidly, with normal firing rates observed after 4–5 days of daily morphine administration. Using a microiontophore technique, a withdrawal response (> 100% activation of LC-neuronal firing) in tolerant rats was then observed with the direct application of the competitive opioid antagonist naloxone. When clonidine was applied to the LC neurons, inhibition of firing comparable to that observed with morphine alone was demonstrated. Finally, Aghajanian in the same set of experiments demonstrated that piperoxane, an α-adrenergic receptor antagonist, blocked clonidine, but not morphine-induced LC neuronal activation. Thus, these data suggest that stimulation of opiate and α_2-adrenergic receptors inhibits in parallel, but not independently, activation of neurons in the LC. Withdrawal of opiates, possibly resulting from or potentiated by an increased number of unbound α_2-adrenergic receptor sites, causes activation of neurons in the LC, leading to manifestations of the narcotic withdrawal syndrome. The effect of naloxone alone on LC neurons was not determined, however, and as a result, a direct effect of naloxone rather than induction of a narcotic withdrawal response cannot be excluded as a possible reason for the heightened activation of LC neurons following naloxone administration. These observations of Aghajanian (21) also offer a cellular basis for the efficacy of clonidine in suppressing some of the symptoms of opiate withdrawal.

A spinal cord effect of opioid withdrawal may account for other symptoms of the withdrawal syndrome, such as hyperreflexia and hyperalgesia. Substance P (SP) is thought to be the neurotransmitter responsible for nociceptive input into the spinal cord (22,23), and its release from the spinal cord is inhibited by opioids in rats and cats (24,25). Vacca et al. (26) observed an increase in SP concentrations in the dorsal horn of rat spinal cords following chronic morphine administration. Bergstrom et al. (27) reported similar findings in rats and suggested that release of accumulated SP or supersensitivity of postsynaptic SP receptors following opioid withdrawal is responsible for the hyperreflexia seen during the narcotic withdrawal syndrome. Bell and Jaffe (28), in a study evaluating dorsal and ventral root depolarization responses in neonatal rat spinal cords, provide evidence supporting a presynaptic mechanism of morphine withdrawal (i.e., presynaptic accumulation of SP and then release) rather than a postsynaptic mechanism. Of interest, Gintzler and Scalisi (29) demonstrated that morphine inhibits and SP induces noncholinergic-mediated contraction of isolated guinea pig ileum. Further studies in the isolated guinea pig ileum strongly suggested that naloxone reversed the effects of morphine by releasing SP (29). Previously, Schulz and Herz (30) had shown that naloxone-precipitated enteric withdrawal from opiates is mediated, at least in part, by excitation of postganglionic cholinergic neurons with release of acetylcholine and activation of smooth muscle muscarinic receptors. Although these preliminary data on the neurohumoral effects of narcotic withdrawal are encouraging, further research in primates is needed to elucidate the mechanism of opiate withdrawal in human infants.

Clinical Manifestations of Opiate Withdrawal
Characteristics at Birth

The incidence of premature birth among heroin-addicted women ranges from 17 to 30% (31–34). Zelson et al. (31) reported more than a twofold increase in premature deliveries over a 10-year period in 384 infants born to heroin-addicted mothers compared with the overall premature birthrate at their institution over the same time period. In contrast to heroin-addicted mothers, women enrolled in methadone treatment programs appear to be at only slightly increased risk of premature delivery. Newman et al. (35) reported a 7% incidence of deliveries prior to 8 months gestation in a large series of methadone-maintained women. Of interest, Olofsson et al. (32)

observed younger mean gestational ages in infants whose mothers had been acutely withdrawn from methadone within a month of delivery, compared with mothers who were maintained on methadone until the time of delivery.

Low birth weight (< 2500 g) is a common sequela among newborns of heroin addicts, as well as the infants of women who use both heroin and methadone and women who enter methadone treatment programs during their third trimester (36–39). Naeye et al. (36) reviewed postmortem data in infants born to heroin addicts and demonstrated that growth retardation had been due mainly to a decreased number of cells in various organs, including the heart, pancreas, adrenal glands, spleen, thymus, and kidneys. Brain specimens were not available. Not all cases of growth retardation could be attributed to poor nutrition during pregnancy. Kandall et al. (37) reported mean birth weights of 2490 and 2535 g (mean gestational age of 38 weeks for both groups) among infants born to heroin- and combined heroin- and methadone-addicted mothers, respectively, compared with a mean birth weight of 3176 g in the control group. Finnegan (38) identified a strong relationship between prenatal care and birth weight among infants born to heroin addicts. Birth weight under 2500 g was observed in 47.6% of infants born to drug-dependent women with no prenatal care compared with an 18.8% incidence for women with good prenatal care. By comparison, Finnegan reported a 20% incidence of low birth weight in a control group of nonaddicts who received no prenatal care.

In contrast to the infants mentioned above, several investigators have observed higher birth weights among infants born to women addicted to methadone than to infants of heroin addicts (32,37,39,40). Kandall et al. (37) reported a mean birth weight of 2961 g (mean gestational age of 39.4 weeks) for 108 infants born to women who used methadone as their sole or major nacrotic during pregnancy compared with a mean birth weight of 2490 g (mean gestational age 38 weeks) for 61 infants born to heroin addicts. The effect of methadone on birth weight was independent of maternal age, race, or prenatal care. The same investigators also observed a direct relationship between methadone dose during the first trimester and birth weight in a subgroup of infants born to mothers registered in a methadone maintenance program where complete records of drug dosages and urinalyses were available. The investigators suggest that methadone may promote fetal growth during the first trimester in a dose-dependent fashion. Although methadone-addicted women have larger babies than women addicted to heroin, both groups have an increased risk of delivering small-for-gestational-age (SGA) infants. Zelson et al. (39) reported incidences of SGA infants of 35 and 22% among babies born to heroin- and methadone-addicted women, respectively. Klenka (34) confirmed the high incidence of SGA infants born to heroin-addicted mothers when he described this finding in eight of 32 infants. On the other hand, Ostrea and Chavez (41) reported a lower incidence of 16.5% in 830 infants born to drug-dependent women.

Head circumference and birth length are also significantly reduced among infants born to narcotic-addicted mothers compared with controls (42,43), although the incidence of head circumference below the 10th percentile did not differ between the two groups (42).

A high incidence of low Apgar scores in infants born to narcotic addicts has also been reported by Olofsson et al. (32) and Ostrea and Chavez (42). Both groups of investigators found a 20% incidence of Apgar scores less than 7 at 1 minute, double the incidence observed by Ostrea and Chavez in their control infants. Ostrea and Chavez (41) also reported more than a two-fold greater incidence of low 5-minute Apgar scores ($\leqslant 6$) in infants born to drug-dependent women compared with controls (7 vs. 3.2%).

Infants born to heroin addicts appear to be less at risk of developing severe hyperbilirubinemia. In a prospective study, Nathenson et al. (44) reported significantly higher mean total bilirubin concentrations in control infants compared with infants born to heroin-addicted women during each of the first 3 days of life. Upon excluding factors predisposing infants to hyper-bilirubinemia, such as hemolytic disease, the elevated bilirubin concentrations were found to be due mainly to an increase in the indirect fraction. The lower bilirubin concentrations observed in the heroin-addicted group most likely resulted from increased activity of bilirubin glucuronyl trans-ferase. This effect of heroin has been demonstrated in animals (43). Marked hypertrophy of the smooth endoplasmic reticulum has also been described in liver biopsies from heroin-addicted adults (45). Zelson et al. (31) reported the occurrence of jaundice in only 24 of 384 infants born to heroin-addicted mothers. Of these 24 infants, 6 had an ABO incompatibility, and 1 was sep-tic. In contrast, limited data are available on the incidence of hyperbilirub-inemia among infants born to women maintained on methadone during pregnancy. Harper et al. (46) reported "clinical jaundice" in approximately half of their group of infants born to women in a methadone treatment pro-gram. However, only five of these infants had serum bilirubin concentrations exceeding 10 mg/dL, and all these babies had mild ABO incompatibilities. more data are required to ascertain the effect of methadone on serum bili-rubin concentrations in newborn infants.

Whether maternal narcotic addiction is associated with congenital defects is unknown. Zelson et al. (31) reported congenital abnormalities in only 4 of 384 infants born to heroin-addicted mothers. In contrast, the data of Ostrea and Chavez (41) reveal a statistically significant increased incidence of congenital malformations in their cohort of 830 newborns. Among the 37 infants with congenital defects, 20 (2.4%) had major malformations, including hydrocephalus, heart disease, and genitourinary tract abnormalities.

Only 0.5% of their control population had major malformations. Harper et al. (46) reported congenital defects in 3 of 51 infants born to women maintained on methadone; however, only one would be considered a major malformation.

Hyaline membrane disease (HMD) appears to occur less frequently among infants born to heroin addicts. Glass et al. (47) reported no cases of HMD in 33 premature infants born to heroin addicts compared with 26 cases in 123 premature infants born to nonaddicted mothers. The findings of this study are supported by the data generated by Gluck and Kulovich (48) and Taeusch et al. (49). Gluck and Kulovich reported mature lecithin/sphingomyelin ratios in fetuses of narcotic addicts at an earlier gestational age than would be expected in fetuses of nonaddicted women, whereas Taeusch and coworkers demonstrated accelerated lung maturation in fetal rabbits injected with heroin compared with fetal rabbits injected with saline. However, Ostrea and Chavez (41) observed no difference in the incidence of HMD between narcotic-addicted and control infants. In summary, in utero narcotic exposure may have profound effects on the developing fetus, effects that may increase perinatal morbidity and mortality. The birth characteristics of infants born to narcotic-addicted women are summarized in Table 1.

Signs and Symptoms of Withdrawal

Overt symptoms of narcotic withdrawal occur in 67–90% of infants born to narcotic-addicted women whether the additive drug is heroin or methadone

Table 1   Birth Characteristics of Infants Born to Narcotic-Addicted Women

Characteristic	Addiction[a]
Birth weight	H < M < N
Premature infants (frequency)	H > M > N
Small for gestational age	H > M > N
Birth length	H = M < N
Head circumference at birth	H = M < N
1 minute Apgar score <7 (frequency)	H, M > N[b]
Hyperbilirubinemia (frequency)	H < N[c]
Congenital malformations	± H, M > N

[a]H, Heroin; M, methadone; N, nonaddicted.
[b]Data comparing Apgar scores in infants born to heroin- and methadone-addicted mothers are not available.
[c]No data available evaluating the incidence of hyperbilirubinemia among infants born to methadone-addicted mothers.
Source: Modified from Ref. 53; used with permission.

(31-33,35,39,40,46,50). Although the incidence of individual symptoms is similar between the heroin and methadone groups, infants born to methadone-addicted mothers appear to experience more symptoms (39), and the withdrawal syndrome appears to be more severe (39,40). Rahbar (40) reported moderate and severe symptoms associated with withdrawal in 50 and 18% of symptomatic infants, respectively, born to methadone-addicted women compared with 14 and 7% of infants born to heroin-addicted mothers.

The severity (50,51) and possibly the duration of the withdrawal syndrome (32) have been shown to correlate directly with the amount of methadone, but not heroin, taken during pregnancy. Ostrea and colleagues (51) observed a milder course among infants whose mothers took less than 20 mg/day of methadone during pregnancy. Olofsson et al. (32), in a similar study, reported withdrawal symptoms lasting longer than 5 days in 20 of 37 infants whose mothers were taking 20 mg or more per day of methadone at the time of delivery compared with 10 of 41 infants whose mothers took less than 20 mg/day.

The onset of narcotic withdrawal symptoms varies tremendously from minutes after delivery to 1-2 weeks of age. However, the majority of infants will develop withdrawal symptoms by 48 h of life (33,39,40,46). Methadone withdrawal, owing to its longer elimination half-life ($t_{1/2\beta}$) of approximately 35 h (52), may be delayed compared with heroin but usually manifests itself within 48 h (46). Harper et al. (46) reported the onset of withdrawal symptoms within 24 h of birth in 42%, 48 h in 73%, and 72 h in 87% of symptomatic infants born to mothers in a methadone treatment program. Late-onset symptoms of withdrawal developed between 7 and 14 days of life in only 2% of these infants. The timing of the last maternal dose of narcotic with respect to birth also appears to influence the time to onset of symptoms (38,53).

The neonatal narcotic withdrawal syndrome is characterized by signs and symptoms of central nervous system excitation, altered gastrointestinal function, respiratory distress, and vague autonomic symptoms. The signs and symptoms of withdrawal have been represented by the mnemonic withdrawal (1):

W — wakefulness
I — irritability
T — tremulousness, temperature variation, tachypnea
H — hyperactivity, high-pitched cry, hyperacusia, hyperreflexia, hypertonus
D — diarrhea, diaphoresis, disorganized suck
R — rub marks (excoriations of knees and face), respiratory distress, rhinorrhea
A — apneic spells, autonomic dysfunction
W — weight loss or failure to gain weight
A — alkalosis (respiratory)
L — lacrimation

Other symptoms include hiccups, vomiting, stuffy nose, sneezing, yawning, photophobia, twitching, myoclonic jerks, opisthotonos, and seizures (1,53). Irritability is the most common manifestation of narcotic withdrawal, appearing in 45 to as many as 100% of symptomatic infants (31,33,39,50). Other symptoms that have been reported in more than half of symptomatic infants include tremors and hypertonicity (31,33,39,50). Vomiting occurs in one-quarter to one-third of infants. The frequency, if reported, of withdrawal manifestations is summarized in Table 2.

Signs and symptoms of central nervous system hyperexcitability, such as irritability, restlessness, and tremors, appear early in the clinical course. Primitive reflexes, such as the Moro reflex, are exaggerated, as are deep tendon reflexes. Fist sucking is common and is reported in up to 80% of narcotic-addicted infants (51). Poor oral intake, regurgitation of feeds, vomiting, and diarrhea are frequently observed upon initiation of oral feedings (33). Feeding difficulties are most likely the result of an uncoordinated and ineffective sucking reflex (54,55). Excessive weight loss or the failure to gain weight, which is commonly observed in narcotic-addicted infants, is due to both poor caloric intake and to an increased tissue oxygen consumption (56).

Abnormalities in ventilation also exist in infants whose mothers abuse narcotics. Glass et al. (57) reported tachypnea with a concomitant primary respiratory alkalosis in 22 infants born to heroin addicts compared with 19

Table 2   Incidence of Withdrawal Manifestations in Symptomatic Infants Born to Narcotic-Addicted Women[a]

Signs and symptoms	% with Manifestation	Ref.
Irritability	45–100	31,33,39,50,51
Tremors	65–86	31,33,39,50,51
Hypertonicity	20–86	31,39,50,51
Vomiting	8–37	31,39,50,51
High-pitched cry	17–45	31,39,50,51
Respiratory distress[b]	9–30	31,33,39,50
Diarrhea	7–22	31,50,51
Fever	6–16	31,33,39,50
Convulsions	3–21	31,32,39,50,61
Diaphoresis	6	31
Yawning	3	31
Sneezing	<1–65	31,51
Hiccups	<1	31

[a]Incidence is reported as percentage of infants with clinical manifestations, not as percentage of all infants born to narcotic-addicted women.
[b]Respiratory distress due to etiologies other than hyaline membrane disease.

normal infants. Olsen and Lees (58) demonstrated a blunted ventilatory response to increasing concentrations of inspired carbon dioxide in 9 infants born to methadone addicts. This depressed response lasted for an average of 15 days, but persisted for 31 days in one infant. Davidson et al. (59) reported abnormal sleeping ventilatory patterns in 27 infants born to substance-abusing mothers, many of whom abused opiates, compared with 43 control infants. These abnormalities included more frequent apneic episodes (≥ 6 s), longer duration of apneic events, and more periodic breathing. The significance of these findings is presently unknown. Follow-up data have not disclosed a relationship in these infants between abnormal ventilatory patterns and future problems, such as the sudden infant death syndrome (SIDS) (60).

Seizures have been reported in up to 21% of infants exhibiting narcotic withdrawal. The onset of seizure activity is usually delayed. Rosen and Pippenger (50) observed seizures in 5 of 18 symptomatic infants born to narcotic addicts. These infants developing seizures between the sixth and eighth days of life. Infants receiving paregoric for withdrawal symptoms had a significantly lower incidence of developing seizures than infants being treated with other drug combinations. These seizures were difficult to control with phenobarbital, diazepam, and paraldehyde alone, but responded to paregoric alone or in combination with diazepam or phenobarbital. Herzlinger et al. (61) reported the occurrence of seizures at a mean age of 10 days (range 3–34 days) in 18 narcotic-addicted infants. Seven infants experienced generalized seizures, seven myoclonic seizures, three had seizure activity manifested as automatisms (staring, blinking, lip smacking or abnormal sucking), and one infant exhibited multifocal clonic seizures. Paregoric was more effective than diazepam in controlling seizures. Interictal electroencephalograms (EEGs) were interpreted as normal in 12 of 13 infants in whom an EEG was obtained. Olofsson et al. (32), who found that seizures were statistically more frequent in infants with 1-minute Apgar scores below 7, inferred that birth asphyxia may predispose infants born to narcotic-addicted women to convulsions. In summary, seizures should be anticipated in infants born to narcotic-addicted mothers and should be treated with either paregoric or a parenteral narcotic agonist, such as morphine, until controlled. Maintenance therapy with paregoric appears to be effective in preventing the recurrence of seizures.

The clinical course of the narcotic-addicted newborn can be extremely variable, ranging from only mild symptoms of brief duration, to a crescendo in severity, to intermittent symptomatology. A protracted clinical course with symptoms lasting 4–6 months has also been described (62). Wilson et al. (63) observed a biphasic course in 82% of symptomatic infants born to heroin-addicted mothers. These infants had an exacerbation or recurrence of symptoms upon discharge to the home environment. Symptoms included restlessness, agitation, tremors, wakefulness, hyperphagia, colic, and vomiting. These symptoms persisted for 3–6 months, and in some infants mandated resumption of therapy. Therefore, close outpatient follow-up to evaluate these infants for a recurrence of signs or symptoms of drug withdrawal is essential. Factors affecting the timing and severity of the withdrawal syndrome are summarized in Table 3.

Although mortality from neonatal narcotic withdrawal approaches 0 with appropriate treatment, these infants may be at increased risk of dying from SIDS. Chavez et al. (64) compared the incidence of SIDS in 688 infants born to narcotic-addicted women with a control group of 388 randomly selected infants born to nonaddicted mothers of similar socioeconomic backgrounds. A fivefold increased incidence of SIDS (2.5 vs. 0.5%) was observed in the group of infants born to narcotic-addicted mothers. Of interest, more deaths were observed in infants who exhibited moderate to severe withdrawal compared with infants who manifested only minor or mild symptoms. The difference achieved significance at the $p < 0.01$ level. The mean age at the time of death was 9.2 weeks. Pierson et al. (65) also reported two confirmed and one possible case of SIDS among 14 infants whose mothers received methadone during pregnancy.

Signs and symptoms of narcotic withdrawal resulting from maternal use of propoxyphene (3–5), codeine (6,7), and pentazocine (8–10) are similar and may be as severe as those described in heroin or methadone withdrawal. In these cases, the majority of infants manifested symptoms within the first 24 h of life but were asympatomatic by 10 days of age. One infant developed seizures at 36 h of life (4), and one infant died of SIDS at 14 weeks of age (10).

Treatment

Some infants exhibiting signs or symptoms of narcotic withdrawal can be effectively managed utilizing conservative measures such as holding, swaddling, minimal stimulation, and demand feedings using a hypercaloric formula (24 cal/oz). However, the majority of symptomatic infants require pharmacological therapy. Finnegan et al. (66) developed a neonatal narcotic abstinence

Table 3   Factors Influencing the Onset and Severity of the Neonatal Narcotic Withdrawal Syndrome

Addictive drug used
Drug dose during pregnancy and at time of delivery
Timing of last dose prior to delivery
Type and amount of analgesia/anesthesia given during labor

scoring system in order to assess the severity of withdrawal and to guide therapy. They ranked 20 common symptoms of narcotic withdrawal, giving each symptom 1 to 5 points based on its clinical significance. The least significant symptoms, such as yawning, receive 1 point, whereas seizures receive 5 points (Table 4). This scoring system assumes that the greater the number of symptoms and the greater their severity, the higher the associated morbidity and mortality. According to Finnegan's guidelines, babies are scored at birth and then hourly for 24 h, every 2 h during the second day of life, and every 4 h thereafter. Infants with abstinence scores of 8 or more received pharmacotherapy, whereas those with scores less than 8 were treated conservatively. Finnegan and her coinvestigators then compared data from a group of 37 infants born to narcotic-addicted women prior to the development of the scoring system with a group of 37 infants born after the institution of the scoring system. The groups were similar with respect to severity of symptoms. Utilization of the scoring system not only increased the number of infants managed conservatively (46 vs. 30%), but also reduced the duration of pharmacological therapy from an average of 8 to 6 days. The mean length of hospitalization was also shortened from 21 to 15 days.

Lipsitz (67) has developed a similar scoring system evaluating 11 signs and symptoms of narcotic withdrawal. This scoring system, while concentrating on the more common symptoms of withdrawal such as tremors, irritability, muscle tone, hyperreflexia, and tachypnea, does not emphasize several clinically important symptoms that may increase morbidity from narcotic withdrawal, such as vomiting, dehydration, seizures, and postprandial sleep. Although we feel the Lipsitz scoring system reliably identifies infants with a drug withdrawal syndrome, Finnegan's scoring system is more detailed, has a greater emphasis on symptoms likely to correlate with morbidity and mortality, and therefore is better suited to quantify the severity of withdrawal and to guide pharmacological therapy. Also, to the best of our knowledge, the Lipsitz scoring system has not been rigorously evaluated as a means for identifying infants requiring pharmacotherapy or to guide ongoing therapy.

Many drugs, including paregoric, tincture of opium, morphine, methadone, diazepam, chlorpromazine, phenobarbital, and clonidine, have been used to treat neonatal narcotic withdrawal (1,2,68). We discuss therapy with paregoric and phenobarbital in detail, since these drugs are the most popular agents used and represent the two important classes of compounds for treatment. Treatment with other drugs has been reviewed (1,2).

Paregoric, a camphorated opium tincture, contains 0.4 mg/mL anhydrous morphine. Since the turn of the century it has been used successfully for the treatment of the neonatal narcotic withdrawal syndrome (69). The recommended dose for full-term infants is 0.2–0.5 mL (0.08–0.20 mg anhydrous

Table 4 Neonatal Narcotic Withdrawal Score

Sign or symptom	Possible score
1. High-pitched cry	
Intermittent	2
Continuous	3
2. Postprandial sleep	
<3 h	1
<2 h	2
<1 h	3
3. Moro reflex	
Hyperactive	2
Markedly hyperactive	3
4. Tremors	
Mild when disturbed	1
Marked when disturbed	2
Mild when undisturbed	3
Marked when undisturbed	4
5. Tone	
Increased	2
Seizures	5
6. Frantic sucking of fists	1
7. Poor feeding	2
8. Vomiting	
Regurgitation	2
Projectile	3
9. Stools	
Loose	2
Watery	3
10. Dehydration	2
11. Frequent yawning	1
12. Sneezing	1
13. Nasal stuffiness	1
14. Sweating	1
15. Mottling	1
16. Fever	
38–38°C	1
>38°C	2
17. Respiratory rate	
>60	1
>60 with retractions	2
18. Excoriation of nose	1
19. Excoriation of knees	1
20. Excoriation of toes	1
Total maximum	40

Source: From Ref. 66; used with permission.

morphine) administered orally every 3–4 h (q4h) until symptoms are controlled (1). In general, we select our initial dose depending on the severity of withdrawal symptoms (Table 5). If no clinical improvement is observed within 4 h after the initial dose, we increase the paregoric dose by 0.05 mL q4h until symptoms are controlled (Finnegan score ≤4).

When the withdrawal score has remained stable for 48 h the total daily dose may be tapered by 10% each day while maintaining the dosage interval constant. If symptoms recur, the dose should be increased to the previous dose which effectively controlled symptoms. Paregoric has the advantage of being a narcotic, so treatment should be more physiological than with nonnarcotic agents; and indeed, treated neonates have a more physiological sucking pattern, higher caloric intake, and more weight gain than infants treated with phenobarbital (55). Also, dosing of paregoric is easily titratable. Disadvantages of paregoric are mainly attributable to the other constituents present in the preparation. Camphor, a central nervous system (CNS) stimulant, is eliminated slowly owing to its high lipid solubility and dependence on glucoronidation for elimination. Paregoric also contains alcohol and anise oil, which may cause dependency (1). Benzoic acid, an oxidative metabolite of benzyl alcohol, is also present in paregoric: circumstantial, but not conclusive, evidence has linked benzyl alcohol, when administered in excessive doses, to the "gasping syndrome" described in premature infants (70–72). Our initial dosing recommendation for paregoric in premature infants is 0.05 mL/kg q4h with increments of 0.02 mL/kg q4h until symptoms are controlled.

Although paregoric may be more physiological, phenobarbital and its analogs have also been employed successfully in the treatment of the neonatal narcotic withdrawal syndrome. Most physicians feel comfortable with using phenobarbital, which has the added advantage of mitigating symptoms

Table 5 Initial Paregoric Dose in Full-Term Infants Based on Withdrawal Score

Withdrawal score[a]	Dose (mL)[b]
<8	None
8–10	0.2
11–13	0.3
14–16	0.4
≥17	0.5

[a]Based on Finnegan Scoring System (66).
[b]See text for dosing interval and guidelines for chronic therapy.

referrable to the central nervous system. Kundstadter et al., in 1958 (73), commented that when sedation is required, phenobarbital is a safer drug than an opiate. This belief is still held by many physicians today. However, phenobarbital will not relieve gastrointestinal symptoms, such as vomiting or diarrhea (69), and may cause significant central nervous system depression. Also, phenobarbital is not a suitable drug for dose titration owing to its prolonged elimination half-life. Other disadvantages of phenobarbital relate to other chemicals present in the formulation; the elixir contains alcohol, whereas the parenteral formulation contains propylene glycol, ethyl alcohol, and benzyl alcohol (1). Finally, there are no standard dosing guidelines for phenobarbital therapy, nor is the therapeutic serum concentration necessary to control withdrawal known.

Two studies have compared the efficacy of treatment with paregoric and phenobarbital (74,75). Kandall et al. (74) prospectively randomized infants to receive paregoric or phenobarbital if their withdrawal score (modified Lipsitz scoring system) was 7 or greater, or if any infant developed excessive severity of any sign. Serum phenobarbital concentrations were not monitored. The drugs were considered by the investigators to be comparable in their ability to control gastrointestinal, CNS, and autonomic symptoms. However, 7 of 62 infants receiving phenobarbital developed seizures, compared with none of 49 infants maintained on paregoric ($p < 0.025$). Carin et al. (75) failed to demonstrate a difference in weight gain between infants treated with paregoric and those treated with phenobarbital. Paregoric-treated newborns received therapy for a longer period of time (median duration 22 days vs. 17 days) compared with phenobarbital-treated infants. This is most likely due to two factors: paregoric therapy was not discontinued until the daily dose had been weaned to 0.1 mL/kg, whereas once phenobarbital administration was stopped, effective serum concentrations were probably maintained for an extended period of time owing to the markedly prolonged $t_{1/2\beta}$ of phenobarbital.

Carin's study has several major flaws, which cast concerns on the validity of the data and conclusions. Among the mothers of infants treated with paregoric, 4 of 16 admitted to using heroin in addition to methadone, and 3 of 16 mothers used cocaine concomitantly. This is in contrast to the mothers whose infants were treated with phenobarbital, who had not used heroin or cocaine. Also, control of withdrawal symptoms and initial and subsequent withdrawal scores were not reported. Therefore, the severity of withdrawal was not controlled for in the treatment randomization process, nor was the efficacy of therapy in controlling withdrawal symptoms reported.

In a more critical evaluation, Kaltenbach and Finnegan (76) demonstrated the superiority of paregoric in a study designed to determine whether there was a relation between pharmacotherapy and developmental outcome. Of

23 infants treated initially with paregoric, treatment was effective with this drug alone in 21. By comparison, only 17 of 36 infants were treated effectively with phenobarbital alone. The remaining 19 infants required the addition of paregoric to their phenobarbital regimen. Finnegan and Ehrlich (77) also reported that paregoric was more effective than phenobarbital or diazepam in controlling symptoms of narcotic withdrawal, whereas phenobarbital was more effective in controlling symptoms associated with nonopiate withdrawal.

In summary, clinical manifestations occur in most infants of narcotic-addicted women. The Finnegan scoring system is a useful tool for assessing the severity of withdrawal and in guiding therapy. However, we would initiate pharmacological therapy with paregoric regardless of the infant's withdrawal score if presenting symptoms included seizures, vomiting, or severe and persistent diarrhea resulting in weight loss or dehydration, or inability

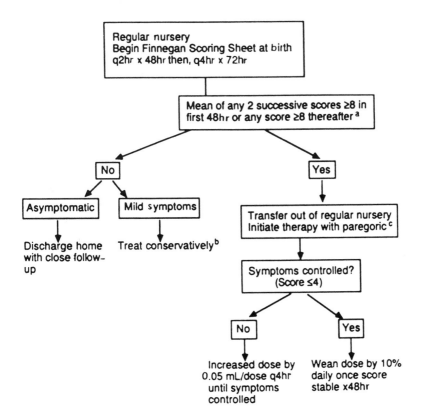

Figure 1 Management approach for the infant born to a narcotic-addicted mother.

to sleep. Figure 1 outlines our treatment approach to infants of narcotic-addicted mothers.

Outcome

Interpreting follow-up data in infants born to narcotic-addicted mothers is very difficult owing to the paucity of studies, lack of adequate control populations, and the chaotic home environment into which these children are returned.

Several studies have revealed marked behavioral abnormalities in narcotic-addicted infants (55,78–80). Strauss et al. (78) used the Brazelton Neonatal Behavioral Assessment Scale to evaluate 44 infants born to narcotic-addicted mothers. Testing was done during the first 48 h of life. Addicted infants spend less time in an alert state and became less responsive to social and nonsocial stimuli over the first 2 days of life. The investigators suggested that this behavior may adversely affect development of infant-caregiver interaction patterns. This speculation is supported by a subsequent study by Kaltenbach et al. (79), who investigated the ability of the infants born to a narcotic-dependent mother to interact with their environment. These infants were evaluated on days 1 and 30 of life. All infants who would eventually require pharmacological therapy had a deficient interaction score on day 1. By day 30, only a subset of infants still receiving treatment demonstrated poor interaction skills. Interestingly, these were the infants whose mothers rarely visited them while hospitalized. The investigators theorized that poor interaction skills on day 1 may have alienated mothers, or conversely, maternal attention may have improved the infant's interaction. Olofsson et al. (80) corroborated the data from these two studies. Of 72 infants born to narcotic addicts who were reinvestigated between 1 and 10 years of life, 21% had moderate or severe psychomotor retardation primarily attributable to a deprivation syndrome. In addition, both Olofsson et al. (80) and Wilson et al. (63) observed hyperactive and aggressive behavior with a decreased attention span and lack of social inhibition in more than half of infants followed through infancy and early childhood.

In contrast to the behavioral abnormalities described above, conflicting data regarding motor and mental development in infants of narcotic-addicted mothers have been reported. Rosen and Johnson (81) observed significantly lower mental and psychomotor developmental indices by the Bayley Scales of Infant Development at 12 and 18 months of age, though all scores were within normal limits. Lifschitz et al. (42) reported a higher incidence of low average and mildly retarded intellectual performance in children between 3 and 6 years of age who were born to narcotic-addicted mothers. Analysis of the data suggested that environmental and prenatal factors, not intrauterine exposure to narcotics, were responsible for the lower scores. By comparison, Wilson et al. (82) found no difference in mental or psychomotor developmental indices by the Bayley Scale at 9 months of age. Fine motor coordination was poorer, however, in infants born to narcotic addicts, supporting a similar observation by Rosen and Johnson (81). Finally, Kaltenbach and Finnegan found no evidence of impaired cognitive function in infants at 6 months of age (83), or in children between 3.5 and 4.5 years of age (84) who were born to narcotic-addicted women.

Kaltenbach and Finnegan (76) reported no differences in mental development at 6 months of age between infants who demonstrated severe withdrawal symptoms at birth and those with mild symptoms not requiring pharmacological therapy. They suggest that appropriate therapeutic intervention may obviate adverse cognitive sequelae. However, prenatal or environmental factors were not analyzed.

As stated previously, infants born to narcotic-addicted women have low measurements on mean birth weight, length, and head circumference. The growth curve in early infancy follows the percentiles noted at birth for these three parameters. However, after 4–6 months of age, some infants appear to have an accelerated growth pattern (62). Chasnoff et al. (62) followed the growth patterns of 15 infants whose mothers were maintained on a low dose of methadone (14 of 15 mothers received < 20 mg/day) during their third trimester of pregnancy. At birth and 4 months of age, the mean birth weight, length, and head circumference lay at the 10th, 10th, and 5th percentiles respectively. However, at 7.5 months, these infants lay at the 40th, 25–50th, and 25th percentiles, respectively.

The excellent outcome for growth noted by Chasnoff et al. may be due to the low dose of methadone administered to the pregnant women. Olofsson et al. (80) demonstrated a correlation between maternal methadone dose and weight, height, and head circumference at a mean age of 3.5 years. Of mothers receiving less than 20 mg/day at birth, none of 33 infants were below the 10th percentile for weight, height, or head circumference, compared with 6 of 31 children whose mothers received 20 or more mg/day of methadone. Unfortunately, growth parameters at birth were not compared between the two groups. Overall, the heights of these children were statistically below the mean for age, a finding similar to those of Wilson et al. (85).

While Lifschitz et al. (42) did not show impaired head growth, Rosen and Johnson (81) reported that head circumferences remained below the 3rd percentile in 63% of infants followed up at 18 months of age whose head circumference at birth was below the 3rd percentile. Wilson et al. (85) reported that 14% of heroin-exposed children had a head circumference below the third percentile when examined between 3 and 6 years of age. Again, the head circumference at birth was not reported. In summary, brain growth may be blunted long term subsequent to in utero narcotic exposure.

Infants born to narcotic-addicted women may also be at increased risk of developing strabismus. Nelson et al. (86) and Rosen and Johnson (81) observed strabismus in 24 and 21% of narcotic-exposed infants, respectively, compared with a reported incidence of 2.8–5.3% in the general population. Therefore, these infants should be evaluated for the presence of strabismus as part of their outpatient follow-up care.

In summary, follow-up studies of narcotic-exposed infants have revealed significant behavioral abnormalities, but not long-term cognitive deficits.

STIMULANTS

Adverse effects on the fetus and newborn attributable to maternal cocaine use during pregnancy are now being appreciated. It is not clear, however, whether infants of cocaine-abusing mothers manifest symptoms from drug withdrawal. Madden et al. (87) reported no overt symptoms of withdrawal in eight infants whose mothers abused cocaine during pregnancy. Infants whose urine screens were positive for other abusive drugs were excluded from their study. Ryan et al. (88) recently compared three groups of infants; one group was born to mothers who used cocaine in addition to methadone and/or other drugs, another group of infants was born to mothers whose drug-use patterns were similar to the first group except they did not use cocaine, and the third group was a control population of non-drug-dependent women. The frequency of drug withdrawal symptoms was comparable between the cocaine/methadone- and methadone-exposed infants, implying that cocaine does not increase the risk of neonatal drug withdrawal. In contrast, other investigators have observed mild "withdrawal" syndromes consisting of abnormal sleep/wake patterns, poor feeding, irritability, tremulousness, hypertonia, and hyperreflexia (89–93). However, these symptoms are similar to those reported by Chasnoff et al. (94) in a 2-week-old cocaine-intoxicated infant. This child manifested symptoms for 48 to 72 h.

Cocaine should readily cross the placenta owing to its high lipid solubility. Since cocaine is primarily eliminated by hepatic metabolism and by plasma cholinesterases (95), which have low activity in the fetus and newborn (96), accumulation of cocaine in the fetus and subsequent toxic manifestations are not surprising. Owing to an expected slow elimination phase for cocaine by the fetus and newborn, we would anticipate withdrawal signs and symptoms to be delayed from birth, if they occur at all. These pharmacokinetic/pharmacodynamic predictions are supported by the data presented by Chasnoff et al. (97). These investigators reported the presence of cocaine or its metabolites in a newborn's urine for at least 4 days after delivery. Therefore, we feel symptoms previously ascribed to "cocaine withdrawal" may in fact represent cocaine intoxication.

Oro and Dixon (92) reported similar symptoms of CNS hyperexcitability among infants born to amphetamine-abusing mothers. However, some of these infants exhibited marked lethargy and required tube feedings when their hyperexcitable state subsided. This state of pronounced lethargy most likely represents a true withdrawal syndrome comparable to that observed during cocaine and methamphetamine withdrawal in adults (98). Other investigators have reported similar observations in infants born to mothers abusing amphetamines (99,100). Ramer (99), in 1974, reported the case of a full-term infant born to a mother using parenterally administered amphetamines during pregnancy. She was admitted to the maternity hospital 4 days prior to delivery. Episodes of diaphoresis, restlessness, and moitic pupils were observed in the newborn during the first day of life. By the third day of life, the infant was listless, with decreased muscle tone, and was observed to have a peculiar glassy-eyed stare. These symptoms abated by the nineth day of life.

In summary, infants born to mothers abusing central nervous system stimulants may exhibit signs or symptoms of intoxication or withdrawal. Similar to the case of narcotic-addicted infants, the temporal relationship between the last maternal dose and delivery appears to be a major factor in the timing of neonatal symptoms and in determining whether the newborn manifests symptoms attributable to intoxication or withdrawal. Marked symptoms of CNS hyperexcitability can be controlled with the administration of benzodiazepines as needed (101), whereas withdrawal symptoms should be managed supportively.

Although infants born to cocaine users may not manifest symptoms of drug withdrawal, cocaine clearly affects pregnancy and neonatal outcome adversely. Women who use cocaine during pregnancy are at increased risk for spontaneous abortion (88,89,102), premature labor (89), precipitous delivery (89), abruptio placentae (89,92,102), and meconium staining (89). Cocaine may also be teratogenic. Bingol et al. (103) reported a significantly higher congenital malformation rate in cocaine-using mothers compared with a non-drug-using control group. Affected infants presented with congenital heart disease or skeletal defects. Chasnoff et al. (104) observed genitourinary tract malformations in 3 of 23 infants born to women who only used cocaine during the first trimester of pregnancy, and in 6 of 52 infants whose mothers used cocaine throughout pregnancy. The genitourinary tract malformations included prune belly syndrome (2), hydronephrosis (4), secondary hypospadias (2), and female pseudohermaphroditism (1). Two additional infants who were exposed to cocaine throughout pregnancy had ileal atresia. These clinical reports of the teratogenic potential of cocaine are supported by the work of Mahalik and coworkers (105), who described skeletal and genitourinary tract malformations in the offspring of gravid mice administered cocaine early in pregnancy. However, in none of these reports did a homogeneous pattern of malformations emerge, and the data should be interpreted cautiously. For example, during embryonic life the genitourinary system does not develop from one origin, and it is impossible to trace the malformations described above to one etiological factor.

Although conflicting data initially appeared in the literature regarding the effect of maternal cocaine use on intrauterine growth (87,89,102), more recent investigations have observed a significant effect on growth (90,103, 106). Bingol et al. (103) reported mean birth weight, length, and head circumference of 2276 g, 46.2 cm, and 32 cm in 50 full-term infants born to women who abused only cocaine during pregnancy, whereas Fulroth et al. (90) discovered a 20% incidence of growth retardation and a 29% incidence of microcephaly in prenatally exposed infants. Most recently, Chasnoff et al. (104) reported lower mean birth weights, lengths, and head circumferences among term infants born to mothers who used cocaine throughout pregnancy compared with control infants. In contrast, no differences in intrauterine growth parameters existed between infants born to mothers who used cocaine only during the first trimester and control infants.

Another adverse neurological outcome described in infants exposed in utero to cocaine is cerebral infarction. Chasnoff et al. (97) reported an infant with a right hemiparesis and right-sided focal seizures on the first day of life born to a mother who used excessive amounts of cocaine for 3 days prior to delivery. Computed tomography of the brain demonstrated a cerebral infarction within the distribution of the left middle cerebral artery, and a lumbar puncture revealed 1800 red blood cells and 5 white cells. The cerebrovascular accident may have resulted from intrauterine hypertension or hypotension due to the vasoconstrictor effects of cocaine on placental blood vessels.

Furthermore, neurobehavioral effects similar to those observed in narcotic-exposed infants have been reported in infants born to cocaine users (90,91, 102,104). Besides being more irritable, these infants demonstrate depressed interactive behavior and impaired responses to environmental stimuli. Chasnoff et al. (104), utilizing the Neonatal Behavioral Assessment Scale between 12 and 72 hours of life, observed significant deficiencies in orientation, motor ability, and state regulation among cocaine-exposed infants. In addition, Dixon et al. (91) observed very poor visual attention and abnormal flash-evoked visual potentials in 11 of 12 infants studied. Of concern are persistent visual disturbances at 4–6 months of age, as revealed by preliminary data. Such neurobehavioral abnormalities may impede the establishment of appropriate caretaker-infant relationships. Abnormal electroencephalograms featuring bursts of sharp wave-and-spike patterns and bursts of theta rhythm have also been seen in newborns of cocaine users (91,93). Doberczak et al.

(93) reported an abnormal EEG during the first week of life in 17 of 38 infants studied. Although the EEG was still abnormal in 9 of 14 infants in whom the test was repeated between days 9 and 14 of life, all but one EEG had normalized by 3 to 12 months of age.

These infants may also be at increased risk of SIDS (88,89). Chasnoff et al. (89) reviewed the histories of 66 cocaine-exposed infants born to women enrolled in perinatal drug programs in San Francisco or Chicago. Ten of these infants died of SIDS. This 15% incidence of SIDS is significantly greater than the risk previously reported for narcotic-exposed infants and for the general population (64). In contrast, however, Bauchner et al. (106) did not detect an increased risk of SIDS among 175 infants exposed to cocaine in utero.

In summary, cocaine intoxication should be anticipated in infants born to mothers abusing cocaine. Signs and symptoms of CNS hyperexcitability may persist for several days. Distinct neurobehavioral and EEG abnormalities have been attributed to in utero cocaine exposure. Long-term studies are required to determine whether these abnormalities will increase the infant's risk for future developmental, cognitive, or behavioral sequelae.

SEDATIVE-HYPNOTICS

Alcohol

Jones et al. (107) first recognized malformations among eight infants born to alcoholic mothers and termed this pattern the fetal alcohol syndrome (FAS). Characteristic features of this syndrome include intrauterine growth retardation, slow postnatal growth, microcephaly, developmental delay, impaired intellectual performance, and craniofacial and musculoskeletal anomalies (107–109). Other reported abnormalities include cardiac defects (mostly septal defects), ear and external genitalia anomalies, and cutaneous anomalies such as hemangiomas, pigmented nevi, and hirsutism (108). Several of the functional and anatomical derangements observed in these infants most likely result from brain dysmorphogenesis. Jones and Smith (109) reported the results of an autopsy performed in one patient with the fetal alcohol syndrome. Histopathology of the brain revealed small size, incomplete development of the cerebral cortex, agenesis of the corpus callosum, and disorganization of neural and glial elements.

Although the fetal alcohol syndrome is well recognized, symptoms of alcohol withdrawal in newborns have not been fully appreciated. Schaefer (110) published the first reported case of alcohol withdrawal in an infant born to an intoxicated American (Yukon) Indian woman. Symptoms appeared by 18–24 h of life and included irritability, coarse tremors of the hands and feet, restlessness, sleepiness, and excessive crying. An "alcoholic fetor" was apparent up to 12 h of life. By the sixth day of life, the infant was still irritable and easily startled; however, other clinical manifestations had resolved. Since the report by Schaefer, other cases of alcohol withdrawal in neonates have been published (111,112). Central nervous system manifestations of alcohol withdrawal develop within 24 h of birth and may include tremors, irritability, hypertonicity, muscle twitching, hyperventilation, hyperacusia, opisthotonos, and seizures (111,112). Gastrointestinal symptoms such as abdominal distention and vomiting are less frequent (111). Symptoms of alcohol withdrawal may be severe but appear to be of brief duration. Infants born to alcoholic mothers may be at a higher risk of seizures than narcotic-exposed infants; three of six newborns reported by Pierog et al. (111) and the neonate described by Nichols (112) developed seizures.

Infants manifesting signs or symptoms of alcohol withdrawal require pharmacological intervention. The infants described above were treated with chlorpromazine or phenobarbital. Such interventions do not appear to be mechanistically based, and these drugs may not prove to be optimal therapy. Phenothiazines reduce the seizure threshold and thus may enhance the risk of seizures in these infants. Phenobarbital has been effective in adult cases of alcohol withdrawal, but it is not easily titrated. Our drug of choice is diazepam. Benzodiazepines demonstrate a cross-tolerance with alcohol and have a wider therapeutic index than phenothiazines or barbiturates (114). In adults, benzodiazepines are as effective as barbiturates in alleviating symptoms of alcohol withdrawal, and they can prevent withdrawal seizures (113). Several dosing regimens of diazepam have been used in adults (114). One such regimen, the diazepam-loading technique, appears to be both safe and effective (115). This technique relies on the slow clearance of diazepam and its active metabolites from the body. After effective loading with diazepam, the therapeutic effect usually persists longer than the duration of the withdrawal syndrome, obviating the need for additional pharmacological therapy. We would recommend administering 0.25 mg/kg IV of diazepam q2h until symptoms are controlled. Sellers et al. (115) reported successful responses to the diazepam-loading technique in a median time of 7.6 h in 36 adults with acute alcohol withdrawal. Only three patients required therapy beyond 24 hours.

In summary, alcohol withdrawal should be considered in the differential diagnosis of the irritable newborn, particularly when characteristic features of the fetal alcohol syndrome are present. Signs and symptoms of neonatal alcohol withdrawal are remarkably similar to those observed in the neonatal narcotic withdrawal syndrome except that seizures may be more frequent in the former, and gastrointestinal symptoms are more prevalent in the latter.

Barbiturates

Signs and symptoms of drug withdrawal have also been described in infants born to mothers receiving barbiturates (116–118). Desmond et al. (116) reported their observations on 15 infants born to mothers who either were addicted to barbiturates or were receiving phenobarbital for sedation, hypertension, or as part of an anticonvulsant regimen. Phenobarbital dosages ranged from 60 to 180 mg qd. Symptoms were similar to those observed in narcotic-exposed infants: all displayed hyperactivity, restlessness, disturbed sleep, and excessive crying, with the majority of infants also noted to be tremulous, hyperreflexic, and hyperphagic. Clinical manifestations of drug withdrawal appeared later in these infants compared with infants born to narcotic addicts. Most of the infants reported by Desmond et al. (116) became symptomatic toward the end of the first week of life, although the age at onset of barbiturate withdrawal was delayed up to 2 weeks in some infants. This delay should not be unexpected, considering the long $t_{1/2\beta}$ of barbiturates. Most infants were symptomatic for 2–6 weeks.

Bleyer and Marshall (117) and Ostrea (118) also reported barbiturate withdrawal in infants born to mothers receiving secobarbital and butalbital, respectively. both these infants developed generalized seizures in addition to other symptoms of neuromuscular excitability.

Infants demonstrating signs or symptoms of barbiturate withdrawal may be effectively treated with phenobarbital. Table 6 lists our indications for initiating therapy. We would administer a loading dose of 20 mg/kg IV or IM, and start maintenance therapy with 4 mg/kg/day IV or PO. Higher maintenance doses may be required to control symptoms (117). Serum phenobarbital concentrations should be monitored to avoid toxicity. When symptoms have been controlled for a week, we decrease the daily dose by 25% of the original dose very week.

Benzodiazepines

Symptoms indistinguishable from narcotic or barbiturate withdrawal, including seizures, have also been observed in infants born to mothers receiv-

Table 6 Indications for Initiating Pharmacological Therapy in Barbiturate Withdrawal

Seizures
Signs or symptoms interfering with normal caretaker–infant interactions, such as moderate to severe hyperactivity or irritability
Poor feeding or failure to gain weight

ing therapeutic doses of chlordiazepoxide (119,120) and diazepam (121, 122). The onset of symptoms may appear shortly after birth or be significantly delayed; Athinarayanan et al. (119) reported the onset of withdrawal at 21 days of age in twin infants born to a mother receiving 30 mg/day of chlordiazepoxide during pregnancy. Withdrawal symptoms persisted for long periods of time in several of these infants.

We recommend initiating treatment of benzodiazepine withdrawal with 0.1 mg/kg diazepam q12h IV. More frequent dosing or larger doses may be required to control symptoms. When symptoms have been well controlled for approximately a week, we recommend weaning diazepam over 3–4 weeks by gradually reducing a given dose each day. Indications for initiating therapy are similar to those for barbiturate withdrawal (see Table 6).

Case reports describing neonatal withdrawal from hydroxyzine (123), ethchlorvynol (124), and glutethimide (125) have also appeared in the literature. Although an abstinence syndrome from these agents would not be surprising, withdrawal from the concomitant use of phenobarbital, diazepam, and heroin, respectively, in these cases cannot be excluded.

In summary, neonatal withdrawal from sedative hypnotics may occur and should be anticipated in infants born to mothers chronically receiving this class of drugs toward the end of pregnancy. Signs and symptoms of neuromuscular excitability predominate and may be delayed from birth in onset and may follow a protracted course. Treatment should be initiated when symptoms are life threatening or interfere with caretaker-infant interactions or when a potentially adverse effect on the growth of the infant is perceived.

MISCELLANEOUS DRUGS

Other classes of drugs reported to be associated with a withdrawal syndrome in the newborn are tricyclic antidepressants (TCAs) (124–126) and phenothiazines (127). Webster (126) observed breathlessness, cyanosis, tachypnea, tachycardia, and irritability in a 1-day-old infant born to a mother receiving desmethylimipramine during pregnancy. Gradual improvement in the infant's condition was noted by 10 days of life. Eggermont (127) noted similar symptoms in three infants whose mothers took imipramine during pregnancy. Ben Musa and Smith (128) described an infant with hypothermia and jitteriness born to a mother receiving clomipramine. Symptoms were present by 12 h of life and persisted for 4 days. More data are required to permit us to appreciate the effect of maternally administered TCAs on the newborn and to decide whether these symptoms result from drug intoxication or drug withdrawal.

O'Conner et al. (129), in 1981, reported an interesting case of late-onset neurological dysfunction in a 3-week-old infant born to a mother who had received intramuscular injections of fluphenazine decanoate daily throughout her last two trimesters of pregnancy. The infant developed choreiform and dystonic movements, primarily of the upper extremities, associated with irritability, hypertonicity, and sleep disturbance. Diphenhydramine hydrochloride administration did little to alleviate the symptoms. The infant gradually improved and by 9 months of age was asymptomatic. This report illustrates a case of drug withdrawal following material administration of a high potency, long-acting phenothiazine. We feel that these symptoms may be analogous to a phenomenon known as withdrawal-emergent dyskinesias, a variant of tardive dyskinesias (130). This phenomenon most likely results from disuse supersensitivity of dopaminergic pathways in the brain. Treatment with phenothiazines may mask the dyskinesias. However, administration of phenothiazines or antimuscarinic agents may also worsen the underlying condition. Therefore, the aim of management should be supportive care with avoidance of neuroleptic and anticholinergic agents.

SUMMARY

Neonatal drug withdrawal syndromes have been reported following chronic maternal administration of many classes of agents. Withdrawal from narcotics has been studied most intensely in newborns and is associated with both short- and long-term morbidity. Although infants born to mothers abusing stimulants may manifest symptoms of drug withdrawal, perinatal complications such as abruptio placentae and cerebrovascular accidents appear to be more worrisome. Neonatal withdrawal from sedative-hypnotics may also occur, with signs and symptoms of neuromuscular hyperexcitability predominating. Finally, the timing of the last maternal dose of a drug, with respect to delivery, as well as a given agent's pharmacokinetic properties, may influence the time to onset of a neonatal abstinence syndrome following delivery. Symptoms may be delayed from birth; they may be severe and life threatening, and the clinical course may be protracted.

Answer

Drug withdrawal occurs when there is little or no drug in the system, therefore the negative neonatal urine test is consistent with the diagnosis. Although other diagnostic options must be carefully ruled out, the baby should benefit from oral paregoric acid treatment or other forms of sedation (e.g., phenobarbital).

REFERENCES

1. Committee on Drugs. Neonatal drug withdrawal. Pediatrics 1983; 72:895–902.
2. Marx CM, Cloherty JP. Drug withdrawal. In Manual of Neonatal Care, 2nd ed (Cloherty JP, Stark AR, eds), Little Brown, Boston, 1985, pp 17–28.

3. Tyson HK. Neonatal withdrawal symptoms associated with maternal abuse of propoxyphene hydrochloride. J Pediatr 1974; 85:684–685.
4. Klein RB, Blatman S, Little GA. Probable neonatal propoxyphene withdrawal: A case report. Pediatrics 1975; 55:882–884.
5. Quillan WW, Dunn CA. Neonatal drug withdrawal from propoxyphene. JAMA 1976; 235:2128.
6. Mangurten HH. Neonatal codeine withdrawal in infants of nonaddicted mothers. Pediatrics 1980; 65:159–160.
7. Van Leeuwen G, Guthrie R, Stange F. Narcotic withdrawal reaction in a newborn infant due to codeine. Pediatrics 1965; 36:635–636.
8. Scanlon JW. Pentazocine and neonatal withdrawal symptoms. J Pediatr 1974; 85:735–736.
9. Kopelman AE. Fetal addiction to pentazocine. Pediatrics 1975; 55:888–889.
10. Goetz RL, Bain RV. Neonatal withdrawal symptoms associated with maternal use of pentazocine. J Pediatr 1974; 84:887–888.
11. Rivers RPA. Neonatal opiate withdrawal. Arch Dis Child 1986; 61:1236–1239.
12. Redmond DE Jr, Huang YH, Snyder DR, Maas JW. Behavioral effects of stimulation of the nucleus locus coeruleus in the stump-tailed monkey *Macaca arctoides*. Brain Res 1976; 116:502–510.
13. Redmond DE Jr. Alterations in the function of the nucleus locus coeruleus: A possible model for studies of anxiety. In Animal Models in Psychiatry and Neurology (Hanin I, Usdin E, eds), Pergamon Press, New York, 1977, pp 293–304.
14. Cedarbaum JM, Aghajanian GK. Catecholamine receptors on locus coeruleus neurons: Pharmacological characterization. Eur J Pharmacol 1977; 44:375–385.
15. Pert CB, Kuhar MJ, Snyder SH. Opiate receptor: Autoradiographic localization in rat brain. Proc Natl Acad Sci USA 1976; 73:3729–3733.
16. Atweh SF, Kuhar MJ. Autoradiographic localization of opiate receptors in rat brain II. The brain stem. Brain Res 1977; 129:1–12.
17. Bird SJ, Kuhar MJ. Iontophoretic application of opiates to the locus coeruleus. Brain Res 1977; 122:523–533.
18. Cedarbaum JM, Aghajanian GK. Noradrenergic neurons of the locus coeruleus: Inhibition by epinephrine and activation by the α-antagonist piperoxane. Brain Res 1976; 112:413–419.
19. Korf J, Bunney BS, Aghajanian GK. Noradrenergic neurons: Morphine inhibition of spontaneous activity. Eur J Pharmacol 1974; 25:165–169.
20. Hamburg M, Tallman JF. Chronic morphine administration increases the apparent number of α_2-adrenergic receptors in rat brain. Nature 1981; 291:493–495.
21. Aghajanian GK. Tolerance of locus coeruleus neurons to morphine and suppression of withdrawal response by clonidine. Nature 1978; 276:186–188.
22. Henry JL. Effects of substance P on functionally identified units in cat spinal cord. Brain Res 1976; 114:439–451.
23. Jessell TM. Substance P in nocioceptive sensory neurons. In Substance P in the Nervous System, Ciba Foundation Symposium 1982; 91:225–248.
24. Yakish TL, Jessell TM, Gamse R, Mudge AW, Leeman SE. Intrathecal morphine inhibits substance P release from mammalian spinal cord in vivo. Nature 1980; 286:155–157.

25. Lembeck F, Donnerer J. Opioid control of the function of primary afferent substance P fibres. Eur J Pharmacol 1985; 114:241–246.

26. Vacca LL, Abrahams SJ, Naftchi NE. Effect of morphine on substance P neurons in rat spinal cord: A preliminary study. Brain Res 1980; 182:229–236.

27. Bergstrom L, Sakurada T, Terenius L. Substance P levels in various regions of the rat central nervous system after acute and chronic morphine treatment. Life Sci 1984; 35:2375–2382.

28. Bell JA, Jaffe JH. Electrophysiological evidence for a presynaptic mechanism of morphine withdrawal in the neonatal rat spinal cord. Brain Res 1986; 382: 299–304.

29. Gintzler AR, Scalisi JA. Effects of opioids on noncholinergic excitatory responses of the guinea-pig isolated ileum: Inhibition of release of enteric substance P. Br J Pharmacol 1982; 75:199–205.

30. Schulz R, Herz A. Aspects of opiate dependence in the myenteric plexus of the guinea pig. Life Sci 1976; 19:1117–1128.

31. Zelson C, Rubio E, Wasserman E. Neonatal narcotic addiction: 10 year observation. Pediatrics 1971; 48:178–189.

32. Olofsson M, Buckley W, Andersen GE, Friis-Hansen B. Investigation of 89 children born by drug-dependent mothers. I. Neonatal course. Acta Paediatr Scand 1983; 72:403–406.

33. Reddy AM, Harper RG, Stern G. Observations on heroin and methadone withdrawal in the newborn. Pediatrics 1971; 48:353–358.

34. Klenka HM. Babies born in a distinct general hospital to mothers taking heroin. Br Med J 1986; 293:745–746.

35. Newman RG, Bashkow S, Calko D. Results of 313 consecutive live births of infants delivered to patients in the New York City methadone maintenance treatment program. Am J Obstet Gynecol 1974; 121:233–237.

36. Naeye RL, Blanc W. Leblanc W, Khatamee MA. Fetal complications of maternal heroin addiction: Abnormal growth, infections and episodes of stress. J Pediatr 1973; 83:1055–1061.

37. Kandall SR, Albin S, Lowinson J, Berle B, Eidelman AI, Gartner LM. Differential effects of maternal heroin and methadone use on birthweight. Pediatrics 1976; 58:681–685.

38. Finnegan LP. Effects of maternal opiate abuse on the newborn. Fed Proc 1985; 44:2314–2317.

39. Zelson C, Lee SJ, Casalino M. Comparative effects of maternal intake of heroin and methadone. N Engl J Med 1973; 289:1216–1220.

40. Rahbar F. Observations on methadone withdrawal in 16 neonates. Clin Pediatr 1975; 14:369–371.

41. Ostrea EM Jr, Chavez CJ. Perinatal problems (excluding neonatal withdrawal) in maternal drug addiction: A study of 830 cases. J Pediatr 1979; 94:292–295.

42. Lifschitz MH, Wilson GS, O'Brian-Smith E, Desmond MM. Factors affecting head growth and intellectual function in children of drug addicts. Pediatrics 1985; 75:269–274.

43. Lifschitz MH, Wilson GS, O'Brian-Smith E, Desmond MM. Fetal and postnatal growth of children born to narcotic-dependent women. J Pediatr 1983; 102:686–691.

44. Nathenson G, Cohen MI, Litt IF, McNamara H. The effect of maternal heroin addiction on neonatal jaundice. J Pediatr 1972; 81:899–903.
45. Holmes AW, Rosenblate H, Einstein R, Baldwin D. The liver disease of heroin addiction (abstr). Gastroenterology 1970; 58:310.
46. Harper RG,Solish GI, Purow HM, Sang M, Panepinto WC. The effect of a methadone treatment program upon pregnant heroin addicts and their newborn infants. Pediatrics 1974; 54:300–305.
47. Glass L, Rajegowda BK, Evens HE. Absence of respiratory distress syndrome in premature infants of heroin-addicted mothers. Lancet 1971; 2:685–686.
48. Gluck R, Kulovich MV. Lecithin/sphingomyelin ratios in amniotic fluid in normal and abnormal pregnancy. Am J Obstet Gynecol 1973; 115:539–546.
49. Taeusch HW Jr, Carson SH, Wang NS, Avery ML. Heroin induction of lung maturation and growth retardation in fetal rabbits. J Pediatr 1973; 82:869–875.
50. Rosen TS, Pippenger CE. Pharmacologic observations on the neonatal withdrawal syndrome. J Pediatr 1976; 88:1044–1048.
51. Ostrea EM, Chavez CJ, Strauss ME. A study of factors that influence the severity of neonatal narcotic withdrawal. J Pediatr 1976; 88:642–645.
52. Gilman AG, Goodman LS, Rall TW, Murad F, eds. The Pharmacologic Basis of Therapeutics, 7th ed, Macmillan, New York, 1985, Appendix II, p 1695.
53. Sweet AY. Narcotic withdrawal syndrome in the newborn. Pediatr Rev 1982; 3:285–291.
54. Kron RE, Litt M, Finnegan LP. Effect of maternal narcotic addiction on sucking behavior of neonates (abstr). Pediatr Res 1974; 8:364.
55. Kron RE, Litt M, Eng D, Phoenix MD, Finnegan LP. Neonatal narcotic abstinence: Effects of pharmacotherapeutic agents and maternal drug usage on nutritive sucking behavior. J Pediatr 1976; 88:637–641.
56. Hyde WH, Scharnberg JT, Rudolph AJ. Oxygen consumption in infants of narcotic addicts (abstr). Pediatr Res 1980; 14:467.
57. Glass L, Rajegowda BK, Kahn EJ, Floyd MV. Effects of heroin withdrawal on respiratory rate and acid-base status in the newborn. N Engl J Med 1972; 286:746–748.
58. Olsen GD, Lees MH. Ventilatory response to carbon dioxide of infants following chronic prenatal methadone exposure. J Pediatr 1980; 96:983–989.
59. Davidson SL, Schuetz S, Krishna V, Bean X, Wingert W, Wachsman L, Keens TG. Abnormal sleeping ventilatory pattern in infants of substance-abusing mothers. Am J Dis Child 1986; 140:1015–1020.
60. Checola RT, Prybylski D, Senie R, Kandall SR. Cardiorespiratory patterns in passively addicted (PA) neonates (abstract). Pediatr Res 1986; 20:345A.
61. Herzlinger RA, Kandall SR, Vaughan HG Jr. Neonatal seizures associated with narcotic withdrawal. J Pediatr 1977; 91:638–641.
62. Chasnoff IJ, Hatcher R, Burns WJ. Early growth patterns of methadone-addicted infants. Am J Dis Child 1980; 134:1049–1051.
63. Wilson GS, Desmond MM, Verniaud WM. Early development of infants of heroin-addicted mothers. Am J Dis Child 1973; 126:457–462.
64. Chavez CJ, Ostrea EM, STryker JC, Smialek Z. Sudden infant death syndrome among infants of drug dependent mothers. J Pediatr 1979; 95:407–409.

65. Pierson PS, Howard P, Kleber HD. Sudden deaths in infants born to methadone-maintained addicts. JAMA 1972; 220:1733-1734.
66. Finnegan LP, Kron RE, Connaughton JF Jr, Emich JP. A scoring system for evaluation and treatment of the neonatal abstinence syndrome: A new clinical and research tool. In Basic and Therapeutic Aspects of Perinatal Pharmacology (Morselli PL, Garattini S, Serini F, eds), Raven Press, New York, 1975, pp 139-153.
67. Lipsitz PJ. A proposed narcotic withdrawal score for use with newborn infants. Clin Pediatr 1975; 14:592-594.
68. Hoder EL, Leckman JF, Ehrenkranz R, Kleber H, Cohen DJ, Poulsen JA. Clonidine in neonatal narcotic-abstinence syndrome (letter). N Engl J Med 1981; 305:1284.
69. Cobrink RW, Hood T Jr, Chusid E. The effect of maternal narcotic addiction on the newborn infant: Review of literature and report of 22 cases. Pediatrics 1959; 24:288-304.
70. Brown WJ, Buist NRM. Cory Gipson HT, Huston RK, Kennaway NG. Fatal benzyl alcohol poisoning in a neonatal intensive care unit (letter). Lancet 1982; 1:1250.
71. Gershanik J, Boecler B, Ensley H, McCloskey S, George W. The gasping syndrome and benzyl alcohol poisoning. N Engl J Med 1982; 307:1384-1387.
72. Committee on Fetus and Newborn, Committee on Drugs. Benzyl alcohol: Toxic agent in neonatal units. Pediatrics 1983; 72:356-358.
73. Kunstadter RH, Klein RI, Lundeen EC, Witz W, Morrison M. Narcotic withdrawal symptoms in newborn infants. JAMA 1958; 168:1008-1010.
74. Kandall SR, Koberczak TM, Mauer KR, Strashun RH, Korts DC. Opiate v. CNS depressant therapy in neonatal drug abstinence syndrome. Am J Dis Child 1983; 137:378-382.
75. Carin I, Glass L. Parekh A, Solomon N, Steigman J, Wong S. Neonatal methadone withdrawal: Effect of two treatment regimens. Am J Dis Child 1983; 137: 1166-1169.
76. Kaltenbach K, Finnegan LP. Neonatal abstinence syndrome, pharmacotherapy and developmental outcome. Neurobehav Toxicol Teratol 1986; 8:353-355.
77. Finnegan LP, Ehrlich S. Maternal drug abuse during pregnancy and pharmacotherapy for neonatal abstinence syndrome (NAS). Pediatr Res (abstr) 1987; 21: 234A.
78. Strauss ME, Lessen-Firestone JK, Starr RH, Ostrea EM. Behavior of narcotics-addicted newborns. Child Dev 1975; 46:887-893.
79. Kaltenbach K, Finnegan LP, Frankenfield M. Neonatal abstinence syndrome (NAS) and interactive behaviors at 1 and 30 days of life. Pediatr Res (abstr) 1981; 15:450.
80. Olofsson M, Buckley W, Andersen GE, Friis-Hansen B. Investigations of 89 children born by drug-dependent mothers: Follow-up 1-10 years after birth. Acta Paediatr Scand 1983; 72:407-410.
81. Rosen TS, Johnson HL. Children of methadone-maintained mothers: Follow-up to 18 months of age. J Pediatr 1982; 101:192-196.

82. Wilson GS, Desmond MM, Wait RB. Follow-up of methadone-treated and untreated narcotic-dependent women and their infants: Health, developmental and social implications. J Pediatr 1981; 98:716–722.
83. Kaltenbach K, Finnegan LP. Perinatal and developmental outcome of infants exposed to methadone in utero. Neotoxicol Teratol 1987; 9:311–313.
84. Kaltenbach K, Finnegan LP. Children exposed to methadone in utero: Cognitive ability in the preschool years (abstr). Pediatr Res 1987; 21:181A.
85. Wilson GS, McCreary R, Kean J, Baxter JC. The development of preschool children of heroin-addicted mothers: A controlled study. Pediatrics 1979; 63: 135–141.
86. Nelson LB, Ehrlich S, Calhoun JH, Matteucci T, Finnegan LP. Occurrence of strabismus in infants born to drug-dependent women. Am J Dis Child 1987; 141:175–178.
87. Madden JD, Payne TF, Miller S. Maternal cocaine abuse and effect on the newborn. Pediatrics 1986; 77:209–211.
88. Ryan L, Ehrlich S, Finnegan L. Cocaine abuse in pregnancy: Effects on the fetus and newborn. Neurotoxicol Teratol 1987; 9:295–299.
89. Chasnoff IJ, Burns KA, Burns WJ. Cocaine use in pregnancy: Perinatal morbidity and mortality. Neurotoxicol Teratol 1987; 9:291–293.
90. Fulroth RF, Phillips BL, Trueax RE, Durand DJ. Description of 72 infants exposed to cocaine prenatally. Pediatr Res (abstr) 1987; 21:361A.
91. Dixon SD, Coen RW, Crutchfield S. Visual dysfunction in cocaine-exposed infants (abstr). Pediatr Res 1987; 21:359A.
92. Oro AS, Dixon SD. Perinatal cocaine and methamphetamine exposure: Maternal and neonatal correlates. J Pediatr 1987; 111:571–578.
93. Doberczak TM, Shanzer S, Senie RT, Randall SR. Neonatal neurologic and electroencephalographic effects of intrauterine cocaine exposure. J Pediatr 1988; 113:354–358.
94. Chasnoff IJ, Lewis DE, Squires L. Cocaine intoxication in a breast-fed infant. Pediatrics 1987; 80:836–838.
95. Stewart DJ, Inaba T, Lucassen M, Kalow W. Cocaine metabolism: Cocaine and norcocaine hydrolysis by liver and serum esterases. Clin Pharmacol Ther 1979; 25:464–468.
96. Echobichon DJ, Stephens DS. Perinatal development of human blood esterases. Clin Pharmacol Ther 1973; 14:41–47.
97. Chasnoff IJ, Bussey ME Savich R, Stack CM. Perinatal cerebral infarction and maternal cocaine use. J Pediatr 1986; 108:456–459.
98. Weiner N. Norepinephrine, epinephrine and the sympathomimetic amines. In The Pharmacological Basis of Therapeutics, 7th ed (Gilman AG, Goodman LS, Rall TW, Murad F, eds), Macmillan, New York, 1985, pp 145–180.
99. Ramer CM. The case history of an infant ;born to an amphetamine-addicted mother. Clin Pediatr 1974; 13:596–597.
100. Eriksson M, Larsson G, Windlbadh B, Zetterstrom R. The influence of amphetamine addiction on pregnancy and the newborn infant. Acta Paediatr Scand 1978; 67:95–99.

101. Gay GR. You've come a long way baby! Coke time for the new American lady of the eighties. J Psychoactive Drugs 1981; 13:297–318.
102. Chasnoff IJ, Burns WJ, Schnoll SH, Burns KA. Cocaine use in pregnancy. N Engl J Med 1985; 313:666–669.
103. Bingol N, Fuchs M, Diaz V, Stone RK, Gromisch DS. Teratogenicity of cocaine in humans. J Pediatr 1987; 110:93–96.
104. Chasnoff IJ, Griffith DR, MacGregor S, Kirkes K, Burns KA. Temporal patterns of cocaine use in pregnancy: Perinatal outcome. JAMA 1989; 261:1741–1744.
105. Mahalik MP, Gautieri RF, Mann DE Jr. Teratogenic potential of cocaine hydrochloride in CF-1 mice. J Pharmacol Sci 1980; 69:703–706.
106. Bauchner H, Zuckerman B, McClain M, Frank D, Freid LE, Kayne H. Risk of sudden infant death syndrome among infants with in utero exposure to cocaine. J Pediatr 1988; 113:831–834.
107. Jones KL, Smith DW, Ulleland CN, Streissguth AP. Pattern of malformation in offspring of chronic alcoholic mothers. Lancet 1973; 1:1267–1271.
108. Hanson JW, Jones KL, Smith DW. Fetal alcohol syndrome: Experience with 41 patients. JAMA 1976; 235:1458–1460.
109. Jones KL, Smith DW. Recognition of the fetal alcohol syndrome in early infancy. Lancet 1973; 2:999–1001.
110. Schaefer O. Alcohol withdrawal syndrome in a newborn infant of a Yukon Indian mother. Can Med Assoc J 1962; 87:1333–1334.
111. Pierog S, Chandavasu O, Wexler I. Withdrawal symptoms in infants with the fetal alcohol syndrome. J Pediatr 1977; 90:630–633.
112. Nichols MM. Acute alcohol withdrawal syndrome in a newborn. Am J Dis Child 1967; 113:714–715.
113. Devenyi P, Harrison ML. Prevention of alcohol withdrawal seizures with oral diazepam loading. Can Med Assoc J 1985; 132:798–800.
114. Sullivan JT, Sellers EM. Treating alcohol, barbiturate and benzodiazepine withdrawal. Rational Drug Therapy 1986; 20:1–8.
115. Sellers EM, Naranjo CA, Harrison M, Devenyi P, Roach C, Sykora K. Diazepam loading: Simplified treatment of alcohol withdrawal. Clin Pharmacol Ther 1983; 34:822–826.
116. Desmond MM, Schwanecke RP, Wilson GS, Yasunaga S, Burgdorff I. Maternal barbiturate utilization and neonatal withdrawal symptomatology. J Pediatr 1972; 80:190–197.
117. Bleyer WA, Marshall RE. Barbiturate withdrawal syndrome in a passively addicted infant. JAMA 1972; 221:185–186.
118. Ostrea EM Jr. Neonatal withdrawal from intrauterine exposure to butalbital. Am J Obstet Gynecol 1982; 143:597–599.
119. Athinarayanan P, Pierog S, Nigam SK, Glass L. Chlordiazepoxide withdrawal in the neonate. Am J Obstet Gynecol 1976; 124:212–213.
120. Bitnum S. Possible effect of chlordiazepoxide on the fetus (letter). Can Med Assoc J 1969; 100:351.
121. Mazzi E. Possible neonatal diazepam withdrawal: A case report. Am J Obstet Gynecol 1977; 129:586–587.

122. Rementeria JL, Bhatt K. Withdrawal symptoms in neonates from intrauterine exposure to diazepam. J Pediatr 1977; 90:123–126.
123. Prenner BM. Neonatal withdrawal syndrome associated with hydroxyzine hydrochloride. Am J Dis Child 1977; 131:529–530.
124. Rumack BH, Walravens PA. Neonatal withdrawal following maternal ingestion of ethchlorvynol (Placidyl). Pediatrics 1973; 52:714–716.
125. Reveri M, Pyati SP, Pildes RS. Neonatal withdrawal symptoms associated with glutethimide (Doriden) addiction in the mother during pregnancy. Clin Pediatr 1977; 16:424–425.
126. Webster PAC. Withdrawal symptoms in neonates associated with maternal antidepressant therapy (letter). Lancet 1973; 2:318–319.
127. Eggermont E. Neonatal effects of maternal therapy with tricyclic antidepressant drugs (letter). Arch Dis Child 1980; 55:81.
128. Ben Musa A, Smith CS. Neonatal effects of maternal clomipramine therapy (letter). Arch Dis Child 1979; 54:405.
129. O'Conner M, Johnson GH, James DI. Intrauterine effects of phenothiazines. Med J Aust 1981; 1:416–417.
130. Baldessarini RJ. Drugs and the treatment of psychiatric disorders. In The Pharmacologic Basis of Therapeutics, 7th ed. (Gilman AG, Goodman LS, Rall TW, Murad F, eds), Macmillan, New York, 1985, pp 387–445.

16

Relationship Between Gestational Cocaine Use and Pregnancy Outcome

A Meta-Analysis

Beatrix Lutiger, Thomas R. Einarson, and Gideon Koren
The Hospital for Sick Children, Toronto, Ontario, Canada

Karen Graham
McMaster University, Hamilton, Ontario, Canada

Clinical Case

Cocaine is detected in the urine of one of your patients, as well as in her baby's urine at birth. Which congenital malformations should you be considering as associated with cocaine?

INTRODUCTION

During the last decade there has been a sharp increase in the recreational use of cocaine in North America, with women of reproductive age showing the greatest increment. In Ontario, Canada, 11.5% of women aged 18 to 29 years reported lifetime use of cocaine in 1987, compared to only 3.5% in 1984 (Smart and Adlaf, 1987). A recent report from a large inner city hospital in California determined that cocaine was the drug most often detected in maternal and neonatal urine, being present in 46 and 41% of samples tested of suspected mothers and babies, respectively (Osterloh and Lee, 1989).

The increase in cocaine use among women of reproductive age has caused concern about the potential fetal effects of the drug taken during pregnancy.

Reprinted with permission of Wiley Liss from Teratology 1991; 44:405–414.

Over the last several years a growing number of studies investigating the effects of maternal cocaine use on the course of pregnancy and fetal outcome have been published. However, a homogeneous pattern of fetal effects has not been established and there is little consensus on the adverse effects of the drug. The wide variety of endpoints reported by different studies has made it difficult to define the risks that cocaine may pose to the pregnant woman and her baby. It is essential that physicians be provided with the best possible estimate of the risk of cocaine exposure in pregnancy so that proper counseling of the pregnant patient can take place. Overestimation of the reproductive risk of cocaine may lead to termination of an otherwise wanted pregnancy, whereas underestimation of the risk does not allow for proper medical approach to the woman and her baby, including appropriate maternal counseling and neonatal follow-up.

Using the statistical approach of meta-analysis (Glass, 1976; Einarson, 1988), it is possible to pool data from studies of similar design to arrive at an overall quantitative estimate of the effect of a drug on pregnancy outcome. The method has recently been applied by us to the field of human reproductive toxicology with examination of Bendectin (Einarson et al., 1988) and spermicide (Einarson et al., 1990) use by the pregnant woman. The objective of the present study was to quantitatively assess the relationship between gestational cocaine use and subsequent pregnancy complications and fetal outcome, using meta-analysis.

METHODS

The medical literature published between January 1975 and August 1989 was searched for papers dealing with the outcome of pregnancy following gestational cocaine exposure, using the National Library of Medicine's bibliographic database. Key words searched were combinations of *cocaine* or *crack*, and *pregnancy, maternal, fetus, newborn, neonate,* and *infant.* All references in the retrieved articles were followed up for further papers. As well, the Index Medicus was searched through this same time period. Journals with at least one previous article on cocaine in pregnancy were searched manually during the time period April 1989 through August 1989 to identify articles not yet included in the indexes.

The criteria for inclusion of papers in this analysis were human exposure to any amount of cocaine during any or all trimesters of pregnancy, as evidenced by drug history or urine test, and report of outcome of pregnancy or fetal development. Only case control or cohort studies with at least one control group were included. Use of other drugs is common among cocaine users and was not an exclusion criterion. Case reports, reviews, and editorials were excluded.

Table 1 Criteria for Inclusion of
Articles in This Meta-Analysis

Cocaine use in pregnancy
Pregnancy or fetal outcomes studies
Human studies
Original work
Cohort of case control
Control group present
English language

The "Methods" section of each paper was evaluated using a scoring sheet, prepared a priori, listing the inclusion criteria (Table 1). Studies fulfilling all inclusion criteria were accepted for analysis. These papers were read, and information was extracted using a data abstraction form. The information collected included the size and selection of the cocaine and control groups, and the pregnancy and fetal outcome measurements studied.

The investigator was blinded to the name of the journal, the authors of the paper, the hospital or site of the study, and the funding agency supporting the study. This blinding was accomplished by removing all identifying statements and titles prior to photocopying the papers for review by another investigator. Without this identification the prestige, reputation, or standards for the journal or author cannot interfere with the selection or analysis of articles. Although journals have a typeset style that theoretically could identify them, the junior investigator who conducted this search was not familiar with the different styles.

STATISTICAL METHODS

For continuous variables (e.g., occipitofrontal circumference, gestational age, etc.) the effect size (*es*) for individual studies and pooled *ES* for overall effects was computed using the Cohen's d (Cohen, 1977). Confidence intervals (CI) for Cohen's d were computed using the Macintosh Statview 512 program (Cohen, 1977). This program assumes a t distribution and uses a 95% confidence interval. The Cohen's d is based on the t test and represents the quantitative difference between two groups. It differs from the t test in that the influence of sample size has been removed. To calculate t, we divide the difference between group means by the standard error (SE), but we use the standard deviation (SD) to calculate d. The values are closely related, since SE = SD/degrees of freedom. However, t increases with sample size, whereas d remains constant. Thus, d represents the standardized difference between group means. Cohen describes $d = 0.2$ as small, 0.5 as medium, and 0.8 as large. For dichotomous variables the odds ratio were calculated using the Mantel-Haenszel formula (Mantel and Haenszel, 1959). Overall odds ratios and d values were calculated from raw data. The pooled mean effect size (ES) and odds ratios were calculated for all eligible reports for the following group comparisons: cocaine alone versus drug-free controls, cocaine in polydrug users versus drug-free controls, and polydrug users using cocaine versus polydrug-no cocaine users.

The *es* for each study and the pooled *ES* for each group comparison are considered significant if the CI for the Cohen's d does not include zero. When the CI includes only negative values, it indicates a positive effect, and when the CI includes only positive values it indicates an adverse effect. The odds ratio is a value ranging from 0 to infinity; a lower limit exceeding unity implies an adverse effect. For an adverse drug effect to be statistically significant, the CI must not contain unity.

For individual odds ratios, 95% confidence intervals were calculated using the Taylor Series method (Kleinbaum et al., 1982). For the overall summary (Mantel-Haenszel, 1959) odds ratio, confidence limits were calculated using the formula developed by Miettinen (1976).

The two statistical methods used in this study, Cohen's d and odds ratio, weight the sample sizes of the studies differently. Cohen's d does not take into account the number of patients per group, whereas the odds ratio does. A level of 0.05 was considered significant for all statistical tests.

RESULTS

A total of 45 scientific papers were identified which dealt with the human effects of cocaine used during pregnancy on pregnancy outcome, with an exponential growth in numbers of papers published in recent years. Based on reading of their Methods sections only, 20 studies met all inclusion criteria and were included in this analysis. Table 2 lists all studies accepted for meta-analysis; 15 were prospective cohort studies, 4 were retrospective cohort studies, and 1 was a case control study.

Table 3 lists all papers rejected from meta-analysis and the reasons for their rejection. Fourteen rejected articles were case reports, seven did not separate cocaine users from other drug users, six did not measure fetal or pregnancy outcome, and four did not have a control group. We noted that several reports were produced by one group of investigators. To avoid duplication of results, we examined them and have found no overlap in the nature of the comparisons.

Table 2 List of Accepted Studies[a]

First author	Study type	Data collection	Study group(s)	Control group(s)
			Sample sizes	
Cherukuri	C	R	55	55
Little	C	R	10	92
Chasnoff, 1985	C	P	12	11;15;15
Shih	C	P	18	18
Chouteau	C	R	124	218
Bauchner	C	P	175	821
Ryan	C	P	50	50;50
Chasnoff, 1987	C	P[b]	52	73
Isenberg	C[c]	P	13	36
Chasnoff, 1988	C	P	50	30
Bingol	C	R	50	110;3340
Chasnoff, 1989a	C	P	23;52	40
Chasnoff, 1989b	C	P	32	18
Zuckerman	C	P	114	1010
Keith	C	R	63;28	27;19;123
Little	C	P	53	100
Fulroth	C	P	35	17;14
Chavez	CC	R	276;791	2835;2973
Hadeed	C	P	56	53
McGregor	C	P	70	70

[a]C, cohort; CC, case control; P, prospective; R, retrospective.
[b]Partly retrospective.
[c]Partly case controlled.

Combinability of Studies

Many meta-analysts such as Rosenthal (1984) and Wolf (1986) recommend calculation of homogeneity before combining results. Chi square for heterogeneity was calculated for all outcomes of interest in this analysis. For outcomes measured on a continuous scale (i.e., head circumference, birth weight, length, and age), Cohen's d was calculated from the reported data and heterogeneity was determined using the method described by Rosenthal and Rubin (1982). For dichotomous variables, heterogeneity of odds ratios was calculated using the method presented by Breslow and Day (1980). When data were not suitable (i.e., cell frequencies of zero when N is not large), as indicated by Breslow and Day (1980, p. 143), Z values were calculated and tested as described by Rosenthal (1984, p. 77).

Table 3 List of Excluded Studies

Ref. reasons for rejection	First author
Cocaine users not separated from other drugs	K.W. Culver
	A.S. Oro
	S.L. Davidson
	M. Shannon
	C.J. Chavez, 1979
	G.M. Tenorio
	B.R. Schwartz
Control group is missing	P.E. LeBlanc
	T.M.Doberczak
	M. Mitchell
	K. Graham
Fetal outcome not studied	C.H. Wang
	D.A. Frank
	D.A. Bateman
	M. Shannon
	M. Mitchell
	C.E. Henderson
Case reports	J.D. Madden
	D.A. Bateman
	A.M. Telsey
	G.M. Tenorio
	R.L. Geggel
	C.E. Henderson
	B.R. Schwartz
	M.P. Teske
	H.O.D. Critchley
	I.J. Chasnoff
	R.R. Townsend
	D. Acker
	E. Collins
	R.E. Mittleman

Three of the 12 continuous variables were heterogeneous (head circumference, birth weight, and length). All three were comparisons between cocaine users and drug-free controls, and a single study was responsible for heterogeneity in all three cases. When that study was removed, chi square was no longer significant in two of the three cases. Removal of a second (outlier) study of birth weight produced homogeneity. In all cases, the effect sizes changed only minimally. When the two discrepant studies of birth weight were removed, the overall effect size was identical to that produced by the original 10 studies. The remaining two effect sizes decreased slightly in value, the largest decrease being from 0.70 to 0.58, the other being from 0.63 to 0.54. Such small changes did not affect the interpretation of the overall effects, which all remained of "medium" magnitude. Glass et al. (1981) are of the opinion that if studies do not differ greatly in their findings, a large database (regardless of quality) is much to be preferred over a small database. Thus, the discrepant study has been retained in this analysis.

Comparison of Cocaine Alone Versus Drug-Free Controls (Table 4)

We analyzed data obtained from studies comparing women who reported cocaine as their only drug of abuse to women who reported no drug abuse. The effect of gestational cocaine use on pregnancy and neonatal complications was commonly investigated (Table 4). Odds ratios computed for likelihood of being small for gestational age (SGA), having low birth weight (< 2500 g), or being premature (< 37 weeks) ranged from 4.31 to 5.31, but none was significantly different from the control group.

The ratio of male to female (m/f) live births was not significant. Similarly, the likelihood of premature rupture of membranes (PROM), abruptio placentae, meconium staining, and fetal distress was not significantly higher in

Table 4 Reproductive Effects of Cocaine in Studies Comparing Those Using Cocaine Alone Versus Drug-Free Controls

Endpoint	n	Odds ratio	95% Confidence interval Lower	Upper
SGA	3	5.31	0.24	118.3
Low birth weight (2500 g)	4	4.40	0.11	175.8
Prematurity	7	4.31	0.13	138.4
m/f	5	1.33	0.007	246.9
PROM	2	2.60	0.06	107.1
Abruptio placentae	8	5.82	0.71	47.8
Meconium	5	2.21	0.03	128.6
Fetal distress	3	2.01	0.11	37.8
Malformation (any)	6	4.08	0.70	23.6
Genitourinary	5	4.97	1.05	23.6
Heart	6	2.36	0.83	6.74
Spontaneous abortion	2	5.32	0.22	125.9
In utero death	2	6.17	1.21	31.5
SIDS	1	4.04	0.18	95.8

babies exposed to cocaine. Due to the very small number of studies investigating most of these endpoints, an adverse effect of cocaine could theoretically become significant with more available studies.

The teratogenic potential of cocaine was investigated in six studies. For malformations in general and for the subgroup of cardiac malformations, the odds ratios were 4.08 and 2.36, with no statistical significance. Conversely, for genitourinary malformations the odds ratio was statistically significant at 4.97 (CI 1.05–23.6).

The odds ratio of cocaine being associated with spontaneous abortions was 5.32 (NS). Two studies investigated rates of intrauterine death, finding a statistically significant odds ratio of 6.17 (CI 1.21–31.5). Only one study compared the frequency of sudden infant death syndrome (SIDS) in women using cocaine alone to those who are drug free, finding an odds ratio of 4.04 (NS).

Comparison of Cocaine/Polydrug Versus Drug-Free Controls (Table 5)

This comparison revealed similar tendencies to those shown above with the cocaine alone versus drug-free controls. In addition to the significantly greater likelihood of neonatal genitourinary malformations (odds ratio 2.79; CI 1.24–62.8), there was a significantly greater likelihood for spontaneous abortions (odds ratio of 10.56; CI 1.74–64.1).

Table 5 Reproductive Effects of Cocaine in Studies Comparing Cocaine/Polydrug Users to Drug-Free Controls

Endpoint	n	Odds ratio	95% Confidence interval Lower	Upper
SGA	3	4.19	0.28	62.16
Low birth weight (< 2500 g)	2	5.23	0.29	95.15
Prematurity (< 37 weeks)	4	5.36	0.35	81.8
Abruptio placentae	5	5.79	0.70	32.1
Meconium	2	1.56	0.04	62.0
Malformation (any)	3	2.83	0.43	18.7
Genitourinary	2	2.79	1.24	6.28
Heart	3	2.32	0.59	9.18
Spontaneous abortion	2	10.56	1.74	64.1
In utero death	2	6.06	0.59	62.6
SIDS	2	3.67	0.93	14.2

Comparison of Cocaine in Polydrug Users Versus Polydrug with No Cocaine (Table 6)

Only the odds ratios for genitourinary malformations was significant (6.08; CI 1.18–31.3). Of interest, several studies reported larger adverse effect sizes for the polydrug controls than for polydrug/cocaine users, making the data more heterogeneous.

The Effect of the Nature of the Comparison on Pooled Effect Size (Table 7)

Analysis of *ES* of the continuous variables (head circumference, gestational age, birth weight and length) reveals that the *ES* is dependent upon the nature of the comparison. Comparison of *cocaine/polydrug users* to *no drug users* consistently yields a medium effect size (0.50 to 0.58); as dose comparison of those using *cocaine alone* to *no drug users* (0.65 to 0.75). The effect sizes when comparing *polydrug/cocaine users* to *polydrug/no cocaine users* were small or nonexistent (0.06–0.37).

Table 6 Reproductive Effects of Cocaine in Studies Comparing Cocaine/Polydrug Users to Polydrug/No Cocaine Controls

Endpoint	*n*	Odds ratio	95% Confidence interval	
			Lower	Upper
SGA	2	2.48	0.12	50.4
Low birth weight (< 2500 g)	1	2.67	0.77	9.27
Prematurity (< 37 weeks)	3	5.37	0.11	15.1
m/f ratio	1	1.44	0.90	2.30
PROM	1	9.00	0.50	161.9
Abruptio placentae	3	5.40	0.97	30.1
Meconium	2	0.55	0.03	9.64
Malformation (any)	3	4.39	0.75	32.4
Genitourinary	3	6.08	1.18	31.3
Heart	3	1.50	0.62	3.63
Spontaneous abortion	2	3.50	0.64	19.2
In utero death	1	2.09	0.40	10.9
SIDS	2	3.58	0.91	14.1

Table 7   Comparison of Fetal Outcomes

	Total studies	Subjects (*n*)	Weighted (*es*)	95% Confidence limit Lower	Upper
A. In infants exposed to cocaine and in drug-free controls					
Occipitofrontal					
circumference, cm	8	2730	0.70	0.32	1.07
Gestational age, weeks	6	594	0.72	0.42	1.01
Birth weight, kg	11	3059	0.71	0.40	1.01
Birth length, cm	6	710	0.63	0.20	1.07
B. In infants with cocaine polydrug exposure and drug-free controls					
Occipitofrontal					
circumference, cm	4	1514	0.35	−0.19	0.89
Gestational age, weeks	3	362	0.43	−0.28	1.15
Birth weight, kg	6	1781	0.69	−0.01	1.37
Birth length, cm	3	514	0.43	−0.68	1.14
C. In cocaine/polydrug vs. polydrug					
Occipitofrontal					
circumference, cm	3	146	0.15	−0.54	0.60
Gestational age, weeks	3	228	0.27	−0.18	0.73
Birth weight, kg	5	281	0.23	−0.03	0.49
Birth length, cm	2	488	0.38	−2.6	3.36

DISCUSSION

Assessing the reproductive risks of cocaine is a complex task because women consuming this compound often abuse other illicit drugs and alcohol, and smoke cigarettes. In addition they tend to be of low socioeconomic class and to have associated risk factors such as sexually transmitted diseases and poor prenatal care. Therefore, comparison of cocaine use to nondrug use during pregnancy is not likely to control for such associated risk factors. Comparison of cocaine users to those who abuse other drugs is also not straightforward because cocaine users may consume higher amounts of cigarettes and alcohol than those who abuse other drugs but not cocaine (Koren and Feldman, 1990).

Another major problem in evaluating drug exposure during pregnancy is the difficulty in ascertaining the exposure. While a positive maternal or neonatal urine test may prove cocaine use during pregnancy, a negative test cannot rule it out as this compound has a short elimination half-life (Chow et al., 1985). Similarly, maternal reports are often negative in the presence of a positive urine test (Zuckerman et al., 1989). Hence a mother-baby pair may often be misclassified as being not exposed to cocaine, and this misclassification may hinder the ability of studies to detect or reject an association with adverse effects. The development of new biological markers that measure cumulative exposure to cocaine, such as neonatal hair (Graham et al., 1989b) or meconium tests (Ostrea et al., 1989), may improve the confirmation of intrauterine exposure.

During the last decade meta-analysis has emerged as a powerful statistical method for combination of similar data obtained from different studies. While this method lends itself to measurement of effects and adverse effects of drugs in general, its use in reproductive toxicology is relatively new (Einarson et al., 1988, 1990).

Meta-analysis does not overcome the limitations of individual studies, but it gives a better estimate of risk because random errors tend to cancel out in the long run, leaving a more clear view of the true trend. Glass (1976) has argued that weaknesses in individual studies do not preclude pooling the results to arrive at an overall conclusion.

Meta-analysis of reproductive outcome in *cocaine/polydrug users* versus *nondrug users* reveals a consistent medium mean effect size for lower head circumference, gestational age, birth weight, and birth length in babies exposed to drugs. This means that children born to cocaine/polydrug users are likely to be different at birth from nonusers in a clinically important way. The likelihood of spontaneous abortion and congenital genitourinary malformations in this comparison is significantly increased for the drug-exposed babies. Considering the clustering of other reproductive risk factors in the cocaine users when compared to nondrug users, one should be extremely careful before attributing these adverse effects to cocaine only. Comparison of the *cocaine alone* group to *nondrug controls* reveals very similar tendencies to the above comparison.

The comparison of reproductive outcome between polydrug users who include cocaine in their repertoire to polydrug users who do not use cocaine may be more appropriate in an attempt to control for other confounding risk factors commonly clustering in cocaine users. Unfortunately, the total number of studies performing such comparisons is small, thus weakening the statistical power. Only the likelihood of genitourinary malformations was increased in babies of polydrug users abusing cocaine when compared to polydrug users not consuming this drug. Even this comparison is not necessarily valid from a methodological standpoint because polydrug users who use cocaine cannot be assumed to be similar to polydrug users who do not. In fact, there is evidence that women using cocaine consume more alcohol, cigarettes, and other drugs than women using other illicit drugs (Koren and Graham, 1991).

Table 7 shows the clear tendency of decreased effect size of changes in growth parameters as the comparison between the cocaine and control groups becomes "cleaner" (namely, with more attempt to control for confouding variables). Of particular interest, there are serious concerns surrounding the effect of cocaine on brain development as may be evidenced by head circumference. Our analysis reveals that upon controlling for polydrug use, this effect disappears (mean ES = 0.17), hence may be attributed to other risk factors clustering in these women (alcohol drinking, cigarette smoking, polydrug use, etc.).

The adverse reproductive effects consistently associated with all comparisons, even after controlling for confounding factors, are genitourinary malformations. This and shorter gestational age may represent a direct effect of the drug on fetal vascularity with resultant vasoconstriction and damage to the genitourinary tract (Chasnoff et al., 1988). The latter may be a direct result of cocaine use, which is known to precipitate labor, and in fact is taken by some women to induce uterine contractions.

Importantly, several adverse effects commonly quoted to be associated with reproductive exposure to cocaine, such as abruptio placentae, cardiac malformations, and the sudden infant death syndrome fail to show by meta-analysis a significantly increased risk despite a large number of studies. This suggests that "positive" studies are quoted more than "negative" studies researching these endpoints. This bias against the null hypothesis was documented by us recently for acceptance, by a large scientific society, of abstracts dealing with reproductive risks of cocaine (Koren et al., 1989).

The failure of meta-analysis to find these associations may indicate that a larger sample size is needed with the possibility of a β error. Furthermore, not enough studies have addressed potential effects of cocaine on the central nervous system to derive a conclusion.

In summary, our analysis reveals very few adverse reproductive effects associated with pregnancy exposure to cocaine when compared to control groups of polydrug users. When the control groups consist of nondrug users, more adverse effects can be associated with cocaine use, indicating that a variety of adverse effects commonly quoted to be associated with cocaine may be caused by confounding factors.

Answer

At present only genitourinary malformations have been significantly associated with cocaine, although even this association is based on very few studies. You may wish to conduct an abdominal ultrasound examination to rule out clinically significant malformations. Head ultrasound testing may help in ruling out intracranial bleeding, described in several case reports to be associated with cocaine.

ACKNOWLEDGMENTS

This study was supported in part by a grant from Health and Welfare Canada, and The Motherisk research fund. KG is supported by Ontario Graduate Studies Scholarship. GK is a Career Scientist of Ontario Ministry of Health.

REFERENCES

Acker D, BP Sachs, KJ Tracey, WE Wise (1983). Abruptio placentae associated with cocaine use. Am J Obstet Gynecol 146(6):220–222.

Bateman DA, MC Heagarty (1989). Passive free-base cocaine ("crack") inhalation by infants and toddlers. AJDC 143:25–27.

Bauchner H, B Zuckerman, M McClain, D Frank, LE Fried, and H Kayne (1988). Risk of sudden infant death syndrome among infants with in utero exposure to cocaine. J Pediatr 113:831–834.

Becker BJ, LV Hedges (1984). Meta-analysis of cognitive gender differences: A comment on an analysis by Rosenthal and Rubin. J Educ Psychol 76:583–587.

Bingol N, M Fuchs, V Diaz, RK Stone, DS Gromisch (1987). Teratogenicity of cocaine in humans. J Pediatr 110:93–96.

Breslow NE, NE Day (1980). Statistical Methods in Cancer Research, Vol 1. The Analysis of Case Control Studies. IARC Scientific Publications No 32, Lyon, France: International Agency for Research on Cancer.

Chalmers TC, H Smith, B Blackburn, et al. (1981). A method for assessing the quality of a randomized control trial. Cont Clin Trials 2:31–49.

Chasnoff IJ, WJ Burns, SH Schnoll, KA Burns (1985). Cocaine use in pregnancy. N Engl J Med 313(11):666–669.

Chasnoff IJ, KA Burns, WJ Burns (1987). Cocaine use in pregnancy: Perinatal morbidity and mortality. Neurotoxicol Teratol 161(9):291–293.

Chasnoff IJ, ME Bussey R Savich, CM Stack (1986). Perinatal cerebral infarction and maternal cocaine use. J Pediatr 108(30):456–459.

Chasnoff IJ, GM Chisum, WE Kaplan (1988). Maternalc ocaine use and genitourinary tract malformation. Teratology 37:201–204.

Chasnoff IJ, Griffith DR, S MacGregor, K Dirkes, K Burns (1989a). Temporal patterns of cocaine use in pregnancy and perinatal outcome. JAMA 261(6):1741–1744.

Chasnoff IJ, CE Hunt, R Kletter, D Kaplan (1989b). Prenatal cocaine exposure is associated with respiratory pattern abnormalities. AJDC 143:583–587.

Chavez CJ, EM Ostrea, JC Stryker, RN Smialek (1979). Sudden infants death syndrome among infants of drug-dependent mothers. J Pediatr 95:407–409.

Chavez GF, J Mulinare, JF Cordero (1989). Maternal cocaine use during early pregnancy as a risk factor for congenital urogenital anomalies. JAMA 262:795–798.

Cherukuri R, H Minkoff, J Feldman, A Parekh, L Glass (1988). A cohort study of alkaloidal cocaine ("crack") in pregnancy. Obstet Gynecol 72(2):147–151.

Chouteau M, Brickner, P Namerow, P. Leppert (1988). The effects of cocaine abuse on birth weight and gestation age. Obstet Gynecol 72(3):351–354.

Chow MF, JJ Ambre, TI Ruo, AJ Atkinson, DJ Bowsher, MW Fischman (1985). Kinetics of cocaine disposition, elimination, and chronotropic effects. Clin Pharmacol Ther 38:318–324.

Cohen J (1977). Statistical Power Analysis for the Behavioral Sciences. Academic Press, Orlando, FL.

Collins E, RJ Hardwick, H Jeffrey (1989). Perinatal cocaine intoxication. Med J Aust 150:331–334.

Critchley HOD, SM Woods, AJ Barson, T Richardson, BA Lieberman (1988). Fetal death in utero and cocaine abuse. Case report. Br J Obstet Gynaecol 95:195–196.

Culver KW, AJ Ammann, JC Partridge, DF Wong, DW Wara, MJ Cowan (1987). Lymphocyte abnormalities in infants born to drug-abusing mothers. J Pediatr 111: 230–235.

Davidson, SL Ward, S Schuetz, V Krishna, X Bean, W Wingert, L Wachsman, T Keens (1986). Abnormal sleeping ventilatory pattern in infants of substance abusing mothers. AJDC 140:1015–1020.

Doberczak TM, S Shanzer, RT Senie, SR Kandall (1988). Neonatal neurologic and electroencephalographic effects of intrauterine cocaine exposure. J Pediatr 113: 354–358.

Einarson TR, JS Leeder, G Koren (1988). A method for meta-analysis of epidemiological studies. Drug Intelligence Clin Pharm 22:813–823.

Einarson TR, G Koren, D Mattice, O Schechter-Tsafriri (1990). Maternal spermicide use and adverse reproductive outcome: A meta-analysis. Am J Obstet Gynecol 162:655–660.

Feldman D, J Gagnon (1986). Abacus Concepts Inc. Brainpower Inc. Statview 512, Version 1.0.

Frank DA, B Zuckerman, H Amaro, K Aboagve, H Bauchner, H Cabral, L Fried, R Gingson, H Kayan, SM Levenson, S Parker, H Reece, R Vinci (1988). Cocaine use during pregnancy: Prevalence and correlates. Pediatrics 82:888–895.

Fulroth R, B Phillips, DJ Durand (1989). Perinatal outcome of infants exposed to cocaine and to heroin in utero. AJDC 143:905–910.

Gegeel RL, J McInerny, NAM Estes (1989). Transient neonatal ventricular tachycardia associated with maternal cocaine use. Am J Cardiol 63:383–384.

Gerbarg ZB, RI Horwitz (1988). Resolving conflict in clinical trials: Guidelines for meta-analysis. J Clin Epidemiol 41:503–509.

Glass GV (1976) Primary, secondary and meta-analysis of research. Educ Res 5:3–8.

Glass GV (1977). Integrating findings: The meta-analysis of research. Rev Res Educ 5:351–379.

Glass GV (1978). In defense of generalization. Behav Brain Sci 3:394–395.

Glass GV, B McGaw, ML Smith (1981). Meta-analysis in Social Research. Sage, Beverly Hills, CA.

Graham K, D Dimitrakoudis, E Pellegrini, G. Koren (1989a). Pregnancy outcome following first trimester exposure to cocaine in social users in Toronto, Canada. Vet Hum Toxicol 31:143–148.

Graham K, G Koren, J Klein, J Schneiderman, M Greenwald (1989b). Determination of gestational cocaine exposure by hair analysis. JAMA 262:3328-3330.

Hadeed AJ, SR Siegel (1989). Maternal cocaine use during pregnancy: Effect on the newborn infant. Pediatrics 84:205-210.

Henderson CE, M Torbey (1988). Rupture of intracranial aneurysm associated with cocaine use during pregnancy. Am J Perinatol 5(2):142-143.

Isenberg SJ, A Spierer, SH Inkelis (1987). Ocular signs of cocaine intoxication in neonates. Am J Ophthalmol 103:211-214.

Keith LG, S MacGregor, S Friedell, M Rosner, IJ Chasnoff, JJ Sciarra (1989). Substance abuse in pregnant women: Recent experience at the Perinatal Center for Chemical Dependence of Northwestern Memorial Hospital. Obstet Gynecol 73: 715-720.

Kleinbaum DG, LL Kupper, H Morgenstern (1982). Epidemiologic Research: Principles and Quantitative Methods. Van Nostrand Reinhold, New York, p 299.

Koren G, Y Feldman (1990). Motherisk, analysis of the first year of counseling women ond rug, chemical and radiation exposure in pregnancy. In: A Clinical Approach to Drug, Chemical, and Radiation Exposure in Pregnancy and Lactation. G Koren, ed. Marcel Dekker, New York.

Koren G, K Graham (1991). Characteristics of pregnant women using cocaine in pregnancy in Toronto. Can Med Assoc J (in press).

Koren G, K Graham, H Shear, T Einarson (1989). Bias against the null hypothesis: The reproductive hazards of cocaine. Lancet 1440-1442.

L'Abbe KA, AS Detsky, K O'Rourke (1987). Meta-analysis in clinical research. Ann Intern Med 107:224-233.

LeBlanc PE, AJ Parekh, B Naso, L Glass (1987). Effect of intrauterine exposure to alkaloidal cocaine ("crack"). Am J Dis Child 141:937-398.

Little BB, LM Snell, MK Palmore, LC Gilstrap (1988). Cocaine use in pregnant women in a large public hospital. Am J Perinatol 5:206-207.

Little BB, L Snell, VR Klein, LC Gilstrap (1989). Cocaine abuse during pregnancy: Maternal and fetal implications. Obstet Gynecol 73:157-160.

MacGregor SN, LG Keith, IJ Chasnoff, MA Rosner, RN Chisum, P Shaw, J Minogue (1987). Cocaine use during pregnancy: Adverse perinatal outcome. Am J Obstet Gynecol 157(3):686-690.

Madden JD, TF Payne, S Miller (1986). Maternal cocaine abuse and effect on the newborn. Pediatrics 77:209-211.

Mantel N, W Haenszel (1959). Statistical aspects of the analysis of data from retrospective studies of disease. J Natl Cancer Inst 22:719-748.

Mantel N, C Brown, DP Byar (1977). Tests for homogeneity of effect in epidemiologic investigation. Am J Epidemiol 106:125-129.

Meijer WS, PIM Schmitz, J Jeekel (1990). Meta-analysis of randomized, controlled trials of antibiotic prophylaxis in biliary tract surgery. Br J Surg 77:283-290.

Miettinen O (1976). Estimability and estimation in case referent studies. Am J Epidemiol 103:226-235.

Mitchell M, RE Sabbagha, L Keith, S MacGregor, JM Mota, J Minoque (1988). Ultrasonic growth parameters in fetuses of mothers with primary addiction to cocaine. Am J Obstet Gynecol 159:1104-1109.

Mittleman RE, JC Cofino, WL Hearn (1989). Tissue distribution of cocaine in a pregnant woman. J Forensic Sci 34:481–486.

Oro AS, SD Dixon (1987). Perinatal cocaine and methamphetamine exposure: Maternal and neonatal correlate. J Pediatr 111:571–578.

Osteroloh JD, BL Lee (1989). Urine drug screening in mothers and newborns. AJDC 143:791–793.

Ostrea E, M Brady, P Parks, D Asensio, A Naluz (1989). Drug screening of meconium in infants of drug-dependent mothers: An alternative to urine testing. J Pediatr 115:474–483.

Ried LD, DA McKenna, JR Horn (1989). Effect of therapeutic drug monitoring services on the number of serum drug assays ordered for patients: A meta-analysis. Ther Drug Monit 11:253–263.

Rosenthal R (1984). Meta-analytic Procedures for Social Research. Sage, Beverly Hills, CA.

Rosenthal R, D Rubin (1982). Comparing effect sizes of independent studies. Psychol Bull 92:500–504.

Ryan L, S Ehrlich, L Finnegan (1987). Cocaine abuse in pregnancy: Effects on the fetus and newborn. Neurotoxicol Teratol 9:295–299.

Sacks HS, J Berrier, D Reitman, VA Ancona-Berk, TC Chalmers (1987). Meta-analysis of randomized controlled trials. N Engl J Med 316:450–455.

Schwartz BR, JM Lage, BR Pober, SG Driscoll (1986). Isolated congenital renal tubular immaturity in siblings. Hum Pathol 17:1259–1263.

Shannon M, PG Lacouture, J Roa, A. Woolf (1989). Cocaine exposure among children seen at a pediatric hospital. Pediatrics 83:337–342.

Shih L, B Cone-Weston, B Reddix (1988). Effects of maternal cocaine abuse on the neonatal auditory system. Int J Pediatr Otorhinolaryngol 15:245–251.

Smart RG, EM Adlaf (1987). Alcohol and Other Drug Use Among Ontario Adults, 1977–1987. Alcoholism and Drug Addiction Research Foundation, Toronto, Ont., Canada, pp 33–37.

Telsey AM, A Merrit, SD Dixon (1988). Cocaine exposure in a term neonate. Necrotizing enterocolitis as a complication. Clin Pediatr 27:547–550.

Tenorio GM, N Mubartz, GH Bickers, RH Hubbrid (1988). Intrauterine stroke and maternal polydrug abuse. Clin Pediatr 27:565–567.

Teske MP, MT Trese (1987). Retinopathy of prematurity-like fundus and persistent hyperplastic primary vitreous associated with maternal cocaine use. Am J Ophthalmol 103:719–720.

Townsend RR, FC Laing, RB Jeffrey (1988). Placental abruption associated with cocaine abuse. AJR 150:1339–1340.

Trock B, E Lanza, P. Greenwald (1990). Dietary fiber, vegetables, and colon cancer: Critical review and meta-analysis of the epidemiologic evidence. J Natl Cancer Inst 82:650–661.

Walker AM, JM Martin-Moreno, FR Artalejo (1988). Odd man out: A graphical approach to meta-analysis. Am J Public Health 78:961–966.

Wang CH, SH Schnoll (1987). Prenatal cocaine use associated with down regulation of receptors in human placenta. Neurotoxicol Teratol 9:301–330.

Wolf FM (1986). Meta-analysis: Quantitative Methods for Research Synthesis. Sage, Beverly Hills, CA.

Zuckerman B, DA Frank, R Hingson, H Amaro, SM Levenson, H Kayne, S Parker, R Vinci, K Aboagye, LE Fried, H Cabral, R Timperi, H Bauchner (1989). Effects of maternal marijuana and cocaine use on fetal growth. N Engl J Med 320: 762–768.

17

Pregnancy Outcome and Infant Development Following Gestational Cocaine Use by Social Cocaine Users in Toronto, Canada

Karen Graham
McMaster University, Hamilton, Ontario, Canada

Annette Feigenbaum, Anne Pastuszak, Irena Nulman, Rosanna Weksberg, Thomas R. Einarson, Stan Ashby, and Gideon Koren
The Hospital for Sick Children, Toronto, Ontario, Canada

Susan Goldberg
The University of Toronto, Toronto, Ontario, Canada

Clinical Case

A young woman in her first trimester of pregnancy used three lines of cocaine weekly before finding out she was pregnant. She discontinued her use of cocaine at 10 weeks of pregnancy. She wants to continue her pregnancy if the teratogenic risk is not high.

INTRODUCTION

Recreational use of cocaine is increasing in Canada and the United States in all age and socioeconomic groups, with women aged 18–29 years showing the greatest rate of increase (1,2). Reports of the effects of cocaine on pregnancy outcome are becoming increasingly common. However, published studies have concentrated on populations of women who have used the drug

---

Reprinted with permission of Toronto University Press from Clin Invest Med 1992; 15:384–394.

Table 1   Comparison of Social Cocaine Users and Cocaine-Dependent Women

Social cocaine users	Cocaine-dependent women
Stop cocaine use when realize pregnant	Use cocaine throughout pregnancy (21)
Rarely use other hard drugs	Frequently use other hard drugs (18)
Generally have good prenatal care	Poor prenatal care (19)
Low incidence of sexually transmitted diseases	High incidence of sexually transmitted diseases (19,21)
Mixed socioeconomic status	Low socioeconomic status (18–21)

frequently throughout pregnancy and had a variety of other risk factors related to use of other drugs, poor prenatal care, and low socioeconomic status. It is evident that these drug-dependent women are the minority of cocaine users, with the vast majority of users consuming the drug less than once monthly (1). Knowledge obtained from studies of drug-dependent women cannot be directly extrapolated to the pregnancies of women who use cocaine occasionally in early pregnancy and generally have few other risk factors (Table 1). The reproductive risks of cocaine use among *social cocaine users* are unknown.

If cocaine causes embryonic damage during the first trimester similar to other classical teratogens, then even a brief exposure during early pregnancy may adversely affect the unborn baby. Conversely, if the effects of cocaine are cumulative and longer exposure is needed to interfere with fetal development, a brief first-trimester exposure to the drug, as is the usually case among women who use the drug before finding themselves pregnant, may not be detrimental. This prospective study was designed to compare outcome of pregnancy and infant well-being following cocaine exposure during early pregnancy by social cocaine users to that of two control groups.

METHODS

Subject Recruitment and Assessments

All women participating in this study were recruited from among those attending the Motherisk Program in Toronto, Canada, between November 1985 and February 1989. The program is an antenatal service that counsels pregnant women and their physicians about concerns related to drug, chemical, and radiation exposure during pregnancy and lactation. The following protocol was approved by The Hospital for Sick Children's Human Experimentation Review Committee.

Social cocaine users, who were selected from all pregnant women admitting to cocaine use in early pregnancy, were defined as women who were not chemically dependent and stopped cocaine use soon after the discovery of pregnancy. Subjects were excluded if cocaine exposure occurred only before conception or continued after the Motherisk Clinic visit despite our recommendation to cease this drug use, or if there were other exposures or medical conditions thought to increase the risk for adverse outcome.

Two control groups were chosen prospectively from among women attending the Motherisk Clinic during the study period and followed in a similar manner to the social cocaine users. One group consisted of women admitting the use during pregnancy of cannabis but not cocaine. This *cannabis user* control group was deemed necessary because many of the social cocaine users admitted using cannabis as well. Subjects were excluded if cannabis exposure occurred only before conception, or if medical conditions or additional exposures placed a given pregnancy at increased risk for adverse outcome. The second control group consisted of women who came to the clinic for exposures to compounds and environmental agents believed to be safe during pregnancy (e.g., oral penicillins, video display terminals, acetaminophen), and reported no exposure to cocaine, cannabis, or other illicit recreational drugs. Subjects were excluded from this *recreational drug-free control group* if they had medical conditions or additional exposures that placed the pregnancy at increased risk for adverse outcome. This group was matched to the social cocaine user group for maternal factors thought to influence pregnancy outcome or infant development, including marital status, cigarette and alcohol consumption, obstetric history, and ethnic background.

Assessment of pregnancy course and infant development was conducted at three time points. During the initial interview in the Motherisk Clinic, early in pregnancy, a detailed history of known reproductive hazards was obtained from each woman, including medical, obstetric, and genetic background, as well as a history of drug, chemical, and radiation exposure. The amount(s) of drug(s) used and the time period of exposure(s) were recorded based on the patient's report. No urinalysis for cocaine or other drugs was routinely performed because these women voluntarily approached the clinic to inquire about their reproductive risks following cocaine exposure during early gestation. Second, by the time of the clinic appointment 1–2 weeks after discontinuing cocaine, urine is not likely to be positive, as verified by us in several cases. Details concerning time of exposure are critical for determining the temporal relation to conception; therefore, in addition to requesting details on last menstrual period, we performed an ultrasound examination if there were doubts about the gestational age. In addition, the women provided personal data about themselves and the father of the baby. Socioeconomic status was estimated using the occupational status titles and the scales of Blishen and Carroll for females (3) and of Blishen and McRoberts for males (4).

Six to ten months after the expected date of confinement, the women were contacted and administered a standard telephone questionnaire. The course of pregnancy, labor and delivery, perinatal period, and the health and development of the infant were assessed. Developmental milestones were recorded and compared with the screening norms of the Denver Developmental Screening Test to identify any areas of developmental delay (5). The interviewer was not blinded to the gestational exposure of the subjects at this time, since follow-up stems from the initial intake form, filled out during the initial visit to the Motherisk Clinic. Obstetric and pediatric records were obtained from appropriate medical centers, and additional medical information was obtained for birth weight, head circumference, gestational age, Apgar scores, and perinatal complications.

At approximately 18 months of age, infant developmental status was assessed during a visit of the mother and infant to the Motherisk Clinic, using the Bayley Scales of Infant Development (BSID) mental and psychomotor scales (MDI and PDI) (6) and the Vineland Adaptive Behavior Scales (7). At this visit, the interviewer was blinded to the in utero exposure of the child. Current marital status, occupations, and education levels of the prospective parents were obtained. Maternal IQ was assessed by the Raven's Standard Progressive Matrices, a language and culturally independent test (8).

During this visit, a detailed physical examination of the infant was performed by one of two clinical geneticists, each of whom was blinded to the in utero exposure. Measurements of current weight were recorded and plotted on standard Tanner-Whitehouse charts (9). In addition, a general physical examination was performed to document any minor or major malformations. Family history and previous medical and surgical history were taken. Where possible, this history was verified by requesting records from the child's primary care physician.

Statistical Analysis

Comparisons of continuous variables between the cocaine, cannabis, and recreational drug-free groups were performed using one-way analysis of variance (ANOVA). The Scheffe F test was used to identify differences between subsets.

Noncontinuous variables measured at nominal level were compared individually using the chi-square test and those in a ranked order by Kruskal-Wallis one-way ANOVA followed by a Mann-Whitney U test when post-hoc analysis was required. Least-squares regression analysis was performed to investigate correlations between variables.

Sample Size

The primary end point in this study is the score of the Bayley Scales of Infant Development, which has a coefficient of variation (CV) between 10 and 15%. If one considers a large effect size (≥ 0.8 SD) to be clinically significant, then between 25 and 54 patients in each group would be required (the smaller number corresponds to 10% and the larger to 15%) (10). Substantially larger numbers would be required to reject the null hypothesis if medium or small effect sizes are considered to be clinically relevant. Because upon starting the study it was evident that between 20 and 30 babies exposed to cocaine would have completed the study within 3 years, and because there were no previous studies on developmental effects of cocaine in social users, we decided to study all available children and subsequently to perform a power analysis to address the possibility of a Type II error (see Results).

RESULTS

Maternal Demographic Characteristics

Six percent ($n = 51$) of all women attending the Motherisk Clinic during the study period reported use of cocaine during or just prior to pregnancy. Fifty-one of them (89%) met our criteria for social cocaine users. Of these, nine relocated and were lost to follow-up, four had elective abortions, three refused to participate, two had spontaneous abortions, two were exposed to cocaine only before conception, and one infant was too young for follow-up. Hence the study group consisted of 30 social cocaine users who completed all assessments (Table 2).

Table 2 Subject Exclusion in the Social Cocaine Users Group

Number of subjects	Description
51	Social cocaine users attending the Motherisk Program
−9	Subject relocated and not found
−4	Elective abortion
−3	Refused to participate in follow-up
−2	Spontaneous abortion
−2	Preconception cocaine exposure only
−1	Infant too young for complete assessment
30	= Number of social cocaine users with complete assessment

All subjects reported stopping cocaine use before coming to the Motherisk Clinic, soon after discovering that they were pregnant. Eighty-seven percent ($n = 26$) of the subjects used less than a total of 10 g of cocaine during early pregnancy; only four women used more than 10 g. Most women snorted cocaine as the sole route of drug intake ($n = 24$); intravenous cocaine use ($n = 4$) and smoking crack ($n = 3$) were less common.

Cannabis use was common among social cocaine users, occurring in 50% ($n = 15$) of the cases. All women reported stopping cannabis use upon realizing that they were pregnant. Use of other psychoactive drugs, which occurred only to a small extent, included sedatives ($n = 2$), opioids ($n = 2$), lysergic acid diethylamide (LSD) ($n = 1$), amphetamines ($n = 1$), and psilocybin ($n = 1$). These drugs were used infrequently and were discontinued upon realization of pregnancy.

Eight percent ($n = 69$) of the women attending the Motherisk Clinic reported use of cannabis just prior to and/or during pregnancy. Fifty-one of these women reported no cocaine use and were considered for inclusion in the cannabinoid control group. After 31 cases had been excluded for a variety of reasons, 20 cases were assessed completely (Table 3). Other drug use was uncommon among subjects in this group, with only four women reporting use of LSD.

The second control group was comprised of 30 women reporting no exposure to any illicit drug during pregnancy. Upon starting the study it was apparent that the social cocaine users and cannabinoid users had very high rates of single motherhood. Therefore, we matched the drug-free control

Table 3   Subject Exclusion in the Cannabinoid Control Group

Number of subjects	Description
69	Cannabis users attending the Motherisk Program
− 18	Used cocaine as well
− 6	Preconception exposure only
− 6	Subject relocated and not found
− 6	Elective abortion
− 5	Spontaneous abortion
− 3	Not pregnant at the time of Motherisk Clinic visit
− 2	Exposure to known teratogens (phenytoin, isotretinoin)
− 2	Refused to participate in follow-up
− 1	Infant too young for complete assessment
20 =	Number of cannabis users (cocaine-free) with complete assessment

Table 4 Comparison of Maternal and Paternal Characteristics Between Groups

| Demographic variables | Groups[a] | | | |
	Social cocaine (n = 30)	Cannabis (n = 20)	Drug-free (n = 30)	p-value
Age, years (mean ± SD)	26.6 ± 5.5	26.3 ± 5.4	29.3 ± 4.8	0.06*
Single at first Motherisk visit, %	70.4	45	31	0.10**
Single at BSID, %	55	33.3	20	0.14**
Ethnic background, %				
Caucasian	100	100	78.9	0.73**
Black	0	0	10.5	0.10**
Oriental	0	0	10.5	0.10**
Gravidity	1.6 ± 1	1.9 ± 0.9	2 ± 1.2	0.39*
Parity	0.2 ± 0.5	0.6 ± 0.8	0.5 ± 0.7	0.14*
Elective abortion	0.3 ± 0.7	0.3 ± 0.6	0.2 ± 0.5	0.80*
Spontaneous abortion	0.1 ± 0.3	0	0.3 ± 0.7	0.12*
SES, female, %				>0.05***
student, housewife, unemployed	20	25	31	
unskilled	50	30	3.5	
skilled	26.7	35	31	
professionals	3.3	10	34.5	
SES, male, %	A	A	B	<0.005***
student, unemployed	7.4	20	3.3	
unskilled	48.1	20	20	
skilled	40.7	40	33.3	
professionals	3.7	20	43.3	
Years of school				
female	12.9 ± 2.3	10.4 ± 4.4	15.1 ± 2.9	0.004[b]
male	12.7 ± 1.6	12.8 ± 2	15.1 ± 2.6	0.004[c]
Maternal IQ[d]	109.1 ± 12.4	109.1 ± 25.2	114.1 ± 11.7	0.24*
Alcohol use (%)	A	A	B	<0.025***
No use	14.3	25	33.3	
< 1 drink/day	46.4	50	60	
1–2 drinks/day	21.4	20	0	
> 2 drinks/day	10.7	5	6.7	
> 5 drinks/day (binge)	7.1	0	0	
Cigarette use[e]	A	A	B	<0.005***
No use	17.2	35	73.3	
< 1/2 ppd	24.1	25	3.3	
1/2 to 1 ppd	55.2	40	23.3	
> 1 ppd	3.4	0	0	

*ANOVA and post-hoc Scheffe F test if ANOVA significant at $p < 0.05$.
**Chi-square, significant at $p < 0.05$.
***Kruskal-Wallis (KW) test and post-hoc Mann-Whitney U test if KW is significant at $p < 0.05$.
[a]Groups with different letters are significant at $p < 0.05$ (i.e., A and A, B and B are nonsignificant and represent different populations).
[b]Cannabis and control group values differ at $p < 0.05$.
[c]Social cannabis users and drug-free group values differ and cannabis and drug-free group values differ at $p < 0.05$.
[d]One father in each group performed the Raven IQ test.
[e]ppd = package per day.

group according to this parameter, in addition to age, gravidity, parity, and amount of alcohol and cigarettes consumed.

The women of the three groups were similar in age, in marital status during pregnancy and at infant developmental testing, in obstetric history, and in ethnicity (Table 4). However, the social cocaine users used significantly more alcohol and cigarettes than the women of the recreational drug-free control group.

The women were of similar socioeconomic status (SES), and at least 20% in each group either stayed at home with their children or attended school. The cocaine-using women had significantly fewer years of formal education than drug-free controls, although they were of similar IQ. Comparison of demographics of cohabitating male partners, who occasionally were not the fathers of the study infants, shows that these spouses of cocaine users were of significantly lower SES than those of the two control groups and had significantly fewer years of formal schooling than the spouses of the drug-free women.

Pregnancy Outcome

Table 5 presents pregnancy outcome variables for the three groups studied. There were no significant differences in mean pregnancy weight gain, in-

Table 5 Comparison of Obstetrical and Neonatal Information

Obstetric and neonatal variables	Groups			
	Social cocaine ($n = 30$)	Cannabis ($n = 20$)	Drug-free ($n = 30$)	p-value
Pregnancy weight gain, kg	17.3 ± 7.6	16.4 ± 5.5	15.9 ± 5.6	0.73[a]
Emergency cesarean section, %	6.9	0	7.1	0.49[b]
Forceps delivery, %	10.7	21	10.7	0.56[b]
Meconium staining, %	12	15.4	17.6	0.89[b]
Gestational age, weeks	39.4 ± 3.3	39.6 ± 1.5	39.5 ± 3.3	0.97[a]
Premature delivery (< 37 wk), %	6.7	0	6.7	0.51[b]
Birth weight, g	3294.6 ± 677.6	3523.4 ± 377.8	3407.7 ± 703.4	0.45[a]
Low birth weight (< 2500 g), %	10	0	10.3	0.4[b]
Apgar score				
at 1 minute	7.9 ± 1.3	8.5 ± 0.6	7.9 ± 1.9	0.38[a]
at 5 minutes	8.6 ± 1.3	9.1 ± 0.2	8.9 ± 1	0.36[a]

[a]ANOVA.
[b]Chi-square.

cidence of emergency cesarean sections or forceps- or vacuum-assisted delivery, or meconium staining of the amnoitic fluid between the three groups. Similarly, there were no significant differences in gestational age at delivery or birth weight, or in incidences of prematurity or low birth weight. Apgar scores at 1 and 5 minutes were not significantly different between the groups.

Three of the four cocaine users who used more than 10 g of cocaine delivered two premature infants and one normal gestational age infant, each weighing less than 2500 g. Apgar scores for the four infants in this subgroup were 7 and 7, and 7 and 9 for the two premature infants, and 4 and 7, and 6 and 4 after an elective and emergency cesarean section for the third and fourth, respectively.

Developmental Assessment

Developmental milestones of the offspring of the social cocaine users were similar to those of offspring of cannabis users and recreational drug-free subjects (Table 6). In general, most children met all milestones within the normal range of time, as described by the Denver Developmental Screening Test (DDST) norms (5). Seven of 30 children of social cocaine users, eight

Table 6 Developmental Assessment Comparisons

Developmental assessment	Groups			
	Social cocaine ($n = 30$)	Cannabis ($n = 20$)	Drug-free ($n = 30$)	p-value[b]
Milestones, mean months ± SD[a]				
1st smiled (0–2 months)	1.2 ± 0.6	1.2 ± 0.4	1.4 ± 0.8	0.47
1st lifted head (0–3 months)	1.5 ± 0.8	1.8 ± 1.2	2.2 ± 1.3	0.13
1st sat unaided (4.5–7.5 months)	5.9 ± 1.3	6 ± 1.0	6 ± 1.2	0.97
1st crawled (6–8.5 months)	7 ± 1.8	7 ± 1.6	7.2 ± 1.5	0.80
1st stood unaided (9–13 months)	9.7 ± 1.7	8.2 ± 2.1	9.2 ± 1.8	0.06
1st walked unaided (11–14 months)	11.7 ± 1.8	11.4 ± 2.8	11.9 ± 2.1	0.78
1st work spoken (8.5–13.5)	9.3 ± 2.3	11.5 ± 4.4	10.9 ± 2.7	0.07
BSID, MDI (mean ± SD)	110.1 ± 13.8	111.6 ± 17.6	109.0 ± 16.5	0.86
BSID, PDI (mean ± SD)	100.1 ± 20.8	106.4 ± 16.3	103.8 ± 12.4	0.42
Vineland (mean ± SD)	98.4 ± 10.9	96 ± 7.7	96.7 ± 9.4	0.65
Infant age at testing, months	20.2 ± 4.2	19.2 ± 2.4	19.8 ± 3.0	0.56

[a]Range given for each milestone is DDST range of normal values from 25th percentile to 95th percentile.
[b]ANOVA.

of 20 of the cannabis group, and eleven of 30 of the drug-free control group showed delay in attaining one milestone, being 2 or more standard deviations below normal, as determined during the standardization of the DDST. Three infants exposed to cocaine, three infants exposed to cannabis, and five drug-free infants were delayed in reaching two milestones.

A comparison of infant development shows similar, and numerically almost identical, scores achieved on the mental and motor scales of the Bayley Scales of Infant Development and on the Vineland Adaptive Behavior Scales. The four infants of mothers using more than 10 g of cocaine attained normal developmental scores. In the three groups, the age at which developmental testing was performed was similar (Table 6). There was a weak correlation between maternal IQ and infant scores on the Bayley Scales Mental Development Index ($r = 0.22$, $p = 0.06$, Fig. 1).

Power analysis reveals that it would take thousands of cases to verify whether the 1–3 point differences in BSID scores reflect a true but marginal effect size. Such an endeavor cannot be undertaken; moreover, such a small difference in scores is within the margin of error of the test and is not believed to be clinically significant.

Physical assessment at 1.5 years revealed no differences in numbers of malformations among the three groups (Table 7). Several children in each group had minor malformations such as epicanthic folds or relative hypertelorism, but no other physical abnormalities. Review of growth parameters found no group having significant growth retardation. Four infants in the

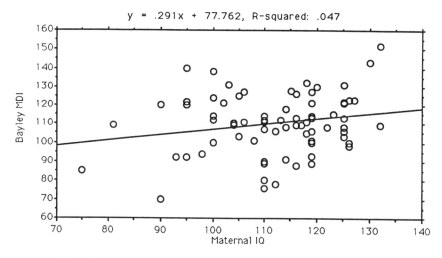

Figure 1 Influence of maternal IQ (Raven) on infant MDI scores for all 80 mother-infant pairs.

Table 7 Infant Abnormalities by Study Group

Study group		Abnormalities documented on examination or from history
Cocaine (*n* = 30)	1	Isolated unilateral 4th–5th finger syndactyly
	1	Ventral septal defect
	1	Functional ejection systolic murmur (ESM)
	1	Intrauterine growth retardation, bilateral hydroceles, phimosis
	1	Prematurity with patent ductus arteriosus
	1	Failure to thrive
Cannabis	1	Intussusception
(*n* = 18)	2	Functional ESM
Drug-free	1	Intrauterine growth retardation, premature thelarche
(*n* = 29)	1	Inguinal hernia (repair)
	1	Dislocated hip
	1	Brachycephaly, speech delay, fine motor incoordination
	1	Nonparalytic strabismus
	2	Small umbilical hernia
	2	Congenital torticollis
	5	Functional ESM

cocaine group, two in the cannabis group, and one in the recreational-drug-free control group were not seen by the geneticists as a result of scheduling difficulties.

Comparison of the children's facial features, both at the follow-up visit and thereafter with the aid of photographs, did not reveal any characteristic or significant dysmorphic features in the cocaine group. In addition, there was no clinical evidence of fetal alcohol syndrome in any infant. Only one child in the cocaine group had mild abnormalities of the external genitourinary system (Table 7). There was no evidence in any child of a vascular disruption event. However, in the absence of any associated alterations in finger size or formation, the case of syndactyly present in one child in the cocaine group could be classified as a vascular disruption.

DISCUSSION

Cocaine use by pregnant women has become a major health issue. To date all reports of effects of cocaine use in pregnancy have dealt with women who use large amounts of cocaine, often throughout pregnancy. These women commonly use other drugs and have poor prenatal care and nutrition, thus making it difficult to determine the independent effect of cocaine on their offspring. It is important to study social cocaine users who stop cocaine use early in pregnancy, because they more closely represent the majority of the cocaine-using population than do cocaine-dependent women. In Ontario, Canada, only 5% of those admitting long-term cocaine use report consuming the drug more than once per month (1). Thus, if social cocaine users expose their fetuses to the drug during embryogenesis, apparent adverse effects consequent to first-trimester cocaine use would suggest that cocaine has embryopathic potential.

It is imperative that the risk of early cocaine exposure in pregnancy be determined so that proper, nonbiased counseling of women can be provided. It is our experience at the Motherisk Program in Toronto that without such information, pregnant social cocaine users often consider termination of pregnancy after extrapolation of information obtained from studies of cocaine-dependent women. The pregnant social cocaine user may learn about the adverse effects of cocaine on pregnancy from the lay media. Newspaper and magazine articles often make such unsubstantiated statements as "a single cocaine hit during pregnancy can cause lasting fetal damage" (11). The tendency to terminate pregnancy based on fear of unknown teratogenic risk was made evident following the Chernobyl radiation incident of 1985. It was estimated that 2500 otherwise wanted pregnancies were terminated in Greece and 100,000–200,000 in all of western Europe, because of scientifically unjustified fear of radiation teratogenicity. At the time, doctors could not allay fears because of lack of data on the degree of exposure and, therefore, on the real teratogenic risk (12).

At Motherisk we rely on self-reporting of exposure to drugs and medications to determine the degree and timing of exposure. It is our experience that these women, who come to the clinic voluntarily and generally before 13 weeks of pregnancy, provide information honestly and to the best of their ability. Temporally then, their report is unlikely to be affected by recall bias. In selected cases, self-reporting was checked against hair accumulation of cocaine with very good correlation (13).

A recognized problem when interviewing female cocaine users is that they often do not have detailed knowledge of the purity of cocaine they used. Based on seized drugs in Toronto in 1987, the Health Protection Branch of Health and Welfare Canada reported that cocaine in Toronto is over 90% pure (14).

An important factor to consider when interpreting our results is that all women themselves requested the clinic visit because of anxiety about their drug use during pregnancy, and all agreed to participate in our follow-up program. In addition, we were able to locate these women over a 2-year period, which reflects a measure of stability in their lives. Therefore, these social cocaine users are a self-selected subset of the population who may be in a better position to provide stable home environments for their infants than the social cocaine users who did not come to our clinic or were lost to follow-up. A child's home environment can influence mental and motor development and performance on standardized developmental tests (15).

Because of the clinical nature of our program, this study could not be blinded during either the initial clinic interview or the telephone follow-up interview. We do not believe that this circumstance has led to any significant bias on the part of the interviewers, since the information collected during these interviews was mainly factual (age, marital status, number of previous pregnancies, drug use, neonatal information, etc.), leaving little room for interpretation. In addition, we verified the women's reports by obtaining the medical records of the deliveries and for the offspring.

The ethnic distribution and ages of women of our three study groups is representative of the distribution of pregnant women attending the Motherisk Program, where 93% were white and the mean age was 29.9 years (16). The social cocaine users in our study are of mixed SES, making this population different from the predominantly lower SES cocaine-dependent women previously studied (17–20). The women studied previously have additional risk factors, including use of other illicit drugs, increased rate of sexually transmitted diseases, and poor prenatal care, which may place the pregnancy at increased risk for complications. All women in our study received good medical care; most came to the Motherisk Clinic in early pregnancy, regularly visited a family doctor, and experienced satisfactory pregnancy weight gain.

The 54% use of cannabis by the social cocaine users in our study is much higher than the 15% prevalence reported for females 18–29, and the 6% incidence reported for those 30–49 years on Ontario (1). This high cannabinoid use among cocaine users has been well described, as cannabinoids "smoothen" some of the undesirable effects of cocaine (20). Alcohol use was also greater among our population of social cocaine users than that reported among Ontario females aged 18–29 or 30–49 years (1) and significantly greater than among the two control groups in this study. Similarly, cigarette use was greater than among the recreational-drug-free control subjects, making it impossible to match for these criteria. These additional drug exposures may potentially affect pregnancy outcome and fetal growth and development, hence are possible confounding variables. However, none of the women consumed alcohol in the teratogenic range (> 2 drinks per day) for more than one week, and almost all stopped their cigarette use during the first trimester before effects on fetal growth are believed to occur. In addition, the cocaine group had fewer maternal and paternal years of schooling and lower parental SES; again, these demographic characteristics may potentially affect an infant's ability to perform during developmental testing.

That the outcome of infants of the social cocaine users was identical to the control infants ruled out major effects of first-trimester cocaine exposure. No differences were found in attainment of developmental milestones or mental and motor functioning as assessed by the Bayley Scales of Infant Development. This test is the most widely used screening tool for cognitive development during the preschool years and has been used to document the teratogenic effects of lead, alcohol, and methadone (21–23). However, longer follow-up is needed to rule out other potential behavioral effects, which cannot be assessed at 1.5 years of life. Children exposed to cocaine in utero were not different from the control groups in incidence of obstetric complications or neonatal adverse effects. However, our sample size was calculated to address the primary end point (the Bayley Scale) and is not sufficient to address differences in obstetric or neonatal complications.

Studies assessing development of infants exposed to cocaine have thus far dealt exclusively with the offspring of drug-dependent women. In one study, children exposed throughout pregnancy to a variety of psychoactive drugs including cocaine scored significantly lower than controls on the Bayley Scales PDI at 3 months and MDI at 6 months, but were within normal limits on both scales by 24 months of age (24). The number of children exposed to cocaine alone or with other drugs was not specified, and the mean scores were not provided. A preliminary report of another study noted that six cocaine-exposed infants tested at 6 months of age had Bayley Scales of Infant Development scores similar to matched controls reporting no drug use (25). The very small sample sizes of both these studies limit the validity of this information.

Only one study has investigated cocaine use occurring in the first trimester of pregnancy. Chasnoff and coworkers compared outcome of pregnancy of 23 women using cocaine only in the first trimester to women using it throughout pregnancy, and to women not using cocaine, cannabis, or alcohol during pregnancy (19). First-trimester cocaine use was associated with an increased rate of abruptio placentae, genitourinary malformations, and neonatal behavioral impairment as compared to the drug-free control group. However, no long-term neurobehavioral assessment was reported on these patients, who were recruited from a drug rehabilitation center and appear to be very different from our social cocaine users.

In summary, in a first study that follows cocaine-exposed infants of social cocaine users into their second year of life, the outcome of pregnancy appears to be within normal limits and identical to two control groups followed prospectively in a similar manner. That the cocaine-exposed infants had normal attainment of milestones and normal scores on their developmental assessment at 1.5 years of age suggests normal brain development. While all women should be encouraged to discontinue cocaine use during gestation, our data indicate that there is no evidence to support women's fears that brief exposure to the drug in early pregnancy warrants termination of pregnancy.

Answer

Our study indicates that babies whose mothers use cocaine have a likelihood of achieving cognitive function comparable to the normal population. It will be important to rule out excessive drinking and smoking, which are commonly combined with cocaine use.

ACKNOWLEDGMENT

This work was supported by a grant from Health and Welfare Canada.

REFERENCES

1. Smart RG, Adlaf EM. Alcohol and Other Drug Use Among Ontario Adults, 1977–1987. Alcoholism and Drug Addiction Research Foundation, Toronto, Ontario, Canada, 1987, pp 33–37.
2. Abelson HK, Miller JP. A decade of trends in cocaine use in the household population. NIDA Research Monograph Series 61. Washington, DC, Government Printing Office, 1985, pp 35–49.
3. Blishen B, Carroll WK. Sex differences in a socioeconomic index for occupations in Canada. Can Rev Sociol Anthopol 1978; 15:352–371.
4. Blishen B, McRoberts H. A revised socioeconomic index for occupations in Canada. Can Rev Sociol Anthropol 1976; 13:71–79.
5. Frankenburg WK, Dodd JB, Fandal A. The Revised Denver Developmental Screening Test Manual. Denver, University of Colorado Press, 1970.
6. Bayley N. Bayley Scales of Infant Development. Psychological Corporation, New York, 1969.
7. Sparrow SS, Balla DA, Cicchetti DV. Vineland Adaptive Behavior Scales. American Guidance Service, Minneapolis, MN, 1984.
8. Raven JC. Standard Progressive Matrices. London, HK Lewis, 1960.
9. Tanner JM, Whitehouse RH, Takaishik M. Standards from birth to maturity for height, weight, height velocity and weight velocity. Arch Dis Child 1966; 41:613–635.
10. Snedecor GW, Cockran WG. Statistical Methods, 7th ed. Iowa State University Press, Ames, 1980.
11. Globe & Mail, Toronto, Ontario, Canada. Babies injured for life by cocaine, study says. September 6, 1988.
12. Trichopoulos D, Zavitsanos X, Koutis C, Drogari P, Proukakis C, Petridou E, et al. The victims of Chernobyl in Greece: Induced abortions after the accident. Br Med J 1987; 295:1100.
13. Forman R, Klein J, Graham K, Greenwald M, Koren G. Cocaine accumulation in maternal and fetal hair: Dose-response characteristics. Life Sci (in press).
14. Health Protection Branch, Ottawa, Canada, 1987 (unpublished).
15. Werner EE, Honzik MP, Smith RS. Prediction of intelligence and achievement at ten years from twenty months pediatric and psychological examinations. Child Dev 1968; 39:1063–1075.

16. Koren G, Feldman Y, MacLeod SM. Motherisk II: The first year of counseling on drug, chemical, and radiation exposure in pregnancy. In Maternal-Fetal Toxicology. A Clinician's Guide, 1st ed. (Koren G, ed). Marcel Dekker, New York, 1990, pp 383–402.

17. MacGregor SN, Keith LG, Chasnoff IJ, Rosner MA, Chisum GM, Shaw P, Minogue JP. Cocaine use during pregnancy: Adverse perinatal outcome. Am J Obstet Gynecol 1987; 157:686–690.

18. Doberczak TM, Shanzer S, Senie RT, Kandall SR. Neonatal neurologic and electroencephalographic effects of intrauterine cocaine exposure. J Pediatr 1988; 113:354–358.

19. Chasnoff IJ, Griffith DR, MacGregor S, Dirkes K, Burnes KA. Temporal patterns of cocaine use in pregnancy: Pregnancy outcome. JAMA 1989; 261:1741–1744.

20. Chasnoff IJ, Lewis DE, Griffith DR, Willey S. Cocaine and pregnancy: Clinical and toxicological implications for the neonate. Clin Chem 1989; 35:1276–1278.

21. Bellinger D, Leviton A, Waternaux C, Needleman H, Rabinowitz M. Longitudinal analysis of prenatal and postnatal lead exposure and early cognitive development. N Engl J Med 19878; 316:1037–1043.

22. O'Connor MF, Brill NF, Sigman M. Alcohol use in primiparous women older than 30 years of age: Relation to infant development. Pediatrics 1986; 78:444–450.

23. Rosen T, Johnson HL. Children of methadone-maintained mothers: Follow-up to 18 months of age. J Pediatr 1982; 101:192–196.

24. Chasnoff IJ, Schnoll SH. Consequences of cocaine and other drug use in pregnancy. In Cocaine: A Clinician's Handbook (Washton AM, Gold MS, eds). Guildford Press, New York, 1987, pp 241–251.

25. Eyler FD, Behnke M, Stewart NJ, Bucciarelli RL. Incidence and effects of cocaine use: Perinatal center experience. Pediatr Res 1988; 22:1468.

18

Biological Markers of Intrauterine Exposure to Cocaine and Cigarette Smoking

Gideon Koren, Julia Klein, Rachel Forman, and My-Khanh Phan
The Hospital for Sick Children, Toronto, Ontario, Canada

Karen Graham
McMaster University, Hamilton, Ontario, Canada

Clinical Case

You suspect that a 4-day-old, 30 weeks gestation baby, with grade III intracranial bleeding, was exposed in utero to cocaine. The mother denies having used this drug, and the baby's urine is negative. How would you proceed?

INTRODUCTION

Almost all xenobiotics circulating in the maternal blood are capable of crossing to the fetus. Thirty years after the thalidomide disaster, only about thirty human teratogens have been identified, whereas a large number of compounds have not been documented to impose fetal risk when used as recommended (1). Even the most potent human teratogens, such as retinoids and thalidomide, adversely affect only some fetuses while sparing many others. This variability in response may stem from pharmacokinetic and/or pharmacodynamic differences.

For most animal and human teratogens dose-response curves can be documented, highlighting the importance of extent of fetal exposure to these

Reprinted with permission of Karger Ltd., Basel, from Dev Pharmacol Ther 1993; 18:228–238.

compounds. However, in recognizing the extent of variability existing in systemic exposure to xenobiotics in adults (in terms of the area under the curve), one can imagine how much larger is the variability of fetal exposure to the same maternal dose by adding known interpatient differences in placental transport and fetal pharmacokinetics.

Consequently, any attempt to explain variability in fetal susceptibility to xenobiotics and their metabolites must incorporate a meaningful measurement of fetal exposure. The most widely used tool for estimation of fetal exposure is measurement of concentrations in umbilical blood in an effort to extrapolate to intrauterine events. However, this can be a useful tool only if the mother has continued her drug consumption, and when the elimination $t_{1/2}$ of the compound in question is long enough. For example, measurement of umbilical carboxyhemoglobin (COHb) may reflect degree of fetal exposure to carbon monoxide. However, the elimination $t_{1/2}$ of CO is around 5 h in maternal serum and 2–3 times longer in the fetal circulation. Hence, if the mother has not smoked during the 10–15 h of the delivery, the baby may have undetectable levels of COHb despite clinically significant exposure throughout pregnancy. The case of cocaine is even more problematic, because the elimination $t_{1/2}$ of this compound is substantially shorter.

In a search for biological markers for fetal exposure to xenobiotics, we have developed during the last few years hair tests for cocaine and its metabolite benzoylecgonine as well as for nicotine and its metabolite cotinine. In this review we wish to describe the rationale for this new approach, some of its technical aspects and, finally, its clinical relevance.

GESTATIONAL COCAINE USE

Recently there has been an increasing use of cocaine in North America (2). In a variety of American inner cities the prevalence of cocaine use among young women has been estimated as high as 40% (3). The potential effects of cocaine on the fetus have raised serious concerns about the short- and long-term health of millions of children exposed in utero to the drug.

To date, the role of cocaine in causing fetal pathology has not been established despite scores of studies comparing such babies to controls (4–14). Because cocaine users tend to be of lower socioeconomic status, maintain poorer prenatal care, and use other recreational drugs, alcohol, and cigarettes, it is almost impossible at present to verify whether cocaine is causing adverse health effects or is only associated with them (4).

One of the main methodological problems in many of the studies addressing fetal effects of cocaine is in the ways cocaine use is ascertained. There is evidence that maternal reports are unreliable (15); similarly blood and urine tests are not sufficiently reliable due to the very short elimination half-life of cocaine.

CIGARETTE SMOKING IN PREGNANCY

Cigarette smoking during gestation is associated with increased risks for low birth weight, prematurity, spontaneous abortions, perinatal mortality, and the sudden infant death syndrome (16–20). Moreover, during the last decade evidence has been accumulated for long-term neurotoxicity affecting neurobehavioral development (21). Fetal concentrations of carboxyhemoglobin are generally higher than maternal levels due to higher affinity of fetal hemoglobin to carbon monoxide (22). Carbon monoxide decreases the amount of oxygen carried to cells but also affects intracellular processes by impairing cytochrome enzymes. In addition to carbon monoxide, other toxins are elicited by cigarette smoke, including nicotine, hydrogen cyanide, and benzopyrene.

HAIR AND MECONIUM AS BIOLOGICAL MARKERS FOR FETAL EXPOSURE

During the last few years the use of hair (23) and meconium (24) has emerged as much more reliable due to the long-term accumulation of cocaine and its major metabolite benzoylecgonine (BZ). While meconium is available only during the first day of life, neonatal hair carries such information until it sheds at 3–4 months of age.

Because neonatal hair grows during the last 3–4 months of pregnancy, measuring cocaine in neonatal hair reflects cocaine use by women who were aware of their pregnancy at the time of drug use. This information is of importance because in our experience many young women who counsel Motherisk in Toronto after they had used cocaine recreationally (and not as part of an addiction pattern) discontinue their habit once pregnancy is detected. Hence, accumulation of cocaine in neonatal hair may detect infants at high risk of being cared for by addicted mothers. There is evidence that maternal addiction put the baby at serious postnatal risks (25).

HAIR ACCUMULATION OF COCAINE: DOSE-RESPONSE STUDIES

To establish the dose-response characteristics of cocaine deposition, the following experiments were carried out. We measured hair concentrations of BZ in adult women who voluntarily admitted cocaine use and recalled their consumption patterns (route of administration and dose). A 10 mg hair sample, corresponding to 8 strands, was cut close to the scalp with scissors. In another three subjects there was a history of an abrupt change in cocaine use. Hair was sectioned to reflect the periods of different consumption, by assuming that adult hair grows at 1–1.5 cm/month. Table 1 shows the data on these three patients.

Table 1 Detection of Changes in Cocaine Use Pattern Through Analysis of Hair

Patients	History	Hair sample (cm)	Time hair represents (months)	BZ (ng/mg hair)
Patient 1	No cocaine use	3–14	3–14	0.056
	Frequent cocaine use	0–3	0–3	6.350
Patient 2	No cocaine use	10–20	10–20	0.191
	Occasional cocaine use	0–10	0–10	0.527
Patient 3	Heavy cocaine use	9–22	9–22	14.575
	Occasional cocaine use	6–9	6–9	6.424
	Occasional cocaine use	1.5–3	1.5–3	3.641

Pregnant guinea pigs purchased from High Oaks (Ontario) were injected subcutaneously with cocaine (4% hydrochloride solution) at daily doses of 5, 7.5, 10, 15, and 20 mg/kg/day between days 40 and 73 of gestation. The normal length of gestation is 66–72 days. After delivery, pup and maternal hair was cut close to the skin at the back using fine scissors.

Hair Analysis

Extraction of BZ from hair samples and subsequent analysis followed a method standardized in our laboratory (23). Briefly, the hair was washed repeatedly with 100% ethanol, and 2 mg hair samples were sonicated with 1 mL methanol for 30 min and subsequently incubated overnight at 45°C. The next day, the methanol was pipetted off and the hair rinsed briefly with an additional 1 mL of methanol. After the methanol had been evaporated at 40°C under a stream of nitrogen, the samples were reconstituted with 0.1 mL phosphate-buffered saline (pH 7.5). For cocaine measurements Coat-A-Count for cocaine metabolite in urine (Diagnostic Products, Los Angeles) was used, but instead of the BZ standards provided with the kit, in-house cocaine hydrochloride standards (1–500 ng/mL) were used. The antiserum used in the method has a much higher affinity for cocaine than for BZ, subsequently the cross-reactivity with BZ is only 0.5%. The sensitivity of the assay is 0.5 ng/mL, which corresponds to 0.025 ng cocaine/mg hair. For the analysis of BZ in the extracts the Roche Abuscreen (Hoffmann-La Roche, Nutley, NJ) for cocaine metabolite in urine was used. The cross-reactivity with cocaine was found to be 4% and the sensitivity of the assay in 5 ng/mL, which corresponds to 0.25 ng BZ/mg hair. Results are expressed in ng cocaine or BZ/mg hair.

Correlation between daily dose of cocaine (in g) consumed by the patients and hair concentrations of BZ was studied by least-squares regression analysis using the Statview 512 program on an Apple Macintosh personal computer. For these calculations we assumed a reported 1 line of cocaine to contain 100 mg of pure cocaine. This estimation is based on a recent analysis revealing that cocaine sold in Toronto is over 95% pure and contains very little adulteration. The correlation between daily dose of cocaine injected to the pups and neonatal hair concentrations was estimated by the above methodology.

A total of eight hair samples from seven adults using cocaine, who volunteered complete history of their cocaine use, were analyzed. Two of these patients reported changes in daily amounts, and their hair was cut to reflect these changes by estimating hair growth of 1 cm/month. The concentrations of BZ ranged between 0.3 and 14.6 ng/mg of hair. There was a significant correlation between reported amounts of cocaine use and hair accumulation ($r = 0.964$, $p < 0.01$).

We subsequently studied the relationship between the cocaine dose given to pregnant guinea pigs and the concentration of BZ in the dams' and their pups' furs. The lower detection limit in our laboratory is 1 ng/g hair. No detectable accumulation was measured in the pups' hair at daily doses of 5 and 7.5 mg/kg, whereas with 10, 15, and 20 mg/kg/day there was a linear correlation in the dams as well as in their pups ($r = 0.867$, $p < 0.0250$ dams; $r = 0.889$, $p < 0.001$ for pups). The same trend was observed when cocaine accumulation in the fur was measured at the daily dose of 15 and 20 mg/kg cocaine hydrochloride.

We then converted the number of lines taken by the women to a daily dose per kilogram in order to compare the human to the animal data. In both species a dose-response curve could be documented. It appears that levels in the tested pregnant guinea pigs were lower than in women taking 10 or 15 mg/kg/day, but at 20 mg/kg/day the human and animal data were similar.

MEASUREMENT OF NICOTINE AND COTININE IN MATERNAL AND FETAL HAIR

Smoking and nonsmoking mothers were identified in two nurseries in Toronto. Detailed history of smoking habits was recorded, and all smoking mothers reported a steady number of cigarettes used daily. Hair samples were obtained by cutting 5-7 hair shafts near the skull using fine scissors.

The hair samples were washed with a detergent, rinsed with water, and dried in a warm (37°C) oven overnight. The following day 2-5 mg hair samples were weighed on an analytical balance and placed in a glass container with 1 mL of 0.6 N NaOH. The samples were digested overnight at 50°C. The following day the solutions were neutralized with 50-70 μL concentrated HCl, and 100 μL aliquots of the neutral solution were used to measure nicotine or cotinine by radioimmunoassay (RIA) described by Langone et al. (26). The RIA materials were obtained from the Department of Biochemistry, Brandeis University, Waltham, Massachusetts. Both nicotine and cotinine assays use the same isogel Tris buffer (0.01 M Tris-HCl, 0.14 rM NaCl, 0.1% gelatin, pH 7.4), [³H]-nicotine or [³H]-cotinine, the respective antiserum raised in rabbits and a goat antirabbit γ-globulin to separate the antibody-bound nicotine or cotinine from the free analyte. For quantification, nicotine standards (0.5–50 ng/mL) or cotinine standards (0.2–20 ng/mL) were used. Results were expressed as nanograms analyte per milligram of hair.

The lowest sensitivity of the assay was 0.25 ng/mg hair for nicotine when 2 mg of hair was used, and 0.1 ng/mg hair for cotinine when 2 mg of hair was used. The cross-reactivity of nicotine in the cotinine assay was 5.0% and that of cotinine in the nicotine assay was 2.0%. The other metabolites, which retain only one of the two ring systems (the pyridine or N-methylpyrolidine rings), did not exhibit any cross-reactivity with either assay.

Pregnant women participating in the study smoked between 5 and 25 cigarettes/day (mean 18 ± 8) during pregnancy. They had a mean of 21.3 ± 18 ng/mg hair of nicotine and 6 ± 9.2 of cotinine; the differences between the concentrations of the drug and its metabolite were significant ($p < 0.01$). There was no correlation between the number of cigarettes smoked daily by the mothers and nicotine or cotinine concentrations in their hair.

Babies of smokers had mean nicotine concentration of 6 ± 9.2 ng/mg (range 0–27.3) and cotinine of 2.1 ± 3.7 ng/mg (range 0–12.2). There was no correlation between number of cigarettes smoked by the mothers and babies' hair concentrations of nicotine or cotinine. Conversely, there was a significant correlation between maternal and neonatal concentration of nicotine ($r = 0.78$, $p < 0.01$ by least-square linear regression) and cotinine ($r = 0.64$, $p < 0.05$, Spearman's correlation). Maternal concentration of nicotine was invariably higher than neonatal levels ($p < 0.01$, Wilcoxon's signed rank test). Conversely, concentrations of cotinine did not differ significantly between mothers and children.

There were 11 pairs of nonsmoking mothers. Their mean hair concentrations of nicotine (0.9 ± 0.8 ng/mg) and cotinine (0.3 ± 0.5 ng/mg) were significantly lower than in smoking mothers ($p < 0.0001$). Similarly, neonatal hair concentrations of nicotine (0.7 ± 0.7 ng/mg) and cotinine (0.3 ± 0.2 ng/mg) were significantly lower in babies of nonsmokers when compared to infants of smokers ($p < 0.001$).

Of the 11 pairs of nonsmokers, 4 mothers were passively exposed to cigarette smoking in the household during pregnancy. Their concentrations of nicotine (0.9 ± 0.9) were not different from those not exposed (0.9 ± 0.9 ng/mg). Conversely, cotinine concentrations in passive smoking mothers

(0.6 ± 0.7 ng/mg) were significantly higher than in those not exposed to any smoke (0 ± 0 ng/mg) ($p < 0.02$). Similar trends were observed in the babies of passive smokers having more cotinine (0.3 ± 0.2 ng/mg) than in nonexposed ones (0.1 ± 0.1 ng/mg; $p < 0.05$), with no differences in nicotine concentrations.

DISCUSSION

The assessment of the reproductive toxicology of cocaine is complex. This drug is a potent vasoconstrictor and it also causes uterine contraction (4); both are mechanisms that may induce fetal damage. However, most women using cocaine have many other risk factors that may cause the reported adverse fetal effects. In a recent meta-analysis we have documented that while a variety of detrimental fetal effects can be associated with cocaine when addicted users are compared to middle-class nonusers, most of these effects are canceled out when women addicted to cocaine are compared to those addicted only to other drugs of abuse (Chapter 16).

Meaningful estimation of fetal toxicity of cocaine must define the dose and time of fetal exposure, because human teratogens invariably follow dose- and time-response curves. A variety of xenobiotics may adversely affect the fetus at high doses, but not in lower doses. The toxicology of human teratogens may follow a dose-response pattern with or without threshold level. The time of exposure may be crucial with some teratogens (e.g., thalidomide), affecting the fetus only during organogenesis, whereas others (e.g., lead) may affect brain development throughout pregnancy (1).

Several studies have revealed that maternal reports of cocaine use are very inaccurate, likely because admitting to drug abuse may result in legal action against women as well as child apprehension by child protection agencies. Similar to nutrients and other small molecules, drugs transfer into the growing hair shaft through the capillaries nourishing it. While the mechanisms governing drug transport into hair are not well understood, it is pharmacokinetically conceivable that systemic exposure to the drug, measured as the area under the concentration-time curve, will dictate the amount of the drug deposited in the hair. The present study reveals an excellent dose-response curve between the dose consumed in humans and animals and their hair concentrations of BZ. Similarly, there is very good correlation between maternal dose and fetal hair concentrations in animals. Recently, meconium has been proposed as an accurate reservoir of fetal exposure to cocaine (24); however, there are several limitations to meconium when compared to hair as a biological marker of intrauterine drug exposure.

1. Meconium is available only during the first day of life, whereas hair will stay positive for several months.

2. At present it is not clear how much cocaine in the meconium stems from swallowing of amniotic fluid versus enterohepatic circulation of the drug, and a dose-response curve has not yet been established.
3. Because hair grows constantly, deposition of cocaine into the shaft yields a rare opportunity to study the time of exposure. As shown in Table 1, sectioning of hair in adults who reported changes in use over time avidly reflects these patterns. Because most women's hair is longer than 10 cm, it should reflect the whole length of gestation.

The initial fetal hair (lanugo) sheds at 5–6 months of gestation, and the hair neonates are born with grew during the third trimester of pregnancy; therefore detection of cocaine in newborn hair reflects maternal use of the drug during the last 3 months of pregnancy. Here again, hair is capable of verifying time of exposure; negative neonatal hair may often confirm maternal reports of stopping cocaine use upon realizing that they were pregnant.

Guinea pigs are optimal for these experiments because their pups are born with abundant fur which develops, similar to humans, during the third trimester of pregnancy. While there are no reported cases of history of second-trimester cocaine exposure and third-trimester nonexposure, we have several such cases in our program, with a corresponding negative cocaine test of neonatal hair. Cocaine elimination in rodents is much faster than in humans, and this may explain why daily doses lower than 10 mg/kg did not result in measurable concentrations in the pups' hair. Similarly, it explains the relatively low accumulation in the adult guinea pig hair as compared to humans. While these preliminary animal studies suggest linearity in cocaine accumulation in hair, larger numbers are needed to address the variability of this phenomenon.

The excellent dose-response curve between amounts used in humans and hair accumulation may be explained by the selection of individuals who voluntarily reported on their use and by the fact that in Toronto most cocaine is more than 95% pure, thus decreasing the potential effect of adulteration. While larger numbers of cases will have to be analyzed, this pilot project emphasizes the promise of hair analysis as a biological marker for maternal and fetal exposure to cocaine.

Being lipid soluble, nicotine has a large distribution volume (2–3 L/kg), and it readily permeates cell membranes. This xenobiotic is absorbed through the lung, skin, gastrointestinal tract, and nasal mucosa and is actively secreted by the renal tubules. Once absorbed, nicotine rapidly disappears from the blood due to both widespread tissue uptake and metabolism (27,28). The elimination half-life of nicotine in man ranges between 1 and 3 h and therefore monitoring this chemical in the blood is not likely to reflect the extent of smoking. Citonine, a major metabolite of nicotine, has a much longer elimination half-life (10–14 h); urinary or salivary measurements of cotinine have been the most accurate estimate to validate self-reported smoking habits (29).

Cigarette smoke enters the body by inhalation; hence estimation of systemic exposure is extremely complicated, as different individuals may have very different modes of smoking in terms of both number and depth of inhalations. Moreover, interindividual variability in distribution and elimination of nicotine and cotinine further makes it difficult to estimate cumulative exposure from single determinations. Our data reveal that the reported number of cigarettes consumed by the pregnant mother does not correlate with hair accumulation of nicotine or cotinine in either mother or fetus. This is not surprising, realizing the large variability in the inhaled dose in addition to the regular sources of pharmacokinetic variability such as distribution and elimination processes. Of importance, there was significant correlation between maternal systemic exposure to nicotine evidenced by hair concentrations of nicotine or cotinine and accumulation of these xenobiotics in fetal hair. This means that like the case of methyl mercury and cocaine, maternal and fetal hair may better estimate long-term systemic exposure to toxic constituents of cigarettes and thereby may yield a better prediction of fetuses at risk.

The concentrations of nicotine and cotinine measured by us in the adult hair agree with those measured in the only two other reports located by us (30,31). During the last years there has been increasing awareness of the serious health risks inflicted by passive exposure to cigarette smoke. Our data suggest that, indeed, women and their unborn babies are accumulating nicotine and cotinine even when they avoid smoking. Although our sample size is too small to draw definite conclusions, of the four babies of nonsmoking women exposed to "passive smoking," three had detectable levels of cotinine in their hair.

A majority of women abusing cocaine also smoke cigarettes (4). Hence it is probable that there are cumulative adverse effects, each one with its own dose-response characteristics. The use of hair test, therefore, may prove to be crucial in explaining why some fetuses are adversely affected in a major way while others escape with no measurable damage.

In summary, we believe that the hair test is likely to develop into a critical tool for assessing the degree and time of fetal exposure to xenobiotics. While our work to date has focused on cocaine and nicotine, other drugs such as opioids, cannabinoids, and amphetamines can already be measured in adult hair, and methodologies for their fetal measurement can be refined.

Answer

At 4 days of life meconium testing is not an option. However, if the mother used cocaine regularly during the last 3–4 months of pregnancy, the infant's hair is likely to be positive for benzoylecgonine.

ACKNOWLEDGMENT

This work was supported by a grant from the Medical Research Council of Canada.

REFERENCES

1. Koren G. Maternal-Fetal Toxicology; a Clinician's Guide [1st ed]. New York, Marcel Dekker, 1990.
2. Abelson HK, Miller JP. A decade of trends in cocaine use in the household populatikon. Natl Inst Drug Abuse Res Monogr Ser 1985; 61:35-49.
3. Shannon MW, Hite C, Woolf A. Detection of in utero drug exposure among term, apparently healthy newborns. Vet Hum Toxicol 1989; 31:347.
4. Lutiger B, Graham K, Einarson TR, Koren G. Relationship between gestational cocaine use and pregnancy outcome: A meta-analysis. Teratology 1991; 44:405-414.
5. Townsend R, Laing FC, Jeffery RB. Placental abruption associated with cocaine abuse. Am J Radiol 1988; 150:1339-1340.
6. Chasnoff IJ, Bussey ME, Savich R, Stack CM. Perinatal cerebral infarction and maternal cocaine use. J Pediatr 1986; 108:456-459.
7. Chasnoff IJ, Griffith DR, MacGregor S, Birkes K, Burns KA. Temporal patterns of cocaine use in pregnancy. Perinatal outcome. JAMA 1989; 261:1741-1744.
8. Oro AS, Dixon SD. Perinatal cocaine and methamphetamine exposure: Maternal and neonatal correlates. J Pediatr 1987; 111:571-578.
9. Chouteau M, Brickner Namerou P, Leppert P. The effect of cocaine abuse on birth weight and gestational age. Obstet Gynecol 1988; 72:351-354.
10. MacGregor SN, Keith LG, Chasnoff IJ, Rosner MA, Chisum GM, Sharo P, Minogue JP. Cocaine use during pregnancy: Adverse perinatal outcome. Am J Obstet Gynecol 1987; 157:686-690.
11. Chasnoff IJ, Burns KA, Burns WJ. Cocaine use in pregnancy: Perinatal morbidity and mortality. Neurotoxicol Teratol 1987; 9:291-293.
12. Chasnoff IJ, Chisum GM, Kaplan E. Maternal cocaine use and genitourinary tract malformations. Teratology 1988; 37:201-204.
13. Little BB, Snell LM, Klein VR, Gilstrap LC. Cocaine abuse during pregnancy: Maternal and fetal complications. Obstet Gynecol 1988; 73:157-160.
14. Brody JE. Widespread abuse of drugs by pregnant women is found. New York Times 1989; 137:1-19.
15. Zuckerman B, Frank DA, Hingson R. Effects of maternal marijuana and cocaine use on fetal growth. N Engl J Med 1989; 320:762-768.
16. The health consequences of smoking: The changing cigarette. Rockville, MD: US Department of Health and Human Services, Public Health Service. Office on Smoking and Health, 1981: DHHS publication No (PHS) 81-501 56:33-61.
17. Triebig G, Zober MA. Indoor air pollution by smoke constituents — A survey. Prev Med 1984; 13:570-581.

18. Martin TR, Bracken ME. Association of low birth-weight with passive smoke exposure in pregnancy. Am J Epidemiol 1986; 124:633–642.
19. Abel EL. Smoking and pregnancy. J Psychoactive Drugs 1984; 16:327–328.
20. Stillman RJ, Rosenberg MJ, Sacks BJ. Smoking and reproduction. Fertil Steril 1986; 46:545–566.
21. Rush D, Callahan KR. Exposure to passive cigarette smoking and child development. Ann NY Acad Sci 1989; 562:74–100.
22. Longo LD. The biological effects of carbon monoxide on the pregnant woman, fetus and newborn infant. Am J Obstet Gynecol 1111; 129:69–103.
23. Graham K, Koren G, Klein J, Schneiderman J, Greenwald M. Determination of gestational cocaine exposure by hair analysis. JAMA 1989; 262:3328–3330.
24. Ostrea EM Jr, Brady M, Gause S, Raymunds AL, Stevens M. Drug screening of newborns by meconium analysis: A large-scale, prospective, epidemiologic study. Pediatrics 1992; 89:107–113.
25. Johnston C. Children of cocaine addicts or study of 25 inner city families. Soc Worker 1990; 58:53–56.
26. Langone J, Gjiba HB, Van Vunakis H. Nicotine and its metabolites: Radio-immunoassay for nicotine and cotinine. Biochemistry 1973; 12:5015–5030.
27. Lenberger L, Rubin A. Physiologic Disposition of Drugs of Abuse. New York, Spectrum, 1978, p 205.
28. Pilotti A. Biosynthesis and mammalian metabolism of nicotine. Acta Physiol Scand 1980; 479:13–17.
29. Haley NJ, Axelrod CM, Tilton KA. Validation of self-reported smoking behavior: Biochemical analysis of cotinine and thiocyanate. Am J Public Health 1983; 73:1204–1207.
30. Haley NJ, Hoffmann D. Analysis for nicotine and cotinine in hair to determine cigarette smoker status. Clin Chem 1985; 31/10:1598–1600.
31. Ishiyama J, Nagai T, Toshida S. Detection of basic drugs (metamphetamines, antidepressants and nicotine) from human hair. J Forensic Sci 1983; 28:380–385.

19

Occupational Exposures Known to Be Human Reproductive Toxins

Yedidia Bentur
Rambam Medical Center, Technion - Israel Institute of Technology, Haifa, Israel

Eli Zalzstein
Soroka Medical Center, Beer-Sheva, Israel

Gideon Koren
The Hospital for Sick Children, Toronto, Ontario, Canada

Clinical Case

A woman working in a battery plant plans pregnancy. Her lead level is 5 μg/dL and she is afraid of adverse effects to her baby.

INTRODUCTION

The latter part of the 20th century has been characterized by a substantial and steady increase in the number of women joining the work force. Moreover, women are taking jobs that were traditionally held by men only. With increased awareness of reproductive toxicology caused by chemicals, women in the reproductive age range and their families are troubled about potential hazards to unborn babies. Moreover, employers are often concerned about their liability in cases of women working with certain chemicals who experience adverse fetal outcome.

Recently, an American battery manufacturer tried to exclude all women of reproductive age from its production line, and a similar thrust has been tried by a Canadian nickel producer. In both cases the workers' unions rejected the manufacturers' attempts.

In comparison to therapeutic agents, our knowledge of reproductive toxicology of industrial chemicals in humans is in most cases sketchy or missing. Before marketing, the teratogenic potential of drugs must be tested in animals; no such data are required for industrial chemicals. In trying to identify adverse reproductive effects in humans of chemicals that have already been introduced into the workplace, one has to struggle with the plethora of methodological problems mentioned in Chapters 3 and 31. Moreover, in most cases workers are exposed to more than one chemical, and often it is impossible to identify a chemical culprit causing reproductive toxicity.

Every chemical used in the workplace has safety exposure limits aimed at protecting the workers from toxicity. However, these standards were not meant to protect the fetus, and it is possible that airborne levels (e.g., of metallic mercury) that are safe for the mother may be hazardous for the developing organism.

It is beyond the scope of this chapter to discuss the toxic potential of every chemical that may be encountered during pregnancy. Because in the vast majority of cases reproductive toxicology has not been proven in women exposed in the workplace, we prefer to include only cases where such evidence is unequivocal. Every case in which a woman experiences clinical symptoms or signs that may be associated with chemical exposure should be investigated in depth. The nature and conditions of the work should be looked into, including ventilation and means of protection, and it should be determined whether a similar clinical picture exists in fellow workers.

If the clinical picture is consistent with the chemical(s) in question, exposure levels must be defined. We often find that women are reluctant to induce such an investigation or even to ask for the installation of recent safety measurements because they are afraid of retaliation by the employer. While there is no simple solution for such a situation, the counselor must explain to such women the seriousness of prolonged exposure. Many large plants have hygienists, safety officers, or physicians on the staff, and these health professionals should assist pregnant workers.

Table 1 is an algorithm of suggested steps in analyzing the reproductive hazard associated with chemicals to which women receive occupational exposure.

DEFINITIONS

The following definitions of workplace standards are commonly employed when discussing occupational standards.

Table 1 A Clinical Approach to Reproductive Hazards of Chemicals

1. Identify the chemicals in question by their safety sheets.[a]
2. Identify symptoms and signs reported to be associated.
3. Rule out underlying conditions that may cause a similar clinical picture (e.g., morning sickness in the first trimester).
4. Obtain a detailed description of the work performed by the woman, length of exposure, and means of protection (ventilation system, respirator, mask, gown, gloves, hood, etc.).
5. Determine whether symptoms and signs are manifest in fellow workers.
6. Obtain the most recent levels of the chemicals in question measured in that particular area.
7. Try to understand the attitude of the woman and her supervisors toward her particular work and toward a possible change of job. Will a change of job affect her income or chances for promotion?
8. Before reporting to the woman on available information, read the data critically and be accurate in your description of what is known.
9. Advise the woman on possible safety measurements to reduce exposure (mask, gloves, ventilation, etc.).

[a]In the United States, a document called a Material Safety Data Sheet is required by law for many chemical agents encountered in the workplace.

PEL: permissible exposure limit set by the U.S. Occupational Safety and Health Administration (OSHA).

TLV: threshold limit value set by the American Conference of Governmental Industrial Hygienists (ACGIH).

Both *PEL* and *TLV* refer to the airborne concentrations of a substance and represent conditions under which it is believed that nearly all workers may be repeatedly exposed, day after day, without adverse effects.

TWA: time-weighted average concentration for a normal 8-hour work day and a 40-hour work week to which nearly all workers may be repeatedly exposed, day after day, without adverse effects.

Usually the values above are expressed as *TLV-TWA* or *PEL-TWA*.

STEL: short-term exposure limit, set by the ACGIH. It refers to the maximum concentration to which workers can be exposed for up to 15 minutes continuously, provided no more than four excursions per day are permitted, but with at least 60 minutes between exposure periods and provided the daily TLV-TWA is not exceeded.

IDLH: immediately dangerous to life or health, a concentration set by the standards completion program of the (U.S.) National Institute of Occupational Safety and Health (NIOSH), in conjunction with OSHA. Represents the maximum concentration from which (in the event of respirator failure), one could escape within 30 minutes without a respirator and without experiencing any escape-impairing symptoms or irreversible health effects.

Ceiling: the concentration that should not be exceeded even for an instant.

The exposure limits are given in parts per million (ppm) or parts per billion (ppb), or as milligrams per cubic meter (mg/m³). The following formula converts these units:

$$mg/m^3 = \frac{ppm \times molecular\ weight}{24.5}$$

It should be noted that all these workplace standards are meant to protect the adult worker; it is unknown whether they also protect the fetus.

Therefore, when counseling the occupationally exposed pregnant woman, the availability of airborne concentrations may be useful mainly in two extreme situations:

1. Concentrations close to or below detectable level, in the absence of adverse effects, may suggest low fetal risk.
2. Concentrations higher than TLV (or PEL) – TWA may suggest that the fetus *is* at risk; the higher the concentration, the larger the possible risk.

This approach needs to be validated by controlled studies.

INTERPRETATION OF ANIMAL STUDIES WHEN NO INFORMATION ON PATIENTS EXISTS

For most of the chemicals in question no epidemiological studies exist. In this case animal studies should not be ignored; rather, they should be continuously interpreted. Parameters that may be of help in this process include molecular similarity of the toxin to a known teratogen, dose, relationship between dose and workplace standards and the "no observable adverse effect level" (NOAEL), route of administration, duration of exposure, gestational age at exposure, species and number of species studied, type of birth defect induced and its incidence, and the greater sensitivity of humans to most developmental toxins.

SUMMARY OF HUMAN DATA

The following short statements summarize published human data on chemicals about which we have been consulted most frequently by pregnant women. Animal studies and chemicals infrequently cited are not included.

Anesthetic Gases

There is no evidence to date that a single course of general anesthesia in early pregnancy is capable of inducing teratogenicity. A large prospective study has shown the safety of nitrous oxide (1). Similarly, thiopental, enflurane, and halothane were not shown to cause untoward embryonic or fetal effects (2). Increased rate of miscarriage among operating room personnel was observed in some studies (3–5). However, methodological problems, mainly response bias, preclude any firm conclusions from their results (6). A recent study showed reduced fertility among female dental assistants exposed to high levels of unscavenged nitrous oxide (7). Most epidemiological studies do not suggest that congenital anomalies occur more often than expected among children of women with occupational exposure to volatile anesthetics during pregnancy. No consistent difference has been observed in the types of patterns of congenital anomalies found in children born to these women when compared with controls (8).

Workplace standards (*nitrous oxide*): TLV-TWA, 50 ppm. Every effort should be made to minimize chronic exposure to nitrous oxide.

Biomonitoring parameters: complete blood count.

Cadmium

There is inconclusive evidence for the adverse effect of cadmium on male fertility (9). In smokers, placental levels were higher (10), and this metal may accumulate in the fetus (11). It may impair placental function by displacing zinc, thereby reducing birth weight (12). Teratogenic effects were not reported in exposed populations (13). Adverse reproductive effects may include low birth weight (14), fewer full-term deliveries, fewer multiple pregnancies, lower birth weight in preterm infants (15), and poorer performance on intellectual and motor skills tests at 6 years of age (16). Cadmium in combination with other heavy metals may have mutagenic effects, but evidence that cadmium alone has cytogenetic effects is as yet inconvincing (17–20). Cadmium may be regarded as a potential workplace carcinogen.

Workplace standards: TLV-TWA, 0.05 mg/m^3; intended change, 0.01 mg/m^3.

Biomonitoring parameters: blood cadmium levels (normal levels differ between smokers and nonsmokers), urinary cadmium-spot or 24-hour collection, urinary metallothionein, and *N*-acetylglucosaminidase.

Carbon Monoxide (CO), Including Methylene Chloride

CO readily crosses the placenta and is eliminated from the fetal circulation more slowly than from the maternal circulation (21). CO poisoning may result in fetal death, stillbirth, or severe neurological deficits (22–24). However, toxicity of this sort has been seen most often in symptomatic maternal poisoning (25). It seems that the fetus is more susceptible than the mother to CO, and some authors believe that there is no margin of safety for CO exposure to the fetus (26). The risk to the fetus from chronic low level exposure is not well documented, and it was suggested that it may pose a risk to the fetus comparable to that from smoking in the mother (27).

Methylene chloride is partially metabolized to CO (25-33%) and may induce CO toxicity. The U.S. Environmental Protection Agency (EPA) regards this substance as having "minimal teratogenic potential" (28). For further discussion of methylene chloride, see "Organic Solvents."

Workplace standards: TLV-TWA, 50 ppm.

Biomonitoring parameters: carboxyhemoglobin (may differ between nonsmokers and smokers). Levels do not necessarily correlate with toxicity.

Cholinesterase Inhibitors

Organophosphates and carbamates are irreversible and reversible cholinesterase inhibitors, respectively. The potential of these pesticides to induce human developmental toxicity is unknown. Rodent studies are of concern, but they involve high doses that are unlikely to be encountered by pregnant women. Several case reports and poorly documented studies described malformations after high acute exposures to organophosphate (29–32) but not in others (33–35). In one case report, a suicide attempt with carbofuran (a carbamate insecticide) resulted in fetal death (36).

Workplace standards: TLV-TWA, 0.1 mg/m³ for parathion.

Biomonitoring parameters: erythrocyte (true) acetylcholinesterase, plasma (pseudo) butirylcholinesterase.

Dibromochloropropane

Occupational exposure to the agricultural nematocide dibromochloropropane has been associated in men with elevated serum gonadotropins, decreased sperm counts, and infertility (37,38). The duration of the exposure may be related to the severity and reversibility of the injury (39–41). A higher percentage of female infants was found after paternal exposure (42,43) but not miscarriages and malformations (44). No chromosomal abnormalities were found in offspring of exposed men (45). Nondisjunction was found in exposed workmen (46). Increased incidence of the frequency of Y chromosomes was not observed in women exposed to dibromochloropropane (37). OSHA determined that this agent may increase the risk of cancer.

Workplace standards: TLV-TWA, not listed; PEL-TWA, 1 ppb.

Biomonitoring parameters: sperm count, serum testosterone, follicle stimulating hormone, luteinizing hormone, as well as liver and kidney function tests.

Epichlorhydrin

Several studies showed epichlorhydrin to be mutagenic in workers; the exposure level in one of these studies was 0.13–1.3 ppm (47,48). However, chromosomal aberrations in lymphocytes were not found in another study involving occupational exposure (49). Epichlorhydrin is a testicular toxicant in animals (50) and is a metabolite of dibromochloropropane, which is also a known testicular toxicant in humans and animals (37,38). An unpublished report of the Shell Oil Company claims no decrease in sperm count or hormonal activity among exposed workers, but no details are available (51). Epichlorohydrin is a suspected human carcinogen.

Workplace standards: TLV-TWA, 2 ppm. Intended change, 0.1 ppm.

Biomonitoring parameters: liver and kidney function tests.

Ethylene Dibromide (Dibromomethane)

Agricultural workers exposed to ethylene dibromide had reduced sperm concentrations and lower percentage of normal cells (52,53). In one study, mean exposure levels were estimated at 88 ppb with peak levels of 262 ppb (52). In the other study marijuana use was more prevalent in the exposed group (53). There was no effect of ethylene bromide on fertility in wives of exposed workers in three chemical plants in southern United States; however, fertility was significantly reduced at the fourth plant (54). Exposure levels in all plants was ≤ 5 ppm. The American Medical Association (AMA) concluded that as of 1980, there was no conclusive human evidence that this agent was a reproductive hazard (55). Ethylene dibromide is a suspected human carcinogen.

Workplace standards: no TLV-TWA; PEL-TWA, 20 ppm.

Biomonitoring parameters: blood bromide levels, complete blood count, liver and kidney function tests.

Ethylene Oxide

Hospital workers exposed to 8-hour weighted mean ethylene oxide concentrations of 0.1–0.5 ppm had a higher incidence of spontaneous abortions (56). However, the rate of miscarriages among controls was lower than expected and not higher than the expected rate among exposed (7.7 vs. 12.7%, respectively). Similar findings, in addition to increased incidence of gynecological problems, were reported in another study (57). These two studies were criticized for their methodology. A case control study did not confirm an association with spontaneous abortions and birth defects (58). Occupational exposure was demonstrated to increase frequency of sister chromatid exchange (59–63). Ethylene oxide is a suspected human carcinogen.

Workplace standards: RLV-TWA, 1 ppm.

Biomonitoring parameters: chest x-ray.

Formaldehyde

No increase in birth defects or spontaneous abortions was observed in women hospital workers occupationally exposed to formaldehyde (56,58). In contrast, a weak association with miscarriages was suggested in another study (64). A Soviet study reported excess menstrual disorders and low birth weight infants, but the women involved had done heavy lifting and the study had methodological problems (65). Occupational exposure at recommended limits is not thought to present a reproductive hazard (66). Formaldehyde is a suspected human carcinogen.

Workplace standards: TLV-TWA, 1 ppm.

Biomonitoring parameters: urine formate; but the use of this agent for biological monitoring is questionable because of large normal variation.

Glutaraldehyde

Miscarriage rate adjusted for possible risk factors was not found to be increased in a questionnaire study of women undergoing surgical sterilization in hospitals (56).

Workplace standards: TLV-ceiling, 0.2 ppm; PEL-TWA, not listed.

Biomonitoring parameters: liver and kidney function tests, chest x-ray, and pulmonary function tests, especially when respiratory tract irritation presents.

Halogenated Hydrocarbon Solvents

The reader is also referred to the discussion on organic solvents (Chapter 20).

Chloroprene

Soviet studies suggested that chloroprene may induce menstrual disorders, decreased sperm motility, and changes in sperm morphology. It seems that high doses are more toxic to the testes, but the effect of near-TLV concentrations is unclear. A threefold increase in abortion rate was reported in wives of workers exposed to 0.3–1.9 ppm, but the significance of this finding is unclear (67). A French study quoted in a NIOSH document observed impotence and reduced libido during overexposure to chloroprene which disappeared after removal from exposure (68). There is limited evidence that this agent may be mutagenic in humans (67).

Workplace standards: TLV-TWA, 10 ppm.

Biomonitoring parameters: liver function tests; chest x-ray in overexposure.

Chloroform (see also organic solvents, Chapter 20)

Chloroform crosses the human placenta (69). In 492 laboratory workers with first-trimester exposure to organic solvents, including chloroform, there was no increased frequency of congenital anomalies (70). Higher frequencies of acquired chromosomal aberrations were observed in women occupationally exposed to organic solvents including chloroform and in the children of these exposed women (71). Chloroform is a potential human carcinogen.

Workplace standards: TLV-TWA, 10 ppm.

Biomonitoring parameters: liver and kidney function tests.

Hexachlorophene

Hexachlorophene was detectable in maternal and cord blood of this bactericidal agent after vaginal use during labor (72). Occupational exposure of women medical personnel during hand washing was suggested to increase the frequency of a heterogeneous group of congenital malformations (73). However, this study was criticized for its methodology, and a more comprehensive and careful epidemiological study could not confirm this association (74). A similar conclusion was achieved in a case control study of children with various anomalies (75). The AMA Council on Scientific Affairs concluded that pregnant women should not use hexachlorophene-containing products (66).

Workplace standards: TLV (or PEL)-TWA, not listed.

Biomonitoring parameters: blood hexachlorophene levels; but correlation with clinical effects is not good.

Tetrachloroethylene (see also organic solvents, Chapter 20)

Women of reproductive age who work in dry-cleaning facilities may receive substantial exposure to tetrachloroethylene, since environmental air levels may range between 200 and 4000 mg/m^3 (30–540 ppm). Sperm from exposed dry-cleaning workers were found to be round, which is believed to be a mark of infertility (76). Wives of dry-cleaning workers required longer periods of time to become pregnant, but they did not have fewer pregnancies or increased spontaneous abortions (77). Although limited epidemiological studies suggest that tetrachloroethylene may induce liver cancer, the data are not satisfactory to reach a definite conclusion on its carcinogenicity in humans (78).

Workplace standards: TLV-TWA, 50 ppm.

Biomonitoring parameters: blood levels, liver and kidney function tests, urinary trichloroacetic acid.

Trichloroethlene (see also organic solvents, Chapter 20)

Trichloroethylene has been reported to cross the placenta (79). An increased incidence of congenital heart disease among offspring of mothers with first-trimester exposure to contaminated groundwater was reported, but a direct cause-and-effect relationship has not been established (80). Another study did not find such an association (81). Although trichloroethylene may be carcinogenic in animals, this effect has not been clearly found in humans (82).

Workplace standards: TLV-TWA, 50 ppm.
Biomonitoring parameters: blood and breath levels.

Lead

For a detailed discussion the reader is referred to Chapter 20. Lead crosses the placenta (83) and accumulates in the fetus (84). It may induce abortions and prematurity (85,86). A dose-related association with minor malformations has been suggested (87). Children with cord blood lead levels exceeding 10 μg/dL scored lower on developmental tests (88). Lead was shown to cause infertility in exposed men (89) and possibly chromosomal aberrations (90). The latter association is still unclear.

Workplace standards: TLV-TWA, 0.15 mg/m^3; PEL-TWA, 0.05 mg/m^3; action level: 0.03 mg/m^3.

Biomonitoring parameters: blood lead levels (if employee's level $\geqslant$40 μg/dL or $\geqslant$30 μg/dL if he or she intends to have children, removal from exposure should be considered), erythrocyte protoporphyrin, and the lead mobilization test may be used to assess total body burden, especially if blood levels are borderline.

Mercury

Elemental (Metallic) Mercury

Occupational male exposure was reported to induce impotence and decreased libido (91) but not infertility (92). Paternal exposure to mercury, confirmed by urinary levels, was suggested to be associated with spontaneous abortions (93). Menstrual disorders were reported in several studies (94,95) as well as infertility (96). Mercury crosses the placenta, and fetal blood levels may be comparable or even higher than maternal level (97–100). No increase in spontaneous abortions was found in female dental assistants exposed to mercury (101,102). Although other authors report more spontaneous abortions (average exposure level 0.08 mg/m^3), it is difficult to separate the effects of other occupational exposures from those of mercury (103,104). There are positive (105) and negative (102,106,107) reports on the ability of metallic mercury to induce birth defects, especially neurological. Fetal and newborn toxic mercury level was estimated to be 3 μg/g (108). Since daily uptake of mercury from dental amalgam is low (2–5 μg), it was suggested that restriction of amalgam therapy in pregnant women is unwarranted (109). In a study of sheep, mercury was shown to be released from maternal dental amalgam fillings and be transferred to the fetus. Although no toxic effects were found, these authors recommended to avoid the use of dental amalgams containing mercury (110).

Workplace standards: TLV-TWA, 0.05 mg/m^3 (skin notation); suggested guideline in pregnancy, 0.01 mg/m^3.

Biomonitoring parameters: blood levels, preshift urine collection, nerve conduction velocities.

Inorganic Mercury

May cross the placenta (111) and effect central nervous system (CNS) development (112). However, a specific embryopathy has not been reported. Indoor exposure to mercury-containing latex paint was shown to result in an increased urine mercury level (113).

Workplace standards: TLV-TWA, 0.05 mg/m^3 (skin notation).

Biomonitoring parameters: as for elemental mercury.

Organic Mercury

Pregnant women treated with mercurials had a higher incidence of spontaneous abortions (114). Methyl mercury may accumulate in the fetus. This is suggested by higher blood mercury level found in infants born to mothers exposed to methyl mercury in contaminated bread (115). Two epidemics of cerebral palsy, microcephaly, and psychomotor retardation were reported after in utero exposure to methyl mercury in Japan (contaminated fish) and Iraq (bread made of contaminated grain) (116–119).

Workplace standards: TLV-TWA: alkyl compounds, 0.01 mg/m^3; aryl compounds, 0.05 mg/m^3 (skin notation).

Biomonitoring parameters: as for elemental mercury.

Organic Solvents

For more detailed discussion the reader is referred to Chapter 20. Because of the complexity and diversity of exposure to organic solvents, adequate epidemiological studies are difficult to conduct and interpret. Several studies suggest these agents to be associated with spontaneous abortions (120–124), especially the aliphatic hydrocarbons (125). Other studies could not confirm this association (126,127). The uncertainty is even larger when congenital malformations are considered (128–131).

Workplace standards: TWA, according to the agents involved.
Biomonitoring parameters: according to the agents involved.

Organochlorine Insecticides

Endosulfan, Dieldrin, Chlordane

No human reproductive information is available.

Lindane

At least 10% can be absorbed through human skin (132). Lindane crosses the human placenta (133), and fetal levels are comparable to maternal level (134, 135). This insecticide may induce menstrual disorders, infertility (136), excess blood loss after delivery, and lower birth weights (137). Although anecdotal reports found higher placenta, fetal, and maternal blood lindane levels in cases of spontaneous abortions and premature deliveries (137,138), other studies could not find a relationship between lindane levels and stillbirth (139) or other pathological conditions of pregnancy (140). Lower levels of testosterone and other sex hormones (141) and reversible oligospermia and high ratio of dead sperm (142) were reported in males occupationally exposed to lindane.

Workplace standards: TLV-TWA, 0.5 mg/m^3.

Biomonitoring parameters: serum levels may be useful in documenting acute toxicity.

DDT

DDT can cross the human placenta at term (143,144). It is unclear whether the insecticide can induce pregnancy complications in humans (133,145–148). Although chlorinated hydrocarbons were found in seminal fluid and cervical mucus of infertility patients (148), their role in reproductive problems is uncertain. The EPA banned the use of DDT because it is stored indefinitely in human tissue.

Workplace standards: TLV-TWA, 0.5 mg/m^3.

Biomonitoring parameters: serum levels may reflect cumulative exposure.

Heptachlor

No increase in the incidence of birth defects was observed in Hawaii in infants exposed in utero to milk contaminated with heptachlor (149). The exposure could not be quantitated in either the study or the control group. After similar incidents in Arkansas, Missouri, and Oklahoma, one report on a neonate who developed gliosarcoma was noted, but heptachlor could not be established as the primary oncogen (150). This agent may be mutagenic in human fibroblasts (151).

Workplace standards: TLV-TWA, 0.5 mg/m^3.

Phenol

No clear association with birth defects was found in women occupationally exposed to phenol among other disinfectants (75). Phenol may induce methemoglobinemia, especially in infants. Based on this possibility, it was suggested in one review that phenol may affect the human fetus (152).

Workplace standards: TLV-TWA, 5 ppm.

Biomonitoring parameters: blood and urine phenol, methemoglobin determination during or at end of shift—nonspecific.

Polychlorinated Biphenyls (PCBs) and Polybrominated Biphenyls (PBBs)

In the Yusho epidemic in Japan (1968), pregnant women were exposed to rice oil contaminated with PCBs. The following adverse pregnancy outcomes were reported: stillbirth; gray-brown discoloration of skin, gingiva, and nails (cola-colored babies); parchmentlike skin with desquamation; exophthalmus; teeth present at birth; conjunctivitis; and low birth weight (153–158). Skin discoloration slowly disappeared after birth, and normal weight was gained afterward (155–158). Persistent signs included recurrent acne and nail pigmentation (159). In a similar epidemic in Taiwan (1979), children exposed in utero had developmental delay in addition to the foregoing abnormalities (160). No association could be demonstrated between cord blood, placenta, and milk PCB levels and birth weight or head circumference (161). Children exposed in these epidemics also scored lower than controls on developmental tests, especially those who had low birth weight and were more severely affected (162). It seems that males were more susceptible to the teratogenic effects of PCBs (153). Small head circumference and low birth weight were found in offspring of women exposed to PCBs contaminated fish in the Great Lakes (163). The children exposed in the Great Lakes region of the United States also had small but significant impairment in short-term memory (164). Workplace exposure was also associated with low birth weight as well as shorter gestation (165). PCBs are considered to be potential human carcinogens (166).

Thirty-three farm children exposed in utero or in early pregnancy to PBBs were normal in growth and in results of physical examination and neurological assessment at the age of 37 months (167).

Workplace standards: TLV-TWA: 42% chlorine, 1 mg/m³ (skin notation); 54% chlorine, 0.5 mg/m³ (skin notation).

Biomonitoring parameters: PCBs can be measured in blood, urine, milk, and adipose tissues. One should consider background levels.

Styrene

The reader is also referred to the discussion on organic solvents, Chapter 20. Two studies from the former Soviet Union showed low concentrations of styrene to be associated with menstrual disorders (168,169). However, a large American study on women exposed to styrene in reinforced plastics companies failed to show this association (170). Styrene has been shown to cross the human placenta (69). In a study on 2209 workers (511 females), again in the reinforced plastics industry, no increase in birth defects was found (171). Chronic occupational exposures to styrene have sometimes been associated with chromosomal damage in germ cells and lymphocytes (172–174).

Workplace standards: TLV-TWA, 50 ppm.

Biomonitoring parameters: urinary mandelic acid; other possible tests include phenylglyoxylic acid in urine and blood styrene level.

2,3,7,8-Tetrachlorodibenzo-*p*-dioxin (TCDD, Dioxins)

There was no increase in malformations following the Seveso dioxin accident (175). Another study suggesting that TCDD may have induced malformations and embryopathy in this accident (176) was shown to have methodological problems that invalidated its finding (177). Offspring of Vietnam veterans exposed to Agent Orange (about 50% 2,4,5-trichlorophenoxyacetic acid contaminated by TCDD) were not found to have increased incidence of malformations (178,179). The data of these studies could not address questions regarding association with defects of rare types or defects in offspring of selected groups of veterans. A study involving 370 men occupationally exposed to TCDD and other dioxins in a Michigan plant did not reveal adverse reproductive outcome (180). TCDD is a potential human carcinogen.

Workplace standards: TLV-TWA: not listed.

Biomonitoring parameters: liver and kidney function tests, complete blood count, serum lipids, prothrombin time, uroporphyrins, fat biopsies.

Vinyl Chloride (Chloroethylene)

Impotence and loss of libido were reported by men occupationally exposed to high levels of vinyl chloride monomer (181,182). Increased rate of miscarriages was found in wives of male vinyl chloride workers (183). This study was criticized for its methodology of data collection and response bias (184, 185). Later studies could not demonstrate such an association (186–188). Although several studies suggested an association between congenital anomalies (especially CNS) and the presence in the community of vinyl chloride industries (189–191), these reports should be considered to be inconclusive. The presence of other pollutants and personal factors were not controlled

(192), and there was no relation between parental occupation with vinyl chloride plant and congenital anomalies in the offspring (191,193). Mutagenicity studies on exposed workers are controversial, but it seem that chromosomal aberrations may be related to duration and extent of exposure, especially if greater than 20 ppm (194). Vinyl chloride is a human carcinogen.

Workplace standards: TLV-TWA: 5 ppm; PEL-TWA: 1 ppm.

Biomonitoring parameters: liver and kidney function tests; complete blood count; other tests may include urinary thiodiglycolic acid and uroporphyrins, as well as pulmonary function tests after exposure to dust.

Radiation

For a detailed discussion on the effects of ionizing and nonionizing radiation and video display terminals on the pregnancy, the reader is referred to Chapter 22.

Answer

Her lead level (5 µg/dL) is below any known teratogenic concentration.

REFERENCES

1. Crawford JS, Lewis M. Nitrous oxide in early human pregnancy. Anaesthesia 1986; 41:900–905.
2. Heinonen OP, Slone D, Shapiro S. Birth Defect and Drugs in Pregnancy. Publishing Sciences Group, Littleton, Ma, 1977.
3. Ferstanding LL. Trace concentration of anesthetic gases. Acta Anesth Scand 1982; 75(suppl):38–43.
4. Tannenbaum TN, Goldberg RJ. Exposure to anesthetic gases and reproductive outcome: A review of the epidemiologic literature. J Occup Med 1985; 27:659–668.
5. Spence AA. Chronic exposure to trace concentration of anaesthetics. In General Anaesthesia, 4th ed (Gray TC, Nunn JS, Utting JE, eds). Butterworths, London, 1980, pp 189–201.
6. Axelsson G, Rylander R. Exposure to anaesthetic gases and spontaneous abortion: Response bias in a postal questionnaire study. Int J Epidemiol 1982; 11: 250–256.
7. Rowland AS, Baird DD, Weinberg CR, et al. Reduced fertility among women employed as dental assistants exposed to high levels of nitrous oxide. N Engl J Med 1992; 327:993–997.
8. Friedman JM. Teratogen update: Anesthetic agents. Teratology 1988; 37:69–77.

9. Schray SD, Dixon RL. Occupational exposures associated with male reproductive dysfunction. Annu Rev Pharmacol Toxicol 1985; 25:567–592.
10. Cadmium and its compounds. In Reproductive Hazards of Industrial Chemicals (Barlow SM, Sullivan FM, eds). Academic Press, London, 1982, pp 136–177.
11. Sikorski R, Radomanski T, Paszkowski T, Skoda J. Smoking during pregnancy and the perinatal cadmium burden. J Perinat Med 1988; 16:225–231.
12. Kuhnert PM, Kuhnert BR, Bottoms SF, Erhard P. Cadmium levels in maternal blood, fetal cord blood and placental tissues of pregnant women who smoke. Am J Obstet Gynecol 1982; 142:1021–1025.
13. Tsvetkova RP. Materials on the study of the influence of cadmium compounds on the generative function. Gig Tr Prof Zabol 1970; 14:31–33.
14. American Medical Association, Council on Scientific Affairs. Effects of toxic chemicals on the reproductive system. AMA, Chicago, 1985.
15. Laudanski T, Sipowicz M, Modzolewski P, et al. Influence of high lead and cadmium soil content on human reproductive outcome. Int J Gynecol Obstet 1991; 36:309–315.
16. Bonithon-Kopp C, Huel G, Moreau T, Wendling R. Prenatal exposure to lead and cadmium and psychomotor development of the child at 6 years. Neurobehav Toxicol Teratol 1986; 8:307–310.
17. Shiraishi Y, Yoshida TH. Chromosomal abnormalities in cultured leucocyte cells from itai-itai disease patients. Proc Jpn Acad Sci 1972; 48:248–251.
18. Shiraishi Y. Cytogenetic studies in 12 patients with itai-itai disease. Hum Gene 1975; 27:31–44.
19. Bui TH, Lindsten J, Nordberg GF. Chromosome analysis of lymphycytes from cadmium workers and itai-itai patients. Environ Res 1975; 9:187–195.
20. Leonard A, Deknudt G, Gilliavod N. Genetic and cytogenetic hazards of heavy metals in mammals. Mutat Res 1975; 29:280–281.
21. Longo LD. The biological effects of carbon monoxide on the pregnant woman, fetus and newborn infant. Am J Obstet Gynecol 1977; 129:69–103.
22. Carbon monoxide. In Reproductive Hazards of Industrial Chemicals (Barlow SM, Sullivan FM, eds). Academic Press, London, 1982, pp 178–199.
23. Caravati EM, McElwee NE, Van Trigt M, Adams C. Carbon monoxide fetotoxicity. Vet Hum Toxicol 1987; 29:460 (abst).
24. Caravati EM, Adams CJ, Joyce SM, Schafer NC. Fetal toxicity associated with maternal carbon monoxide poisoning. Ann Emerg Med 1988; 17:714–717.
25. Koren G, Sharav T, Pastuszak A, et al. A multicenter, prospective study of fetal outcome following accidental carbon monoxide poisoning in pregnancy. Reprod Toxicol 1991; 5:397–405.
26. Waterman FK. Occup Health Ont 1984; 5:10–22. Quoted in Carbon Monoxide Monograph, Reprotext Information System, Micromedex, Denver, CO, 1992.
27. Carbon monoxide. In Reprotext Information System, Micromedex, Denver, CO, 1992.
28. Bayard S, et al. GRA & I (14), 1985. Quoted in Carbon Monoxide Monograph, Reprotext Information System, Micromedex, Denver, CO, 1992.

29. Ogi D, Hamada A. Case reports on fetal deaths and malformations of extremities probably related to insecticide poisoning. J Jpn Obstet Gynecol Soc 1965; 17:569.

30. Romero P, Barnett PG, Midtling JE. Congenital anomalies associated with maternal exposure to oxydemeton-methyl. Environ Res 1989; 50:256–261.

31. Nora JJ, Nora AH, Sommerville RJ, Hill RM, McNamara DG. Maternal exposure to potential teratogens. JAMA 1967; 202:1065–1069.

32. Hall JG, Palliser PD, Clarren SK, et al. Congenital hypothalamic hamartoblastoma, hypopituitarism, imperforate anus, and postaxial polydactyly — A new syndrome? Part I: Clinical, causal and pathogenetic considerations. Am J Med Genet 1980; 7:47–74.

33. Gordon JE, Shy CM. Agricultural chemical use and congenital cleft lip and/or palate. Arch Environ Health 1981; 36:213–220.

34. Midtling JE, Barnett PG, Coye MJ, et al. Clinical management of field worker organophosphate poisoning. West J Med 1985; 142:514–518.

35. Karalliedde L, Senanayaka N, Ariaratnam A. Acute organophosphorous insecticide poisoning during pregnancy. Hum Toxicol 1988; 7:363–364.

36. Klys M, Kosun J, Pach J, Kamenczak A. Carbofuran poisoning of pregnant woman and fetus per ingestion. J Forensic Sci 1989; 34:1413–1416.

37. Whorton D, Krauss RM, Marshall S, Milby TH. Infertility in male pesticide workers. Lancet 1977; 2:1259–1261.

38. Whorton D, Milby TH, Krauss RM, Stubbs HA. Testicular function in DBCP exposed pesticide workers. J Occup Med 1979; 21:161–166.

39. Lanham JM. Nine-year follow-up of workers exposed to 1,2-dibromo-3-chloropropane. J Occup Med 1987; 29:488.

40. Potashnik G, Yanai-Inbar I. Dibromochloropropane: An 8-year reevaluation of testicular function and reproductive performance. Fertil Steril 1987; 47:317–323.

41. Eaton M, Schenker M, Whorton MD, Samuels S, Perkins C, Overstreet J. Seven-year follow-up of workers exposed to 1,2-dibromo-3-chloropropane. J Occup Med 1986; 28:1145–1150.

42. Goldsmith JR, Potashnik G, Israeli R. Reproductive outcomes in families of DBCP-exposed men. Arch Environ Health 1984; 39:85–89.

43. Potashnik G, Goldsmith J, Insler V. Dibromochloropropane-induced reduction of the sex ratio in man. Andrologia 1984; 16:213–218.

44. Potashnik G, Phillip M. Lack of birth defects among offspring conceived during or after paternal exposure to dibromochloropropane. Andrologia 1988; 20: 90–94.

45. Potashnik G, Abeliovich D. Chromosomal analysis and health status of children conceived to men during or following dibromochloropropane-induced spermatogenic suppression. Andrologia 1985; 17:291–296.

46. Kapp RW Jr, Picciano DJ, Jacobson CB. Y chromosomal nondisjunction in dibromochloropropane-exposed workmen. Mutat Res 1979; 64:47–51.

47. Kucerova M, Zhurkova VS, Polivkova Z, Ivanova JE. Mutagenic effect of epichlorhydrin. Mutat Res 1977; 48:355–360.

48. Picciano D. Cytogenic investigation of occupational exposure to epichlorohydrin. Mutat Res 1979; 66:169-173.

49. Sram RJ, Landa L, Samkova I. Effect of occupational exposure to epichlorohydrin on the frequency of chromosome aberrations in peripheral lymphocytes. Mutat Res 1983; 122:59-64.

50. John JA, Quast JF, Murray FJ, Calhoun LG, Staples RE. Inhalation toxicity of epichlorohydrin: Effects on fertility in rats and rabbits. Toxicol Appl Pharmacol 1983; 68:415-423.

51. Epichlorohydrin. In Reproductive Hazards of Industrial Chemicals (Barlow SM, Sullivan FM, eds). Academic Press, London, 1982, pp 287-295.

52. Ratcliffe JM, Elliott MJ, Wyse RK, Hunter S, Alberti KG. Semen quality in papaya workers with long-term exposure to ethylene dibromide. Br J Ind Med 1987; 44:317-326.

53. Takahashi W, Wong L, Rogers BJ, Hale RW. Depression of sperm counts among agricultural workers exposed to dibromochloropropane and ethylene dibromide. Bull Environ Contamin Toxicol 1981; 27:551-558.

54. Wong O, Utidjian HMD, Karten VS. Retrospective evaluation of reproductive performance of workers exposed to ethylene dibromide. J Occup Med 1979; 21:98-102.

55. Ter Haar G. An investigation of possible sterility and health effects from exposure to ethylene dibromide. In Ethylene Dichloride: A Potential Health Risk? (Ames B, Infante P, Reitz R, eds). Cold Spring Harbor Laboratory, Cold Spring Harbor, NY, 1980, pp 167-177.

56. Hemminki K, Mutanen P, Saloniemi I, Niemi ML, Vainio H. Spontaneous abortions in hospital staff engaged in sterilising instruments with chemical agents. Br Med J 1982; 285:1461-1463.

57. Yabukova ZN, Shamova HA, Muftaknova FA, Shilova LF. Gynecological disorders in workers engaged in ethylene oxide production. Kazan Med Zh 1976; 57:558-560.

58. Hemminki K, Kyyronen P, Lindbohm ML. Spontaneous abortions and malformations in the offspring of nurses exposed to anesthetic gases, cytostatic drugs and other potential hazards in hospitals, based on registered information of outcome. J Epidemiol Community Health 1985; 39:141-147.

59. Laurent C, Frederic J, Leonard AY. Sister chromatid exchange frequency in workers exposed to high levels of ethylene oxide, in a hospital sterilization service. Int Arch Occup Environ Health 1984; 54:33-43.

60. Stolley PD, Soper KA, Galloway SM, Nichols WW, Norman SA, Wolman SR. Sister chromatid exchanges in association with occupational exposure to ethylene oxide. Mutat Res 1984; 129:89-102.

61. Yager JW, Hines CJ, Spear RC. Exposure to ethylene oxide at work increases sister chromatid exchanges in human peripheral lymphocytes. Science 1983; 219:1221-1223.

62. Schulte PA, Boeniger M, Walker JT, et al. Biologic markers in hospital workers exposed to low levels of ethylene oxide. Mutat Res 1992; 278:237-251.

63. Lerda D, Rizzi R. Cytogenetic study of persons occupationally exposed to ethylene oxide. Mutat Res 1992; 281:31-37.

64. Savitz DA, John EM. Adverse pregnancy outcomes among cosmetologists. Gov Rep Announce Index (GRA&I) 1991; 21:92.
65. Shumilina AV. Menstrual and child-bearing functions of female workers occupationally exposed to the effects of formaldehyde. Gig Tr Prof Zabol 1975; 19: 18–21.
66. American Medical Association Council on Scientific Affairs. Effects of Toxic Chemicals on the Reproductive System. AMA, Chicago, 1985.
67. Chloroprene. In Reproductive Hazards of Industrial Chemicals (Barlow SM, Sullivan FM, eds). Academic Press, London, 1982, pp 239–252.
68. US Department of Health, Education and Welfare. Criteria document for a recommended standard: Occupational exposure to chloroprene. DHEW (NIOSH) Publication No 77-210, 1977.
69. Dowty BJ, Laseter JL, Storer J. The transplacental migration and accumulation in blood of volatile organic constituents. Pediatr Res 1976; 10:696–701.
70. Axelsson G, Lutz C, Rylander R. Exposure to solvents and outcome of pregnancy in university laboratory employees. Br J Ind Med 1984; 41:305–312.
71. Funes-Cravioto F, Kalmodin-Hedman B, Lindsten J, et al. Chromosome aberrations in chemical laboratories and a rotoprinting factory and in children of women laboratory workers. Lancet 1977; 2:322–325.
72. Strickland DM, Leonard RG, Stavchansky S, Benoit T, Wilson RT. Vaginal absorption of hexachlorophene during labor. Am J Obstet Gynecol 1983; 147: 769–772.
73. Halling H. Suspected link between exposure to hexachlorophene and malformed infants. Ann NY Acad Sci 1979; 320:326.
74. Baltzar B, Ericson A, Kallen B. Pregnancy outcome among women working in Swedish hospitals. N Engl J Med 1979; 300:627–628.
75. Hernberg S, Kurppa K, Ojajavri J, et al. Congenital malformations and occupational exposure to disinfectants: A case-referent study. Scand J Work Environ Health 1983; 9:55. Quoted in Hexachlorophene Monograph, Teris, Micromedex, Denver, CO, 1992.
76. Eskenazi B, Wyrobek AJ, Fenster L, et al. A study of the effect of perchloroethylene exposure on semen quality in dry cleaning workers. Am J Ind Med 1991; 20:575–591.
77. Eskenazi B, Fenster L, Hudes M, et al. A study of the effect of perchloroethylene exposure on the reproductive outcomes of wives of dry-cleaning workers. Am J Ind Med 1991; 20:593–600.
78. Proctor NH, Hughes JP, Fischman ML, eds. Chemical Hazards of the Workplace. Lippincott, Philadelphia, 1988, pp 399–401.
79. Laham S. Studies on placental transfer of trichloroethylene. Ind Med 1979; 39: 46–49.
80. Goldberg SJ, Lebowitz MD, Graver EJ, Hicks S. An association of human congenital cardiac malformations and drinking water contaminants. J Am Coll Cardiol 1990; 16:155–164.
81. Susan SH, Shaw G, Harris JA, Neutra RR. Congenital cardiac anomalies in relation to water contamination, Santa Clara County, California 1981-3. Am J Epidemiol 1989; 129:885–893.

82. Kimbrough RD, Mitchell FL, Houk VN. Trichloroethylene: An update. J Toxicol Environ Health 1985; 15:369–383.
83. Kostrial K, Momcilovic B. Transport of lead-203 and calcium-47 from mother to offspring. Arch Environ Health 1974; 29:28.
84. Rayegowda BK, Glass L, Evans HE. Lead concentration in newborn infants. J Pediatr 1972; 80:116.
85. Fahim MS, Fahim Z, Hall DG. Effects of subtoxic lead levels on pregnant women in the State of Missouri. In Proceedings of the International Conference on Heavy Metals in the Environment, Toronto, Ont, Canada, October 27-31, 1975.
86. Nogaki K. On action of lead on body of lead refinery workers: Particularly conception, pregnancy and parturition in case of females and on vitality of their newborn. Excerpta Med 1958; 4:2176.
87. Needelman HL, Rabinowitz M, Leviton A, Linn S, Schoenbaum S. The relationship between prenatal exposure to lead and congenital anomalies. JAMA 1984; 251:2956-2959.
88. Bellinger D, Leviton A, Waternaux C, Needelman H, Rabinowitz M. Londitudinal analysis of prenatal and postnatal lead exposure and early cognitive development. N Engl J Med 1987; 316:1037-1043.
89. Dekknudt GH, Leonard A, Ivanov B. Chromosome aberrations observed in male workers occupationally exposed to lead. Environ Physiol Biochem 1973; 3:132-138.
90. Rom WN. Effects of lead on the female reproduction: A review. Mt Sinai J Med 1976; 43:542-551.
91. McFarland RB, Reigel H. Chronic mercury poisoning from a single brief exposure. J Occup Med 1978; 20:532-534.
92. Lauwerys R, Roels H, Geret P, Toussaint G, Bouckaret A, De Cooman S. Fertility of male workers exposed to mercury vapor or to manganest dust: A questionnaire study. Am J Ind Med 1985; 7:171-176.
93. Cordier S, Deplan F, Mandereau L, Hemon D. Paternal exposure to mercury and spontaneous abortions. Obstet Gynecol Surv 1992; 47:152-154.
94. Goncharuk GA. Problems relating to occupational hygiene of women in production of mercury. Gig Tr Prof Zabol 1977; 5:17-20.
95. Panaova Z, Dimitrov G. Ovarian function in women having professional contact with metallic mercury. Akus Ginek 1974; 13:29-34.
96. Rachootin P, Olsen J. The risk of infertility and delayed conception associated with exposures in the Danish workplace. J Occup Med 1983; 25:394-402.
97. Lauwerys R, Buchet JP, Roels H, Hubermont G. Placental transfer of lead, mercury, cadmium and carbon monoxide in women. I. Comparison of the frequency biological indices in maternal and umbilical cord. Environ Res 1978; 15:278-289.
98. Lien DC, Todoruk DN, Rajani HR, Cook DA, Herbert FA. Accidental inhalation of mercury vapour: Respiratory and toxicologic consequences. Can Med Assoc J 1983; 129:591-595.
99. Baglan RJ, Brill AB, Schulert A, et al. Utility of placental tissue as an indicator of trace element exposure to adult and fetus. Environ Res 1974; 8:64-70.

100. Wannag A, Skejerasen J. Mercury accumulation in placenta and fetal membranes. A study of dental workers and their babies. Environ Physiol Biochem 1975; 5:348–352.
101. Heidam LZ. Spontaneous abortions among dental assistants, factory workers, painters and gardening workers: A follow-up study. J Epidemiol Community Health 1984; 38:149–155.
102. Brodsky JB, Cohen EN, Whitcher C, Brown BW, Wu ML. Occupational exposure to mercury in dentistry and pregnancy outcome. J Am Dent Assoc 1985; 111:779–780.
103. Goncharuk GA. Effect of chronic mercury poisoning on the immunological reactivity of offspring. Gig Tr (Kiev) 1971; 7:73–75.
104. Panova Z, Ivanova S, Promeni V. Ovarialanta funktsiia: Niakoi funktsionalni pokazateli na chernia drob pri profesionalen kontakt s metalen zhivak (purvo suobshtenie). Akush Ginekol (Sofia) 1976; 15:133–137.
105. Kurppa K, Holmberg PC, Hernberg S, Rantala K, Riala R, Nurminen T. Screening for occupational exposures and congenital anomalies. Scand J Work Environ Health 1983; 9:89–93.
106. Klinkova-Deutschor E. Teratogenni vlivy zerniho prostredi. Cesk Neurol Neurochir 1977; 40:283–291.
107. Ericson A, Kallen B. Pregnancy outcome in women working as dentists, dental assistants or dental technicians. Int Arch Occup Environ Health 1989; 61: 329–333.
108. Koos BJ, Longo LD. Mercury toxicity in the pregnant woman, fetus, and newborn infant. Am J Obstet Gynecol 1976; 126:390–409.
109. Larsson KS, Sagulin GB. Placental transfet of mercury from amalgam. Lancet 1990; 2:1251.
110. Vimy MJ, Takahashi Y, Lorscheider FL. Maternal-fetal distribution of mercury (203-Hg) released from dental amalgam fillings. Am J Physiol 1990; 258: R939–R945.
111. Mercury and its compounds. In Reproductive Hazards of Industrial Chemicals (Barlow SM, Sullivan FM, eds). Academic Press, London, 1982, pp 386–406.
112. Choi BH. Neurobiol Trace Elem 1983; 2:197–235. Quoted in Mercury Monograph, Reprotext Information System, Micromedex, Denver, CO, 1992.
113. Agocs MM, Etzel RA, Parrish RG. Mercury exposure from interior latex paint. N Engl J Med 1990; 323:1096–1101.
114. Alfonso J, DeAlvarez R. Effects of mercury on human gestation. Am J Obstet Gynecol 1960; 80:145–154.
115. Amin-Zaki L, Elhassani SB, Majeed MA, Clarkson TW, Doherty RA, Greenwood MR. Intra-uterine methylmercury poisoning in Iraq. Pediatrics 1974; 54:587–595.
116. Matsumoto H, Koya G, Takeuchi T. Fetal Minamata disease: A neuropathological study of two cases of intrauterine intoxication by a methyl mercury compound. J Neuropathol Exp Neurol 1965; 24:563–574.
117. Muramaki U. The effect of organic mercury on intrauterine life. Acta Exp Biol Med Biol 1972; 27:301–306.

118. Marsh DO, Myers GJ, Clarkson TW, Amin-Zaki L, Tikriti S, Majeed MA. Fetal methylmercury poisoning: Clinical and toxicological data on 29 cases. Ann Neurol 1980; 7:348-353.

119. Amin-Zaki L, Elhassani S, Majeed MA, et al. Perinatal methylmercury poisoning in Iraq. Am J Dis Child 1976; 130:1070-1076.

120. Strandberg M, Sandback K, Axelson O, Sundell L. Spontaneous abortions among women in hospital laboratory. Lancet 1978; 1:384-385.

121. Hemminki K, Franssilla E, Vainio H. Spontaneous abortions among female workers in Finland. Int Arch Occup Environ Health 1980; 45:123-126.

122. Lipscomb JA, Fenster L, Wrensch M, Shusterman D, Swan S. Pregnancy outcomes in women potentially exposed to occupational solvents and women working in the electronics industry. J Occup Med 1991; 33:597-604.

123. Pastides H, Calabrese EJ, Hosmer DW Jr, Harris DR Jr. Spontaneous abortion and general illness symptoms among semiconductor manufacturers. J Occup Med 1988; 30:543-551.

124. Huel G, Mergler D, Bowler R. Evidence for adverse reproductive outcomes among women microelectronic assembly workers. Br J Ind Med 1990; 47:400-404.

125. Lindbohm ML, Taskinen H, Sallmen M, Hemminki K. Spontaneous abortions among women exposed to organic solvents. Am J Ind Med 1990; 17:449-463.

126. Heidan LZ. Spontaneous abortions among factory workers. The importance of gravidity control. Scand J Soc Med 1983; 11:81-85.

127. Axelson G, Liutz C, Rylander R. Exposure to solvents and outcome of pregnancy in university laboratory employees. Br J Ind Med 1984; 41:305-312.

128. Holmberg PC, Nurminen M. Congenital defects of the central nervous system and occupational factors during pregnancy. Am J Ind Med 1980; 1:167-176.

129. Hansson E, Jansa S, Wande H, Kàllén B, Östlund E. Pregnancy outcome for women working in laboratories in some of the pharmaceutical industries in Sweden. Scand J Work Environ Health 1980; 6:131-134.

130. Rantala K, Riala R, Nurminen T. Screening for occupational exposures and congenital malformations. Scand J Work Environ Health 1983; 9:89-93.

131. Tikkanen J, Heinonen OP. Maternal exposure to chemical and physical factors during pregnancy and cardiovascular malformations in the offspring. Teratology 1991; 43:591-600.

132. Feldman RJ, Maibach HI. Percutaneous penetration of some pesticide and herbicides in man. Toxicol Appl Pharmacol 1974; 28:126-132.

133. Saxena MC, Siddiqui MK, Bhargava AK, Seth TD, Krishnamurti CR, Kutty D. Role of chlorinated hydrocarbon pesticides in abortions and premature labour. Toxicology 1980; 17:323-331.

134. Yoshimura M. Kinki Daigaku Igaku Zasshi 1979; 4:209-218. Quoted in Lindane Monograph, Reprotext Information System, Micromedex, Denver, CO, 1992.

135. Saxena MC. Arch Toxicol 1984; 48:127-134. Quoted in Lindane Monograph, Reprotext Information System, Micromedex, Denver, CO, 1992.

136. Ilina VI, Bleckherman NA. Deiaki dani pro stan stetsyfichnykh funktsii zhino-choho orhanizmu v osib iaki pratsiuiut, z heksakhlortsykloheksanom. Pediatr Akush Ginekol 1974; 1:46–49. Quoted in Lindane Monograph, Reprotext Information System, Micromedex, Denver, CO, 1992.

137. Verzhanskii PS. Gumoral n regul rodovoi deyat lech EE. Narushenii 1976; 88–91. Quoted in Lindane Monograph, Reprotext Information System, Micromedex, Denver, CO, 1992.

138. Wassermann M, Ron N, Bercovici B, Wassermann D, Cucos S, Pines A. Premature delivery and organochlorine compounds: Polychlorinated biphenyls and some organochlorine insecticides. Environ Res 1982; 28:106–112.

139. Curley A, Copeland MF, Kimbrough RD. Chlorinated hydrocarbon insecticides in organs of stillborn and blood of newborn babies. Arch Environ Health 1969; 19:628–632.

140. Poradovsky K, Rosival L, Meszarosova A. Transplacentarny prienik pesticidov pocas fuziologickej tehotnosti. Cesk Gynekol 1977; 42:405–410.

141. Tomczak S, Baumann K, Lehnert G. Occupational exposure to hexachlorocyclohexane. IV. Sex hormone alterations in HCH-exposed workers. Int Arch Occup Environ Health 1981; 48:283–287.

142. Cranz C. Contraception Fertil Sex 1981; 9:421–423. Quoted in Lindane Monograph, Reprotext Information System, Micromedex, Denver, CO, 1992.

143. Cariati E, Acanfora L, Branconi F, Bigazzi Grasso C, Capri R, Grasso G, *p,p*-DDT in perinatal samples: Report on maternal and neonatal measurements. Biol Res Pregnancy Perinatol 1983; 4:169–171.

144. Siddiqui MKJ, Saxena MC, Bhargava AK, Murti CRK, Kutty D. Chlorinated hydrocarbon pesticides in blood of newborn babies in India. Pestic Monit J 1981; 15:77–79.

145. Saxena MC, Siddiqui MK, Agarwal V, Kutty D. A comparison of organochlorine insecticide contents in specimens of maternal blood, placenta and umbilical-cord blood from stillborn and live-born cases. J Toxicol Environ Health 1983; 11:71–79.

146. Leoni V, Fabiani L, Marinelli G, et al. PCB and other organochlorine compounds in blood of women with or without miscarriage: A hypothesis of correlation. Ecotoxicol Environ Saf 1989; 17:1–11.

147. Ron M, Cucos B, Rosenn B, Hochner-Colnikier D, Ever-Hadani P, Pines A. Maternal and fetal serum levels of organochlorine compounds in cases of premature rupture of membranes. Acta Obstet Gynecol Scand 1988; 67:695–697.

148. O'Leary JA, Davies JE, Feldman M. Spontaneous abortion and human pesticide residues of DDT and DDE. Am J Obstet Gynecol 1970; 108:1291–1291.

149. LeMarchand L, Kolonel LN, Siegel BZ, Dendle WH. Trends in birth defects for a Hawaiian population exposed to heptachlor and for the United States. Arch Environ Health 1986; 41:145–148.

150. Chadduck WM, Gollin SM, Gray BA, Norris JJ, Araez CA, Tryka AF. Gliosarcoma with chromosome abnormalities in a neonate exposed to heptachlor. Neurosurgery 1987; 21:557–559.

151. Ahmed FE, Hart RW, Lewis NJ. Pesticide induced DNA damage and its repair in cultured human cells. Mutat Res 1977; 42:161–174.
152. Kuntz WD. The pregnant woman in industry. Am J Ind Hyd Assoc 1976; 37: 423–426.
153. Kuratsure M, Yoshimura Y, Matsuzaka J, Yamagushi A. Epidemiologic study on Yusho, a poisoning caused by ingestion of rice oil contaminated with a commercial brand of polychlorinated biphenyls. Environ Health Perspect 1972; 1:119–128.
154. Miller RW. Congenital PCB poisoning: A reevaluation. Environ Health Perspect 1985; 60:211–214.
155. Kodama H, Ota H. Studies on the transfer of PCB to infants from their mothers. Jpn J Hyg 1977; 32:567–573.
156. Funatsu I, Yamashita F, Ito Y, et al. Polychlorbiphenyls (PCB) induced fetopathy. I. Clinical observation. Kurume Med J 1972; 19:43–51.
157. Taki I, Hisanaga S, Amagase Y. Report on Yusho (chlorobiphenyls poisoning) in pregnant women and their fetuses. Fukuoko Acta Med 1969; 60:471–474.
158. Yamashita F. Clinical features of polychlorobiphenyls (PCB)-induced fetopathy. Paediatrician 1977; 6:20–27.
159. Gladen BC, Taylor JS, Wu YC, Ragan NB, Rogan WJ, Hsu CC. Dermatological findings in children exposed transplacentally to heat-degraded polychlorinated biphenyls in Taiwan. Br J Dermatol 1990; 122:799–808.
160. Rogan WJ, Gladen BC, Hung KL, et al. Congenital poisoning by polychlorinated biphenyls and their contaminants in Taiwan. Science 1988; 241:334–336.
161. Rogan WJ, Gladen BC, McKinaly JD, et al. Neonatal effects of transplacental exposure to PCBs and DDE. J Pediatr 1986; 109:335–341.
162. Yu M, Hsu C, Gladen BC, Rogan WJ. In utero PCB/PCDF exposure: Relation of developmental delay to dysmorphology and dose. Neurotoxicol Teratol 1991; 13:195–202.
163. Fein GG, Jacobson JL, Jacobson SW, Schwartz PM, Dowler JK. Prenatal exposure to polychlorinated biphenyls effects on birth size and gestational age. J Pediatr 1984; 105:315–320.
164. Jacobson JL, Jacobson SW, Humphrey HEB. Effects of in utero exposure to polychlorinated biphenyls and related contaminants and cognitive functioning in young children. J Pediatr 1990; 116:38–45.
165. Taylor PR, Lawrence CE, Hwang HL, Paulson AS. Polychlorinated biphenyls' influence on birthweight and gestation. Am J Publ Health 1984; 74:1153–1154.
166. Letz G. The toxicology of PCBs — An overview for clinicians. West J Med 1983; 138:534–540.
167. Weil WB, Spencer M, Benjamin D, Seagull E. The effect of polybrominated biphenyl on infants and young children. J Pediatr 1981; 98:47–51.
168. Polrovskii VA. Gig Tr Prof Zabol 1967; 11:17–20. Quoted in Styrene Monograph, Reprotext Information System, Micromedex, Denver, CO, 1992.
169. Zlobina NS, Izyumora AS, Ragule NY. The effect of low styrene concentrations on the specific functions of the female organism. Gig Tr Prof Zabol 1975; 12:21–25.

170. Lemasters GK, Hagen A, Samuels SJ. Reproductive outcomes in women exposed to solvents in 36 reinforced plastics companies. I. Menstrual dysfunction. J Occup Med 1985; 27:490–494.

171. Harkonen H, Tola S, Korkala ML, Hernberg S. Congenital malformations, mortality and styrene exposure. Ann Acad Med Singaport 1984; 13(2 suppl): 404–407.

172. Meretoja T, Vainio H, Sorsa M, Harkonen H. Occupational styrene exposure and chromosomal aberrations. Mutat Res 1977; 56:193–197.

173. Meretoja T, Jarventaus H, Sorsa M, Vainio H. Chromosome aberrations in lymphocytes of workers exposed to styrene. Scand J Work Environ Health 1978; 4(suppl 2):259–264.

174. Nordenson I, Beckmann L. Chromosomal aberrations in lymphocytes of workers exposed to low levels of styrene. Hum Hered 1984; 34:178–182.

175. Mastroiacovo P, Spagrolo A, Marni E, Meazza L, Bertollini R, Segni G. Birth defects in the Seveso area after TCDD contamination. JAMA 1988; 259:1668–1672.

176. Tognoi G, Bonaccarsi A. Epidemiological problems with TCDD (a critical review). Drug Metab Rev 1982; 13:447–469.

177. Friedman JM. Does agent orange cause birth defects? Teratology 1984; 29:193–221.

178. Donovan JW, MacLennan R, Adena M. Vietnam service and the risk of congenital anomalies. A case-control study. Med J Aust 1984; 140:394–397.

179. Erickson JD, Mulinare J, McClaim PW, et al. Vietnam veterans' risk for fathering babies with birth defects. JAMA 1984; 252:903–912.

180. Townsend JD, Bodner KM, Van Peenen PFD, Olson RD, Cook RR. Survey of reproductive events of wives of employees exposed to chlorinated dioxins. Am J Epidemiol 1982; 115:695–713.

181. Walker AE. A preliminary report of a vascular abnormality occurring in men engaged in the manufacture of polyvinyl chloride. Br J Dermatol 1975; 93:22–23.

182. Walker AE. Clinical aspects of vinyl chloride disease: Skin. Proc R Soc Med 1976; 69:286–289.

183. Infante PF, McMichael AJ, Wagoner JK, Waxweiler RJ, Falk H. Genetic risks of vinyl chloride. Lancet 1976; 1:734–735.

184. Buffer PA. Some problems involved in recognizing teratogens used in industry. Contrib Epidemiol Biostat 1979; 1:118–137.

185. Paddle GM. Genetic risks of vinyl chloride. Lancet 1976; 1:1079.

186. Sanotsky IV, Davtian RM, Glushchenko VI. Study of the reproductive function in men exposed to chemicals. Gig Tr Prof Zabol 1980; 5:28–32.

187. Lindbohm M, Hemminki K, Kyyronen P. Spontaneous abortions among women employed in the plastics industry. Am J Ind Med 1985; 8:579–586.

188. Mur JM, Manderean L, Deplan F, Paris A. Richard A, Hemon D. Spontaneous abortion and exposure to vinyl chloride. Lancet 1992; 339:127–128.

189. Infante PF. Oncogenic and mutagenic risks in communities with polyvinyl chloride production facilities. Ann NY Acad Sci 1976; 271:49–57.

190. Edmonds LD, Falk H, Nissim JE. Congenital malformations and vinyl chloride. Lancet 1975; 2:1098.

191. Edmonds LD, Anderson CE, Flynt JW, James LM. Congenital central nervous system malformations and vinyl chloride monomer exposure: A community study. Teratology 1978; 17:137–142.
192. Hemminki K, Vineis P. Extrapolation of the evidence on teratogenicity of chemicals between humans and experimental animals: Chemicals other than drugs. Teratogen Carcinog Mutagen 1985; 5:251–318.
193. Theriault G, Iturra H, Gingras S. Evaluation of the association between birth defects and exposure to ambient vinyl chloride. Teratology 1983; 27:359–370.
194. Vinyl chloride. In Reproductive Hazards of Industrial Chemicals (Barlow SM, Sullivan FM, eds). Academic Press, London, 1982, pp 566–582.

20

The Common Occupational Exposures Encountered by Pregnant Women

Yedidia Bentur
Rambam Medical Center, Technion–Israel Institute of Technology,
Haifa, Israel

Gideon Koren
The Hospital for Sick Children, University of Toronto, Toronto,
Ontario, Canada

Clinical Case

A woman working in a word processing center was told by her girlfriend that exposure to video terminals may have adverse effects on fetal life. Your patient, who has just learned that she is pregnant, depends very much on this job as her husband is unemployed.

INTRODUCTION

It is clear from animal experiments and human epidemiological studies that industrial chemicals have the potential of being reproductive toxins. However, our knowledge of the reproductive toxicology of industrial chemicals in humans is sparse or absent. Before therapeutic agents are marketed, their teratogenic potential must be tested in animals; these data are not always required for chemicals. Other factors also may differ between medical and occupational exposures. In the workplace the exposure is usually to several chemicals, which may change between working days or even within a single day. In some cases one has to deal with possible unknown by-products. The amounts of the chemicals absorbed are often unclear, and the circumstances

---

Modified from the authors' article in the American Journal of Obstetrics and Gynecology 1991; 165(2):429–437, with permission.

of exposure may vary from plant to plant or even within the same operation. Every chemical in the workplace has safety exposure limits aiming at protecting the worker. However, these standards were not designed to protect the fetus. Hence, even if one can obtain exposure levels, one is never sure whether safe levels to the mother are also safe for her unborn baby; lead is a good example of such a discrepancy (1,2). An interesting attempt to approach this problem is illustrated by a recent study that suggested 20 ppm as a pregnancy guidance value for occupational exposure to toluene (3). This choice was based on "no observable adverse effect level" (NOAEL) of 500, 400, and 200 ppm in pregnant rabbits, rats, and mice and their offspring, respectively, and applying safety factors for interspecies and intraspecies variation.

In approaching the occupationally exposed woman, the following steps are suggested:

1. Obtain medical, obstetric, and genetic history from the patient and her spouse, including the use of cigarettes, alcohol, and drugs.
2. Identify the chemicals in question, if possible, by their material safety data sheets (MSDS).
3. Obtain a detailed description of the process the patient is operating, the work she performs, the length of exposure, and the means of protection used (ventilation system, hood, respirator, mask, gown, gloves, etc.).
4. Obtain information on possible exposure from nearby work stations.
5. Identify symptoms and signs reported to be associated with the chemicals and temporal relationship to the exposure.
6. Rule out underlying conditions that may cause a similar clinical picture (e.g., morning sickness).
7. Determine whether there are symptoms and signs manifest in fellow workers?
8. Ascertain the pregnancy outcome in other workers.
9. Obtain occupational history of the spouse.
10. Obtain the most recent levels of the chemicals in question or radiation measured in that particular area and their relation to the recommended threshold limit value-time-weighted average (TLV-TWA).
11. Find out whether employees are being regularly examined by an occupational physician and whether biological monitoring is done (e.g., blood lead levels, urinary phenol excretion, blood count for benzene, hepatic aminotransferase for carbon tetrachloride).
12. Try to understand the attitude of the woman and her supervisors toward her particular work and toward a possible change of job. Will a change of job affect her income or chances for promotion?
13. Search as many data sources as possible and evaluate the data critically to allow the patient to receive the most accurate information.

14. Convey the information to the patient, estimate the risk (if possible), and advise about ways to assess severity of exposure (environmental and biological measurements) and on possible safety means to reduce exposure (ventilation, mask, gloves, etc.).

The Motherisk Program in Toronto is an antenatal counseling service for health professionals, women, and their families, dealing with exposures to drugs, chemicals, radiation, and infections in pregnancy and lactation. In 1990 between 40 and 50 telephone calls were processed daily. Women are referred to a clinic if they have been exposed to known or suspected teratogens, long-term drug therapy, new drugs on which there is sparse or no information, and drugs of abuse, or if they have experienced occupational exposure. After the expected day of confinement, follow-up of pregnancy outcome is performed, and all data are computerized for clinical and research use. In 1988, 5040 telephone calls were received; 167 (3.3%) of them were due to occupational exposures to video display terminals (Table 1). This exposure is the one most frequently encountered in the workplace. Organic solvents were the concern of up to 150 of the callers, most of them entailing the use of oil-based paints, some of them at home. In 56 the exposure to organic solvents occurred in the workplace, and 24 of them were followed in the clinic (Table 2). Twenty-nine patients were advised for exposure to lead (mostly in the form of paints); six were occupationally exposed, and three were seen in the clinic.

The Drugs and Chemicals in Pregnancy Program in Haifa, Israel, was established in 1991 and is affiliated to the Israel Poison Information Center. Its objectives are similar to those of the Motherisk Program in Toronto; however, it is mainly oriented to poisoning, radiation, chemical, and occupational exposures in pregnancy. An important referring center is the Israel Teratological Counselling Service in Jerusalem. In addition to textbooks, the Drugs and Chemicals in Pregnancy Program uses several computerized databases including Drugdex, Poisindex, Hazardous Substances Data Bank, Registry of Toxic Effects of Chemical Substances, Reprotext, Reprotox, TERIS, Shepard's Catalog of Teratogenic Agents—online, Canadian Centre for Occupational Health and Safety—CCINFO, and Medline. In its first year of operation, 18 occupationally exposed patients were consulted, and

Table 1 Distribution of Telephone Consultations for Occupational Exposures in 1988

Number of consultations	Exposure			
	Video display terminal	Organic solvents	Lead	Miscellaneous
5040	167	56	6	13

Table 2 Distribution of Occupational Exposures with Clinic Follow-Up in 1988

	Number of cases	Total clinic visits (%)[a]	Occupational exposures seen in clinic (%)[b]
Organic solvents[c]	24	6.3	66.6
Video display terminals[d]	5	1.3	13.8
Lead[e]	3	0.8	8.3
Polychlorinated biphenyls	2	0.5	5.5
Miscellaneous[f]	5	1.3	13.8

[a]A total of 380 patients were seen in the clinic.
[b]Thirty-six patients with occupational exposures were monitored in the clinic.
[c]Two patients were exposed to organic solvents and lead.
[d]Four patients came to the clinic because of drug exposure.
[e]Two patients were exposed to lead and organic solvents.
[f]Each patient was exposed to multiple chemicals; no organic solvents.

27 in the first 6 months of 1992. The three most common exposures were organic solvents (42%), ionizing radiation (11%), and pesticides (9%). Most of the women occupationally exposed to organic solvents and all those exposed to ionizing radiation were laboratory technicians (academic or industrial). Those exposed to pecticides were involved in various agricultural tasks.

Different distribution of occupations among women and lack of awareness to reports on the use of video display terminals in pregnancy may explain the different pattern of calls between the programs in the two countries.

This chapter reviews the state of our knowledge on the reproductive hazards of these exposures and gives the clinician up-to-date information with which to advise women.

EXPOSURES

Video Display Terminals

For discussion of this subject, the reader is referred to Chapter 22: Ionizing and Nonionizing Radiation in Pregnancy.

Organic Solvents

In our clinics we often counsel women who are occupationally exposed to numerous chemicals, most of which are organic solvents. A proper consultation in such cases is extremely difficult, because it is hard to estimate the predominant chemicals and their by-products. Even if one identifies the more toxic agents, it is still hard to assess the circumstances of exposure. For many chemicals one can measure neither airborne nor blood levels. Smelling the odor of organic solvents is not indicative of a significant exposure, because the olfactory nerve can detect levels as low as several parts per million, which are not necessarily associated with toxicity. For example, the odor threshold of toluene is 0.8 ppm, whereas TLV-TWA is 100 ppm. Finally, reproductive information on many solvents is at best sparse: either limited to animal studies or nonexistent.

Organic solvents are a structurally diverse group of low molecular weight chemicals that are liquids and are able to dissolve other organic substances (4). They are ubituitous in our industrialized society, both at work and at home, and they may be encountered as individual agents or in complex mixtures such as gasoline. Chemicals in the solvent class include aliphatic hydrocarbons (such as mineral spirits, varnish, and kerosene), aromatic hydrocarbons (benzene, toluene, xylene), halogenated hydrocarbons (carbon tetrachloride, trichloroethylene, methylcellosolve), aliphatic alcohols (acetone), glycols (ethylene glycol), and glycol ethers (methoxyethanol) (5,6). Fuels are mixtures of various hydrocarbons.

The mechanisms by which many solvents exert their toxicity are unclear and may vary from one solvent to another. Halogenated hydrocarbons such as carbon tetrachloride may general free radicals (4). Simple aromatic compounds such as benzene may disrupt polyribosomes (7), whereas some solvents are thought to affect lipid membranes and to penetrate tissues such as the brain.

Incidental exposures may include vapors from gasoline, lighter fluid, spot removers, aerosol sprays, and paints (8). The short duration, low level exposures may go undetected. More serious exposures occur mainly in industrial or laboratory settings during such manufacturing and processing operations as dry cleaning, working with paint removers, thinners, floor and tile cleaners, and glues, and using laboratory reagents. Gasoline or glue sniffing, although not occurring in the occupational setting, is another source of exposure to organic solvents during pregnancy.

Workers with short-term exposure to organic solvents experience fatigue, concentration disorder, feelings of drunkenness, dizziness, pneumonitis, and vomiting (5). Long-term exposure (e.g., to benzene) may irreversibly affect the central nervous system and liver and may cause blood disorders.

Although the toxic effects of organic solvents are relatively well known in the adult, there is a paucity of information on the impact of in utero exposure.

In 1988 the Motherisk patient population included 150 (2.9%) cases of telephone counseling and 24 clinical consultations dealing with organic solvents (Tables 1 and 2). Most of the occupationally exposed women were seen in the clinic, and most of them were involved in manufacturing, processing, and application of paints and glues. Others were machinists, laboratory technicians, and dry cleaners.

It is beyond the scope of this chapter to review all the organic solvents, so we chose toluene as an illustrative example of exposure. This agent is used in a variety of mixtures and products. Also important, it is a common substance of abuse. Toluene is an aromatic hydrocarbon used as a solvent for paints, thinners, coatings, and glues (5). It is a popular replacement for the more chronically toxic benzene solvents. Most exposures involve inhalation; however, absorption is almost complete after oral administration (5). Toluene inhalation by pregnant rats induced decreased fetal weight and retardation of skeletal growth (9,10). No malformations were demonstrated in rats or mice after inhalation (10,11), but oral administration to mice induced cleft palate (12). Fetal neuromotor abnormalities may be induced by inhalation of 800 mg/m^3 of toluene (more than twice the TLV-TWA) by pregnant rats (13). However, subcutaneous injection of toluene (1.2 g/kg) to rats did not result in behavioral changes (10). A study from 1977 compared pregnancy outcomes among 168 women occupationally exposed to varnishes containing toluene (55 ppm) with those of 201 control women (14). While there were twice as many low birth weight infants in the toluene-exposed group, the two groups did not differ with regard to fertility, course of pregnancy, perinatal mortality, or adverse effects in the newborn. Unfortunately, congenital defects were not evaluated. It was suggested that occupational exposure to aromatic solvents, mainly to toluene, may be associated with various birth defects, predominantly renal-urinary or gastrointestinal (15). Toluene-exposed shoe workers had a higher rate of spontaneous abortions: odds ratio 9.3, 95% confidence interval (CI) 1.0–84.7 (16). Chinese shoe workers exposed to toluene and benzene had a significantly higher rate of menstrual disorders and spontaneous abortions (17). Abuse of large quantities of pure toluene by inhalation throughout pregnancy was reported to result in microcephaly, central nervous system (CNS) dysfunction, minor craniofacial anomalies, and variable growth deficiencies in three patients (18). These features resembled the pattern of malformations described in connection with exposure to alcohol or certain anticonvulsant medications and were named "fetal solvent syndrome." More features of toluene embryopathy are discussed at the end of this section.

Many organic solvents are teratogenic and embryotoxic in laboratory animals, depending on specific solvent, dose, route of administration, and animal species (4,7). Malformations described include hydrocephaly, exencephaly, skeletal defects, cardiovascular abnormalities, and blood changes. Other abnormalities include poor fetal development and neurodevelopmental deficits. In some of the studies exposure levels were high enough to induce maternal toxicity.

Because of the complexity and diversity of organic solvents and because exposure usually involves more than one agent and different circumstances, adequate human epidemiological studies are difficult to conduct and interpret. In addition, studies are subjected to recall and response bias and are not always controlled for other risk factors (age, smoking, etc.). Isolated case reports suggesting that solvent-related embryopathy may occur in humans have appeared for many years. In one report five of nine women who gave birth to infants with caudal regression syndrome had been exposed to solvents, including xylene, trichoroethylene, methylchloride, acetone, and gasoline (19). These agents do not belong to the same subgroup of organic solvents, and it is impossible to identify the potential culprit.

Several epidemiological studies suggested association between adverse pregnancy outcome and exposure to organic solvents. Although these solvents may have common chemical features, there is no indication that they were teratogenic as a group or individually. These studies reported esophageal stenosis or atresia in babies of female laboratory workers (20), omphalocele or gastroschisis in offspring of mothers in the printing industry (21), and an association between increased risk of malformations and laboratory work in the pharmaceutical and paper industries (22,23). Case control studies of central nervous system defects in Finland showed an association with organic solvents (24,25). However, when the study was extended for 3 more years the authors could not prove this association (26). A study based on occupational titles in Denmark suggested that malformations of the CNS were related to fathers exposed to solvents and employed as painters (odds ratio 2.8 and 4.9, respectively) (27). A cumulative case referent study covering 3.5 years suggested an association of organic solvents with cleft palate (28). The prevalence of exposure to organic solvents at work during the first trimester was 10.4% among 569 mothers of children with cardiovascular malformation, compared with 7.8% in the control group (29). This retrospective study found an adjusted relative odds ratio of 1.3 for cardiovascular malformations and 1.5 for ventricular septal defects, both probably insignificant. In 1991 this group published assessments of risk factors for cardiovascular defects in general and ventricular septal defect (VSD) specifically in Finland and again found no significant association with exposure at work to organic solvents (30,31). Maternal alcohol consumption during the first trimester was more common among mothers of VSD infants than among controls (47 vs. 38%, respectively, $p < 0.05$) (31). A study from California could not demonstrate any difference in neurobehavioral development and growth between children exposed in utero to organic solvents and a group of matched, unexposed children (32). Another study published by the same group suggested an association between exposure to organic solvents and preeclampsia (33). No correlation was found between laboratory work and sister chromatid exchanges and micronuclei in 59 Canadian laboratory workers (34). There was, however, an association between such exchange and recent or past smoking.

Spontaneous abortions were reported in 262 factory workers in Denmark; when controlled for gravidity, however, there was no longer a statistically significant increased risk (35). No increased risk for miscarriage was found in university laboratory workers exposed to organic solvents (36). Conversely, shift work in these workers was related to a higher miscarriage rate (relative risk 3.2). This study did not demonstrate any differences in perinatal death rates or in the prevalence of malformations among women working with organic solvents when compared with controls. Spontaneous abortions were found among women exposed to organic solvents during their work in a hospital laboratory (37), in electronic plants (38,39), in photolithography areas in the semiconductor industry (40), and in microelectronic equipment assembly plants (41). In the latter study, the odds ratio of spontaneous abortions, which was 0.9 before the women began to assemble microelectronic components, increased to 5.6 after the commencement of this employment. However, many of these studies are limited by recall bias, small sample size, wide confidence intervals, and variable exposures, which in many cases are not quantitated. In this respect, it is interesting to mention Lindbohm's study, which examined the rate of medically diagnosed spontaneous abortions among women occupationally exposed to at least one of six organic solvents (styrene, trichlorothylene, xylene, tetrachlorothylene, toluene and 1,1,1-trichloroethane) who were also biologically monitored (42). Reference values of hygiene standards were exceeded in 38% of styrene exposures and were reached in 15% of tetrachloroethylene exposures. The adjusted odds ratio of spontaneous abortions for solvent exposure was significantly increased (2.2, 95% CI 1.2–4.1), especially for exposure to aliphatic hydrocarbons (3.9, 95% CI 1.1–14.2), for graphics workers (5.5, 95% CI 1.3–20.8), and for toluene-exposed shoe workers (9.3, 95% CI 1.0–84.7). Confounding factors, again, are small sample size and multiple exposures in some cases. Association of spontaneous abortions with exposure to aliphatic hydrocarbons, but not with the use of solvents as a group was also suggested in a large case control study (43). In a case referent study, the odds ratio of spontaneous abortions was increased by paternal exposure to several organic solvents, maternal exposure to organic solvents, and maternal heavy lifting (44). The cohort was too small to permit the evaluation of the effect of these parameters on congenital malformations.

A discussion of organic solvents would be incomplete without mentioning the fetal solvent (or gasoline) syndrome. In 1979 a syndrome of anomalies (hypertonia, scaphocephaly, mental retardation, and other CNS effects) was suggested in two children in a small American Indian community where gasoline sniffing and alcohol abuse are common (45). Four other children had similar abnormalities, but in their cases it was impossible to verify gasoline sniffing. It is unclear what was the contribution of the lead in the gasoline or the alcohol abuse in producing these abnormalities. In another case, a child with nearly classic fetal alcohol syndrome was born to a mother with major addiction to solvents, mainly toluene (46). Heavy alcohol consumption was also reported in that woman, and the authors questioned a possible interaction between solvents and alcohol. Toluene embryopathy was described in two additional children whose mothers probably did not abuse alcohol (47). Paint sniffing, namely toluene, resulted in severe renal tubular acidosis in five pregnant women (48). Fetal heart rate tracing and dynamic ultrasonographic examinations were normal in four of five. Three neonates exhibited growth retardation, and two had anomalies and hyperchloremic acidosis. Renal tubular acidosis was observed in more than half the women who abused toluene, especially in the long duration abusers (48). This study showed that among 21 newborns exposed to toluene in utero, preterm delivery, perinatal death, and growth retardation were significantly increased. Developmental delay was a common finding in these children. Another publication reported on two neonates with transient renal tubular dysfunction due to maternal toluene sniffing throughout the pregnancies. These infants were dysmature and had some dysmorphic features (50). It is important to remember that the mothers in many of these cases showed signs of solvent toxicity, indicating heavy exposure. In our experience this is not the case in most occupational exposures during pregnancy.

In summary, although causation is not fully established, one cannot ignore the relatively large number of studies suggesting that organic solvents may have the potential to induce spontaneous abortions. Two ongoing studies in the semiconductor industry (IBM and Johns-Hopkins Hospital, the Semiconductor Industry Association, and University of Davis, California) may shed more light on this issue. It appears also that congenital malformations cannot be excluded as a reproductive hazard. However, it is hard to prove or quantitate this suspicion, certainly not for solvents as a group. One may even expect that a ubiquitous exposure to solvents would by chance alone be associated with an increase in birth defects, which may differ from one study to another. While fetal toxicity is biologically sensible in cases of intoxicated mothers, the evidence of fetal damage from levels that are not toxic to the mother is scanty, inconsistent, or missing.

Lead

The third most common occupational exposure in pregnancy encountered by the Canadian investigators was lead. It accounted for 29 (0.6%) of the telephone consultations provided by the Motherisk Program during 1988. Three of them were followed up in the Motherisk Clinic (Tables 1 and 2). The vast majority of lead exposures involved artists using glass staining techniques or workers in the paint manufacturing sector of the automotive and aircraft industries. Other occupational sources of lead exposure during pregnancy reported in the literature include the printing, smeltering, and battery industries (51). Not only is lead an occupational hazard, it also can enter the body from contaminated soil and drinking water (52), by residence close to industrial areas or from a lead-exposed spouse (53), and by consumption of moonshine whisky (54).

Although it seems that blood lead levels in the United States are declining (55), levels are now being considered toxic at a much lower range than in the past [$< 10 \mu g/dL$ in children (56); and $< 40 \mu g/dL$ in adults (57)]. Lead intoxication is still a hazard in the industrialized countries, and pregnant women are at risk.

Lead crosses the placenta (58,59), possibly by both passive diffusion and active transport (59), and it is unclear whether placental permeability to lead is constant throughout gestation (58,60–62). Transplacental transfer of lead has been shown in the human fetus as early as 12–14 weeks of gestation, along with increasing amounts of lead in fetal tissues with advancing gestational age (63). Fetal bone and liver may have higher lead concentrations than maternal tissues (64). Calciotropic factors determine the uptake and storage of lead in the bone compartment. Thus, pregnancy-induced changes in calcium-related regulatory factors may result in mobilization of lead from the bone to more bioavailable compartments in the mother and fetus (51,65). Iron deficiency may further increase the susceptibility to lead toxicity.

During the late 19th and early 20th centuries women in the pottery and white lead industries used lead as an abortifacient (51). European studies from that time found infertility, abortion, stillbirth, fetal death, and microcephaly to be associated with industrial lead exposure (53,66–69). Even paternal lead exposure was found as early as 1860 to affect fertility and viability of the offspring (70). Wives of lead workers were reported to have more abortions, stillbirths, and premature births than women in the general population (53,71). Consequently, the employment of women in plants involving a lead hazard was forbidden (72). Although these studies should be evaluated with consideration of the high fetal and neonatal loss for other working women at that time (73), most of the studies from the 1950s and later confirmed the early observations. For example, a study comparing the course and lead values in 249 pregnancies in Columbia, Missouri, with 253 occurring at the center of America's lead belt at Rolla, Missouri, showed that 96% versus only 70% were delivered at term (74). In addition, 17% of the lead-exposed pregnancies had premature rupture of membranes, as compared with only 1% in the non-exposed group. Maternal and fetal blood lead levels in the cases of premature membrane rupture and preterm delivery were higher than in controls. Significantly higher lead concentrations were found in membranes of patients with stillbirths and preterm births, but there was a low correlation between membrane and antenatal blood lead concentrations (75). A detailed Japanese study showed an increase in spontaneous abortions among female lead workers from a prelead rate of 45.6 per 1000 to 84.2 per 1000 (the rate in nonexposed employees was 59.1 per 1000) (76). A Danish study showed that when lead was used as an abortifacient, 60% of the pregnancies in the first trimester ended in abortion (77). Moreover, women with a history of childhood lead poisoning were suggested to be at higher relative risk (RR) for having spontaneous abortions or stillbirths (RR, 1.6; 95% CI, 0.6–4.0) and having children with learning disabilities (RR, 3.0; 95% CI, 0.9–10.2) (78). A dose-dependent decrease in hypothalamic gonadotropin-releasing hormone and somatostatin was found in lead-treated guinea pigs and their fetuses (79). Although the relevance of these changes is unclear, they may partially explain decreased reproductive capacity.

A study from Boston (4354 cases) suggested that lead may be associated, in a dose-related fashion, with an increased risk for minor anomalies (80). The relative risk increased from 1.0 at 0.7 μg/dL to 2.73 at the level of 24 μg/dL. The anomalies discovered did not have a specific pattern and were of little health consequence. They included hemangiomas (14 of 1000 births), hydrocele (27.6 of 1000 male infants), minor skin anomalies (12.2 of 1000 births), and undescended testicles (11 of 1000 male infants).

Lead also affects the male gonads; chromosomal alterations, as well as abnormalities in sperm count, vigor, and morphological features were demonstrated in workers and experimental animals (81–83). Marital life records of lead-exposed men showed 24.7% of the marriages to be infertile compared with 14.8% in the nonlead control group. The rate of prematurity or stillbirth was 8.2%, whereas in the control group it was 0.2% (83). In a case referent study, a significant increase in spontaneous abortions was found in the wives of workers occupationally exposed to lead whose blood level was greater than 1.5 μmol/L (31 μg/dL) during or close to the time of spermatogenesis (84).

Although increased numbers of chromosomal aberrations (gaps, breaks, fragments, chromatid aberrations) have been reported in lead workers, the contribution of lead itself is still unclear (51).

Lead also seemed to have a small but demonstrable association with pregnancy-induced hypertension and elevated blood pressure at the time of delivery, but not with preeclampsia (85,86).

One of the main concerns regarding lead is its ability to cause neuropsychological impairment in children. In the late 1970s half the children in the United States under 5 years of age had blood lead levels exceeding 20 μg/dL, and among urban black children the figure approached 60% (87). At this level a variety of enzymatic and neurophysiological processes are impaired. Until recently, it was unclear at what level deficits in children's learning and behavior become apparent, nor was the contribution of in utero exposure clearly identified. In a series of studies from Boston (1,2), blood lead levels and development were monitored in a group of urban children from birth to the age of 2 years. No infant had a cord blood lead level exceeding 25 μg/dL, the level regarded at that time by the Centers for Disease Control as the upper normal limit for children. At all ages children whose cord level was greater than 10 μg/dL scored lower in the Mental Development Index of the Bayley Scales [4.8-point difference between the low ($<$ 3 μg/dL) and high ($\geq$ 10 μg/dL) groups]. At the age of 6 months, scores on the Psychomotor Development Index were not significantly related to cord blood lead level. Scores were not related to infants' postnatal blood lead levels. At the age of 57 months the performance of these children was tested on the McCarthy Scale of Children's Ability (88). Surprisingly, at this age there was no association between prenatal lead exposure and children's cognitive function, except for children with high postnatal exposure ($>$ 10 μg/dL), particularly at 24 months of age. A study from Cincinnati obtained similar initial results (89). Comparable to the Boston study, neuropsychological follow-up of the Cincinnati cohort, as assessed by the Kaufman Assessment Battery for Children at the age of 4 years, was inversely associated with higher neonatal blood lead level only in children from the poorest families (90). The relationship between prenatal low level lead exposure and neurobehavioral development was not confirmed in another study (91). However, the mean cord lead level was 8.1 μg/dL, which is lower than the cutoff point of 10 μg/dL suggested by the Boston study. It is still unclear at what gestational age the fetus is most sensitive. Since the fetal brain develops throughout gestation, it is conceivable that lead deposition at any stage may be harmful. However, it seems that low level prenatal-lead-induced neurodevelopmental impairment may be reversible, provided the exposure is discontinued.

It has been suggested that cord blood levels above 15 μg/dL induce a modest decrease in fetal growth (92). The on stature effect of lead exposure (in utero as well as during the first year of life) was transient at 33 months of age, if subsequent exposure to lead was not excessive (93). Another study could not confirm an association between prenatal lead exposure and neonatal size (94).

These data suggest that low levels of lead delivered to the fetus may be toxic and may cause behavioral and developmental impairment. It led the Centers for Disease Control to reduce the acceptable level for young children from 25 to 10 μg/dL (56). Animal studies are consistent with these findings (95-99), and it is possible that brain lead levels remain elevated longer than blood levels after short-term exposure (100,101). It is also possible that the fetus is more sensitive to lead than the young child. Possible mechanisms for the brain damage include interference with embryonic nutrition and energy supply, competition with cations such as zinc, iron, or calcium (102), interference with mitochondrial function (103) and synthesis of cytochromes, and effect on deoxyribonucleic acid synthesis (104).

A study in Toronto found that about 90% of newborns had cord blood levels below 3 μg/dL and none above 10 μg/dL (105), whereas in Boston about one-third had such levels and one-third had levels exceeding 10 μg/dL. In Braunschweig, Germany, only 4.7% of the neonates had cord blood lead level above 10 μg/dL (106). This range of results illustrates the difference between different urban environments.

The data above imply that it is important to detect, as early as possible, babies potentially exposed in utero to excess lead. Several studies documented a high correlation between maternal and cord blood lead levels (58,61,107-109). In one of them mean cord levels were 10.1 μg/dL, compared with 10.3 μg/dL in the mother ($r = 0.6377$) (61). However, it is not advisable to assume lead exposure throughout pregnancy from a single blood measurement, because of the changes in maternal blood levels and placental permeability to lead (2). An alternative method of assessing long-term lead exposure and estimating in utero exposure is head hair analysis, which reflects cumulative values (110,111).

On the basis of the higher susceptibility of the fetal brain to lead, it may be argued that treatment should be instituted even when levels are low; however, the effectiveness of this approach has not been studied. More realistically, removal of the woman from the source of exposure is the first step. From the chelating agents available, BAL (dimercaprol) is a very toxic compound that has been shown to induce skeletal abnormalities in fetal mice (112). One woman who was treated for arsenic intoxication, in the sixth month of pregnancy, gave birth to a normal child (113). Ethylenediaminetetraacetate (EDTA) is less toxic, but it can chelate calcium, zinc, and other trace elements and may adversely affect the fetus. In one case it was given at the eighth month of gestation (at maternal level of 240 μg/dL) without complication (73). The infant was normal, with an undetected cord lead level. However, the sensitivity of the assay was very low (< 60 μg/dL was undetectable). This infant had normal mental and developmental assessments at age 4. In another patient treated with calcium EDTA at the same gestational age, it appeared that the treatment did not adequately reduce the infant's lead burden (114); this child had a blood lead level of 60 μg/dL at the time of delivery and radiological evidence of bony changes suggestive of prolonged exposure. A 17-year-old female in her 39th week of pregnancy who had a blood lead level of 79 μg/dL with a corresponding amniotic fluid lead level of 90 μg/dL was treated with 2 g/day Ca-EDTA for 3 days. Eight days later her blood lead level was 26 μg/dL. She delivered a normal-appearing girl, and the cord blood lead concentration was 79 μg/dL. Based on this result, the authors suggested a delay in the crossing of the placental barrier by Ca-EDTA (115). D-Penicillamine is less effective than dimercaprol and Ca-EDTA, and in the doses used in lead poisoning it may cause connective tissue abnormalities (mainly cutis laxa) in human fetuses (116). There is no experience with the use of the new oral chelators 2,3-dimercaptosuccinic acid (DMSA) and dimercaptopropane-1-sulfonate (DMPS) in human pregnancy. At doses between 100 and 1000 mg/kg/day, DMSA induced increases in resorptions and in post-implantation loss, as well as reduced fetal weight, but there was no teratogenicity in rats (117). Changes in mineral metabolism were suggested as one possible mechanism (118). The therapeutic dose in adults is 30 mg/kg/day. Similar effects were observed with DMPS in mice (119). Both chelators prevented arsenic teratogenicity and embryotoxicity in mice (120,121). Since these chelators are less toxic, it is hoped that they will indicate the appropriate cheolators for use in pregnancy. More critical research is needed to assess the need for treatment of low level exposures, to establish the criteria for instituting therapy, to evaluate the response, and to identify the chelator of choice.

In the case of a woman occupationally exposed to lead, it is important to measure her blood lead concentrations and compare them with the mean levels measured in the same city. Several women employed in stained glass workshops had lead levels well below or near the mean recently determined for women in Toronto (105), indicating that their lead load was within the expected range. Should there be a substantially higher lead level in such patients, they would be advised to discontinue their occupational exposure.

SUMMARY

Of the three most common occupational exposures in pregnancy, video display terminals do not represent a reproductive risk. Organic solvents may damage the fetal brain at high exposure levels, such as those encountered in substance abuse. There is no clear evidence to suggest that maternal exposure to allowable levels causes fetal damage. Some risk of spontaneous abortions for certain organic solvents cannot be ruled out, although the claim is not well established at this time. In the case of lead, a dose-response fetal risk appears to have been established, and lead levels should be monitored to avoid fetal risk.

Answer

Video terminals do not emit radiation that can affect the fetus. This has been proved by direct measurements as well as by epidemiological studies in pregnant women.

REFERENCES

1. Bellinger DC, Needelman HL, Leviton A, Waternaux C, Rabinowitz MB, Nichols ML. Early sensory-motor development and prenatal exposure to lead. Neurobehav Toxicol 1984; 6:387–402.
2. Bellinger D, Leviton A, Waternaux C, Needelman H, Rabinowitz M. Longitudinal analysis of prenatal and postnatal lead exposure and early cognitive development. N Engl J Med 1987; 316:1037–1043.
3. Klimisch HJ, Hellmig J, Hoffmann A. Studies on the prenatal toxicity of toluene in rabbits following inhalation exposure and proposal of a pregnancy guidance value. Arch Toxicol 1992; 66:373–381.
4. Fabro S, Brown NA, Scialli AR. Is there a fetal solvent syndrome? Reprod Toxicol Med Lett 1983; 2:17–20.
5. Ellenhorn MJ, Barceloux DG. Medical Toxicology. Diagnosis and Treatment of Human Poisoning. Elsevier, New York, 1988, pp 940–1006.
6. Cornish HH. Solvents and vapors. In Casarett and Doull's Toxicology: The Basic Science of Poisons, 2nd ed (Doul J, Klassen CD, Amdur MO, eds). Macmillan, New York, 1980, pp 468–496.
7. Freedman ML. The molecular site of benzene toxicity. J Toxicol Environ Health 1977; 2(suppl):37–43.
8. Industrial solvents. In Chemically Induced Birth Defects (Schardein JL, ed). Marcel Dekker, New York, 1985, pp 645–658.
9. Hudak A, Rodics K, Stuber I, Ungvary G, Krasznai G, Szomolanyi I, Csonka A. The effects of toluene inhalation on pregnant cfy rats and their offspring. Orsz Munka-Uzemegeszsegugui Intez Munkavedelm 1977; 23(suppl):25–30.
10. da Silva VA, Malheiros LR, Paumgartten FJ, Sa Rego M de M, Riul TR, Golovattei MA. Toxicology 1990; 64:155–158.
11. Hudak A, Ungvary G. Embryotoxic effects of benzene and its methyl derivatives: Toluene, xylene. Toxicoloty 1978; 11:55–63.
12. Nawrot PS, Staples RE. Embryofetal toxicity and teratogenicity of benzene and toluene in the mouse. Teratology 1979; 19:41A.
13. da Silva VA, Malherios LR, Bueno FM. Effects of toluene exposure during gestation on neurobehavioral development of rats and hamsters. Braz J Med Biol Res 1990; 23:533–537.

14. Syrovadko ON. Working conditions and health status of women handling organosilicon varnishes containing toluene. Gig Tr Prof Zabol 1977; 21:15-19.
15. McDonald JC, Lavoie XX, Cote R, McDonald AD. Chemical exposures at work in early pregnancy and congenital defect: A case-referent study. Br J Ind Med 1987; 44:527-533.
16. Lindbohm ML, Taskinen H, Sallmen M, Hemminki K. Spontaneous abortions among women exposed to organic solvents. Am J Ind Med 1990; 17:449-463.
17. Huang XY. Influence on benzene and toluene to reproductive function of female workers in leather shoe-making inductry. Chung Hua Yu Fang I Hsueh Tsa Chin 1991; 25:89-91.
18. Hersh JH, Podruch PE, Rogers G, Weisskopf B. Toluene embryopathy. J Pediatr 1985; 106:922-927.
19. Kucera J. Exposure to fat solvents: A possible cause of sacral agenesis in man. J Pediatr 1969; 72:857-859.
20. Meirik O, Kàllén B, Gauffin U, Ericson A. Major malformations in infants born of women who worked in laboratories while pregnant. Lancet 1979; 2:91.
21. Erickson DJ, Cochran WM, Anderson CE. Birth defects and printing. Lancet 1978; 1:385.
22. Hansson E, Jansa S, Wande H, Kàllén B, Östlund E. Pregnancy outcome for women working in laboratories in some of the pharmaceutical industries of Sweden. Scand J Work Environ Health 1980; 6:131-134.
23. Blomqvist U, Ericson A, Kàllén B, Wasterholm P. Delivery outcome for women working in the pulp and paper industry. Scand J Work Environ Health 1981; 7:114-118.
24. Holmberg PC. Central-nervous-system defects in children born to mothers exposed to organic solvents during pregnancy. Lancet 1979; 2:177-179.
25. Holmberg PC, Nurminen M. Congenital defects of the central nervous system and occupational factors during pregnancy. Am J Ind Med 1980; 1:167-176.
26. Rantala K, Riala R, Nurminen T. Screening for occupational exposures and congenital malformations. Scand J Work Environ Health 1983; 9:89-93.
27. Olsen J. Risk of exposure to teratogens amongst laboratory staff and painters. Dan Med Bull 1983; 30:24-28.
28. Holmberg PC, Hernberg S, Kurppa K, Rantala K, Riala R. Oral clefts and organic solvent exposure during pregnancy. Int Arch Occup Environ Health 1982; 50:371-376.
29. Tikkanen J, Heinonen OP. Cardiovascular malformations and organic solvent exposure during pregnancy in Finland. Am J Ind Med 1988; 14:1-8.
30. Tikkanen J, Heinonen OP. Maternal exposure to chemical and physical factors during pregnancy and cardiovascular malformations in the offspring. Teratology 1991; 43:591-600.
31. Tikkanen J, Heinonen OP. Risk factors for ventricular septal defects in Finland. Public Health 1991; 105:99-112.
32. Eskenazi B, Gaylord L, Bracken MB, Brown D. In utero exposure to organic solvents and human neurodevelopment. Dev Med Child Neurol 1988; 30:492-501.
33. Eskenazi B, Bracken MB, Holford TR, Crady J. Exposure to organic solvents and hypertensive disorders of pregnancy. Am J Ind Med 1988; 14:177-188.

34. Narod SA, Neri L, Risch HA, Raman S. Lymphocyte micronuclei and sister chromatid exchanges among Canadian federal laboratory employees. Am J Ind Med 1988; 14:449–456.

35. Heidan LZ. Spontaneous abortions among factory workers. The importance of gravidity control. Scand J Soc Med 1983; 11:81–85.

36. Axelson G, Liutz C, Rylander R. Exposure to solvents and outcome of pregnancy in university laboratory employees. Br J Ind Med 1984; 41:305–312.

37. Strandberg M, Sandback K, Axelson O, Sundell L. Spontaneous abortions among women in hospital laboratory. Lancet 1978; 1:384–385.

38. Hemminki K, Franssilla E, Vainio H. Spontaneous abortions among female workers in Finland. Int Arch Occup Environ Health 1980; 45:123–126.

39. Lipscomb JA, Fenster L, Wrensch M, Shusterman D, Swan S. Pregnancy outcomes in women potentially exposed to occupational solvents and women working in the electronics industry. J Occup Med 1991; 33:597–604.

40. Pastides H, Calabrese EJ, Hosmer DW Jr, Harris DR Jr. Spontaneous abortion and general illness symptoms among semiconductor manufacturers. J Occup Med 1988; 30:543–551.

41. Huel G, Mergler D, Bowler R. Evidence for adverse reproductive outcomes among women microelectronic assembly workers. Br J Ind Med 1990; 47:400–404.

42. Lindbohm ML, Taskinen H, Sallmen M, Hemminki K. Spontaneous abortions among women exposed to organic solvents. Am J Ind Med 1990; 17:449–463.

43. Windham GC, Shusterman D, Swan SH, Fenster L, Eskenazi B. Am J Ind Med 1991; 20:241–59.

44. Taskinen H, Anttila A, Lindbohm ML, Sallmen M, Hemminki K. Spontaneous abortions and congenital malformations among the wives of men occupationally exposed to organic solvents. Scand J Work Environ Health 1989; 15:346–352.

45. Hunter AGW, Thompson D, Evans JA. Is there a fetal gasoline syndrome? Teratology 1979; 20:75–80.

46. Toutant C, Lippmann S. Fetal solvent syndrome. Lancet 1979; 1:1356.

47. Hersh JH. Toluene embryopathy: Two new cases. J Med Genet 1989; 26:333–337.

48. Goodwin TM. Toluene abuse and renal tubular acidosis in pregnancy. Obstet Gynecol 1988; 71:715–718.

49. Wilkins HL, Gabow PA. Toluene abuse during pregnancy: Obstetric complications and perinatal outcomes. Obstet Gynecol 1991; 77:504–509.

50. Lindemann R. Congenital renal tubular dysfunction associated with maternal sniffing of organic solvents. Acta Paediatr Scand 1991; 80:882–884.

51. Rom WN. Effects of lead on the female reproduction: A review. Mt Sinai J Med 1976; 43:542–551.

52. Baghurst PA, McMichael AJ, Vimpani GV, Robertson EE, Clark PD, Wigg NR. Determinants of blood lead concentrations of pregnant women living in Port Pirie and surrounding areas. Med J Aust 1987; 146:69–73.

53. Hamilton A, Hardy HL. Hereditary lead poisoning. In Industrial Toxicology. Publishing Sciences, Acton, MA, 1974, pp 119–121.

54. Palmisano PA, Sneed RC, Cassady G. Untaxed whisky and fetal lead exposure. J Pediatr 1969; 75:869–872.

55. Annest JL, Pirkle JL, Makuc D, Neese JW, Bayse DD, Kovar MG. Chronological trend in blood lead levels between 1976 and 1980. N Engl J Med 1983; 308: 1373–1377.
56. US Centers for Disease Control. Preventing lead poisoning in children. A statement by the Centers for Disease Control, Atlanta, October 1991. Quoted in Poisondex, Micromedex, Denver, CO, 1992.
57. OSHA.CFR. Code of Federal Regulations 29CFR 1910, 1025. Chap. XVII (7-1-88 ed), 1988, pp 832–870. Quoted in Poisondex, Micromedex, Denver, CO, 1992.
58. Baltrop D. Transfer of lead to the human foetus. In Mineral Metabolism in Pediatrics (Baltrop D, Burland WL, eds). Blackwell Scientific, Oxford, 1969, pp 135–151.
59. Kostial K, Momcilovic B. Transport of lead-203 and calcium-47 from mother to offspring. Arch Environ Health 1974; 29:28.
60. Alexander F, Delves H. Blood lead levels during pregnancy. Arch Environ Health 1981; 48:35–39.
61. Gershanick J, Brooks G, Little J. Blood lead values in pregnant women and their offspring. Am J Obstet Gynecol 1974; 119:508–511.
62. Lubin H, Caffo A, Reece R. A longitudinal study of interaction between environmental lead and blood lead concentrations during pregnancy, at delivery and in the first 6 months of life. Pediatr Res 1978; 12:425.
63. Rajegowda BK, Glass L, Evans HE. Lead concentration in newborn infants. J Pediatr 1972; 80:116.
64. Karlog O, Moller KO. Three cases of acute lead poisoning: Analysis of organs for lead and observations on polarographic lead determinations. Acta Pharm 1958; 15:8–16.
65. Silbergeld EK. Lead in bone: Implication for toxicology during pregnancy and lactation. Environ Health Perspect 1991; 91:63–77.
66. Oliver T. A lecture on lead poisoning and the race. Br Med J 1911; 1:1096–1098.
67. Rennert O. Über eine hereditâre Folge der chronischen Blievergiftung. Arch Gynaecol 1881; 16:109.
68. Chyzzer A. Des intoxications par le plomb se présentant dans le céramique en Hongrie. Natl Acad Sci (Budapest) 1908; 44:906–911.
69. Legge TM. Industrial lead poisoning. J Hyg 1901; 1:96.
70. Paul C. Étude sur l'intoxication lente par les préparations de plomb; de son influence par le produit de la conception. Arch Gen Med 1869; 5:513–33.
71. Deneufbourg H. L'intoxication saturnine dans ses rapports avec la grossesse. Thesis, Université de Paris, 1905.
72. Hamilton A. Industrial Poisons in United States. Macmillan, New York, 1929, pp 8–17, 110–115.
73. Angle CR, McIntire MS. Lead poisoning during pregnancy. Am J Dis Child 1964; 108:436–439.
74. Fahim MS, Fahim Z, Hall DG. Effects of subtoxic lead levels on pregnant women in the state of Missouri. In Proceedings of the International Conference on Heavy Metals in the Environment, Toronto, Ont, Canada, Oct 27–31, 1975.

75. Baghurst PA, Robertson EF, Oldfield RK, et al. Lead in the placenta, membranes, and umbilical cord in relation to pregnancy outcome in a lead-smelter community. Environ Health Perspect 1991; 90:315–320.
76. Nogaki K. On action of lead on body of lead refinery workers: Particularly conception, pregnancy and parturition in case of females and on vitality of their newborn. Excerpta Med 1958; 4:2176.
77. Pindborg S. On solverglodforgifting i Denmark. Ugeskr Lacg 1945; 107:1–6.
78. Hu H. Knowledge of diagnosis and reproductive history among survivors of childhood plumbism. Am J Public Health 1991; 81:1070–1072.
79. Sierra EM, Tiffany-Castiglioni E. Effects of low-level lead exposure on hypothalamic hormones and serum progesterone levels in pregnant guinea pigs. Toxicology 1992; 72:89–97.
80. Needelman HL, Rabinowitz M, Leviton A, Linn S, Schoenbaum S. The relationship between prenatal exposure to lead and congenital anomalies. JAMA 1984; 251:2956–2959.
81. Deknudt GH, Leonard A, Ivanov B. Chromosome aberrations observed in male workers occupationally exposed to lead. Environ Physiol Biochem 1973; 3:132–138.
82. Lancranjan I, Popsecu H, Gavanescu O, Klepsch I, Serbanescu M. Reproductive ability of workmen occupationally exposed to lead. Arch Environ Health 1975; 30:396–401.
83. Stofen D. Less noted European papers on lead. In Proceedings of the International Symposium on Environmental Health Aspects of Lead, Amsterdam, Oct 2–6, 1972, pp 473–485.
84. Lindbohm ML, Sallmen M, Anttila A, Taskinen H, Hemminki K. Paternal occupational lead exposure and spontaneous abortion. Scand J Work Environ Health 1991; 17:95–103.
85. Hardy HL. What is the status of knowledge of the toxic effects of lead on identifiable groups in the population? Clin Pharmacol Ther 1966; 7:713–733.
86. Rabinowitz M, Bellinger D, Leviton A, Needelman H, Schoenbaum S. Pregnancy hypertension, blood pressure during labor and blood lead levels. Hypertension 1987; 10:447–451.
87. Mahaffey KR, Annest JL, Roberts J, Murphy RS. National estimates of blood lead levels: United States, 1976–1980: Association with selected demographic and socioeconomic factors. N Engl J Med 1982; 307:573–579.
88. Bellinger D, Solman J, Leviton A, Rabinowitz M, Needelman HL, Waternaux C. Low-level lead exposure and children's cognitive function in the preschool years. Pediatrics 1991; 87:219–227.
89. Dietrich KN, Kraft KM, Bornschein RL, et al. Low-level fetal lead exposure effect on neurobehavioral development in early infancy. Pediatrics 1987; 80:721–730.
90. Dietrich KN, Succop PA, Berger OG, Hammond PB, Bornschein RL. Lead exposure and the cognitive development of urban preschool children: The Cincinnati Lead Study cohort at age 4 years. Neurotoxicol Teratol 1991; 13:203–211.

91. Cooney GH, Bell A, McBride W, Carter C. Neurobehavioral consequences of prenatal low level exposures to lead. Neurotoxicol Teratol 1989; 11:95–104.
92. Bellinger D, Leviton A, Rabinowitz M, Alfred E, Needelman H, Schoenbaum S. Weight gain and maturing in fetuses exposed to low levels of lead. Environ Res 1991; 54:151–158.
93. Shukla R, Dietrich KN, Bornschein RL, Berger O, Hammond PB. Lead exposure and growth in the early preschool child: A follow-up report from the Cincinnati Lead Study. Pediatrics 1991; 88:886–892.
94. Greene T, Ernhart CB. Prenatal and preschool age lead exposure: Relationship with size. Neurotoxicol Teratol 1991; 13:417–427.
95. Bushness PJ, Bowman RE. Persistence of impaired reversal learning in young monkeys exposed to low levels of dietary lead. J Toxicol Environ Health 1979; 5:1015–1023.
96. Levin ED, Bowman RE. The effect of pre or postnatal lead exposure on Hamilton Search Task in monkeys. Neurobehav Toxicol Teratol 1983; 5:391–394.
97. Mele PC, Bushnell PJ, Bowman RE. Prolonged behavioral effects of early postnatal lead exposure in rhesus monkeys: Fixed-interval responding and interactions with scopolamine and pentobarbital. Neurobehav Toxicol Teratol 1984; 6:129–135.
98. Rice DC, Willes RF. Neonatal low-level lead exposure in monkeys (*Macaca fascicularis*): Effect on two-choice non-spatial form discrimination. J Environ Pathol Toxicol 1979; 2:1195–1203.
99. Rice DC, Gilbert SG, Willes RF. Neonatal low-level lead exposure in monkeys: Locomotor activity, schedule-controlled behavior, and the effects of amphetamine. Toxicol Appl Pharmacol 1979; 51:503–513.
100. Goldstein GW, Asbury AK, Diamond I. Pathogenesis of lead encephalopathy: Uptake of lead and reaction of brain capilaries. Arch Neurol 1974; 31:382–389.
101. Hammond PB. The effects of chelating agents on the tissue distribution and excretion of lead. Toxicol Appl Pharmacol 1971; 18:296–310.
102. Mahaffey K, Michaelson A. Interactions between lead and nutrition. In Low Level Lead Exposure: The Clinical Implications of Current Research (Needelman HL, ed). Raven Press, New York, 1980, pp 159–200.
103. Holzman J, Hsu JS. Early effects of lead on immature rat brain mitochondrial respiration. Pediatr Res 1976; 10:70–75.
104. Choi DD, Richter G. Stimulation of DNA synthesis in rat kidney by repeated administration of lead. Proc Soc Exp Biol Med 1973; 142:446–449.
105. Koren G, Cheng M, Klein J, et al. Lead exposure in mothers and infants in Toronto, 1989. Can Med Assoc J 1990; 142:1241–1244.
106. Meyer J, Genenich HH, Robra BP, Windorfer A. Determinants of lead concentration in the umbilical cord blood of 9189 newborns of a birth cohort in the government district of Braunschweig. Zentralb Hugg Umweltmed 1992; 192:522–533.
107. Angell NF, Lavery JP. The relationship of blood lead levels to obstetric outcome. Am J Obstet Gynecol 1982; 142:40–46.

108. Zetterlund B, Winberg J, Lundgren G, Johansson G. Lead in umbilical cord blood correlated with the blood lead of the mother in areas with low, medium or high atmospheric pollution. Acta Paediatr Scand 1977; 66:169–175.
109. Milman N, Christensen JM, Ibsen KK. Blood lead and erythrocyte zinc protoporphyrin in mothers and newborn infants. Eur J Pediatr 1988; 147:71–73.
110. Laker M. On determining trace element levels in man: The uses of blood and hair. Lancet 1982; 2:260–262.
111. Huel G, Everson RB, Manger I. Increased hair cadmium in newborns of women occupationally exposed to heavy metals. Environ Res 1984; 1:115–121.
112. Schardein JL. Chemical antagonists. In Chemically Induced Birth Defects. (Schardein JL, ed). Marcel Dekker, New York, 1985, pp 534–545.
113. Kantor MI, Levin PM. Arsenical encephalopathy in pregnancy with recovery. Am J Obster Gynecol 1948; 56:370–374.
114. Timpo AE, Amin JS, Casalino MB, Yuceoylu AM. Congenital lead intoxication. J Pediatr 1979; 94:765–767.
115. Peral M, Boxt M. Radiographic findings in congenital lead poisoning. Radiology 1980; 136:83–84.
116. Briggs GG, Freeman RK, Yaffe SJ, eds. Drugs in Pregnancy and Lactation, 2nd ed. Williams & Wilkins, Baltimore, 1986, p 331.
117. Domingo JL, Ortega A, Paternain JL, Llobet JM, Corbella J. Oral *meso*-2,3-dimercaptosuccinic acid in pregnant Sprague-Dawley rats: Teratogenicity and alterations in mineral metabolism. I. Teratological evaluation. J Toxicol Environ Health 1990; 30:181–190.
118. Paternain JL, Ortega A, Domingo JL, Llobolt JM, Corbella J. Oral *meso*-2,3-dimercaptosuccinic acid in pregnant Sprague-Dawley rats: Teratogenicity and alterations in mineral metabolism. II. Effect on mineral metabolism. J Toxicol Environ Health 1990; 30:191–197.
119. Bosque MA, Domingo JL, Paternain JL, Llobelt JM, Crobella J. Evaluation of the developmental toxicity of 2,3-dimercapto-1-propanesulfonate (DMPS) in mice. Effect on mineral metabolism. Toxicology 1990; 62:311–320.
120. Domingo JL, Bosque MA, Piera V. *meso*-2,3-Dimercaptosuccinic acid and prevention of arsenite embryotoxicity and teratogenicity in the mouse. Fundam Appl Toxicol 1993; 17:314–320.
121. Domingo JL, Bosque MA, Llobelt JM, Corbella J. Amelioration by BAL (2,3-dimercapto-1-propanol) and DMPS (sodium 2,3-dimercapto-1-propanesulfonic acid) of arsenite developmental toxicity in mice. Ecotoxicol Environ Safety 1992; 23:274–281.

21

Maternal–Fetal Toxicology of Medicinal Plants: A Clinician's Guide

Samuel Randor, Thomas R. Einarson, Anne Pastuszak, and Gideon Koren
The Hospital for Sick Children, Toronto, Ontario, Canada

Clinical Case

A 25-year-old Chinese woman used comfrey (symphytum) as an anti-inflammatory agent. She wants to know if it may adversely affect her baby.

INTRODUCTION

Millions of people in North America regularly consume medicinal plants, either self-prescribed or with the advice of naturopaths or other individuals. Physicians caring for pregnant women are often faced with very difficult situations of not being able to identify natural remedies taken by expectant mothers, and it is almost never possible for the practicing physician to estimate the risk of such compounds.

Since its inception in 1985, the Motherisk Program in Toronto has counseled increasing numbers of women and health professionals on the safety/risk of natural products. Although these substances constitute only a small percentage of our overall calls on safety of drugs, chemicals, radiation, and infections during pregnancy and lactation, analysis of the safety/risk of natural products is the most difficult. Unlike the makers of medicinal drugs or occupational chemicals, manufacturers of these nondrug materials are not bound by legislation to test their safety. The concept that "natural" means "safe" has been proven erroneous numerous times by cases of poisonings and abuse.

Most medicinal plants contain scores of active ingredients, and unlike the cases of medicinal drugs or industrial chemicals, the concentrations of these principles differ from crop to crop and even within the plant itself.

Presently, there is no clinically relevant source of information for health professionals caring for pregnant women on the safety/risks associated with common medicinal plants. In an attempt to close this gap, 2 years ago the Motherisk Program initiated an in-depth review and analysis of published data on 50 common medicinal plants.

Table 1 identifies each by its various names, including the scientific and common. The column "Purported indications for use" should not be interpreted as suggesting that we believe in or support such use. Rather, it aims at suggesting to the physician why a given patient might have taken a certain remedy. In the column on "Pharmacological and toxicological effects relevant to pregnant women" we have tried to extract from voluminous amounts of data the information that is relevant for the well-being of the mother, hence of her baby. The column entitled "Reproductive pharmacology and toxicology" relates to published information in animals (A) or humans (H) relevant to the reproductive system and its function before, during, or after conception. Here too, the presentation of information should not be interpreted as our support of its validity. For example, while many remedies have been believed traditionally to be abortifacient, modern research has often refuted such claims; absence of such research, however, does not mean that the agent is really abortifacient.

We have chosen only few references for each plant out of the many available.

ACKNOWLEDGMENT

This work was supported by the Motherisk Research Fund, Toronto, Ontario, Canada.

Answer

Confrey has been associated in animal studies and human case reports with hepatic veno-occlusive disease. It should be avoided during pregnancy.

Table 1 Safety Risks for Pregnant Women of 50 Common Medicinal Plants

Name of plant	Purported indications for use	Pharmacological and toxicological effects relevant to pregnant women	Reproductive pharmacology toxicology in humans (H) and animals (A)	Ref.
1. Algae (marine) spp. Common name: seaweeds [Rhodophyceae, Phaeophyceae, Cyanophyta] Kelp is a common name for brown, giant algae; particularly *Laminaria* spp.; kelp is also a common name for *Fucus vesiculosis* L. (bladderwrack)	Nutritive; demulcent/ emolient; antiulcerogenic; laxative; connective tissue protective/promoter; immune modulator; antimicrobial; cardio- vascular stimulant/ depressant; anticoagulant, fibrinolytic; thyroidal stimulant; CNS sedative; hypolipemic; hypo- glycemic	Particularly rich in various micronutrients, most notably iodine (see below) in seawater (as opposed to freshwater) algae; also found are a large variety of bioactive com- pounds, some of which are frank toxins in some algae, others being potent (estab- blished or experimental) pharmaceuticals, including agar (syn. agar-agar, vege- table gelatin), alginic acid salts (algn.), and carrageenin (cargn.), which are hydro- colloidal substances with wide-ranging use in the phar- maceuticals (as excipients) cosmetic, and food industries (as processants), in addition to their direct nutritional and clinical roles (e.g., agar as Oriental food and as bulk laxative).	*Fucus vesiculosus* L. was touted as remedial for, and normalizer of, the ovary, uterus, testis, and prostate. Traditional ecbolic use of *Codium fragiles.* High iodine intake in preg- nancy may result in congeni- tal goiter and hypothyroid- ism (H). *Laminaria* sp. have been widely used intravaginally for thera- peutic abortion in the first and second trimester, via uterine cervical osmotic rip- ening and dilatatory effect. Normal pregnancy outcomes were reported following cer- vical dilatation with *Lamin- aria* tents. Teratogenicity (mostly CNS and skeletal) was reported for cargn. and agar, respectively, in some species (A).	1–18

(continues)

449

Table 1 Continued

Name of plant	Purported indications for use	Pharmacological and toxicological effects relevant to pregnant women	Reproductive pharmacology toxicology in humans (H) and animals (A)	Ref.
1. Algae (marine) spp. (continued)		Large dietary intake of iodine in the form of seaweed can induce goiter. Iodine-induced hypothyroidism is not uncommon (12 of 23 in one series, including 2 patients who digested 25-45 mg/day from seaweed preparations) and may revert to normal upon iodine restriction alone. Thyroidal stimulatory effects that may lead to thyrotoxicosis are also possible (the Job Basidow phenomenon). Prostatic cancer was epidemiologically linked to chronic large consumption of seaweeds.	No information could be found regarding reproductive effects of extracts of fresh-water algae.	
		The degraded form is ulcerogenic in some species but not in others. Humans appear to be resistant to this intestinal ulcerogenicity, but cargn. (found in many infant formulas) might be hazardous to premature babies because of their proneness to necrotizing enterocolitis.		

Dietary seaweeds in large amounts were implicated as risk factors in cerebrovascular disease mortality (H).

Agar, a bulk laxative, and other poorly absorbed high molecular weight constituents (including undegraded cargn.), may affect absorption of nutrients or drugs. Serum cholesterol was reduced by cargn. and algn. via inhibition of its absorption in the gut, but elevated in the case of agar. Undegraded cargn. were shown to selectively induce drug-metabolizing enzyme systems in intestine, including increased cytochrome P-450 levels.

A reproducible inflammatory reaction to injection of cargn. to a rodent paw has been extensively used in experimental screening of anti-inflammatory drugs.

The λ-cargn. variety is the most toxic variety and single IP injection has caused acroneurosis and 90% mortality within a month.

(continues)

Table 1 Continued

Name of plant	Purported indications for use	Pharmacological and toxicological effects relevant to pregnant women	Reproductive pharmacology toxicology in humans (H) and animals (A)	Ref.
1. Algae (marine) spp. (continued)		Many instances of contamination of algal products by heavy metals (arsenic, mercury, etc.).		
2. *Allium sativum* L. [Amaryllidaceae] Garlic, stinky rose, camphor of the poor, poor man's treacle	Antimicrobial; anti-inflammatory; spasmolytic; immune stimulant; hypotensive; hypoglycemic; hypolipemic; antithrombotic; antineoplastic; expectorant; diuretic; carminative; stomachic	GI, skin, and eye irritation. Large amounts of chronic use may cause gastroenteritis, kidney irritation, asthmatic reactions, dizziness, sweating. Chronic ingestion was associated with arrhythmia, hemolytic anemia, dehydration, weakness, lethargy, weight loss, or failure to thrive, including with amounts within therapeutic range. Inhibits thyroid iodine uptake. Additive hypotensive effect with *Viscum album*. Contains substantial amounts of oxalate and sulfur compounds (notably allicin, the major odor principles), particularly in the essential oil extract.	Reports of (H) and (A) in vitro oxytocicity, but not embryotoxic or abortifacient effects could be demonstrated in vivo, nor anti-implantation in (A); conflicting reports on antispermatogenic effect (A); documented equipotent estrogenic and androgenic activity as well as gonadotropic effect (A). Conflicting reports on mutagenicity in short-term genotoxicity assays. Potential fetal and neonatal hypothyroidism in pregnancy and lactation, with resultant complications.	19–33

34-39

3. *Aloe vera* L.
A. barbadensis Miller,
A. ferox Miller,
A. perryi Baker, and
related spp.
[Liliaceae]
Aloe vera; Barbados
or Curaçao aloa;
Cape aloe; Zanzibar
or Socotrine aloe,
respectively

Cathartic; laxative; emollient; moisturizer; antipruritic analgesic; antiinflammatory; antimicrobial; antineoplastic; hypoglycemic

Anthraquinone glycosides (and free forms) are colonic irritants, hence potent cathartics in large doses, with severe cramping and at times, bloody diarrhea; hemorrhagic gastritis reported; kidney irritation and sometime nephritis; acute and chronic toxicity may lead to serious electrolyte disturbances. Chronic use for relief of constipation or as drug of abuse (mostly in eating disorders) may lead to the cathartic colon syndrome.

Interference with absorption of nutrients and drugs.

Rare contact dermatitis with gel. Contains tannins, antiprostaglandin, and antihistamine compounds.

Contains glucomannan (a polysaccharide similar to guar), which has been used as bulk laxative; several cases of esophageal obstruction were reported in individuals without underlying esophageal pathology due to glucomannan rapid swelling in water.

Traditional contraceptive, emmenagogue, and abortifacient, but also clinical reports on use in functional sterility (latex).

Abortifacient (H), possibly via GI irritation, which may lead to pelvic congestion. In addition, oxytocicity was demonstrated in vitro (A) models

Conflicting reports of antiimplantation and abortifacient effects in (A), reported estrogenic effects in (A).

Increased meconium release and neonatal nephropathy in humans.

Contraindicated in pregnancy.

(continues)

453

Table 1 Continued

Name of plant	Purported indications for use	Pharmacological and toxicological effects relevant to pregnant women	Reproductive pharmacology toxicology in humans (H) and animals (A)	Ref.
4. *Ananas comosus* L. Mezz. [Bromeliaceae] Pineapple, ananas	Digestive aid; laxative; spasmolytic; anti-inflammatory; antimicrobial; antineoplastic; for wound debridement	Broad margin of safety in experimental (A). In therapeutic doses may cause nausea, vomiting, diarrhea, rash, menorrhagia, and tachycardia. Allergic reactions, including rare fatalities reported. Contains a proteolytic enzyme, bromelain, which is substantially absorbed from the GI tract with multiorgan/tissue distribution (A) (H) in spite of molecular weight of 18,000–31,000. Anticoagulation effect of bromelain is via inhibition of platelet aggregation and increased serum fibrinolytic activity (A), (H). Also contains coumarins; oxalic acid, serotonin, essential oil, salicylates.	Traditional antifertility effects. Uterine relaxing effect of bromelaine in (H). Antifertility including abortifacient effects in (A). Contains steroidal phytoestrogens (e.g., β-sitosterol; antiimplantation, antigonadotropism, oxytocicity, cytotoxicity, and other concerns).	27,40–47
5. *Angelica sinensis* (oliv.) Diels (syn. *A. polymorpha*), *A. arachangelica* L. (syn. *A. officinalis* (Moench) Hoffm.),	Estrogenic/antiestrogenic; anti-inflammatory; antimicrobial; immune-stimulant/suppressive; anticoagulant; analgesic; antiulcerogenic; spasmo-	*Angelica* species and their crude extracts exhibit very low toxicity in (A) and (H) (except the ether extract of *A. sinensis*, which was reported to be very toxic, doses	Traditional emmenagogue and abortifacient. Extensive clinical use in menstrual, menopausal, and other gynecological disorders and in obstetrical situations (e.g.,	48–55

454

A. sylvestris L, and related spp. Chinese angelica or Dong-quai (or Danggui), European angelica, wild angelica, respectively

lytic; sedative; hypotensive; bradycardic; antiarrhythmic; antilipemic; antineoplastic; diuretic; antianemic

of 0.06 and 0.02 mL/kg were fatal to dogs and cats, respectively. There are surprisingly few reports of human adverse effects considering the extensive use of these agents, particularly in the Orient. Numbness of the tongue, gastric discomfort, nausea, and vomiting were noted with some patients treated with *A. pubescens* Maxim. for bronchitis; in combination with another remedy, *A. sinensis* was implicated in cases of lassitude, drowsiness, and urticaria.

All parts are rich in coumarins—some of the constituent furocoumarin are highly photosensitizing in (A) and (H), including by internal application. Photocarcinogenicity and mutagenicity were demonstrated in (A) (e.g., bergapten or 5-methoxypsoralen). Hepatotoxicity (xanthotoxin) or convulsions and paralysis (angelicotoxin) were noted with high doses of such coumarins.

toxemia), in the Orient. Reputation as a "female remedy." Both estrogenic and progestogenic effects were reported (H).

Successful treatment of uterine prolapse by an injectable preparation was reported; in vitro oxytocicity and extracts were used as ecbolic (labor inducer) as part of a multicomponent remedy, but the overall uterine effect of oral crude extracts decreases myometrial sensitivity in pregnancy.

No abortifacient or other toxic effects were noted in pregnant women who ingested angelica compound (containing additional ingredients) for several days. Estrogenic, anti-, or pro-progesterone, gonadotropin stimulant, and antiluteinizing hormone effects were noted in some (A) in vivo, and luteotropic effects in vitro; some of the data derive from mixed compounds.

(continues)

Table 1 Continued

Name of plant	Purported indications for use	Pharmacological and toxicological effects relevant to pregnant women	Reproductive pharmacology toxicology in humans (H) and animals (A)	Ref.
5. *Angelica sinensis* (continued)			Abortifacient effects were noted in (A). In some (A), long-term administration of extracts were reported to increase uterine weight, DNA content, and glucose utilization; in vivo oxytocicity (up to tonic contractions with multiple medication or high dosage).	
6. *Arctium lappa* L. (syn. *A. majus* Bernh.) [Compositae (Asteraceae)] Burdock, great burr, love leaves, cockle buttons, etc.	Immune-stimulant; antimicrobial; hypoglycemic; antineoplastic; diuretic	Several cases of atropine poisoning from commercial preparations; likely a contamination. Allergenicity, as with other Compositae via sesquiterpene lactones, mostly contact dermatitis. Very rich (up to 50%) in inulin; also contains tannins and polyphenolic acids. Aggravation of experimental diabetes was reported.	Oxytocicity (A); no antifertility effects demonstrated (A); presence of steroidal phytoestrogens. Sesquiterpene lactones are excreted in breast milk.	56–58

| 7. *Arctostaphylos uva-ursi* (L.) Sprengel (syn. *Arbutus uva-ursi* (L.)) [Ericaceae] Bearberry, uva-ursi, kinnikinik, manzanita | Diuretic; antimicrobial; astringent; anti-inflammatory; choleretic; laxative; hypoglycemic; antineoplastic | The constituent hydroquinone glycosides (up to 18% in leaves by weight, mostly arbutine) are hydrolyzed in the stomach to hydroquinone, one gram of which, per se, was shown to cause tinnitus, nausea, vomiting, cyanosis, convulsions, and collapse; fatal acute cases were reported with amounts equal to or greater than 5 g. Other symptoms associated with hydroquinone (mostly exposure via skin-lightening creams or soaps and industrially) include eye and lung irritation up to serious injury, various cutaneous manifestations (inflammation, hypopigmentation but also paradoxical hyperpigmentation, leukoderma, eruptions, allergic contact dermatitis), headache, dizziness, delirium, jaundice, albuminuria, hematuria, hemolytic anemia. In (A) studies various other hematological changes, hyperreflexia and | Oxytocic effects in large doses (H), possibly via tannins and flavonoids. Antifertility effect via cytotoxicity as well as antigonadotropin in (A). No teratogenicity elicited in partial (A) studies by gestational hydroquinone. Hydroquinone was positive in the *E. coli* Po/A DNA repair test, but inactive in the Ames and other genotoxicity assays. | 59–63 |

(continues)

Table 1 Continued

Name of plant	Purported indications for use	Pharmacological and toxicological effects relevant to pregnant women	Reproductive pharmacology toxicology in humans (H) and animals (A)	Ref.
7. *Arctostaphylos uva-ursi* (L.) Sprengel (continued)		hypoglycemia were also demonstrated. Hydroquinone appear to be oxidized to quinone prior to bioaction. Such symptoms are noted only rarely in users of uva-ursi preparations in reasonable amounts. Doses up to 20 g of the leaves were pharmacologically inactive in healthy individuals. Consumption of bearberry and related hydroquinone-yielding plants may well result in systemic toxicity. Contains very high level of phenolic acids and tannins (up to 40% in leaves); also contains flavonoids (e.g., quercetin) volatile oil, and the triterpene ursolic acid (antineoplastic). Imparts green color to urine.		

No.	Plant	Uses	Adverse reactions/toxicity	Comments	Ref.
8.	*Calendula officinalis* L. [Compositae (Asteraceae)] Garden marigold, calendula, gold-bloom, holligold	Wound-healing promoter; topical anti-inflammatory; analgesic; astringent; antimicrobial; immune-stimulant; antineoplastic	Hypersensitivity reactions via sesquiterpene lactones, including anaphylactic shock. Cross-sensitivity with other Compositae. Contains triterpene saponins, with a strong hemolytic activity in (A), flavonoids (e.g., quercetin), volatile oils, salicylates, mucilage.	Traditional oxytocic and emmenagogue. Antispermatic effect, demonstrated in vitro in (A) and (H). Estrogenic activity by some extracts was noted in (A). Oxytocity, antigonadotropism, cytotoxicity, and other effects of constituent steroidal phytoestrogen and flavonoids (e.g., quercetin, rutin).	64,65
9.	*Capsicum frutescense* L.; *C. annuum* var. *conoides* [Solanaceae] Cayenne pepper, capsicum, African chillies; paprika, pimento, Mexican chillies, tabasco pepper, respectively	Laxative/antidiarrheal; appetite stimulant; diaphoretic; hypoglycemic; hypolipemic; hypotensive; cardio-stimulant; CNS stimulant; anticoagulant; antimicrobial; topical analgesic (counterirritant)	Various external and internal irritative adverse reactions via oleoresin, capsaicin; gastric irritation. Potential carcinogenicity via metabolites of capsaicin; implicated in (A) jejunal adenocarcinoma, hepatoma, and as gastric cocarcinogen, and in (H) precancerous oral submucosal fibrosis. Capsaicin-treated newborn (A) exhibited sensory neuronal damage and growth retardation. Capsaicin stimulates liver cytochrome P-450 dependent arylhydroxylase (A).	Oxytocity of extracts in (A). Solanine is a teratogen in some (A) models. Female (A) treated neonatally with capsaicin displayed fewer mating and pregnancies; male fertility decreased as well; mechanism unclear.	37,66–70

(continues)

Table 1 Continued

Name of plant	Purported indications for use	Pharmacological and toxicological effects relevant to pregnant women	Reproductive pharmacology toxicology in humans (H) and animals (A)	Ref.
9. *Capsicum frutescense* L. (continued)		Contains solanidan alkaloids (e.g., solanine, an anticholinesterase inhibitor, among other properties). In high doses, toxic in (A) and (H), as with consumption of green potatoes. In vitro inhibition of mitochondrial oxidative phosphorylation and ATPase activity in high doses (A).		
10. *Carica papaya* L. [Caricaceae] Papaya, pawpaw, melon tree	Digestive aid; debridement agent; anti-inflammatory; antimicrobial; hypoglycemic; antineoplastic	Allergic reactions to the major constituent proteolytic enzymes papain and chymopapain, including fatal anaphylaxis, with cross-sensitivity with pineapple's bromelaine. The latex is irritative and vesicant externally and may induce severe gastritis internally. Ingestion of large amounts of papaya or papain may cause esophageal perforation particularly when used clinically to treat food (e.g., meat) impaction.	Traditional contraceptive, abortifacient, and ecbolic (including via cervical application of latex). (H) uterine relaxing effect, intravaginally and PO, particularly in habitual aborters possibly via carpaine. Anti-implantation, male contraceptive (without affecting spermatogenesis). Oxytocic, tocolytic, abortifacient, embryotoxic, and teratogenic effects reported in several (A) species; there are negative reports as well for all of the above	32,42, 71–75

	Uses	Pharmacology/Toxicity	Notes	Ref.
		Decreased iron absorption by concomitant papaya juice. Contains carpaine (alkaloid), with cardiac and CNS depressant activity up to paralysis (A), (even in concentration of only 0.02%). Contains considerable amounts of benzylglucosinalates (a source of nitriles), isocyanates and some free thiocyanate, and serotonin.	Contains steroidal phytoestrogens. Potential oxytocicity via β-sitosterol, serotonin, and tannins. Contains suspected teratogenic piperidine alkaloids.	
11. *Cassia acutifolia* Del. (syn. *C. senna* L.) *C. angustifolia* Vahl. [Leguminosae] Alexandrine or Khartoum senna; Tinnevelly or Indian senna, respectively	Cathartic; laxative; antineoplastic; antimicrobial	In small amounts causes mild abdominal discomfort, but sometimes severe catharsis. Acute overdose and chronic use may result in serious (H) GI irritation by anthraquinone glycosides (e.g., sennosides) and free anthroquinones (e.g., aloe-emodin), including gripping, diarrhea, dehydration; prolonged use may also result in weight loss, protein-losing enteropathy, steatorrhea, acid-base and electrolyte imbalance, mostly hypokalemia; also hypocalcemia, hypomagnesemia; may	No oxytocicity or teratogenicity demonstrated so far in (A) and (H) in usual doses; overdose may cause abortion (H). Gestational and lactational implication of anthraquinone glycosides (large doses): see above, *Aloe vera*, No. 3. Contains steroidal phytoestrogens (e.g., β-sitosterol).	76-82

(continues)

Table 1 Continued

Name of plant	Purported indications for use	Pharmacological and toxicological effects relevant to pregnant women	Reproductive pharmacology toxicology in humans (H) and animals (A)	Ref.
11. *Cassia acutifolia* Del. (continued)		lead to dependence (atonic syndrome (also known as cathartic colon syndrome). Imparts red color to urine. A phenomenon described in chronic senna users but not with other cathartic laxatives is reversible finger clubbing (hypertrophic osteopathy). Hypersensitivity reactions described. Rare instances of colonic perforation, including fatalities, with senna use for bowel preparation prior to barium enema. Controversial toxic destruction of colonic myenteric neurons. Monoamine oxidase (MAO) inhibition by senna and sennoides (A).		
12. *Centella asiatica* L. (syn. *Hydrocotyle asiatica* L.) [Umbelliferae or Apiaceae]	Connective tissue protector/promoter (particularly veins, in autoimmune disorders); wound-healing promoter;	Occasional contact dermatitis; very rare systemic reactions with moderate oral use; large dose may cause headache, stupor, dizziness, and coma;	Traditional emmenagogue. Spermicidal effects of saponin fraction could not be demonstrated in (H).	83–90

Plant	Uses/Activity	Notes	Toxicity	Ref.
Gotu kola, Indian or South African pennywort	antiulcerogenic; sedative/stimulant; hepatoprotective	dizziness and diarrhea reported with chronic use. Triterpene glycoside (asiaticoide) constituent is a skin carcinogen in (A) by repeated application. Cholinergic activity by the extract.	No anti-implantation effects or teratogenicity, but questionable antifertility and uterine relaxation demonstrated in some (A).	
13. *Crataegus oxycanthus* L.; *C. monogyna* Jackin [Rosaceae] Hawthorn	Hypotensive; cardiotonic; coronary vasodilator; hypolipemic; sedative; spasmolytic; collagen stabilizer; antimicrobial	Low toxicity in (A) and (H); large doses may cause hypotension, arrhythmias, and sedation. Likely interaction with concurrent cardioactive drugs; documented facilitation of hypotensive effects by mistletoe. Rich in flavonoids (e.g., quercetin, anthrocyanidines), with particular affinity for the heart, its vessels, and the aorta. A commercial preparation of anthrocyanidines of hawthorn origin (Catergen) has been incriminated in cases of hemolytic anemia. Rich in cardiotonic amines (e.g., phenylethylamine, tyramine), choline, acetylcholine, and cyanogenic glycosides (e.g., amygdalins).	Teratogenicity and fetotoxicity of phytocyanogens in (A). Potential oxytocicity by quercetin and tyramine. However, in vivo (A) studies failed to elicit antiovulatory, anti-implantation, and embryotoxic effects and anthrocyanidines from other sources are devoid of fetotoxic or teratogenic effects and have been advocated for their protective action both on the maternal capillaries and those of the placenta and neonate. Mutagenicity was demonstrated in some short-term genotoxicity systems.	91-94

(continues)

Table 1 Continued

Name of plant	Purported indications for use	Pharmacological and toxicological effects relevant to pregnant women	Reproductive pharmacology toxicology in humans (H) and animals (A)	Ref.
13. *Crataegus oxycanthus* L. (continued)		Several proanthrocyanidines in hawthorn exert specific inhibition of angiotensin-converting enzyme, similar to that of captopril.		
14. *Dioscorea villosa* L.; *D. allata* L.; *D. nipponica* Makino; *D. composita* Heml. and related spp. [Dioscoraceae] Wild or bitter yam, colic or rheumatic root; greater yam, guoshanlong; bar-basco; respectively	Source of steroidal hormones; anti-inflammatory; antiallergic; anti-rheumatic, expectorant, hypoglycemic, hypolipemic, cardiotonic, coronary vasodilator, laxative	Mild (H) adverse reactions with moderate nutritional and medicinal use, most commonly diarrhea; serious poisonous species. For example, *D. dumetorum*, used traditionally in Africa as hypoglycemic and as famine food, contains tropane alkaloids (e.g., dioscorine and the hypoglycemic dumetorine), both CNS depressants and convulsants in (A). In (H), overconsumption may result in burning sensation in mouth and throat, GI upset, speech disturbances, followed by vertigo, salivation, lacrimation, sensation of heat, deafness, and delirium; can be fetal within hours or days.	Traditional contraceptive. Emmenogogue effects described. The saponin glycosides are a substrate for industrially derived, active steroids, particularly sex hormones, via chemical and microbiological processes. No information regarding steroidal hormonal effect of the plant itself or its extracts in (A) and (H), although the presence of steroidal phytoestrogens (e.g., sitosterol, stigmasterol) is known. Teratogenicity could not be demonstrated in (A) studies; oxytocic effect of saponin extracts at low dose, tocolytic in high doses in (A).	52,54,55, 78,95–97

		The major active constituents are saponin glycosides (e.g., diosgenin, dioscin). Most edible yams are low saponin or require special preparation to avoid toxicity. Dioscin is convulsant and anticoagulant and contains a powerful trypsin inhibitor. GI spasmodic effects in small doses, relaxant in large doses (A). Sweet yam has been confused with glory lilly (*Gloriosa superba*), with resulting colchicine poisoning.	Purported luteotropic anti-LH antiprogesterone effects in (A) and emmenagogue effects in (H).
15. *Echinacea angustifolia* Dc; *E. purpurea* L. and related spp. [Compositae] Echinacea, American or purple cone flower, scurvy root	Immune stimulant; anti-inflammatory; antimicrobial; wound-healing agent; antineoplastic	Little known about toxicity. No (H) reports; (A) toxicity studies are very scant and so far encouraging. Potential allergenicity as for other Compositae. The plant increases properidin levels, and inulin, the major component, activates the alternative complement pathway, thus promoting several immune and inflammatory reactions; other polysaccharide components bind to	Weak oxytocic effect in (A). Hyaluronidase-inhibiting activity; may interfere with implantation.
			5,98–100

(continues)

465

Table 1 Continued

Name of plant	Purported indications for use	Pharmacological and toxicological effects relevant to pregnant women	Reproductive pharmacology toxicology in humans (H) and animals (A)	Ref.
15. *Echinacea angusti-folia* Dc (continued)		receptors on T lymphocytes, with resulting nonspecific T-cell activation. Allergy- and autoimmune-prone individuals might be at risk by such concerted immune stimulation. Single dose weekly of extracts promoted cell-mediated immunity, while daily higher doses depressed it, in (H) clinical studies. Cortisone-like activity reported in (A).		
16. *Ephedra sinica* Stapf.; *E. mevadensis* Watson (syn. *E. viridis*); *E. gerardiana* Wall ex. Stapf. and related spp. [Ephedraceae (Gnetaceae)] Ma-huang; Mormon, squaw, or teamster's tea; Pakistani ephedra; respectively	Cardiostimulant; hypo-tensive/hypertensive; decongestant (mucous tissues); bronchodilator; GI relaxant; diuretic/antidiuretic; CNS stimulant; astringent; antimicrobial	Overdose reactions to ephedra or its major sympathomimetic alkaloids (e.g., ephedrine, pseudoephedrine) include headache, restlessness, dizziness, tinnitus, insomnia, numbness or tingling of extremities, skin flushing, chest and/or upper abdominal discomfort, hypertension, palpitations, tachycardia, extrasystoles (but bradycardia and cardiosedation in larger doses),	Anti-implantation, equivocal embryotoxic, unspecified antifertility, but not abortifacient effects were demonstrated in (A). Oxytocity of crude extracts of various spp. and of ephedrine was demonstrated in (A) despite evidence of anti-serotonin activity at the uterine level, enhanced by cocaine, blocked by ergot-amine. In (H), however,	101–106

nausea, vomiting, lacrimation, and rhinorrhea, but xerostomia, fever, and psychosis. Immediate or delayed contact dermatitis and allergy to pollen were noted in sensitive individuals. Chronic exposure (such as in antiasthma or antiobesity products) is usually free of cumulative effects in therapeutic doses but tolerance with dependence (likely due to the tachyphylactic propensity of ephedra alkaloids) was reported, as were cases of chronic excessive intake of ephedrine resulting in cardiomyopathy with clinical, hemodynamic, and ECG findings resembling those of pheochromocytoma.

The effect on blood pressure of crude plant material may be very variable depending on the part (roots are usually hypotensive; aerial parts, hypertensive) and the relative concentrations of hypertensive (ephedrine and its

ephedrine is considered to be tocolytic, as are crude extracts in some (A) studies. Sympathomimetics, as a class, were shown to be teratogenic in some (A) but not in (H). Late gestational and prepartum exposure to ephedrine was associated with fetal tachycardia and/or increased beat-to-beat variability and with neonatal CNS irritability.

Table 1 Continued

Name of plant	Purported indications for use	Pharmacological and toxicological effects relevant to pregnant women	Reproductive pharmacology toxicology in humans (H) and animals (A)	Ref.
16. *Ephedra sinica* Stapf. (continued)		congeners, L-tyrosine betaine) and hypotensive (macrocyclic spermine alkaloids – ephedradines, feruloylhistamine) agents in different species. Edible *Ephedra* fruits are usually devoid of sympathomimetic alkaloids; their presence in most North American *Ephedra* species is in dispute. Crude plant materials are hyperglycemic (mostly due to ephedrine), but a hypoglycemic fraction is present as well (A). The constituent volatile oil has potent CNS depressant effect in (A), including generalized muscular paralysis antagonized by ephedrine. Contains phenolic acids (e.g., gallic acid), (+)-catechin (a flavonoid) and its polymerization products (condensed tannins), as well as a saponin.		

17. *Equisetum arvense* L.; *E. hyemale* L. [Equisetaceae] Horsetail, field horsetail; shavegrass, bottle brush, scouring rush, respectively	Diuretic; astringent	Nicotine-like intoxications in (A) and in children using the stems as whistles or blow guns. Seborrheic dermatitis. Contains several potentially toxic compounds besides nicotine (which is present at <1 ppm), including aconitic acid (neurotoxic), the saponin equisitonine (neurotoxic), 3-methoxypyridine (antivitamin B_6), palmitic acid and silica (5–8%; abrasive). Also contains phenolic acids (e.g., caffeic, ferulic, tannins, and oxalic acid. Contains an antithiaminase that was implicated in poisoning (equisetosis) in grazing (A); may be hazardous in alcoholic and other conditions associated with low thiamine.	Nicotine is a teratogenic in some (A) but not in (H). Contains steroidal phytoestrogens (e.g., β-sitosterol), and nicotine itself is estrogenic; but no estrogenicity in an (A) in vivo study. Demonstrated in vitro oxytocicity, likely via nicotine, β-sitosterol, and palmitic acid.	107–109
18. *Eupatorium perfoliatum* L. [Compositae (Asteraceae)] Boneset, Indian sage, feverwort, sweating plant	Anti-inflammatory; antipyretic; diaphoretic; immune stimulant; antimicrobial; laxative	In large doses may be cathartic and emetic. Allergenicity via sesquiterpene lactones; cross-reactivity with other Compositae spp. Contains toxic pyrrolyzidine alkaloids, tannins, polysaccharides (e.g., inulin),	Contains steroidal phytoestrogens (e.g., β-sitosterol). Toxic pyrrolizidines (see *Symphytum*, below, No. 39) and sesquiterpene lactones exert reproductive effects, including potential fetoembryotoxicity and teratogenesis.	64, 100,110

(continues)

Table 1 Continued

Name of plant	Purported indications for use	Pharmacological and toxicological effects relevant to pregnant women	Reproductive pharmacology toxicology in humans (H) and animals (A)	Ref.
18. *Epatorium perfoliatum* L. (continued)		flavonoids (e.g., quercetin), cytotoxic flavones (e.g., eupatorin), and high levels of nitrates.	Oxytocity of tannins, β-sitosterol, and quercetin; however, a tocolytic effect was noted in (A) by a crude extract. High nitrate content (300–1000 ppm), probably responsible for abortion in grazing (A).	
19. *Gentiana lutea* L. *G. acaulis* L. (syn. *G. crassicaulis* Dutt.) *G. manshurica* Kitag.., and related spp. [Gentianaceae] Gentian, yellow gentian, bitter root; stemless gentian, ginjiao; longdan; respectively	Appetite stimulant; choleretic; anti-inflammatory; antihistaminic; analgesic; antimicrobial; hepatoprotective; cardiodepressant (hypotensive, bradycardic); sedative/stimulant; diuretic	May cause gastric irritation via bitter glycosides, with nausea and vomiting even in small doses in sensitive persons; moderately toxic in (A). Contains tannins; the related *G. lactea* contains an MAO inhibitor. Hyperglycemic activity reported (A). May be confused with *Veratrum album* L. (see below, No. 47), which is often adjacent in the field, with resulting serious toxicity.	Folkloric emmenagogue. Larval insecticide. No antiovulating, antifertilization, uterine, or embryotoxic effects were reported in some (A) studies.	111–116

| 20. *Ginkgo biloba* L. [Ginkgoaceae] Ginkgo, maidenhair tree, kew tree | Vasodilator; antithrombotic; anti-inflammatory; antiallergic; spasmolytic; antineoplastic | Mild side effects with therapeutic doses, mostly dizziness, headache, irritability, chest discomfort, and GI discomfort; severe external irritant, vesicant and allergen (pulp), similar to and cross-reactive with poison ivy and related plants. Systemic intoxications following large doses of extracts or small amounts of pulp, including perioral edema, gastroenteritis, senation of rectal burning, tenesmus, nephritis, and pulmonary edema.

Overdose of the kernel may cause additional toxicity including foaming, salivation, and florid neurological symptoms up to convulsions, coma, and death. May induce vasoconstriction particularly in fully dilated vessels.

The major constituents, flavonoids (e.g., quercetin, ginkgogenin, proanthroacyanidines), have a strong affinity for CNS, adrenal, and thyroid tissue. Reported pharmacological actions include | Was used during pregnancy and in labor to improve placental circulation and fetal oxygenation.
Without affecting maternal blood flow or amniotic pressure; increases fetal pH and Po_2 in experimental circulatory insufficiency (A).
Quercetin inhibits estrogen synthetase.
Cyanogenicity. |

(continues)

471

Table 1 Continued

Name of plant	Purported indications for use	Pharmacological and toxicological effects relevant to pregnant women	Reproductive pharmacology toxicology in humans (H) and animals (A)	Ref.
20. *Ginkgo biloba* L. (continued)		antiprostaglandin, antihistamine, antiserotonin, antiplatelet aggregation, calcium channel blocker, free radical scavenger, and antidepressant effects. Different doses may have opposite effects (e.g., small doses of extract, 0.25–4.0 mg/L in vitro activated phosphodiesterase, thus increased cyclic AMP, while higher doses, 5–250 mg/L, exhibited a dose-dependent inhibition).		
21. *Glycyrrhiza glabra* L.; *G. uralensis* Fisch. and related spp. [Leguminosae (Favaceae)] Licorice, Spanish or Russian licorice; gancao, respectively	Anti-inflammatory; antiallergic; antiarthritic; antimicrobial; demulcent; gastroprotective and antiulcerogenic; expectorant; spasmolytic; antidiuretic; antineoplastic; hepatoprotective; antitoxicant	A triterpene glycoside, glycyrrhizine, inhibits steroid dehydrogenase and reductase enzymes, particularly in the liver, thereby increasing the half-life of cortisol, aldosterone, and progesterone in (A) and (H). Acute or chronic overdose or, in some cases, small amounts in remedies, foods,	Traditional emmenagogue and abortifacient. Reported cases of (H) amenorrhea, hyperprolactinemia, loss of libido, and impotence with chronic use; no spermicidal effect observed in (H). Reports of estrogenicity in (A) in vivo, via constituent steroidal phytoestrogens (estradiol, estrone, β-sitosterol),	123–135

or beverages, or in chewing tobacco, may often lead to a well-documented syndrome of pseudohyperaldosteronism with hypertension and hypokalemia.

In (A), administration of extracts may lead to adrenal atrophy.

Both cortisol-like and cortisol-antagonist; evidence of inhibition of 11-β-hydroxy-steroid dehydrogenase by acute and chronic licorice exposure, thereby inhibiting the conversion of the active steroid cortisol to the inactive cortisone.

Attenuates actions of a variety of substances, including poisons (e.g., strychnine, tetrodoxine), drugs (e.g., nicotine, cocaine), and medicinals (e.g., barbiturates, pilocarpine, urethan). Mechanism unclear, possibly including glucuronic-like conjugation action. Enhances toxicity of epinephrine and various botanical compounds including ephedrine.

isoflavones, and coumestans. Glycyrrhizine binds weakly to estrogen and androgen receptors in (A) with likely antihormonal effects. Others report a normalizing of endogenous estrogen regardless of the direction of change.

Oxytocity (including via the constituent alkaloid licorine), tocolysis, or no uterine effects; equivocal or no embryotoxicity; weak anti-implantation; no antiovulatory or antifertilization effects in (A).

Increased progesterone and cortisol half-life.

(continues)

Table 1 Continued

Name of plant	Purported indications for use	Pharmacological and toxicological effects relevant to pregnant women	Reproductive pharmacology toxicology in humans (H) and animals (A)	Ref.
21. *Glycyrrhiza glabra* L. (continued)		Extracts possess anticholinergic activity. Contains tannins, coumarins, flavonoids, salicylates.		
22. *Humulus lupulus* L. [Cannabacea or Moraceae] Hops, lupuline	Sedative/hypnotic; spasmolytic; antimicrobial	Low toxicity in (A) and (H). Therapeutic doses can cause GI irritation, anorexia. Prolonged use may lead to GI upset, dizziness, intoxication, and jaundice. Has been classified as narcotic by some. Contact dermatitis, upper respiratory allergy, and anaphylaxis. Acute intravascular hemolysis was reported, with in vitro confirmation in (H). Hypoglycemia; smoked as marijuana substitute. Contains tannins, flavonoids (e.g., rutin).	Contains phytoestrogens, including estrone and estradiol, but questionable estrogenicity; some reports of high level effects, but no estrogenicity noted so far in beer (contains hops). Tocolysis by extracts was reported. Reduced sensitivity of ovaries to gonadotropins in (A) by extracts. Mutagenicity of crude extracts. Rutin is antigonadotropic (A). Potential oxytocity via constituents tannins and rutin in (A).	5, 136–142
23. *Hydrastis canadensis* L. [Ranunculaceae] Goldenseal, Indian tumeric, yellow root, eye balm	Antimicrobial; immune stimulant; antipyretic; astringent; spasmolytic; choleretic; hypoglycemic; antineoplastic	Overdose may cause mucous hypersecretion, nausea, vomiting and diarrhea, ulcerations of any surface; hypertension or hypotension, myocardiac depression, dyspnea, hyper-	Increases myometrial tonus and stimulates uterine contractions in (A) and (H); had been used as postpartum uterine hemostatic prior to the advent of the more re-	142–148

liable ergot alkaloids. Larger doses are tocolytic.

reflexia, paresthesia, convulsions, and death through respiratory failure. Chronic ingestion of moderate amounts may inhibit vitamin B absorption.

The isoquinoline alkaloids (e.g., bereberine, hydrastine) are of moderately acute (A) toxicity parenterally but have little effect orally and no cumulative chronic toxicity. The alkaloids have at times opposite or dual effect (e.g., hypertension by hydrastine overriding hypotensivity of berberine when testing crude materials in small or moderate dosages). In high dosage hydrastine is hypotensive as well. Notable actions of berberine (A) include respiratory stimulation in therapeutic doses; CNS effects such as paralysis of the respiratory center, ataxia, motor inhibition, and flaccidity; a dose-dependent biphasic effect on acetylcholine (low dosage potentiated and high dosage antagonized it);

(continues)

Table 1 Continued

Name of plant	Purported indications for use	Pharmacological and toxicological effects relevant to pregnant women	Reproductive pharmacology toxicology in humans (H) and animals (A)	Ref.
23. *Hydrastis canadensis* L. (continued)		negative or positive ionotropic and negative chronotropic cardiac effects; hypotensive effect via cholinergic, vasodilation, and inhibition of the pressor reflex of the vasomotor center; antihistamine; cytotoxicity, including via inhibition of the biosynthesis of DNA, RNA, proteins and lipids, and the oxidation of glucose; antimicrobial. Rare cases of allergy to berberine. Contains tannins, volatile oil. Imparts dark appearance to urine; can interfere with urinalytical detection of some illicit drugs.		
24. *Hypericum perforatum* L. [Hyperiaceae (or Guttiferae)] St. John's wort, Klamath weed, devil's scourge, etc.	Anxiolytic/antidepressant; antimicrobial; wound healing; antiulcerogenic; astringent; antineoplastic; diuretic	Appears safe, in limited (H) studies, in usual doses. Extensive phototoxicity in various grazing (A) species, including blindness and often fatal anorexia due to constituent naphthodianthrons	Traditional oxytocic, emmenagogue, abortifacient. Oxytocity reported in (H) in vitro. Oxytocic and tocolytic effects reported in (A). Potential reproductive effects of the constituent MAO	41, 149–151

| 25. *Juniperus communis* L.; *J. sabina* (syn. *J. scropularium*) [Cupressaceae] Common or ground or dwarf juniper; Rocky Mountain or Western juniper; respectively | Diuretic; antimicrobial; astringent; hypoglycemic | (e.g., hypericine), which are powerful MAO inhibitors; no phototoxic effects were reported in (H). Contains tannins and flavonoids (e.g., quercetin, rutin). Kidney irritant (via 4-terpineol) in therapeutic doses; hazardous in the presence of nephritis or other nephropathies. Large or even small repeated doses may cause GI irritation, nephrotoxicity, metrorrhagia, tachycardia, hypertension, psychiatric changes, and seizures. Contact dermatitis and other allergic reactions.

Juniper tar, used dermatologically, contains polycyclic aromatic hydrocarbons, likely carcinogen in (H) skin. Contains phenolic (gallic) acid and tannins, essential oil [with several (A) carcinogenic components], podophyllotoxin (antimitotic, antineoplastic). Smoked as strong hallucinogen. Imparts violet color to urine. | inhibitors (increase uterine serotonin—oxytocity, teratogenicity); steroidal phytoestrogens.

Traditional emmenagogue and abortifacient, but does not stimulate in vitro (H) uterine muscle; uterine excitation following kidney and bladder irritation. Anti-implantation, embryotoxic, oxytocic or tocolytic, and abortifacient effects were noted in some (A), but negative results were reported as well. Podophyllotoxin is a strong embryocidal and growth retardant agent, with questionable teratogenicity (A). Mutagenicity in several bacterial systems. | 20,70, 106, 152–162 |

(continues)

Table 1 Continued

Name of plant	Purported indications for use	Pharmacological and toxicological effects relevant to pregnant women	Reproductive pharmacology toxicology in humans (H) and animals (A)	Ref.
26. *Lobelia inflata* L.; *L. radicans* Thunb. (syn. *L. chinesis* Lour.) [Lobeliaceae or Campanulaceae] Lobelia, Indian tobacco, asthma weed, etc.; Bambianlian, respectively	Expectorant; antitussive; respiratory stimulant; spasmolytic; emetic; tobacco smoking deterrent	Usually safe in therapeutic oral amounts; nicotine-like effects in small or moderate doses of the constituent pyridine alkaloids (particularly lobeline), with CNS stimulation followed by depression, nausea, tremors, dizziness, bradycardia, hypertension, euphoria, and rare contact dermatitis. In large doses, curarelike effects; diaphoresis, emesis, tachycardia, hypotension, hypothermia, paresis, convulsions, coma, medullary paralysis, and death. In susceptible individuals as little as 50 mg of the dried herb, or 1 cc of the tincture has produced adverse effects.	No direct information on reproductive effects; however, lobeline-derived products are considered to be potential teratogens on grounds of structural similarity to known pyridine (piperidine) alkaloids (A). The related plant *Nicotiana tabacum* is a known fetal resorption inducer and teratogen in several (A) species via nicotine; also teratogens are the related *Nicotiana glauca* Graham (via anabasine) and *Conium maculatum* L. (via coniine) (A). Nicotine is estrogenic and oxytocic in (A) studies. Nicotine in lactation may be antigalactogogue.	70,94
27. *Matricaria chamomilla* L.; *Anthemis nobilis* L. (syn. *Chamaemelum nobilis* L.) [Compositae (Asteraceae)]	Spasmolytic; sedative; antimicrobial; anti-inflammatory; antipyretic; antiulcerogenic	Allergic reactions as Compositae with cross-sensitivity. Contact dermatitis, anaphylaxis, and other serious hypersensitivity reactions, via sesquiterpene lactones. In large quantities, can be emetic.	Folkloric emmenagogue and abortifacient. Reproductive safety established for an active constituent α-bisabolol (a sesquiterpene alcohol) and for extracts (regarding embryotoxicity, fertilization, and ovulation).	114, 163–166

| German or Hungarian or wild chamomile; common or English chamomile; respectively | | Sesquiterpene lactones are cytotoxic. | Implicated (indirectly) in a case of hepatic veno-occlusive disease but is not known to contain toxic pyrrolizidines. | |
| 28. *Medicago sativa* L. [Leguminosae] Alfalfa, Lucerne | Nutritive; hypolipemic; antimicrobial; anti-inflammatory | A nonprotein amino acid, L-canavanin—an arginine analog—is found in high concentrations in seeds and sprouts; it inhibits arginine-dependent enzymes; its metabolite canaline is an ornithine analog; may inhibit pyridoxal phosphate and dependent enzymes. Reactivation of systemic lupus erythematosus (SLE) in (H)—linked to *L. canavaline*; also pancytopenia and hypocomplementemia in normal subjects; SLE-like syndrome was induced in monkeys fed alfalfa seeds. Allergenicity: exposure may intensify or exacerbate symptoms caused by sensitivity to other substances (e.g., grass pollen, wheat, etc.). | High content of phytoestrogens including steroidal (including β-sitosterol), coumestans (coumarin derivative), and isoflavones, probably accounting for reproductive disturbances in grazing (A); both estrogenic and anti-estrogenic activities of different extracts; and in different species and experimental conditions; anti- or proluteinizing hormone and prolactine, antigonadotropin, anti-androgenic, antiovulatory, estrus cycle disruptive, contraceptive or interceptive, and equivocal embryotoxic effects were noted in various (A) species; oxytocity in (A) including via the presence in seeds of lactogenic and emmenagogue alkaloids (e.g., | 1, 167–177 |

(continues)

479

Table 1 Continued

Name of plant	Purported indications for use	Pharmacological and toxicological effects relevant to pregnant women	Reproductive pharmacology toxicology in humans (H) and animals (A)	Ref.
28. *Medicago sativa* L. (continued)		High level dietary alfalfa induced intestinal changes in (A) possibly related to an increased susceptibility to colon cancer, including via fermantation products. May cause phototoxicity in (A). Extracts exhibited anti-vitamin E activity. Conflicting reports regarding safety in grazing and experimental (A) including in terms of growth and development. High phenolic fractions (including tannins) inhibited trypsin, amylase, and lipase (A). High saponin content (hypolipemic), hemolytic in vitro but negligibly in vivo under normal conditions. Stimulation of intestinal microsomal mixed function oxidase reactions, and increased rate of hepatic drug metabolism, were demonstrated in (A) with possible effects of drug metabolism.	linolenic, linoleic, palmitic), tannins, β-sitosterol, etc.	

| 29. *Mentha pulegium* L.; *Hedeoma pulegioides* (L.) Pers. (syn. *Cunilia pulegioides* L.) [Labiatae] Pennyroyal, stinkweed; American pennyroyal, squawmint, mosquito plant, respectively | Emmenagogue; abortifacient; antineoplastic; spasmolytic; analgesic; antimicrobial | The active component, a volatile oil (composed of up to 96% monoterpene pulegium) has been associated with severe CNS, liver, GI, kidney, lung, and hematological complications including fatalities in (H) in doses advocated for abortifacient effect (1–2 tbsp). Toxicity, including GI upset, hematemesis, peripheral vascular collapse, confusion, delirium, twitching, seizures, and coma, has been manifested with less than 1 tsp of oil. Neurotoxic and hepatotoxic effects of large doses of oil in (A). Ingestion of small amounts of leaves is probably safe, but long-term use may be harmful. | Traditional and equivocally substantiated emmenagogue and abortifacient application of the oil in (A) and (H), probably via reflex excitation of the uterus following kidney or bladder irritation; no (H) oxytocity was demonstrated in vitro, nor in gravid or nongravid experimental (A). The tea or tablets (leaves) too are hazardous in pregnancy due to potential emmenagogue effect and general toxicity. Out of 21 reported cases of attempted abortion with pennyroyal preparations (mostly oil), 5 were effective, with stated doses of 0.8–15 cc essential oil per person, but always with moderate to serious systemic toxicity. Doses in ineffective cases ranged up to 30 cc/person; however, actual gestation was not ascertained in some of the reports. | 161, 178–180 |

(continues)

481

Table 1 Continued

Name of plant	Purported indications for use	Pharmacological and toxicological effects relevant to pregnant women	Reproductive pharmacology toxicology in humans (H) and animals (A)	Ref.
30. *Mentha x piperata* L.; *M. arvensis* (L.) var. *piperascens* Malinv.; *M. spicata* L. (syn. *M. viridis* L.) [Labiatae] Peppermint; Japanese peppermint, corn mint, bohe; spearmint, respectively	Carminative, choleretic; antiulcerogenic; spasmolytic; sedative/stimulant; anti-inflammatory; antipyretic; antimicrobial; antineoplastic	Peppermint oil, the active constituent (mostly menthol) may cause GI reflux and heartburn in therapeutic (few drops) doses, particularly in cases of hiatus hernia; also hemolysis and jaundice in cases of G6PD deficiency; allergic reactions including to mentholated cigarettes and toothpaste, ranging from contact dermatitis and urticaria, to headache and flushing, to epiglottal spasm and asphyxiation. Larger doses (usually > 5 cc), may produce GI upset, bradycardia, atrial fibrillation, dizziness, ataxia, blurred vision, palindromic rheumatism. Menthol has a calcium channel blocking effect. Several components of the essential oil are (A) carcinogenic. Contains flavonoids (e.g., rutin, hesperidin), tannins, and salicylates.	Traditional emmenagogue and abortifacient. Spermicidal activity noted in (H) in vitro. Conflicting information regarding anti-ovulatory, antiimplantation, oxytocic, embryotoxic, and abortifacient effects by extracts, particularly the essential oil. Young leaves are high in pulegiol, a known (A) and (H) abortifacient. Mutagenicity of menthol but not of the crude oil. Potential antigonadotropism, oxytocity etc., via constituent flavonoids and tannins.	181–190

| 31. *Panax ginseng* C.A. Mayer; *P. quinti-folium* L.; *P. pseu-doginseng* Wall, and related *Panax* spp.; *Eletheuro-coccus senticosus* (Rupr. and Maxim.) Maxim. [(syn. *Acan-thopanax senticosus* (Rupr. and Maxim.) Maxim.)] [Araliaceae] Korean ginseng; American ginseng; Sanchi ginseng; Siberian ginseng or wild pepper or touch-me-not, respectively | Adoptogen (i.e., pro-moter of nonspecific increased resistance to various stressors and pathogenic insults); CNS stimulant; antipsy-chotic; antidepressant; anticonvulsant; cardio-arrhythmic; hypotensive/hypertensive; anti-inflammatory; antialler-gic, immune-stimulant; analgesic; spasmolytic; hypoglycemic; hypolipe-mic; antidiuretic, anti-toxicant, particularly antihepatotoxic; antineoplastic | Low toxicity in (A), relatively free of adverse effects in small and moderate doses in (H); occasional GI upset and hemorrhagic tendencies were noted. Chronic use of larger doses (> 3 g/day) has led to ginseng abuse syndrome in 15% of users: hypertension, tonic; antianginotic; anti-nervousness, insomnia, skin eruptions; also noted: head-ache, precordial pain, edema, palpitations, hypotension, bleeding disorders; anorexia and weight loss, euphoria or depression, restlessness, vertigo, increased or decreased sexual potency. Higher amounts (> 15 g/d) may lead to cardiodepression, CNS depression, confusion, and feelings of depersonali-zation; very large doses have caused fatalities. Withdrawal from long-term use was re-ported to result in hypoten-sion, weakness, and tremor in some individuals. Several cases of neonatal in-toxication (with 0.3–0.6 mL decoction), including one fatality. |

(continues)

Table 1 Continued

Name of plant	Purported indications for use	Pharmacological and toxicological effects relevant to pregnant women	Reproductive pharmacology toxicology in humans (H) and animals (A)	Ref.
32. *Passiflora incarnata* L.; *P. laurifolia* L., and related spp. [Passifloraceae] Passion flower, passiflora, grandilla, maypop, etc.; Jamaican honeysuckle, respectively	Sedative/hypnotic; spasmolytic; analgesic; anticonvulsant; hypotensive; antimicrobial; anti-inflammatory	In large doses, reports of complex, dose-related CNS stimulant/depressant effects in (A) and (H), related to constituent indole (harmala) alkaloids (e.g., harmine and harmaline, which are MAO inhibitors in large doses); a maltol-containing fraction, and flavonoids (e.g., quercetin). Classified by some as a narcotic. Contains coumarins and cyanogenic glycosides. Harmaline is more hallucinogenic than mescaline.	Contains steroidal phytoestrogens (e.g., β-sitosterol). Conflicting reports about oxytocity by crude preparations in (A); the constituent harmala alkaloid (via serotonin accumulation in uterus by MAO inhibition; quercetin, and other flavonoids, e.g., rutin; phytosterols, and fatty acids, e.g., linoleic) are oxytocic in (A). Reproductive concerns regarding coumarins, cyanogenic glycosides, and flavonoids, particularly quercetin and phytoestrogens, include teratogenicity and embryotoxicity in (A).	4,47,56, 210–212
33. *Phytolacca americana* L. (syn. *P. acinosa* Roxb.) [Phytolaccaceae] Pokeweed, inkberry, American nightshade, Shanglu	Immune stimulant; anti-inflammatory; antimicrobial (mostly viral); emetic; expectorant	Highly toxic in (H) mainly via triterpene saponins (e.g., phytolaccine); GI irritant and five nonspecific mitogens with symptomatology ranging from gastroenteritis (including hemorrhagic), burning sensation of mouth	Traditional abortifacient. Spermaticidal and blastocidal in some (A) by extracts of the related *P. decandra* L.; a report on such contraceptive use in (H). Oxytocic and abortifacient in (A).	12, 213–217

and stomach, headache and dizziness in mild cases, including in "therapeutic" doses, to lethargy, weakness, sweating, salivation, urgency, blurred vision, paresthesia, vertigo, syncope, hypotension, respiratory depression, and convulsions in severe cases. Ingestion of fewer than 10 uncooked berries in adults is usually harmless; the root, shoots and leaves are toxic as well. Fatalities reported, particularly in children; central and peripheral cholinergic mechanisms are suggested in severe toxicity. The mitogens have hemagglutinating as well as mitogenic activities; plasmacytosis, thrombocytopenia, and other hematological abnormalities noted, possibly related to immune or hypersensitivity mechanisms. In therapeutic amounts, stimulates corticosteroid release via central mechanisms (A). Contains tannins, oxalic acid.

Potential oxytocicity via tannins.

(continues)

485

Table 1 Continued

Name of plant	Purported indications for use	Pharmacological and toxicological effects relevant to pregnant women	Reproductive pharmacology toxicology in humans (H) and animals (A)	Ref.
34. *Plantago ovata* Forsks.; *P. psyllium* L.; *P. indica* L. (syn. *P. arenaria* Walds. and Kit.) and related spp. [Plantaginacea] Blond or Indian psyllium, ispagula, psyllium, ispagula, etc.; French, Spanish, or brown psyllium; black psyllium, respectively; all are also known as plantago, plantain (there is considerable confusion in the literature regarding common names (e.g., compare).	Laxative; antidiarrheal; demulcent/emolient; hypolipemic; hypoglycemic; antiulcerogenic; anti-inflammatory; expectorant; antitussive; respiratory depressant; antimicrobial; hepatotonic	Generally safe in (H) experience. Allergenicity mostly occupational (e.g., considerable risk to respiratory health of personnel in chronic care hospitals); there is a case of anaphylactic shock with medicinal (laxative) use. Reports of esophageal and intestinal (bezoar) impaction. Contains a nephrotoxic pigment (H), which is removed from commercial preparations. May interfere with absorption of concurrent medication and nutrients. Reports of both carcinogenic and antitumor effects in (A). Causes epithelial cell loss and muscle layer hypertrophy in the jejunum and ileum after prolonged use in monkeys. Contains several alkaloids including plantagin, a car-	Traditional contraceptive and abortifacient, including intravaginally. Clinical abortifacient in (H) by dilatory intravaginal application. Estrogenic and progestogenic (H); also an ovulation-inducing effect. No estrogenicity, but antiandrogenic effects were noted in (A). Sperm coagulation and spermicidal studies were negative, as were studies of milk production. Contains steroidal phytoestrogens (e.g., β-sitosterol); tannins; fatty acids (e.g., linoleic). Issues of oxytocicity, also antigonadotropism, antiimplantation cytotoxicity, etc. (e.g., β-sitosterol).	1, 218–235

	Uses	Toxicity	Comments	Ref.
		diovascular stimulant and de-pressant in small and large doses, respectively, in (A). Contains tannins. Inhibits (A) and (H) pancreatic proteolytic enzymes and lipase. May inhibit absorption of vitamin B_1 in (H).		1,236
35. *Rhamnus purshianus* DC [Rhamnaceae] Cascara sagrada, sacred bark, chittem bark	Cathartic laxative; emetic; antineoplastic	Relatively mild irritant laxative via anthraglycosides (e.g., cascaroides) and free anthraquinones (e.g., emodin), but severe intoxications including fatalities have been reported. Symptoms include dizziness, nausea, emesis, abnormal pain, watery or bloody diarrhea (drastic catharsis) with further complications. If enough is absorbed, kidney damage is possible. Chronic use may deplete potassium and magnesium and may cause colonic melanosis and other features of cathartic colon syndrome. Contains tannin and phenols. Imparts red color to urine.	Folkloric abortifacient; reports of severe intoxications when used. Probably safe as an occasional laxative during pregnancy but possible fetal adverse effects with large or extended dose. Potential oxytocicity and other effects via tannin.	

(continues)

Table 1 Continued

Name of plant	Purported indications for use	Pharmacological and toxicological effects relevant to pregnant women	Reproductive pharmacology toxicology in humans (H) and animals (A)	Ref.
36. *Rubus idaeus* L. [Rosaceae] Raspberry, American raspberry, hindberry, bramble of Mount Ida	Uterine contractility modulator; astringent; antidiarrheal; hypoglycemic	May cause contact dermatitis via constituent linolenes. Contains coumarins, phenolic acids, and tannins. "Lithospermic acid" was reported to inhibit thyrotropin.	Uterine relaxant effects of extracts were demonstrated in pregnant but not in nonpregnant (H) uterus. Contains fragarine and other substances that can act as either uterine stimulants or relaxants as demonstrated in various (A) species in vitro and/or in vivo, as well as for crude extracts, but not in others. Contains "lithospermic acid" (a mixture), which was shown to inhibit effects of gonadotropin (pituitary and chorionic) and prolactin in (A) in vitro and in vivo.	237–241
37. *Scutellaria laterifolia* L.; *S. baicalensis* Georgi [Labiatae]	Sediative/hypnotic; spasmolytic; hypotensive; anti-inflammatory; antiallergic;	Low toxicity in (H) with conventional doses; rare GI tract upset. Overdoses may cause giddiness, confusion, stupor,	Potential reproductive implications of coumarins, tannins, and of the hypoglycemic effect. Traditional remedy for abnormal fetal movements. Contains steroidal phytoestrogens (e.g., β-sitosterol: con-	1,37, 242–246

Plant	Activity	Comments	Ref.
Skullcap, helmet flower, mad dog weed; huangquin, respectively	antimicrobial; diuretic	cerns of oxytocicity, cyto-toxicity, antigonadotropism, etc.). Potential reproductive implications of the constituent tannin and volatile oil. twitching, and epilepsy according to old reports. Several cases of hepatitis associated with ingestion of a preparation containing skullcap and valerian. Low toxicity in (A) PO; high toxicity IV. Anti-inflammatory via potent inhibition of sialidase by flavonoids (e.g., baicalein) and antihistamine effect. Drug-metabolizing enzyme inhibitor (A). Contains volatile oils, tannin, a bitter glycoside, etc.	
38. *Silybum marianum* (L.) Gaertn. (syn. *Caardus marianus* L.) [Compositae] Milk thistle, silybum	Hepatoprotective/ promotive choleretic; hypolipemic	Remarkable safety of the flav-olignan active constituents (e.g., silymarin or silibin) in experimental (A) and clinical studies. Diarrhea reported with high doses. Poisoning reported in grazing (A) due to high nitrate content. High doses are hepatotoxic in vitro in (A) and (H). Silymarin inhibits prostaglandin synthetase and cyclic AMP phosphodiesterase. Traditional emmenagogue. Contains tyramine, an (A) oxytocic; however, no uterine effects were observed in pregnant (A) by crude extracts. Potential reproductive implications of antiprostaglandin effects.	1,247

(continues)

Table 1 Continued

Name of plant	Purported indications for use	Pharmacological and toxicological effects relevant to pregnant women	Reproductive pharmacology toxicology in humans (H) and animals (A)	Ref.
38. *Silybum marianum* (L.) Gaertn. (continued)		Enhancement of mixed function oxidase systems (A), but in (H) there was no change in the half-life of concomitant phenazone and phenylbutazone.		
39. *Symphytum officinale* L.; *S. asperum* Lepechin; *S. x uplandicum* Nyman (a hybrid of the preceding spp.) [Boraginaceae] Common comfrey, knitbone, bruisewort, ass-ear, bum plant; prickly comfrey; Russian comfrey, respectively	Anti-inflammatory; astringent; demulcent/emolient; wound-healing promoter (in various tissues); hemostatic; expectorant; antineoplastic	Several cases of (H) poisoning by comfrey (particularly roots and young leaves) preparation (teas, tablets, fresh leaves), including fatalities. Many more toxicities to *Senecio*, *Crotalaria* and *Heliotropium* genera. The most common finding is hepatic veno-occlusive disease, usually presenting with dull ache in the upper abdomen, hepatomegaly, or hepatosplenomegaly, ascites, pedal edema, decreased urinary output, headache, apathy, and quasipathognomonic histology, which can develop within days or even weeks after a short-term large dose exposure. More frequently daily	Some comfrey preparations reported to exhibit antigonadotropin effects in vitro and in vivo (A). Cases of fatal (H) neonatal veno-occlusive hepatic disease consequent to gestational exposure to moderate daily amounts (beverage of uncertain identity) throughout the pregnancy, without apparent ill effect on the mother. Transplacental liver necrosis in (A) was found in dosage regimen that failed to affect the maternal liver. Various fetotoxicities and structural terata (mostly skeletal, also visceral) (A), possibly due to the alkylating properties of the toxic metabolites.	1, 248–259

		amounts of 1–3 cups of comfrey root tea over many months or a few years prior to diagnosable pathology. Hepatocellular and renal tumors were noted in (A) fed diet rich in comfrey for 2 years. Large doses (A) led to lesions to the renal glomeruli, pancreas, and GI tract; metabolic and hematological alterations; right ventricular hypertrophy; pulmonary arterial hypertension; and endothelial lesions. Roots and young leaves are richest in P/A, and cooking destroys much of their toxic propensity.	Oxytocic in (A). Production of toxic pyrroles from P/A was noted in embryos (H).	
40. *Tanacetum parthenium* Sch-Bip. (syn. *Chrysanthemum parthenium* L. Bernh.) [Compositae (Asteraceae)]	Analgesic; anti-inflammatory; antipyretic; antipsoriatic	Potentially toxic tannins; choline; the treterpene sabaurenol.

In long-term (H) users: reports of oral inflammation and ulcerations, nausea, vomiting, tachycardia, sedative and tranquilizing effects, and visual disturbances. Withdrawal syndrome: rebound migraine, anxiety, | Traditional emmenagogue, abortifacient and acbolic oxytocic and for threatened miscarriage. Teratogenicity in (A). Mutagenicity in bacteria but no genotoxic effects in (H) chronic consumption. | 58, 260–265 |

(continues)

Table 1 Continued

Name of plant	Purported indications for use	Pharmacological and toxicological effects relevant to pregnant women	Reproductive pharmacology toxicology in humans (H) and animals (A)	Ref.
40. *Tanacetum parthenium* Sch-Bip. (continued) Feverfew, featherfew, midsummer daisy, Santa Maria		sleep disturbance, muscle and joint stiffness, and fatigue. Contact dermatitis via sesquisterpene lactones; cross-sensitivity with other Compositae (e.g., ragweed, chamomile) and with plants from other families containing chemically related lactones. Extracts exhibit pronounced antiprostaglandin, antileuko-trienes, antihistamine, and antiserotonin action in (A) and (H), with antithrombotic and antiplatelet aggregation consequences.		
41. *Taraxacum officinalis* Wiggers; *T. mongolicum* Hand.-Mazz. [Compositae (Asteraceae)] Dandelion, lion's tooth etc.; pugongying, respectively	Diuretic; laxative/anti-diarrheal; choleretic; hepatoprotective; immune-stimulant; anti-inflammatory, antimicrobial; hypoglycemic	In therapeutic doses, occasional nausea, vomiting, diarrhea; contact dermatitis in sensitive individuals as with other Compositae, via sesquiterpene lactones, with common cross-sensitivity; infrequent systemic hypersensitivity reactions.	In (A) studies, no demonstration of estrogenic, oxytocic, embryotoxic, fertilization inhibition, or antiovulatory effects, despite the presence of phytoestrogenic compounds (e.g., β-sitosterol, coumestrol) tannins, and sesquiterpene lactones.	58, 109,114, 266–268

42. *Trifolium pratense* L.; *T. repense* [Leguminosae] Red clover, meadow clover, cow clover, white clover, respectively	Antineoplastic; antimicrobial; antithrombotic; spasmolytic; expectorant; nutritive	Low toxicity in (A). Contains inulin (40% in root), tannins, and phenols. In (A) potent diuretic effect. Rich in coumarins. A case of hemorrhagic illness was associated with a multi-ingredient remedy containing clover and other coumarin-bearing plants. Contains cyanogenic glycosides; responsible for toxicity in grazing (A). Photodermatitis (A). The seeds contain trypsin and chymotrypsin inhibitors. Considerable content of saponins; also presence of phenolic acids, salicylates, chloramide (L-dopa conjugated with caffeic acid).	Rich source of vitamin A (14,000 IU/100 g). In excess, vitamin A is a teratogen in (A) and (H). Estrogenic activity in several studies but negative reports as well (A); contains pignan (equol), isoflavones and coumestrol phytoestrogens; crude extracts stronger than components. Reported substantial antifertility effect in grazing (A), tocolytic (A) and questionable antispermatic effects. Congenital joint laxity and dwarfism in (A) fed clover silage during gestation, related to low manganese bioavailability in such silage. Teratological and other implications of coumarins and cyanogenic glycosides.	1,4,109, 269–275
43. *Tussilago farfara* L. [Compositae] Coltsfoot, coughwort, horse-hoof, kuandong Hua	Expectorant; antitussive; antiasthmatic; demulcent	Weak allergen via sesquiterpene lactones, compared to other Compositae. Contains toxic pyrrolizidine alkaloids (e.g., tussilagine), phenolic acids and tannins,	Reproductive hazards of pyrrolizidine alkaloids (see *Symphytum* above, No. 39). One case of purported coltsfoot consumption during pregnancy resulting in fatal	257,276

(continues)

Table 1 Continued

Name of plant	Purported indications for use	Pharmacological and toxicological effects relevant to pregnant women	Reproductive pharmacology toxicology in humans (H) and animals (A)	Ref.
43. *Tussilago farfara* L. (continued)		flavonoids (e.g., quercetin), choline, inuline, essential oils. Rats fed diets rich in coltsfoot developed liver tumors, likely via the constituent pyrrolizidine alkaloids. Respiratory and cardiovascular stimulatory action of the constituent sesquiterpene, tussilagone. Potent platelet aggregation suppression by extract; also, a calcium channel blocker.	neonatal hepatoveno-occlusive disease attributed to pyrrolizidine alkaloids; however, questionable botanical identity on chemoanalytical grounds. Small doses of an extract are oxytocic in vitro and in vivo (A). Large doses: tocolysis inhibition or initial stimulation followed by inhibition. Contains steroidal phytoestrogens (e.g., sitosterol, stigmasterol) Potential oxytocicity via quercetin, phytoestrogens, and tannins.	
44. *Ulmus fulva* Michx. (syn. *U. rubra* Muhle) [Ulmaceae] Slippery elm, red elm	Demulcent/emollient; GI anti-inflammatory; antimicrobial; expectorant	Contact dermatitis and pollen allergenicity; no systemic reactions reported. Contains cyanidanol glycosides and calcium oxalate.	Traditional abortifacient and ecbolic. Contains steroidal phytoestrogens (e.g., β-sitosterol). Concerns of oxytocicity, cytotoxicity, and antigonadotropism.	1,277
45. *Urtica diorca* L. [Urticaceae]	Antiallergic; immune-stimulant;	Contact urticaria (H) likely by leukotrienes, histamine, and	Traditional emmenagogue and abortifacient.	1, 278–285

Stinging or common or greater nettle	antirheumatic; diuretic; astringent; antineoplastic; nutritive	serotonin existing in plant hairs and extracts, via direct inflammatory effects and secondary release of tissue mediators. Ingestion of hot water extract (tea) may cause gastric irritation, burning sensation of skin, edema, and oliguria, likely reflecting hypersensitivity reactions. Hyperglycemic effects in (A). Contains a mitogenic lectin, stimulating (H) lymphocytic proliferation; a spasmolytic coumarinic glycoside scopoletin; tannins.	Reports of weak anti-implantation activity, both in vitro and in vivo oxytocicity, but no abortifacient effect and equivocal embryotoxicity in (A). Potential antigonadotropic cytotoxic/neoplastic, oxytocic agent. Structural teratogenicity and functional fetal and/or neonatal toxicity via the presence of steroidal phytoestrogen (e.g., β-sitosterol), serotonin coumarins, tannins, flavonoids, fatty acids (e.g., linoleic, palmitic), betaine, and leukotrienes.	
46. *Valeriana officinalis* L.; *V. wallichii* DC; *V. edulis* Mayer and related spp. [Valerianaceae] Valerian, all-heel; Indian valerian; Mexican valerian, respectively	Sedative/hypnotic; spasmolytic; anticonvulsant; hypotensive; antidiuretic; hepatoprotective; antineoplastic; antimicrobial	Very low oral toxicity in (A) and (H) including in controlled short-term trials. Active ingredients, the valepotriates (iridoids) exhibit cytotoxic and antineoplastic effects in (A) in vitro, with alkylating activity comparable to mustardlike agents; substantially less in vivo activity. Concern has been raised about long-term use	Studies failed to show anti-ovulation, antifertilization, and embryotoxic effect (A). Oxytocic, tocolytic, or no uterine effects were reported for various crude extracts, including essential oil, in vitro, and in vivo. Contains steroidal phytoestrogens (e.g., β-sitosterol). Issues of antigonadotropism, anti-implantation, cytotoxicity,	1,58,114, 286-290

(continues)

Table 1 Continued

Name of plant	Purported indications for use	Pharmacological and toxicological effects relevant to pregnant women	Reproductive pharmacology toxicology in humans (H) and animals (A)	Ref.
46. *Valeriana officinalis* L. (continued)		in (H). Classified by some as a narcotic. A preparation consisting of valerian and skullcap (see *Scutellaria*, above, No. 37) was implicated in several cases of (H) hepatitis. Contains tannins and essential oils, flavonoids, choline. Acts as sedative in states of agitation and as a stimulant in cases of fatigue.	oxytocity, etc. (A); potential oxytocity via tannins. Mutagenic activity in bacterial models.	
47. *Veratrum album* L.; *V. viride* L. [Liliaceae] White (European or American) hellebore; green or false hellebore, respectively	Hypotensive; sedative; spasmolytic; antineoplastic	Highly toxic in (A) and (H) via glycoalkaloids (e.g., veratrine). (H) symptoms include nausea, vomiting, abdominal pain, salivation, bradycardia, hypotension, respiratory depression, confusion, syncope, and seizures. Rarely fatal because of early emesis and poor GI absorption. Has been used as sneezing powder with resulting toxicity.	Traditional abortifacient. Early embryonic death and teratogenicity in some (A). Mostly craniofacial, cephalic, and limb defects in several species, with different terata with different stages of exposure. Oxytocic in vitro and estrogenic in some (A); no oxytocicity in vivo (A), and abortifacient effect could not be demonstrated.	108,218

48. *Verbascum thapsus* L. [Scrophulariaceae] Mullein, candleflower, longwort, etc.	Demulcent (mostly respiratory); astringent; antimicrobial	Cases of occupational dermatitis. Contains tannins, saponins, hydrocarbons, and triterpenic alcohol.	The related *V. lasianthum* yields a steroidal phytoestrogen (β-sitosterol); potential oxytocicity. Potential reproductive implications of tannins.	1, 295–296
49. *Viscum album* L.; *Phoradendron serotinum* (Ref.) M.C. Johns. and related spp. [Loranthaceae] European and American mistletoe, respectively	Hypotensive; cardiodepressant; sedative; spasmolytic; immunostimulatory; antineoplastic	Large ingestion may cause gastroenteritis leading to dehydration, bradycardia, hypotension/hypertension, delirium, hallucinations, and cardiac arrest; fatalities reported, particularly in children (it is a common intoxicant in this age group). In most cases, up to 3 berries or 2 leaves are innocuous. Contains toxic proteins (viscotoxins, pharotoxins) that interfere with DNA and RNA synthesis), lectins [in minute amounts, yet highly cytotoxic in (H); comparable to ricin and abrin; increase secretion of interleukins and tumor necrosis factor (TNF) in (A) and in (H)], pressor amines (e.g., β-phenylhydramine,	Traditional contraceptive and abortifacient; fatalities reported following such use. Several reports from nineteenth century on (H) labor induction and abortion. Extracts are oxytocic in vitro and in vivo in (A). Contains steroidal phytoestrogens (e.g., β-sitosterol); issues of antigonadotropism, antiimplantation, and cytotoxicity. Constituent amines, fatty acids (e.g., linoleic, palmitic), and β-sitosterol are oxytocic in (A). Potential reproductive implication of potent antineoplastic effects in vitro and in vivo in (A) and encouraging (H) safety.	297–300

(continues)

497

Table 1 Continued

Name of plant	Purported indications for use	Pharmacological and toxicological effects relevant to pregnant women	Reproductive pharmacology toxicology in humans (H) and animals (A)	Ref.
49. *Viscum album* L. (continued)		tyramine, histamine), GI irritative alkaloids, acetylcholine, complex (tannins) and simple phenolics, flavonoids (e.g., quercetin), a wide range of carbohydrates, and fatty acids. Pilocarpine-like effect reported; may interfere with asthma treatment and anticholinergic drugs. Hypoglycemic (A). Lethal doses (A) were associated with hemorrhagic manifestations (liver, GI) and fatty degeneration of the thymus.		

| 50. *Zingiber officinalis* Rosc. [Zingiberaceae] Ginger, shengjiang | Anti-inflammatory; antirheumatic; immunestimulant; antimicrobial; analgesic; antiemetic; antiulcerogenic; hypolipemic; hypoglycemic; cardiotonic; antineoplastic | Devoid of toxicity in usual amounts (A), (H); large overdose may cause CNS depression, hallucinations, and cardiac arrhythmias. Potent inhibitor of prostaglandins, thromboxane and leukotriene synthesis, platelet aggregation, and histamine release. Contains essential oils, cytotoxic compounds, salicylates, monoterpenes. Stimulates liver cytochrome P-450 and other drug-metabolizing enzymatic systems; may affect concomitant medication. | Traditional abortifacient. Extracts of related *Curcurma longa* L. (tumeric), *Curcurma zedoaric* Rosc., and *Alpinia* spp. exhibit anti-implantation, oxytocic, and abortifacient activities (A). No pertinent studies specific to ginger could be found except as part of multi-ingredient compounds implicated as a tocolytic (A); an extract of the related *Z. cassumunar* Roxb. exhibited a dose-related uterine-relaxing effect in pregnant and nonpregnant (A). Contains both mutagenic and antimutagenic constituents as determined in short-term genotoxicity essays. | 70,218, 301–305 |

Randor et al.

REFERENCES

1. OTA Workshop Staff on Plants. Plants—The Potentials for Extracting Protein, Medicines, and Other Useful Chemicals. Workshops Proceedings. Congress of the United States Office of Technology Assessment, Washington, DC, 1984, pp 1-252.
2. Tajiri J, Higashi K, Morita M, Umeda T, Sato T. Studies of hypothyroidism in patients with high iodine intake. J Clin Endocrinol Metab 1986; 63(2):412-417.
3. Severson RK, Nomura AM, Grove JS, Stemmermann GN. A prospective study of demographics, diet, and prostate cancer among men of Japanese ancestry in Hawaii.
4. Harmon NE, Blackburn JL. Herbal Products: A Factual Appraisal for the Health Care Professional. Context Publications, Winnipeg, 1985.
5. Reddy BS, Numoto S, Choi CI. Effect of dietary *Laminaria angustata* (brown seaweed) on azoxymethane induced intestinal carcinogenesis in male F344 rats. Nutr Cancer 1985; 7(1-2):59-64.
6. Omura T, Hisamatsu S, Takizawa Y, Minowa M, Yanagawa H, Shigematsu I. Geographic distribution of cerebrovascular disease mortality and food intake in Japan. Soc Sci Med 1987; 24(5):401-407.
7. Cardellina JH, Marner FJ, Moore RE. Seaweed dermatitis: Structure of lyngbyatoxin A. Science 1979; 204:193-195.
8. Yamamoto I, Maruyama H, Moriguchi M. The effect of dietary seaweed on 7,12-dimethyl-benz[a]anthracene-induced mammary tumorigenesis in rats. Cancer-Lett 1987 May; 35(2):109-118.
9. Kemper K, Horwitz RI, McCarthy P. Decreased neonatal serum bilirubin with plain agar: A meta-analysis. Pediatrics 1988; 82(4):631-638.
10. Pintauro SJ, Gilbert SW. The effects of carrageenan on drug-metabolizing enzyme system activities in the guinea-pig. Food Chem Toxicol 1990; 28(12):807-811.
11. Olms G, *Fucus. Fucus vesiculosus.* 1991; 140-146.
12. Kong YC, Xie J, But PP. Fertility regulating agents from traditional Chinese medicines. J Ethnopharmacol 1986; 15:1-44.
13. Galina MP, Avnet NL, Einhorn A. Iodides during pregnancy. An apparent cause of neonatal death. N Engl J Med 1962; 22(267):1124-1127.
14. Krishna U, Gupta AN, Ma HK, Manuilova I, Hingorani V, Prashad RN, Bygdeman M, Herczeg J, Obersnel KD, Losa A, et al. Randomized comparison of preoperative cervical dilatation. World Health Special Programme of Research, Development and Research Training in Human Research: Task Force on Prostaglandins for Fertility Regulation. Contraception 1986; 34(3):237-251.
15. Van LL, Darney PD. Successful pregnancy outcome after cervical dilatation with multiple *Laminaria* tents in preparation for second-trimester elective abortion: A report of two cases. Am J Obstet Gynecol 1987; 156(3):612-613.
16. Thangam TS, Kathiresan K. Toxic effect of seaweed extracts on mosquito larvae. Indian J Med Res 1988; 88:35-37.
17. Rovasio RA, Monis B. Teratogenic effect of lambda carrageenan on the chick embryo. Teratology 1981; 23:273-278.

18. Bologa-Campeanu M, Koren G, Rieder M, McGuigan ??. Prenatal adverse effects of various drugs and chemicals. A review of substances of frequent concern to Canadian mothers. Med Toxicol 1988; 3:307-323.
19. Hamon NW. Garlic and the genus *Allium*. Can Pharmaceut J 1987; 120:492-498.
20. Caporaso N, Smith SM, Eng RHK. Antifungal activity in the human urine and serum after ingestion of garlic (*Allium sativum*). Antimicrob Agents Chemother 1983; 23:700.
21. Fedder SL. Spinal epidural hematoma and garlic ingestion (letter). Neurosurgery 1990; 27(4):659.
22. Stallbaumer M. Onion poisoning in a dog. Vet Rec 1981; 108:523-524.
23. Willis JA Jr. Goitrogens in foods. Intoxicants occurring in fods. Natl Acad Sci Nat Res Council 1966; 3-17.
24. Backon J. Predicting new effective treatments of alcohol addiction on the basis of their properties of inhibition of noradrenergic activity and/or thromboxane or on the activation of the dopamine reward system and/or the β-endorphin. Med Hypotheses 1989; 29:237-239.
25. Lorenzo VB, Sanchez B, Murias F, Dominguez MC. Garlic extract as an oxytocic substance. Arch Inst Farmacol Exp 1958; 10:10-14.
26. Sharaf A. Food plants as a possible factor in fertility control. Qual Plant Mater Veg 1969; 17:153.
27. Prakash AO, Mathur R. Screening of Indian plants for antifertility activity. Indian J Exp Biol 1976; 14:623-626.
28. Prakash AO, Gupta RB, Mathur R. Effect of oral administration of forty-two indigenous plant extracts on early and late pregnancy in albino rats. Probe 1978; 17:4 315-323.
29. Kamboj VP. A review of Indian plants with interceptive activity. Indian J Med Res 1988; 4:336-355.
30. Dixit VP, Joshi S. Effects of chronic administration of garlic (*Allium sativum* Linn.) on testicular function. Indian J Exp Biol 1982; 20:534-536.
31. Tokin IB. The effect of phytoncides on spermatozoa and spermatogenesis in mammals. Dokl Akad Nauk SSSR 1953; 93:567-568.
32. Lafont P, Lafont J. Genotoxicity of spices and flavors: Determination by three different methods. Boll Chim Farm 1987; 126:133-135.
33. Stacchini A, Mangegazzini C. Aromatic plants used in foods: Criteria for evaluating their safety. Boll Chim Farm 1987; 126:88-92.
34. The Lawrence Review of Natural Products. Aloe. Monograph. Pharmaceutical Information Associates, Levittown, PA, 1988.
35. Grindlay D, Reynolds T. The aloe vera phenomenon: A review of the properties and modern uses of the leaf parenchyma gel. J Ethnopharmacol 1986; 16: 117-151.
36. Hogan DJ. Widespread dermatitis after topical treatment of chronic leg ulcers and stasis dermatitis. Can Med Assoc J 1988; 138:336-338.
37. Boyd LJ. The pharmacology of the homeopathic drugs. J Am Inst Homeopathy 1928; 21:7-15.
38. Goswami CS, Bokadia MM. The effects of extracts of *Aloe barbadensis* leaves on the fertility of female rats. Indian Drugs 1979; 16:124-125.

Randor et al.

39. Tewari PV, Mapa HC, Chaturvedi RR. Experimental study on estrogenic activity of certain indigenous plants. J Res Indian Med Yoga Homeopathy 1976; 11:7–12.

40. Taussig SJ, Bakin S. Bromelain, the enzyme complex of pineapple (*Ananas comosus*) and its clinical application. An update. J Ethnopharmacol 1988; 22: 191–203.

41. Lots-Winter H. On the pharmacology of bromelain: An update with special regard to animal studies on dose-dependent effects. Planta Med 1990; 56(3): 249–253.

42. Hunter RG, Henry GW, Civin WH. The action of papain and bromelain on the uterus. Am J Obstet Gynecol 1957; 73(2):875–880.

43. Yagami Y, Aoyama T. Action of bromelain on the uterine cervix. Acta Obstet Gynaecol Jap 1969; 16(1):12–16.

44. Garg SK, Saksena SK, Chaudhury RR. Antifertility screening of plants. Part VI. Effects of five indigenous plants on early pregnancy in albino rats. Indian J Med Res 1970; 58:1285–1289.

45. Pakrashi A, Basak B. Abortifacient effect of steroids from *Ananas comosus* and their analogues on mice. J Reprod Fertil 1976; 46:461–462.

46. Maurer HR, Hozumi M, Okabe-Kado J. Bromelain induces the differentiation of leukemic cells in vitro: An explanation for its cytostatic effects? Planta Med 1988; ?:377–806.

47. The Lawrance Review of Natural Products. *Ananas comosus*. Monograph System. Pharmaceutical Information Associates, Levittown, PA, 1988.

48. Murakami S, Kijima H, Isobe Y, Muramatsu M, Aihara H, Otomo S, Baba K, Kozawa M. The inhibition of gastic H^+, $K(^+)$-ATPase by chalcone derivatives, xanthoangelol and 4-hydroxyderricin, from *Angelica keiskei* Koidzumi. J Pharm Pharmacol 1990; 42(10):723–726.

49. Woo WS, Lee CK, Shin KH. Isolation of drug metabolism modifiers from roots of *Angelica koreana*. Part IV. Planta Med 1982; 45:234–236.

50. Guo TL, Zhuo XW. Clinical observations on the treatment of the gestational hypertension syndrome with *Angelica* and *Paeonia* powder. Chin J Mod Dev Tradit Med 1986; 6(12):714–716.

51. Kurmukov AG, Akhmedkhodzhaeva KS, Sidyakin VG, Syrov VN. Phytoestrogens from plants of Central Asia. Rast Resur 1976; 12:515–525.

52. Usuki S. Effects of hachimijiogan, tokishakuyakusan, and keishibukuryogan on the corpus luteum function and weights of various organs in vivo. Am J Chin Med 1987; 15(3/4):99–108.

53. Usuki S. Effects of tokoshakuyakusan and its components on rat corpus luteum function in vitro. Am J Chin Med 1988; 16(I–2):11–19.

54. Usuki S. Effects of hachimijiogan, tokishakuyakusan, and keishibukuryogan on estrogen and progesterone secretions by rat preovulatory follicles. Am J Chin Med 1986; 14:161–170.

55. Usuki S. Effects of hachimijiogan, tokishakuyakusan, and keishibukuryogan on progesterone secretions by corpus luteum. Am J Chin Med 1987; 15(3/4): 117–125.

56. The Lawrence Review of Natural Products. Burdock. Monograph. Facts and Comparisons. Lippincott, St Louis, MO, 1986.

57. Matsui ADS, Rogers J, Woo YK, Cutting WC. Effects of some natural products on fertility in mice. Med Pharmacol Exp 1967; 16:414.
58. Panter KE, James LF. Natural plant toxicants in milk: A review. J Anim Sci 1990; 68:982–994.
59. The Lawrence Review of Natural Products. *Uva ursi.* Monograph Systems. Pharmaceutical Information Associates, Levittown, PA, 1987.
60. Matsuda H, Nakata H, Tanaka T, Kubo M. Pharmacological study on 3*Arctostaphylos uva-ursi* (L.) Spreng II combined effects of arbutin and prednisolone or dexamethasone on immunoinflammation. Yakugakn Zassui 1990; 110(1):68–76.
61. American Conference of Governmental Industrial Hygienists. Threshold Limit Values and Biological Exposure Indices for 1989–90. ACGIH, Cincinnati, OH, 1989.
62. Deichmann WB, Keplinger ML. Hydroqinones. In Patty's Industrial Hygeine and Toxicology, 3rd ed, Vol 2A (Clayton GD, Clayton FE, eds), John Wiley and Sons, New York, 1981.
63. Hazardous Substances Data Bank. National Library of Medicine, Bethesda, MD (CD-ROM version). Microdex, Denver, CO, 1990.
64. The Lawrence Review of Natural Products. *Calendula.* Monograph Systems. Pharmaceutical Information Associates, Levittown, PA, 1987.
65. Banaszkiewicz W, Kowalska M, Mrozokiewizc A. Determination of the estrogenic activity of *Calendula officinalis* flowers in biological units. Poznan Towarz Pryjaciol Nauk, Wydzial Lekar, Prace Komisji Far 1963; 14:53–633.
66. Locock RA. Herbal medicines. Capsicum. RPC 1985; 517–519.
67. Tominack RL, Spyker DA. Capsicum and capsaicin—A review: Case report of the use of hot peppers in child abuse. Clinical Toxicol 1987; 25(7):591–601.
68. Traurig H, Saria A, Lembeck F. The effects of neonatal capsaicin treatment on growth and subsequent reproductive function in the rat. Nauyn-Schmiedeberg's Arch Pharmacol 1984; 327:254–259.
69. The Lawrence Review of Natural Products. Capsicum peppers. Facts and Comparisons. St Louis, MO, 1989.
70. Sambaian K, Srinivasan K. Influence of spices and spice principles on hepatic mixed function oxygenase system in rats. Indian J Biochem Biophys 1989; 26(4): 254–258.
71. Ballot D, Baynes RD, Bothwell TH, Gillooly M, MacFarlane BJ, MacPhail AP, Lyons G, Derman DP, Bezwoda WR, Torrance JD, et al. The effect of fruit juices and fruits on the absorption of iron from a rice meal. Br J Nutr 1987; 57(3):331–343.
72. Jamwal KS, Anand KK. Preliminary screening of some abortifacient indigenous plants. Indian J Pharm 1962; 24:218–220.
73. Das RP. Effects of papaya seed on the genital organs in female albino rats. Indian J Exp Biol 1980; 18:408–409.
74. Chinoy NJ, Verma RJ, Sam MG, D'Souza OM. Reversible antifertility effects of papaya seed extract in male rodents. J Anrol 1985; 6:2 Abstra-M10.
75. Sareen KN, Misra N, Varma DR, Amma MKP, Gujral ML. Oral contraceptives. V. Anthelmintics as antifertility agents. Indian J Med Res 1970; 59:302.
76. The Lawrence Review of Natural Products. Senna. Monograph System. Pharmaceutical Information Associates, Levittown, PA, 1989.

77. Beuers U, Spengler U, Pape GR. Hepatitis after chronic abuse of senna. Lancet 1991; 337(8737):372–373.
78. Jagjivan B, Morcos SK, Liddell H. Adverse reaction to X-Prep. Br J Radiol 1988; 61(729):853–854.
79. Ralevic V, Hoyle CH, Burnstock G. Effects of long-term laxative treatment on rat mesenteric resistance vessel responses in vitro. Gastroenterology 1990; 99(5): 1352–1357.
80. Heinicke ER, Kiernan JA. Resistance of mysenteric neurons in the rat's colon to depletion by 1,8-dihydroxyanthraquinone. J Pharm Pharmacol 1990; 42(2): 123–125.
81. Hiraoka A, Koike S, Sakaguchi S, Masuda Y, Terai F, Muira I, Kawasaki T, Kawai H, Sakaibara M. The sennoside of constituents of *Rhei rhizoma* and *Sennae folium* as inhibitors of serum monoamine oxidase. Chem Pharm Bull (Tokyo) 1989; 37(10):2744–2746.
82. Aldridge JFL. Visual display units and health. Practitioner 1985; 229:539–545.
83. Kartnig T. Clinical applications of *Centella asiatica* (L.) Urb. Herbs Spices Med Plants 1988; 3:146–173.
84. The Lawrence Review of Natural Products. *Centella asiatica* (L.) Urb. Phrmaceutical Information Associates, Levittown, PA, 1988.
85. Lindberg JF. Kola, ginseng, and mislabeled herbs (letter). JAMA 1977; 237(1): 24–25.
86. Siegel RK. In reply—Kola, ginseng, and mislabeled herbs (letter). JAMA 1977; 237(1):25.
87. Setty BS, Kamboj VP, Garg HS, Khanna NM. Spermicidal potential of saponins isolated from Indian medicinal plants. Contraception 1976; 14(5):571–578.
88. Dutta T, Basu UP. Crude extracts of *Centella asiatica* and products derived from its glycosides as oral antifertility agents. Indian J Exp Biol 1968; 6:181–182.
89. Ramaswamy AS, Periyasamy SM, Basu NK. Pharmacological studies on *Centella asiatica*. J Res Indian Med 1970; 4:160.
90. Matsui ADS, Hoskin S, Kashiwagi M, Aguda BW, Zebart BE, Norton TR, Cutting WC. A survey of natural products from Hawaii and other areas of the Pacific for an antifertility effect in mice. Int Z Klin Pharmakol Ther Toxikol 1971; 5:65.
91. The Lawrence Review of Natural Products. Hawthorne. Pharmaceutical Information Associates, Levittown, PA, 1987.
92. Hamon NW. Herbal medicine. Hawthorns. The genus *Crataegus*. DPJ.RPC 1988; 708–724.
93. Del Vecchio A, Senni I, Cossu G, Molinaro M. Effects of *Centella asiatica* on biosynthetic activity in cultured fibroblasts. Farmaco 1984; 39(10):355–364.
94. Leslie GB, Salmon G. Repeated dose toxicity studies and reproductive studies on nine Bio-strath herbal remedies. Swiss Med 1979; 1(1/2):1–3.
95. Briggs CJ. Herbal medicine. Dioscorea: The yams—A traditional source of food and drugs. CPJ. RPC 1990; 413–415.
96. Dai SJ, Chen YH. Healing of ten-year amenorrhea with traditional herbal drugs. Shang-Hai Chung I Tsa Chih 1982; 5:17.
97. Stohs SJ, Wegner CL, Rosenberg H. The presence of stigmasterol, sitosterol, campesterol, diosgenin and 25D-spirostan-3,5-diene were found in undifferen-

tiated suspension cultures of *D. deltoidea* by gas liquid chromatography and mass spectrometry. Planta Med 1975; 28:101–105.

98. The Lawrence Review of Natural Products. *Echinacea*. Pharmaceutical Information Associates, Levittown, PA, 1990.

99. Coeugniet EG, Elek E. Immunomodulation with *Viscum album* and *Echinacea purpurea* extracts. Onkologie 1987; 10(3 suppl):27–33.

100. Boyd LJ. Pharmacology of the homeopathic drugs. 2. J Am Inst Homeopathy 1928; 21:209.

101. The Lawrence Review of Natural Products. The Ephedras. Pharmaceutical Information Associates, Levittown, PA, 1989.

102. Li WK, Wang CS. Survey of airborne allergic pollens in North China: Contamination with ragweed. N Engl Registry Allergy Proc 1986; 7(2):134–143.

103. Hikino H, Ogata M, Konno C. Structure of feruloylhistamine, a hypotensive principle of *Ephedra* roots. Planta Med 1983; 48:108–110.

104. Prakash AO. Potentialities of some indigenous plants for antifertility activity. J Crude Drug Res 1986; 24(1):19–24.

105. Lee EB. Teratogenicity of the extracts of crude drugs. Korean J Pharmacog 1982; 13:116–121.

106. Prakash AO. Biological evaluation of some medicinal plant extracts for contraceptive efficacy. Contracep Del Syst 1984; 5(3):9–10.

107. Sankawa U. Screening of bioactive compounds in Oriental medicinal drugs. Korean J Pharmacog 1980; 11:125–132.

108. Keeler RF. Livestock models of human birth defects, reviewed in relation to poisonous plants. J Anim Sci 66:2414–2427.

109. Bergeron JM, Gouler M. Study on the phytoestrogenic and phytogenic effects of open-land plants on the laboratory mouse. Can J Zool 1980; 58:1575–1581.

110. Locock RA. Herbal Medicine. Boneset. Eupatorium. CPJ.RPC 1990; ?:229–233.

111. The Lawrence Review of Natural Product;s. Gentian. Pharmaceutical Information Associates, Levittown, PA, 1990.

112. Schaufelberger D, Hostettmann K. Chemistry and pharmacology of *Gentiana lactea*. Planta Med 1988; 54(3):219–221.

113. Garnier R, Carlier P, Hoffelt J, Savidan A. Acute dietary poisoning by white hellebore (*Veratrum album* L.). Clinical and analytical data. À propos of 5 cases. Ann Med Intern (Paris) 1985; 136(2):125–128.

114. Leslie GB, Salmon G. Repeated dose toxicity studies and reproductive studies on nine Bio-strath herbal remedies. Swiss Med 1979; 1(1/2):1–3.

115. Lee EB. The screening of biologically active plants in Korea using isolated organ preparations. IV. Anticholinergic and oxytocic actions in rat's ileum and uterus. Korean J Pharmacog 1982; 13:99–101.

116. Lee EB. The screening of biologically active plants in Korea using isolated organ preparation. IV. Anticholinergic and oxytocic actions in rat's ileum and uterus. Annu Rep Nat Prod Res Inst Seoul Natl Univ 1981; 20:1–3.

117. Itokawa H, Totsuka N, Nakahara K, Takeya K, Lepoittevin J-P, Asakawa Y. Antitumor principles for *Ginkgo biloba* L. Chem Pharm Bull 1987; 35(7):3016–3020.

118. Macovschi O, Prigent AF, Nemoz G, Pacheco H. Effects of an extract of *Ginkgo biloba* on the 3′,5′-cyclic AMP phosphodiesterase activity of the brain of normal and triethyltin-intoxicated rats. J Neurochem 1987; 49(1):107–114.
119. Wada K, Ishigaki S, Ueda K, Sakata M, Haga M. An antivitamin B_6, 4′-methoxypyridoxine, from the seed of *Ginkgo biloba* L. Chem Pharm Bull (Tokyo) 1985; 33(8):3555–3557.
120. Saponaro A. Minerva Med 1973; 79:4194.
121. Gebner B, Voelp A, Klasser M. Study of the long-term action of a *Ginkgo biloba* extract on vigilance and mental performance as determined by means of quantitative pharmaco-EEG and psychometric measurements. Arzneim Forsch 1985; 35:1459–1465.
122. Anon. Therapeutic uses of *Ginkgo*. Lawrence Rev 1985; 6(6).
123. Chandler RF. Licorice, More than just of flavour. CPJ. RPC 1985; 118:421–424.
124. The Lawrence Review of Natural Products. Licorice. Pharmaceutical Information Associates, Levittown, PA, 1989.
125. Monder C, Stewart PM, Lakshmi V, et al. Liquorice inhibits corticosteroid 11-β-dehydrogenase of rat kidney and liver: In vivo and in vitro studies. Endocrinology 1989; 125:1046–1053.
126. Latif SA, Conca TJ, Morris DJ. The effects of the liquorice derivative, glycyrrhetinic acid, on hepatic 3α- and 3β-hydroxysteroid dehydrogenases and 5α- and 5β-reductase pathways of metabolism of aldosterone in male rats. Steroids 1990; 55:52–58.
127. Farese RV, Biglieri EG, Shackleton CHL, Irony I, Gomez-Fontes R. Licorice-induced hypermineralocorticoidism. N Engl J Med 1991; 325(17):1223–1227.
128. Roussak NJ. Fatal hypokalemic alkalosis with tetany during liquorice and PAS therapy. Br Med J 1952; 1:360–361.
129. Tamaya T, Sato S, Okada H. Inhibition by plant herb extracts of steroid bindings in uterus, liver and serum of the rabbit. Acta Obstet Gynecol Scand 1986; 65:839–842.
130. Edwards CRW. Lessons from licorice. N Engl J Med 1991; 325(17):1242–1243.
131. Setty BS, Kamboj VP, Garg HS, Khanna NM. Spermicidal potential of saponins isolated from Indian medicinal plants. Contraception 1976; 14(5):571–578.
132. Sharaf A, Goma N. Phytoestrogens and their antagonism to progesterone and testosterone. J Endocrinol 1965; 31:289.
133. Holler H, Huckel H, Schneider W. Does licorice possess estrogenic properties? Sci Pharm 1960; 28:33.
134. Shihata M, Elghamry MI. Experimental studies in the effect of *Glycyrrhiza glabra*. Planta Med 1963; 11:37.
135. Sharma BB, Varshney MD, Gupta DN, Prakash AO. Antifertility screening of plants. Part I. Effect of ten indigenous plants on early pregnancy in albino rats. In J Crude Drug Res 1983; 21(4):183–187.
136. The Lawrence Review of Natural Products. Hops. Pharmaceutical Information Associates, Levittown, PA, 1989.

137. Materia Medica—Botanical Research Summaries. *Humulus lupulus* (hops) flower cones. Eclectic Dispensatory of Bot Ther ????; 5-17-5-18.
138. Li WK, Wang CS. Survey of air borne allergic pollens in North China: Contamination with ragweed. N Engl Reg Allergy Proc 1986; 7(2):134-143.
139. Anorve-Lopez E, Reed CE. Food skin testing in patients with idiopathic anaphylaxis. J Allergy Clin Immunol 1986; 77(3):516-519.
140. Prinlas RJ, Jacobs DR, Gow RS, Blackburn H. Coffee, tea and VPB. J Chronic Dis 1979; 33:67-72.
141. Ho PS. Hypoglycaemia. Diabetes Res 1989; 10(20):69-73.
142. Kumai A, Okamoto R. Extraction of hormonal substance from hops. Toxicol Lett 1984; 21(2):203-207.
143. The Lawrence Review of Natural Products. Goldenseal. Monograph System. Pharmaceutical Information Associates, Levittown, PA, 1987.
144. Hamon NW. Goldenseal. Herbal medicine. CPJ.RPC. 1990;
145. Williams WW. The effects of hydrastis and its alkaloids on blood pressure. JAMA 1908; 50:26-30.
146. Lieb CC. Pharmacologic action of ecbolic drugs. Am J Obstet 1914; 69:1-32.
147. Mikkelsen SL, Ash KD. Adulterants causing false negatives in illicit drug testing. Clin Chem 1988; 34(11):2333-2336.
148. Osol A, Farrar CF, eds. The dispensary of the United States of America, 25th ed. Lippincott, Philadelphia, 1953, pp 660-661.
149. The Lawrence Review of Natural Products. St John's wort. Monograph, Facts and Comparisons. St Louis, MO, 1989.
150. Awang DVC. St John's wort. Herbal Medicine. CPJ.RPC 1991; 124:33-35.
151. Jayasuriya H, McChesney JD, Swanson SM, Pezzuto JM. Antimicrobial and cytotoxic activity of rottlerin-type compounds from *Hypericum drummondii*. J Nat Prod 1989; 52:325-331.
152. Mishra MB, Tewari JP, Bapat SK. A preliminary pharmacological screening of *Hypericum perforatum*. Labdev 1965; 3:272.
153. Chandler RF. An inconspicuous but insidious drug. Herbal medicine. Rev Pharm Can 1986; 563-566.
154. The Lawrence Review of Natural Products. Juniper. Monograph System. Pharmaceutical Information Associates, Levittown, PA, 1987.
155. Swanston-Flatt SK, Day C, Bailey CJ, Flatt PR. Traditional plant treatments for diabetes. Studies in normal and streptozotocin diabetic mice. Diabetologia 1990; 33(8):462-464.
156. Phillips DH, Scohket B, Hewer A, Grover PL. DNA adduct formation in human and mouse skin by mixtures of polycyclic aromatic hydrocarbons. IARC Sci Publ 1990; 104:223-229.
157. Prochnow L. Experimental contribution to the knowledge of the activity of folkloric abortifacients. Arch Int Pharmacol Ther 1911; 21:313-319.
158. Patoir A, Patoir G, Bedrine H. Toxic action of wormwood and essential oil of Savin in animals. C R Seances Soc Biol Ses Fil 1938; 127:1325.
159. Kagaya Y. Pharmacology of Savin. Neunyn-Schmiedebergs Arch Exp Pathol Pharmacol 1927; 124:245-247.
160. Gunn JWC. The action of the emmenagogue oils on the human uterus. J Pharmacol Exp Ther 1921; 16:485.

161. Datnow MW. An experimental investigation concerning toxic abortion produced by chemical agents. J Obstet Gynecol Br Emp 1928; 35:693.
162. Lafont P, Lafont J. Genotoxicity of spices and flavours: Determination by three different methods. Boll Chim Farm 1987; 126:133–135.
163. Hamon NW. The chamomiles. Herbal medicine. Can Pharm J 1989; 122: 612–615.
164. The Lawrence Review of Natural Products. Chamomile. Monograph, Facts and Comparisons. St Louis, MO, 1991.
165. Feigen M. Fatal veno-occlusive disease of the liver associated with herbal tea consumption and radiation. Aust NZ J Med 1984; 14:61–62.
166. Habersang S, Leuschner F, Isaac O, Thiemer K. Pharmacological studies with compounds of Camomille IV. Studies on toxicity of α-bisabolol. Planta Med 1979; 37:115–132.
167. The Lawrence Review of Natural Products. Alfalfa. Monograph, Facts and Comparisons. Lippincott Company, St Louis, MO, 1986.
168. Cheeke PR. Nutr Rep Int 1976; 13:315.
169. Malinow MR, et al. Food Cosmet Toxicol 1981; 19:443.
170. Wattenberg LW. Cancer Res 1975; 35:3326.
171. Chury J. Antigonadotropic action of Lucerne, '*Medica sativa*'. Ann Endocrinol 1968; 29:699.
172. Hettle JA, Kitts WD. Effects of phytoestrogenic alfalfa consumption on plasma LH levels in cycling ewes. 1983; 6(3):233–238.
173. Sakaguchi E, Matsumoto T. Effects of estrogenic substances in herbage in plasma levels of growth hormone and prolactin of the lactating hamster. Nippon Chikusan Gakkaiho 1979; 50:753–755.
174. Morley JE, Meyer N, Pekary AE, Briggs JE, Melmed S. A prolactin inhibitory factor with immunocharacteristics similar to thyrotropin releasing factor (TRH) is present in the rat pitutary tumors (GH3 and W5) testicular tissue and a plant material, alfalfa. Abstracts of the Endocrine Society's 62nd Annual Meeting, Washington, DC, 1980, pp 18–20.
175. Willet EL, Quisenberry JH, Henke LA, Maruyama C. Koa haole as a roughage for nonruminants. Bienn Rep Agric Exp Sta 1947; 1944–46:46.
176. Chury J, Crha J, Panek K. The influence of feeding Lucerne to bucks on fertilizing and development of the ovum in rabbits. Vet Med 1970; 15:147.
177. Fredricks GR, Kincaid RL, Wright RW, Bondioli K. Reproductive effects of some factors on the estrogen activity of Lucerne. Fed Proc 1980; 39:432.
178. Briggs CJ, Pennyroyal A. Traditional medicinal herb with toxic potential. Can Pharm J 1989; 122:369–372.
179. Macht D. The action of the so-called emmenagogue oils on the isolated uterus with a report of a case of Pennyroyal poisoning. JAMA 1913; 61:105–107.
180. Gold J, Cates JR, W. Herbal abortifacients. JAMA 1980; 243:1;365–1366.
181. The Lawrence Review of Natural Products. Peppermint. Monograph. Facts and Comparisons, Lippincott Company, St Louis, MO, 1990.
182. Olowe SA, Ransome-Kuti O. The risk of jaundice in glucose-6-phosphate dehydrogenase deficient babies exposed to menthol. Arch Toxicol 1984; 7(suppl): 408.

183. Thomas JG. Peppermint fibrillation. Lancet 1962; 1:222.
184. Luke E. Addiction to metholated cigarettes. Lancet 1962; 1:110–111.
185. Williams B. Palindronic rheumatism: A request. Med J Aust 1972; 2:390–391.
186. Buch JG, Dikshit RK, Mansuri SM. Spermicidal effect of certain volatile oils on human spermatozoa in vitro. J Anrol 1985; 6(2):Abstr-M41.
187. Kholkute SD, Mudgal V, Deshpande PJ. Screening of indigenous medicinal plants for antifertility potentiality. Planta Med 1976; 29:151–155.
188. Kanjanapothi D, Smitasiri Y, Panthong A, Taesotikul T, Rattanapanone V. Postcoital antifertility effect of *Mentha arvensis*. Contraception 1981; 24:559–567.
189. Bodhankar SL, Garg SK, Mathur VS. Antifertility screening of plants. Part IX. Effect of five indigenous plants on early pregnancy in female albino rats. Indian J Med Res 1974; 62:831–837.
190. Croteau R, Venkatachalam KV. Metabolism of monoterpenes: Demonstration that (+)-*cis*-isopulegone, not piperitenone, is the key intermediate in the conversion of (−)-isopipertitenone to (+)-pulegone in peppermint (*Mentha piperita*). Arch Biochem Biophys 1986; 249(2):306–315.
191. Chandler RF. Ginseng—An aphrodisiac? Can Pharm J 1988; 121:36–38.
192. Shibata S, Tanaka O, Shoji J, Saito H. Chemistry and pharmacology of *Panax*. Econ Med Plant Res 1985; 1:218–284.
193. Farnsworth NR, Kinghorn DA, Soejarto DD, Walker DP. Siberian ginseng (*Eleutherococcus senticosus*): Current status as an adaptogen. Econ Med Plant Res 1985; 1:155–215.
194. The Lawrence Review of Natural Products. *Eleutherococcus*. Monograph System. Pharmaceutical Information Associates, Levittown, PA, 1988.
195. The Lawrence Review of Natural Products. Ginseng. St Louis, MO. Lippincott Co, 1990; 1–3.
196. Siegel RK. Ginseng abuse syndrome. JAMA 1979; 241(15):1614–1615.
197. Odani T, Ushio Y, Arichi S. The effect of ginsenosides on adrenocorticotropin secretion in primary culture of rat pituitary cells. Planta Med 1986; 177–179.
198. Fulder SJ. The growth of cultured human fibroblasts treated with hydrocortisone and extracts of the medicinal plant *Panax ginseng*. Exp Gerontol 1977; 12:125–131.
199. Odashima S, Ota T, Fujikawa-Yamamoto K, Abe H. Induction of phenotypic reverse transformation by plant glycosides in cultured cancer cells. Gan To Kagaku Ryoho 1989; 16(4 Pt 2-2):1483–1489.
200. Gao Q-P, Kiyohara H, Cyong J-C, Yamada H. Chemical properties and anti-complementary activities of polysaccharide fractions from roots and leaves of *Panax ginseng*. Planta Med 1989; 55:G1–G9.
201. Jones BD, Runikis AM. Interaction of ginseng with phenelzine (letter). J Clin Psychopharmacol 1987; 7(3):201–202.
202. Hopkins MP, Androff L, Benninghoff AS. Ginseng face cream and unexplained vaginal bleeding. Am J Obstet Gynecol 1988; 159:1121–1122.
203. Chung KY, Kim SJ. Inhibitory effect of Korean *Panax ginseng* extract on secretion of pituitary prolactin in normal puerperal women. K'at'ollik Taehak Uihakpu Mommunjip 1976; 29:313.

204. Palmer VBV, Montgomery ACV, Monteiro JCMP. Ginseng and mastalgia. Br Med J 1978; ?:1284.
205. Hess Jr, FG, Parent RA, Cox GE, Stevens KR, Becci PJ. Food Chem Toxicol 1982; 20:189–192.
206. Ge R, Pu H. Effects of ginsenosides and pantocrine on the reproductive endocrine system in male rats. Chung I Tsa Chih 1986; 64:301–304.
207. Baik DW, Lee SY, Chi HJ. The effects of ginseng saponin on prolactin secretion in rats. Korean J Biochem 1979; 9:33–39.
208. Fahim MS, Fahim Z, Harman JM, Clevenger TE, Mullins W, Hafez ESE. Effect of Panax ginseng on testosterone level and prostate in male rats. Arch Androl 1982; 8:261–263.
209. Himi T, Saito H, Nishiyama N. Effect of ginseng saponins on the survival of cerebral cortex neurons in cell cultures. Chem Pharm Bull (Tokyo) 1989; 37(2): 481–484.
210. The Lawrence Review of Natural Products. Passion flower. JB Lippincott Co., St. Louis, MO, 1989.
211. Farnsworth NR. Hallucinogenic plants. Science 1968; 162:1086–1092.
212. Pilcher JD. The action of various "female" remedies on the excised uterus of the guinea pig. JAMA 1916; 67:490.
213. The Lawrence Review of Natural Products. Pokeweed. JB Lippincott Co., St. Louis, MO, 1991; 1–2.
214. Barker BE, Farnes P, LaMarche PH. Haematological effects of pokeweed (letter). Lancet 1967; ?:437.
215. Mamo E, Worku M. Oral administration of a water extract of Phytolacca dodecandra L'Herit in mice—Effects on reproduction. Contraception 1987; 35(2): 155–161.
216. Stolzenberg SJ, Parkhurst RM. Spermicidal actions of extracts and compounds from Phytolacca dodecandra. Contraception 1974; 10(2):134–143.
217. Yeung HW, Feng Z, Li WW, Cheung WK, Ng TB. Abortifacient activity in leaves, roots and seeds of Phytolacca acinosa. J Ethnopharmacol 1987; 21: 31–35.
218. Woo WS, Lee EB. The screening of biological active plants in Korea using isolated organ preparations. II. Anticholinergic and oxytocic actions in the ileum and uterus. Korean J Pharmacog 1979; 10(1):27–30.
219. Sayed MD. Traditional Medicine in health care. J Ethnopharmacol 1980; 2: 19–22.
220. The Lawrence Review of Natural Products Monograph System. Plantain. Pharmaceutical Information Associates. Levittown, PA, 1988.
221. Frati-Munari AC, Flores-Garduno MA, Ariza-Andraca R, Islas-Andrade S, Chavez-Negrete A. Efecto de diferentes dosis de mucilago de Plantago psyllium en la prueba de tolerancia a la glucosa. [Effect of different doses of Plantago psyllium mucilage on the glucose tolerance test.] Arch Invest Med Mex 1989; 20(2):147–152.
222. Malo J-L, Cartier A, L'Archevêque, Ghezzo H, Lagier F, Trudeau C, Dolovich J. Prevalence of occupational asthma and immunologic sensitization to psyllium among health personnel in chronic care hospitals. Am Rev Respir Dis 1990; 142:1359–1366.

223. Hansen WE. Effect of dietary fiber on proteolytic pancreatic enzymes in vitro. Int J Pancreatol 1986; 1(5–6):341–351.
224. Roe DA, Kalkwarf H, Stevens J. Effect of fiber supplements on the apparent absorption of pharmacological doses of riboflavin. J Am Diet Assoc 1988; 88(2):211–213.
225. Nordstrom M, Melander A, Robertsson E, Steen B. Influence of wheat bran and of bulk-forming ispaghula cathartic on the bioavailability of digoxin in geriatric in-patients. Drug Nutr Interact 1987; 5(2):67–69.
226. Jacobs LR. Relationship between dietary fiber and cancer: Metabolic, physiologic, and cellular mechanisms. Proc Soc Exp Biol Med 1986; 183(3):299–310.
227. Friedman E, Lightdale C, Winawer S. Effects of psyllium fiber and short-chain organic acids derived from fiber breakdown on colonic epithelial cells from high-risk patients. Cancer Lett 1988; 43(1–2):121–124.
228. Prior A, Whorwell PJ. Double blind study of ispaghula in irritable bowel syndrome. Gut 1987; 28(11):1510–1513.
229. Paulini I, Mehta T, Hargis A. Intestinal structural changes in African green monkeys after long-term psyllium or cellulose feeding. J Nutr 1987; 117(2):253–266.
230. Khanna NM, Sarin JPS, Nandi RC, Singh S, Setty BS, Kamoj VP, Dhawan BN, Singh L, Kutty D, Engineer AD, et al. Isaptent – A new cervical dilator. Contraception 1980; 21:29–40.
231. Fazal U. Preliminary clinical study of the treatment of Kasarat-E-Tams (menorrhagia) with Tikhm-E-Bartang (*Plantago major* Linn.). J Res Indian Med Yoga Homeopathy 1979; 14:1–6.
232. Ge QS, Zhang YW, Shen LZ. Induction of ovulation with kidney-replenishing herbal drugs: Analyses of 95 cases. Chung I Tsa Chih 1982; 23(5):95–97.
233. Bergeron JM, Gouler M. Study on the phytogenic effects of open-land plants on the laboratory mouse. Can J Zool 1980; 58:1575–1581.
234. Jiu J. A survey of some medicinal plants of Mexico for selected biological activities. Lloydia 1966; 29:250–259.
235. Shukla PC, Desai MC, Purohit LP, Desai HB. Use of isabgul (*Plantago ovata* Forsk.) gola in the concentrate mixture of milk cows. Gujarat Agric Univ Res J 1983; 9(1):33–36.
236. Lampe KF, Fagerstrom R. Plant Toxicity and Dermatitis. Williams & Wilkins, Baltimore, 1968.
237. Reid TM, Robinson HG. Frozen raspberries and hepatitis A. Epidemiol Infect 1987; 98(1):109–112.
238. De Vincenzi M, Badellino E, Di Folco S, Dracos A, Magliola M, Stacchini A, Stacchini P, Silvano V. A basis for estimation of consumption: Literature values for selected food volatiles. Food Addit Contam 1989; 6(2):235–267.
239. Bamford DS, Percival RC, Tothill AU. Raspberry leaf tea: A new aspect to an old problem. Br J Pharmacol 1970; 40:161P.
240. Burn JH, Withell ER. A principle in raspberry leaves which relaxes uterine muscle. Lancet 1941; 2:1.
241. Beckett AH, Belthle FW, Fell KR, Lockett MF. The active constitutents of raspberry leaves. A preliminary investigation. J Pharm Pharmacol 1954; 6:785.

242. The Lawrence Review of Natural Products. Scullcap. JB Lippincott Co., St. Louis, MO, 1990; 1–2.
243. Harvey J. Mistletoe hepatitis. Br Med J Clin Ed 1981; 282(6259):186–187.
244. Liu ML, Li ML. Studies on flavonoids of Likiang skullcap (*Scutellaria likiangensis*). Chin Tradit Herbal Drugs 1988; 19:50–52.
245. MacGregor FB, Abernethy VE, Dahabra S, Cobden I, Hayes PC. Hepatotoxicity of herbal remedies. Br Med J 1989; 299:1156–1157.
246. Razina TG, Udintsev SN, Tiutrin II, Borovskaia TG, Iaremenko KV. The role of thrombocyte aggregation function in the mechanism of the antimetastatic action of an extract of Baikal skullcap. Vopr-Onkol 1989; 35(3):331–335.
247. Pilcher JD, Durman GE, Delzell WR. The action of the so-called female remedies on the excised uterus of the guinea-pig. Arch Intern Med 1916; 18:557.
248. Awang DVC. Herbal medicine: Comfrey. Can Pharm J 1987; 120:100–104.
249. The Lawrence Review of Natural Products. Comfrey. Pharmaceutical Information Associates, Levittown, PA, 1990.
250. Bach N, Thung SN, Schaffner F. Comfrey herb tea-induced hepatic venoocclusive disease. Am J Med 1989; 87(1):97–99.
251. Smith LW, Culvenor CCJ. Plant sources of hepatotoxic pyrrolizidine alkaloids. J Nat Prod 1981; 44(2):129–152.
252. Roitman JN. Comfrey and liver damage. Lancet 1981; i:944.
253. Mohabbat O, Younos MS, Merzad AA, Srivastava RN, Sediq GG, Aram GN. An outbreak of hepatic veno-occlusive disease in North-Western Afghanistan. Lancet 1976; 269–272.
254. Anderson C. Comfrey toxicity in perspective. Lancet 1981; 1424.
255. Blaskó G, Cordell GA. Recent developments in the chemistry of plant-derived anticancer agents. Econ Med Plant Res 1988; 2:123–129.
256. Wagner H, Horhammer L, Frank U. Constituents of medicinal plants with hormone and antihormone activity. Arzneim-Forsch 1970; 20:705–713.
257. Roulet M, Laurini R, Rivier L, Calame A. Hepatic veno-occlusive disease in newborn infant of a woman drinking herbal tea. J Pediatr 1988; 112(3):433–436.
258. Newbezne PM. The influence of low lipotrotrophic diet or response of maternal and fetal rats to lasiocarpine. Cancer Res 1966; 28:2327.
259. Armstrong SJ, Zuckerman AJ. Production of pyrroles from pyrrolizidine alkaloids by human embryo tissue. Nature 1970; 228:569.
260. Awang DVC. Herbal medicine: Feverfew. Can Pharm J 1989; 122:266–270.
261. The Lawrence Review of Natural Products. Feverfew. Monograph Facts and Comparisons. Lippincott Co., St. Louis, MO, 1990.
262. Cooper MR, Johnson AW. Poisonous plants in Britain. Ministry of Agriculture Fisheries and Food, 1984, p 161.
263. Baldwin CA, Anderson LA, Phillipson JD. Herbal remedies: What pharmacists should know about feverfew. Pharm J 1987; 2:237.
264. Warren RG. Current drug information: The anti-migraine activity of feverfew (*Tanacetum parthenium*). Aust J Pharm 1986; 67:475–477.
265. Berry MI. Herbal remedies: Feverfew faces the future. Pharm J 1984; 611–614.

266. Zeller W, De Gols M, Hausen BM. The sensitizing capacity of Compositae plants. VI. Guinea pig sensitization experiments with ornamental plants and weeds using different methods. Arch Dermatol Res 1985; 277(1):28–35.

267. Racz-Kotilla, et al. Planta Med 1974; 26:212.

268. Dhar ML, Dhar MM, Dhawan BN, Metrotra BN, Ray C. Screening of Indian plants for biological activity: Part I. Indian J Exp Biol 1968; 6:232–247.

269. Cassady JM, Zennie TM, Chae YH, Ferin MA, Portuondo NE, Baird WM. Use of a mammalian cell culture benzo(*a*)pyrene metabolism assay for the detection of potential anticarcinogens from natural products: Inhibition of metabolism by biochanin A, an isoflavone from *Trifolium pratense* L. Cancer Res 1988; 48(22):6247–6261.

270. Hogan RP. Hemorrhagic diathesis caused by drinking an herbal tea. JAMA 1983; 249(19):2679–2680.

271. Chury J. Phytoestrogen content of plants. Experientia 1960; 16:194.

272. Ostrovsky D, Kitts WD. Estrogen-like substances in legumes and grasses. The influence of fractionation and route of administration on the estrogenic activity of plant materials. Can J Biochem 1962; 40:159.

273. Gil LA, Ramirez J, Diaz JC. Estrogen activity of four clover (*Trifolium* sp.) varieties with grasses and study of isoflavones in *T. repens* var. Ladino. Turrialba 1984; 34(4):437–444.

274. Dhawan BN. Screening of Indian plants for biological activity. Indian J Exp Biol 1977; ?:208.

275. Hidiroglou M, Ivan M, Bryan MK, Ribble CS, Janzen ED, Proulx JG, Elliot JI. Assessment of the role of manganese in congenital joint laxity and dwarfism in calves. Ann Rech Vet 1990; 21(4):281–284.

276. The Lawrence Review of Natural Products. Coltsfoot. Monograph. Facts and Comparisons. Lippincott Co., St. Louis, MO, 1989; 1–2.

277. The Lawrence Review of Natural Products. Slippery Elm. Monograph. Facts and Comparisons. Lippincott Co., St. Louis, MO, 1991; 1–2.

278. Ye G, Cao Q, Chem X, Li S, Jia B. *Ulmus macrocarpa* Hence for the treatment of ulcerative colitis: A report of 36 cases. J Tradit Chin Med 1990; 10(2): 97–98.

279. The Lawrence Review of Natural Products. Nettles. Monograph. Facts and Comparisons. Pharmaceutical Information Association, Levittown, PA, 1989; 1–2.

280. Mittman P. Randomized, double-blind study of freeze-dried *Urtica dioica* in the treatment of allergic rhinitis. Planta Med 1990; 56(1):44–47.

281. Wagner H, Willer F, Kreher B. Biologically active compounds from the aqueous extract of *Urtica dioica*. Planta Med 1989; 55(5):452–454.

282. Czarnetzki BM, Thiele T, Rosenbach T. Immunoreactive leukotrienes in nettle plants (*Uritica urens*). Int Arch Allergy Appl Immunol 1990; 91(1):43–46.

283. Sharma BB, Varshney MD, Gupta DN, Prakash AO. Antifertility screening of plants. Part I. Effect of ten indigenous plants on early pregnancy in albino rats. Int J Crude Drug Res 1983; 21(4):183–187.

284. Aswal BS, Bhakuni DS, Goel AK, Kar K, Mehrotra BN, Mukherjee KC. Screening of Indian plants for biological activity. Part X. Indian J Exp Biol 1984; 22(6):312–332.

285. Safin VA, Petrov MI. Action of nettle preparations on smooth muscles of the uterus and small intestine. Tr Perm Farm Inst 1969; 3:281.
286. The Lawrence Review of Natural Products. Valerian. 1986; 1–2.
287. Béliveau J. Herbal medicine: *Valeriana officinalis.* Can Pharm J 1986; 119: 24–27.
288. Houghton PJ. The biological activity of valerian and related plants. J Ethnopharmacol 1988; 22:121–142.
289. Ren SL, Yu LS, Pei N, Zhao GJ. Pharmacological actions of kuanyexiecao (*Valeriana officinalis*) on smooth muscles and cardiovascular system. Chung Ts'ao Yao 1982; 13:119–18.
290. Pilcher JD, Mauer RT. The action of "female remedies" on intact uteri of animals. Surg Gynecol Obstet 1918; 27:97.
291. Jaffe AM, Gephardt D, Courtemanche L. Poisoning due to ingestion of *Veratrum viride* (false hellebore). J Emerg Med 1990; 8:161–167.
292. The Lawrence Review of Natural Products. White Hellebore. Monograph. Pharmaceutical Information Association, Levittown, PA, 1987.
293. Carlier P, Efthymiou M-L, Garnier R, Hoffelt J, Fournier E. Poisoning with veratrum-containing sneezing powders. Hum Toxicol 1983; 2:321–325.
294. Omnell ML, Sim FRP, Keeler RF, Harne IC, Brown KS. Expression of veratrum alkaloid teratogenicity in the mouse. Teratology 1990; 42:105–119.
295. The Lawrence Review of Natural Products. Mullein. Monograph Facts and Comparisons. Lippincott Co., St. Louis, MO, 1989; 1–2.
296. Romaguera C, Grimalt F, Vilaplana J. Occupational dermatitis from *Gordolobo* (mullein). Contact Dermatitis 1985; 12(3):176.
297. Anderson LA, Phillipson JD. Mistletoe – The magic herb. Pharm J 1982; ?: 437–439.
298. The Lawrence Review of Natural Products. Mistletoe. Monograph. Facts and Comparisons. Lippincott Co., St. Louis, MO, 1990; 1–2.
299. Howard HP. Mistletoe as an oxytocic. Med News (Philadelphia) 1892; 60: 547.
300. Kochmann M. The pharmacology of mistletoe. Naunyn-Schmiedebers Arch Exp Pathol Pharmakol 1931; 161:553.
301. Mascolo N, Jain R, Jain SC, Capasso F. Ethnopharmacologic investigation of ginger (*Zingiber officinale*). J Ethnopharmacol 1989; 27:129–140.
302. Srivastava KC, Mustafa T. Ginger (*Zingiber officinale*) and rheumatic disorders. Med Hypotheses 1989; 29:25–28.
303. Hong ND, Chang IK, Kim NJ, Lee IS. Studies of the efficacy of combined preparations of crude drug. (XXXIX). Effects of hyangsayangwee-tang on the stomach and intestinal disorder. Korean J Pharmacog 1989; 20(3):188–195.
304. Kanjanapothi D, Soparat P, Panthong A, Tuntiwachwuttikul P, Reutrakul V. A uterine relaxant compound from *Zingiber cassumunar.* Planta Med 1987; 329–332.
305. Nagabhushan M, Amonkar AJ, Bhide SV. Mutagenity of Gingerol and shogaol and antimutagenicity of zingerone in *Salmonella* microscome assay. Cancer Lett 1987; 36:221–233.

22

Ionizing and Nonionizing Radiation in Pregnancy

Yedidia Bentur
Rambam Medical Center, Technion–Israel Institute of Technology, Haifa, Israel

Clinical Case

You sent a female patient for thyroid scan, suspecting hyperthyroidism. She returns to your office a few days later in panic because she had not known she was pregnant when the scan was performed. She has been told by several people, including one physician, that the radioactive iodine will cause thyroid damage to her 6-week fetus. What would be your advice?

INTRODUCTION

Radiation is an anxiety-provoking term. In the minds of many, it is impossible to separate the psychological and physical effects of the atomic bomb from the effects of low dose ionizing radiation. This anxiety is only aggravated by our knowledge of the carcinogenic effects on people (e.g., radium dial workers, uranium miners, patients who receive radiotherapy or isotope therapy, and the victims of high exposures following the bombings of Hiroshima and Nagasaki and the Chernobyl accident) of high exposures to radiation. Such discomfort may explain in part the ignorance of the public and many scientists and physicians regarding the qualitative and quantitative effects of ionizing radiation in spite of the extensive studies that have been carried out. Another source of confusion is the fact that the term "radiation" is applied to x-ray, ultrasound, microwave, and other forms. Therefore, it has even been suggested that *radiation* should be applied to high energy ionizing radiation (x-rays, gamma rays, radionuclides), whereas radar, FM broadcast range radio waves, diathermy, and microwaves should be termed *long-wavelength electromagnetic waves* or, in the case of ultrasound, *sound waves* (1).

Despite the increase in concern regarding the effects of ionizing radiation on health and reproduction, the medical use of x-rays has continued to grow. In 1980 the number of x-ray procedures in the United States was 225 million (roughly equal to the total population) (2). Approximately 80 million fertile men and women were exposed to x-ray procedures in that year. About 30,000 fertile women may have been exposed to abdominal x-rays in early pregnancy (3). In the United Kingdom, approximately 12% of the total radiation dose to the population is due to man-made irradiation, and from that about 94% is due to medical procedures (4). About 21 million radiodiagnostic studies were carried out annually in 1977 in the United Kingdom, of which about 6% were fluoroscopic investigations (5). Although fluoroscopies involve mainly the abdominal region and are associated with high dose exposure, the use of gonadal shields is still low (6).

It is in this context of anxiety, ignorance, and confusion and, on the other hand, increasing medical use of ionizing radiation, that the reproductive effects of diagnostic and therapeutic uses of ionizing radiation are reviewed here.

HISTORY

Until 1895, when Wilhelm Roentgen devised a method to generate x-rays, human beings were exposed only to natural sources of ionizing radiation. *Background radiation*, as this form of energy is also called, consists of electromagnetic and particulate forms of ionizing radiation coming from the sun and the stars; radionuclides in the soil; and gamma rays, x-rays, and alpha and beta particles from rocks and air. Roentgen's invention introduced to science and medicine an enormous new source of ionizing radiation. The diagnostic uses of x-rays were developed rapidly following this discovery. In addition, this radiation was used for cancer therapy and also for tinea capitis (7), enlarged tonsils and adenoids (8), thymic enlargement (9), and infertility (10). In 1896 Antoine Becquerel discovered that certain elements emit radiation. It was not until 1906, after the French physicist accidentally burned himself while carrying a radioactive compound in his pocket, that the possible therapeutic uses of radioisotopes were conceived.

Only after the bombings of Hiroshima and Nagasaki in World War II had provided live evidence of the hazards posed by radiation were serious studies conducted regarding its delayed genetic effects and somatic damage. The medical uses of x-rays were intensely scrutinized, with a particular focus on what harm might be done to developing humans, including the mutagenic and carcinogenic effects of ionizing radiation.

DEFINITIONS

Ionizing radiation can be expressed in units of exposure (roentgen), its absorbance into human tissue (rad, gray), and as the biological effectiveness of absorbed radiation (rem) (11).

The *roentgen* (R) is the international unit of x- or gamma radiation equal to the amount of radiation that produces, in one cubic centimeter of dry air at 0°C and standard atmospheric pressure, ionization of either sign equal to one electrostatic unit (esu) of charge.

The *rad* is a unit of absorbed dose of ionizing radiation equal to an energy of 100 ergs/s of irradiated material: 100 rad = 1 Gy (gray) = 1 J/kg.

The *rem* (roentgen-equivalent man) is the dosage of an ionizing radiation that will cause the same biological effect as 1 R of x-ray or gamma ray dosage; 100 rem = 1 Sv (sievert).

The relationship between the absorbed energy (in rad or Gy) and the effectiveness of that energy in causing damage incorporates a factor called the *relative biological effectiveness* (*RBE*): 1 rem = 1 rad/RBE or 1 Sv = 1 Gy/RBE. Thus, RBE is a correction factor for predicting the biological effect of absorbed radiation. For radiation in soft tissue, RBE is about 1; hence rad and rem (or Gy and Sv) are often used interchangeably.

The density of the radiation-induced ionizations in any tissue is directly related to the energy transferred to the irradiated substance, which is expressed as the *linear energy transfer* (LET).

MECHANISM OF ACTION

X-rays and gamma rays are short-wavelength electromagnetic rays. Ionizing radiation in the form of high energy photons in gamma rays and lower energy x-ray photons can alter the normal structure of the biochemical components of a living cell through direct and indirect mechanisms.

The direct mechanism involves disrupting the atom's structure of biological molecules by adding sufficient energy to incite electron shells to free an electron from its atomic orbit and produce a charged or ionized compound and a free electron. The indirect mechanism involves the radiolysis of water (which makes up more than 60% of the content of living cells) to form radicals like OH^-, H^+, H_2, and H_2O_2. These reactive compounds can attack and disrupt neighboring molecules.

Particulate radiation is generated from the spontaneous disintegration of radioactive compounds, which results in the emission of alpha particles (helium nuclei), beta particles (electrons), and other forms of energy. Nuclear fission generates a variety of heavy charged particles, fission fragments, and uncharged neurons. These subatomic particles can also disrupt the atomic structure of biological molecules by inducing ionizations.

Particulate radiation does not penetrate tissues deeply, but it does generate ions densely along a short path (high LET). X-rays and gamma rays penetrate tissues deeply but generate ions sparsely along their path (low LET). The harm that follows from a single, random modification in a cell component (such as the genetic structure of stem cells) as a result of ionizing radiation (or any other toxin), termed a *stochastic effect*, may still allow the cells to proliferate. A nonstochastic effect is produced by numerous and/or repeated instances of damage. Stochastic effects can theoretically originate in a single deleterious effect, which can be associated with extremely low levels of radiation. Thus, an experimentally derived dose-response curve for effects such as carcinogenesis, mutagenesis, and maybe even abortions may not include a threshold dose below which no adverse effects occur. On the other hand, the dose-response curve for nonstochastic effects (e.g., cataract formation) would be expected to show a threshold dose, which defines the smallest dose of radiation that induces detectable harm.

Similarly, Smith (12) separates the harmful effects of ionizing radiation into two classes:

1. *Deterministic effects*, which result in loss of tissue function, usually at doses in excess of a few hundred millisieverts (tens of rems). Its dose-frequency relationship is sigmoid, and a tissue-specific dose threshold exists. This type of injury may also involve various compensatory and repair mechanisms. When the radiation dose is fractionated, there is greater repair and proliferation, hence increasing the tolerance of the tissue. This radiobiological observation of tolerance dose for most tissues guides the radiotherapist in judging the regimen to avoid unwanted side effects.

2. *Stochastic effects*, as discussed earlier. Since no dose threshold is assumed for these effects, there is great uncertainty as to how best to predict unavoidable injurious effects that may result, for instance, from exposure to an ionizing radiation dose equivalent to the natural background levels.

BIOLOGICAL EFFECT

Before discussing the biological effect of ionizing radiation, it is important to refer to some of the findings of the review of the 30-year study of the survivors of the Hiroshima and Nagasaki bombings (13). It was clearly shown in this study that radiation effects are dose dependent. More than 90% of survivors received much less than 10 rad from the atomic bombs. The possibility that such survivors will develop any disease from atomic bomb exposure is no greater than those of nonexposed individuals. Those who received higher doses have greater risks.

Testes

In various animal experimental studies, it was shown that prenatal doses of ionizing radiation between 50 and 500 rad can induce testicular hypoplasia and sterility (11). This radiosensitivity differed among different animal species (14) and according to the gestational state (15). Fertility data from radiotherapy patients (16) is often of limited value, because illness and simultaneous administration of cytotoxic agents can also alter sperm production.

In a study sponsored by the U.S. Atomic Energy Commission (AEC), normal men received large, defined doses of x-irradiation to the testes and were monitored for alterations in testicular cell populations, spermatogenesis, and fertility (17,18). Testicular radiation doses of 15–100 rad caused a decline in the sperm count about 50 days after irradiation, probably through an effect on the spermatogonia. A 15-rad dose caused only oligospermia. Doses of 50–80 rad and higher produced aspermia within 2–6 months. A decline in the sperm count was produced in less than 50 days after a single dose of 400 rad. It seems that this higher dose affected the spermatids, which are produced in the later stages of spermatogenesis. This finding in humans of increased radiosensitivity at earlier stages of cell division is consistent with findings in experimental models (19,20). The findings of the recovery phase in the AEC study suggested that repopulation of germinal cells becomes less and less efficient as radiation exposures increase (18). Histological recovery (increasing number of spermatogonia) was observed about 7 months postirradiation doses of 100–600 rad. After 100 rad the appearance of sperm in seminal fluid coincided with the earliest sign of histological recovery (7 months). But sperm production was not detectable until 11 and 24 months after doses of 200 and 600 rad. Similar findings were observed in the mouse (21), but its testicular tissue is significantly less radiosensitive than that of the human (22). It was also suggested in the human study (18) that radiation interfered with normal gonadotropin production by Leydig cells, thereby causing an increase in their number as a compensatory mechanism. The complete recovery of normal sperm concentrations after doses of between 100 and 600 rad took between 9 months and 5 years (18). Some men who had been accidentally exposed to large doses of radiation fathered children after even longer periods of time (23). Mouse experiments suggest that fertility can return when the sperm count is only 10% of its normal density (24).

Ovaries

In the prenatal period, radiation sensitivity is high in oogonia that are undergoing mitosis (11). The mammalian primary oocyte arrested in meiosis has been found to have varying radiosensitivity, depending on the subject's age and the species studied (25,26). In vitro studies indicate that the human oocyte may be among the most radioresistant (27), whereas other studies show the mouse's oocyte to be among the most radiosensitive (28,29). Irradiation was shown in animals to cause rapid changes in germ cell structure characterized by a condensation of the chromosomes and damage to the nuclear envelope (28,30). Damaged oocytes either undergo repair (31) or are eliminated from the ovary within days or weeks (28,29). Doses of radiation sufficient to destroy most of the small primordial follicles have little effect on oocytes in Graafian follicles (27). The radiation dose administered influences mainly the proportion of oocytes affected, but not the time course of degenerative changes (32).

It seems that exposure in utero to low dose radiation has little effect on human fertility, although the data are very limited. A fertility study on 180 women showed that 1-5 rad of gonadal radiation during infancy did not significantly affect the number of children born or the age distribution of births when compared with control data (33). Brent has estimated that acute doses below 25 rad absorbed by the fetus during gestation are unlikely to result in sterility in the human female or male (14).

The observation in animals that moderate doses of radiation (50 rad) increased litter size, probably owing to superovulation (28,34,35), may have provided the empirical basis for the treatment of infertile women with x-rays in the past (10).

Other human data showed that radiotherapy involving 600 rad in women over 40 years of age induced permanent menopause (16). Younger women exposed to this dose of radiation are likely to recover normal menstrual function and fertility. A fractionated dose of 2000 rad over 5-6 weeks is considered likely to produce complete sterility in 95% of girls and young women (16). An extended period of amenorrhea is expected after radiation doses that are inadequate to cause complete sterility (11). Young women with post-irradiation amenorrhea were reported to resume their menstrual cycle only after a successful pregnancy (27,36,37).

Gestation

In a study looking at the outcome of pregnancy in survivors of Wilms' tumor, it was suggested that radiation induces somatic damage to abdominopelvic structures (38). This type of radiotherapy involves gonadal exposure of about 900 rad (one exposure) or 1100-1600 rad in fractionated doses (11). Among 114 pregnancies in women who had received abdominal radiotherapy for Wilms' tumor, an adverse outcome occurred in 34 (30%) in the form of perinatal deaths (17 pregnancies) and low birth weight infants (18 pregnancies).

In comparison, only in two (3%) out of 77 pregnancies in nonirradiated females with Wilms' tumor and in the wives of male patients with Wilms' tumor was there an adverse outcome. The absence of adverse outcomes in the pregnancies fathered by irradiated males suggests that radiation-induced germinal mutation is an unlikely explanation. This is supported by similar findings in other studies (39,40). In addition, shortened trunk, scoliosis, fibrosis of the abdominal musculature, and functional impairment of visceral organs have been reported in women who received curative radiation for Wilms' tumor in childhood (41–43). Possible mechanisms for this impaired gestation are reduced distensibility of the irradiated uterine musculature and the abdominal cavity as well as uterine vascular insufficiency (11). This high risk of adverse pregnancy outcome should be considered in the counseling and prenatal care of women who have received abdominal radiotherapy for Wilms' tumor.

A British study showed that female survivors of childhood cancer who had been given abdominal or gonadal irradiation had excessive miscarriages (19%) compared with a control group of females with similar neoplasms who were not irradiated (9%) (44).

Leukemic children who received prophylactic irradiation of the central nervous system had in adulthood lower fertility expressed as a lower first-birth rate (rate ratio 0.39) than those without radiation, indicating that doses of 18–24 Gy to the brain may possibly be a risk factor (45). Hypothalamic or pituitary injury is a suggested mechanism. In both these studies (44,45), there was no increased risk for congenital anomalies.

Genetic Disorders

Demonstrating the genetic effects of ionizing radiation in humans is limited by the difficulty in establishing a causal link between chromosomal damage and radiation exposure in the presence of other environmental mutagens. Chromosomal abnormalities are believed to be associated with 50% of spontaneous abortions and 8–10% of stillbirths (46). Radiation genetic damage cannot be distinguished from this high natural occurrence of human genetic disorders.

Animal studies have shown that radiation can induce subtle genetic abnormalities in small, short-lived organisms (47) and that repeated small doses of radiation caused fewer mutations than the equivalent amount of radiation administered as a single dose (20,48). Animal data also suggest that radiation-induced point mutations could not account for even a small proportion of radiation-induced teratogenicity unless it simply involves cell death (1). Upon looking at children born to radiation-exposed and unexposed survivors of the bombings of Hiroshima and Nagasaki, no significant difference was found regarding the incidence of stillbirths, congenital abnormalities, and neonatal fatalities (49). An apparent increase in abnormal pregnancies that correlated with increasing radiation dose was not found to be statistically significant. The data also suggested an increase in congenital problems when either mother or father had been exposed to ionizing radiation, but no cumulative effect was present in the data collected for births in which both parents had been exposed to radiation.

A case control study of 67 infants with trisomy 21 and their matched controls showed no association with medical radiography. The relative risk of trisomy for a radiographic examination involving direct irradiation of the ovaries prior to conception (mean ovarian dose 2.19 and 2.41 mGy for case and controls, respectively) was 0.8; the 95% confidence interval (CI) was 0.34–1.83 (50). There are no reports of excessive genetic disorders in geographical areas where the annual background radiation is known to be as high as 1.3 rem (10 times the average background exposure in the United States) (51,52). The Committee on the Biological Effects of Ionizing Radiation of the U.S. National Academy of Sciences has estimated that 50–250 rem would be the dose of radiation sufficient to double the natural human mutation rate (47).

Table 1 shows the known spontaneous incidence of genetic disorders causing serious handicaps per million liveborn, together with estimates of additional radiation-induced defects.

It seems that no correlation has been demonstrated between exposure to ionizing radiation and the incidence of genetic disorders in any human population at any dose level (47,53). If medical and occupational exposures are kept within recommended limits, radiation is responsible for few, if any, of the genetic disorders occurring spontaneously (54).

Table 1 Estimated Genetic Effects of Radiation per Million Liveborn Offspring

Genetic disorders	Incidence	Additional effects of exposure of 1 rem/30-year generation	
		First generation	At equilibrium[a]
Recessive	1,000	Very few	Very slow increase
Autosomal dominant and X-linked	10,000	5–65	40–200
Irregularly inherited	90,000	Very few	20–900
Chromosomal aberrations	6,000	10	Slight increase

[a]Refers to later generations when the rate of elimination of defective genes is balanced by the rate of additional mutations.
Source: Modified from Ref. 47.

Teratogenesis

During the preimplantation period of gestation (0–2 weeks), the embryo is most sensitive to the lethal effect of radiation (55,56), probably owing to genetic damage (11,55), and is insensitive to its growth-retarding and teratogenic effects (1). During early organogenesis the embryo is very sensitive to the growth-retarding, teratogenic, and lethal effects of irradiation but can recover somewhat from the growth-retarding effects in the postpartum period (1). It seems that the time period for radiation-induced multiple malformations other than of the central nervous system is the second to fourth week of gestation, representing 5% of the length of pregnancy, versus, for instance, 14% of the pregnancy in rat (11). During the early fetal period the fetus exhibits central nervous system sensitivity to radiation, and it can be growth retarded at term, from which it recovers poorly in the postpartum period; at the same period, however, the fetus has diminished sensitivity to multiple-organ teratogenesis (57,58). During the later fetal stages, the fetus will not be grossly deformed by radiation. If the radiation exposure is high enough, it will sustain permanent cell depletion of various organs and tissues (14,59). Cell death, mitotic delay, and disturbances of cell migration are among the mechanisms postulated for the irradiation effects, but it is difficult to determine which of them are most important in radiation-induced embryopathology. In addition, the same mechanism may not have the same importance in different stages of the pregnancy. For instance, cell death may be of minimal importance in the preimplantation period because of the embryo's capacity for repair and the pluripotent nature of each remaining viable cell at this early stage (1,60,61). In later stages of the pregnancy, the fetus loses this ability and cell death then becomes a primary factor.

Tables 2 and 3 summarize the effects of different radiation doses at various stages of the pregnancy.

The classic effects of radiation on the developing mammal are gross congenital malformations, intrauterine growth retardation, and embryonic death. Central nervous system effects and growth retardation are the cardinal effects. Each of these effects has a dose-response relationship and a threshold exposure below which there is no difference between the irradiated population and the control population (1).

Microcephaly and Mental Retardation

Many studies indicate that microcephaly is the most common malformation observed in human beings randomly exposed to high doses of radiation during pregnancy (62–69). In Goldstein and Murphy's studies, where the radiation dose was greater than 100 rad, out of 75 pregnancies, there were 16 microcephalic children, and almost all were developmentally delayed (63,64). A total of 28 children had severe disturbances of the central nervous system.

Table 2 A Compilation of the Effects of 10 Rad or Less Acute Radiation at Various Stages of Gestation in Rat and Mouse[a]

	Stage of gestation (days)				
Feature	Preimplantation	Implantation	Early organogenesis	Late organogenesis	Fetal stages
Mouse	0–4.5	4.5–6.5	6.5–8.5	8.5–12.0	12–18
Rat	0–5.5	5.5–8.0	8–10	10–13	13–22
Corresponding human gestation period	0–9	9–14	15–28	28–50	50–280
Lethality	+[b]				
Growth retardation at term	–	–	–	–	–
Growth retardation as adult	–	–	–	–	–
Gross malformations (aplasia, hyperplasia, absence or overgrowth of organs or tissues)	±[c]	–	–	–	–
Cell depletions, minimal but measurable tissue hypoplasia[d]	–	–	–	–	–
Sterility	–	–	–	–	–
Significant increase in germ cell mutations[e]	±	±	±	±	±
Cytogenic abnormalities	–[c]	–	–	–	–
Neuropathology		–	–	–	–

Tumor induction[e,f]	−	−	−	±	±	±
Behavior disorders[g]	−	−	−	−	−	−
Reduction of life span[e]	−	−	−	−	−	−

[a] Dose fractionation or protraction effectively reduces the biological results of all the pathological effects reported to this table. (−) indicates no observed effect; (±) questionable but reported or suggested effect; (+) demonstrated effect.

[b] At this stage the murine embryo is most sensitive to the lethal effects of irradiation. With 10 rad in the mouse, Rugh reports a slight decrease in litter size in the mouse (57).

[c] Rugh reports exencephalia with 15 and 25 rad in a strain of mice with a 1% incidence of exencephalia. Others have not been able to repeat these results (54).

[d] Recent reevaluation of the atomic bomb victims data suggests the possibility that mental retardation is a risk in the 10- to 20-rad range. This is not supported by most other data.

[e] The potential for mutation induction exists in the embryonic term cells or their precursors. Several long-term studies indicate that considerably greater dose in mice and rats do not affect longevity, tumor incidence, incidence of congenital malformations, litter size, growth rate, or fertility.

[f] Stewart and others have reported that 2-rad increases the incidence of malignancy by 50% in the offspring. See text for discussion.

[g] Piontkovskii (1) reports behavioral changes in the rat after 1 rad daily irradiation. This work has not been reproduced.

Source: From Ref. 1, used with permission.

Table 3 A Compilation of the Effects of 100-Rad Acute Radiation on Embryonic Development at Various Stages of Gestation in Rat and Mouse[a]

Feature	Stage of gestation (days)				
	Preimplantation	Implantation	Early organogenesis	Late organogenesis	Fetal stages
Mouse	0–4.5	4.5–6.5	6.5–8.5	8.5–12.0	12–18
Rat	0–5.5	5.5–8.0	8–10	10–13	13–22
Corresponding human gestation period	0–9	9–14	18–36	36–50	50–280
Lethality	+++[b,c]	+	++	±	–
Growth retardation at term	–	+	+++	++	+
Growth retardation as adult	–	+	++	+++	++
Gross malformations (aplasia, hyperplasia, absence or over-growth of organs or tissues)	–	–	+++	±[d]	–[d]
Cell depletions, minimal but measurable tissue hypoplasia	–	–	±	++	+[k]
Sterility	–	–	±	–	++[e]
Significant increase in germ cell mutations[f]	±	±	±	±	±
Cytogenic abnormalities[c,g]	±	–	+++	+[a]	+[a]
Cataracts	–	–	++	++	+[a]
Neuropathology[h]	–	–	+++	+++	++
Tumor induction[h]	–	±	±	±	±

Behavior disorders[i]	–	–	–
Reduction of life span[j]	–	±	±	±
(in nonmalformed embryos)			

[a] Dose fractionation or protraction effectively reduced the biological result of all the pathological effects reported in this table.

[b] (–) no observed effect; (±) questionable but reported or suggested effect; (+) demonstrated effect; (+ +) readily apparent effect; (+ + +) occurs in high incidence.

[c] Russell (cited in Ref. 1) reported that 200 rad increased the incidence of XO aneuploidy in 2–5% of offspring in mice with a spontaneous incidence of 1%. A dose of 100 rad kills substantial numbers of mouse and rat embryos at this stage, but the survivors appear and develop normally.

[d] One hundred rad produces changes in the irradiated fetus that are subtle and necessitate detailed examination and comparison with comparable controls.

[e] The male gonad in the rat can be made extremely hypoplastic by irradiation in the fetal stages with 15 rad. In the mouse the newborn female is most sensitive to the sterilized effects of radiation. Much of this research on other animals cannot be applied to the human.

[f] The potential for mutation induction exists in embryonic germ cells or their precursors. The relative sensitivity of the embryonic germ cells when compared to adult germ cells is not known. Several long-term studies in animals do not indicate any exceptional differences.

[g] Footnote refers to the aneuploidy produced in a strain of mice with a 1% incidence of spontaneous XO aneuploidy. Bloom (cited in Ref. 1) has reported a much higher percentage of chromosome breaks in human embryos receiving 100–200 rad in utero than in adults receiving the same dose of irradiation. As yet there have been no diseases associated with this increase in frequency of chromosome breaks.

[h] Animal experiments and the data from Hiroshima and Nagasaki do not support the concept that in utero irradiation is much more tumorigenic than extrauterine irradiation, on the other hand, Stewart and colleagues (96,97,99) and many others report that irradiation from pelvimetry (2 rad) increases the incidence of leukemia and other tumors.

[i] A statistically significant increase in percentage of mental retardation occurs with this dose of radiation. On the other hand, normal intelligence has been found in children receiving much higher doses in utero.

[j] Animal experiments indicate that survivors of in utero irradiation have a life span that is longer than that of groups of animals given the same dose of radiation during their extrauterine life and the same life expectancy as nonirradiated controls.

[k] There is a consensus that the brain maintains a marked sensitivity to radiation throughout all of gestation. Mental retardation is a serious risk at this dose.

Source: From Ref. 1, used with permission.

In another study, Dekaban reported that 22 of 26 infants exposed to hundreds of rad between the third and twentieth week of human gestation were microcephalic, developmentally delayed, or both (62). Severe mental retardation following in utero exposure to the atomic bombs was not observed in any patient receiving in utero less than 50 rad (70). It has also been documented that 10–20 rad of low-LET radiation will not increase the incidence of microcephaly in experimental animals (14). Analysis of the data on survivors of atomic bombings in Japan using refined estimates of the obsorbed dose in fetal tissues demonstrated that the highest risk for forebrain damage occurred at 8–15 weeks' gestational age (71). These data were consistent with a linear dose-response model, which did not indicate the existence of a threshold dose. The authors estimated the probability of increasing the incidence of mental retardation was 0.4% rad of radiation (i.e., four additional cases of mental retardation for each 1000 births). In contrast, the data collected for in utero exposures after the fifteenth week of gestation were not linearly related to dose, suggesting that a nonlinear model with a threshold dose for radiation effects best fits the data for this period of gestation. During 8–15 weeks of gestation, the risk of impaired central nervous system development was five times greater than that estimated for 16–25 weeks. Radiation exposure before the eighth week of gestation and after the twenty-fifth week was not associated with an increased risk of mental retardation. In a recent study, Yoshimaru et al. assessed school performance of prenatally exposed survivors of the atomic bombings using the DS86 dosimetry system instituted in 1986. They found that damage to the fetus exposed at 16–25 weeks after fertilization appeared similar to that seen in the 8–15 week group (72). Otake et al. reviewed 45 years' study on brain damage among prenatally exposed survivors of Hiroshima and Nagasaki (73). Again, they noted an increased frequency of severe mental retardation, a diminution in IQ score and school performance, and increased occurrence of seizures among individuals exposed in the eighth through twenty-fifth week postconception, especially in the 8–15 week period. Sixty percent of those with severe mental retardation had small heads, and 10% of survivors with small head size were mentally retarded. A linear dose-response model fitted the data. There was strong evidence of threshold at 0.12–0.23 Gy (12–23 rad) at 8–15 weeks exposure (when two probably non-radiation-related cases of Down's syndrome were excluded) and a 0.21-Gy (21-rad) threshold at 16–25 weeks exposure. Regression analysis of IQ scores and school performance showed greater linearity with the new dosimetry system (DS86) than with the old (T65DR). These two parameters were similar to those in a control group for those exposed in utero to doses under 0.1 Gy (10 rad).

Other studies of this population also suggest that in utero radiation may affect intelligence test scores, with the greatest sensitivity during the eighth to fifteenth week of gestation (2,74). One estimate of the dose-response relationship was a 20-point loss on IQ tests for each additional Gy (100 rad) of exposure. The relationship between dose and intelligence test scores is not yet well established, and the findings have to be refined to a demonstrable level of statistical significance or clinical relevance (2,74). Smith quotes two studies that demonstrated a downward shift in the Gaussian distribution of IQ with an estimated probability coefficient indicating a loss of 30 IQ points per sievert (100 rem) fetal dose at 8–15 weeks after conception (12). A similar, but smaller, shift to lower intelligence was detectable following exposure through the period from 16 to 25 weeks, but not at other periods of pregnancy.

The estimates above are associated with numerous uncertainties (11): the number of subjects in each age-defined exposure group was small, and estimates of fetal absorbed dose and prenatal age at exposure cannot be confirmed.

During the eighth to fifteenth week of human fetal development, there is a well-characterized period of neuronal proliferation and migration in which cells that begin in the ventricular regions of the growing brain migrate into the various layers of the emerging cerebral cortex (75). The apparent absence of an effect prior to the eighth week suggests that neuronal proliferation is capable of adequately replacing lost cells, or the effects on cell migration during weeks 8–15 postconception may be the crucial component of cerebral damage caused by radiation (11). The finding of a small head size in the populations of affected neonates (76) is related to a reduction in cell number, which in turn could be due to impairment of neuronal proliferation and/or massive cell killing (71).

The finding of mental retardation in infants with normal head size (63,64,74) could be explained by glial cell proliferation after irradiation, as shown in animal studies (77).

Other Malformations

In two studies from 1929 on 75 pregnancies, quoted above, besides microcephaly and mental retardation (16 infants), two children were born with hypoplastic genitalia, one with cleft palate, and one with hypospadias, an abnormality of the large toe, and an abnormality of the ear (63,64). There were various abnormalities of the eyes, including microphthalmia, cataracts, strabismus, retinal degeneration, and optic atrophy. In a study of 26 infants exposed to radiation between the third and twentieth week of gestation, 22 were seriously affected. The most frequent abnormalities reported were small size at birth and stunted growth, microcephaly, mental retardation, microphthalmia, pigmentary changes of the retina, genital and skeletal malformations, and cataracts (62). All the malformed children exhibited growth retardation. The estimated protracted exposure was 250 rad. The patients were irradiated for dysmenorrhea, menorrhagia, myomata, arthritis or tuberculosis of the sacroiliac joint, and malignant tumors of the uterus or cervix. In 1930 a typical camptomelic dwarf was born to a woman who had received high dose radiation from the second to the fifth month of gestation (78). This rare syndrome had not been described prior to 1930, and the authors were not in a position to recognize its possible genetic cause.

Growth Retardation

Growth retardation, microcephaly, and mental retardation are predominant observable effects following acute exposures to exceeding 50 rad (low-LET radiation) (1). Radiation-induced morphological malformations have never been reported in humans without the coexistence of growth retardation or a central nervous system abnormality (mainly microcephaly, mental retardation, and readily apparent eye malformations) (1). In a study mentioned above, growth retardation was reported in all children malformed in utero following large doses of maternal pelvic x-irradiation (62). Impairment of growth was also detected among adolescents who had been exposed in utero to gamma and neutron radiation in Hiroshima and Nagasaki (79). The abnormal findings in this population included reduced height and weight (67, 80) and reduced head and chest circumference (76,81).

Diagnostic irradiation involving less than 5 rad to the human fetus has not been observed to cause congenital malformations or growth retardation (82–88), but not all such studies are negative (89). Animal studies support the contention that gross congenital malformations will not be increased in a human pregnant population exposed to 5 rad or less (1,90). In addition, most human exposures to extensive diagnostic radiation studies are fractionated and/or protracted. The likelihood of producing malformations with this type of radiation is lower than with an acute exposure to low-LET radiation (91,92). One might suggest that functional or biochemical changes may be produced at low levels and with low incidence; so far it has not been proven, at least not regarding thyroid function, liver function, and fertility (1).

Oncogenesis

Epidemiological studies involving adults and children have established the potential of ionizing radiation to induce leukemia and solid tumors (47,93). It has also been shown that carcinoma of the thyroid was more prevalent in infants irradiated for thymic hyperplasia (94). Einhorn has suggested the period of organogenesis may be highly resistant to carcinogenesis, possibly because of the existence of highly active regulators influencing development which may control cancer (95). However, a few studies have suggested that in utero radiation may be leukemogenic and may even induce other cancers (96–99). The present estimate is that a 1– to 2–rad in utero radiation exposure increases the chance of leukemia developing in the offspring by a factor of 1.5–2.0 over the natural incidence (1). In comparison, a 2–rad dose delivered to an adult population would not make a perceptible change in the incidence of leukemia even for very large population groups (100,101). An investigation utilizing data on the incidence of neoplastic disease in twins exposed in utero to diagnostic obstetrical x-ray examinations suggested a 2.4–fold risk of childhood cancer (102). Based on this finding and earlier estimates, the increase in neoplastic diseases associated with low dose ionizing radiation is believed to range between 100 and 240 cases per million persons exposed per rad (98,103,104). The British Oxford Survey of Childhood Cancer estimates the risk following human in utero irradiation for cancer induction, including leukemia, to be 0.022/Gy (0.00022/rad) (105). This risk, based on a survey of the doses (mean fetal dose 6 mGy or 0.6 rad) associated with United Kingdom routine obstetric radiology in late pregnancy in the period 1958–1961, was estimated to be 0.04–0.05/Gy or 0.004–0.005/ rad (95% CI, 0.008–0.095/Gy) (106).

Among the survivors of the atomic bombings exposed in utero, there were only 18 incident cases of cancer in the years 1950–1984, five of them in the zero-dose group (107). Two of these patients had childhood cancer during the first 14 years of life; both were exposed to 0.30 Gy (30 rad) or more. All other cases developed cancer in adulthood. The estimated relative risk for cancer at 1 Gy (100 rad) uterine dose was 3.77. The Life Span Study from Japan, based on the new DS86 dosimetry system, indicates an upper bound of risk on 95% CI of 0.028/Gy (0.00028/rad) (108). In a review of several studies dealing with this issue, it has been noted that when considering the variety of control groups and the sampling variability, the results are remarkably consistent in showing an excessive frequency of leukemia among children whose mothers were exposed to radiation during pregnancy (109).

A major criticism of these studies has focused on the possible confounding effects of selection factors leading to prenatal x-ray, and the possibility that these selection factors may be independently related to increased risk of malignancy (47). In some studies, the number of patients was small, whereas other studies could not demonstrate any increase in leukemia following in utero diagnostic radiological procedures (85,110) or exposure to higher doses, including the atomic bomb (111,112). An identical increased risk of leukemia was reported whether the mother had received radiation from diagnostic procedures shortly before or after conception (113), but this was not proven in another study (114). It should be pointed out that siblings of leukemic children have an incidence of leukemia of 1:720 per 10 years, which is greater than the 1:2000 risk of leukemia following pelvimetric exposure and the 1:3000 probability of leukemia in the general population of children followed for 10 years (Table 4) (1). In addition, several animal studies could not demonstrate a significant increase in the incidence of cancer after in utero irradiation (115–117).

At present, it is not clear whether radiation exposure during either preconception or postconception is a causative or associative factor in the increased incidence of leukemia (1,118). Genetic or other environmental factors may be more important than prenatal diagnostic radiation in the production of leukemia. That Japanese bomb survivors exposed in utero to up to 500 rad apparently did not experience a significant increase in carcinogenesis proves the complexity of this tissue. Smith, from the International Commission on Radiological Protection, concludes that in utero irradiation is not considered likely to significantly influence the lifetime risk of a person living to old age who is irradiated throughout life (12).

Although it seems that a dose of less than 10 rad to the implanted embryo does not result in a significant increase in the incidence of congenital malformations, growth retardation, or fetal death, low risk tumorigenic or genetic hazards cannot be ruled out (1). It is one thing to avoid radiation because

Table 4 Risk of Leukemia in Various Groups with Specific Epidemiological and Pathological Characteristics in Populations Followed up for 10–30 Years

Group	Approximate risk	Increased risk over control population	Occurrence
Identical twin of leukemic twin	1/3	1000	Weeks to months
Irradiation-treated polycythemia vera	1/6	500	10–15 years
Bloom's syndrome	1/8	375	< 30 years old
Hiroshima survivors who were within 1000 m of the hypo-center	1/60	50	Average, 12 years
Down's syndrome	1/95	30	< 10 years old
Irradiation-treated patients with ankylosing spondylitis	1/270	10	15 years
Siblings of leukemic children	1/720	4	To 10 years
Children exposed to pelvimetry in utero (gestational exposure)	1/2000	1.5	< 10 years
U.S. white children < 15 years old	1/2800	1	To 10 years

Source: From Refs. 1 and 115 used with permission.

of a potential hazard, but it is another matter to recommend therapeutic abortion on this basis.

RADIODIAGNOSIS IN PREGNANCY

Diagnostic radiology usually involves a radiation dose of 0.02–5.0 rad. Thus, from a clinical standpoint, estimating the risk of gestational effects from a dose of x-ray radiation smaller than 5 rad is of primary importance. The radiation risk, especially in diagnostic radiation, should always be evaluated with consideration of the significant normal risks of the pregnancy. Spontaneous risks of pregnancy are 2 orders of magnitude greater than the theoretical risks of diagnostic radiation. Table 5 lists an estimation of the risks of radiation in the human embryo based on human epidemiological studies and mouse and rat radiation embryological studies. As can be seen from Tables 6 and 7, the maximum theoretical risk to the human embryos exposed to doses of 5 rad or less is extremely small.

Extrapolation of risk estimates after intrauterine exposures to the atomic bomb may not be applicable to low level radiodiagnostic exposures. For instance, an analysis of data from Hiroshima and Nagasaki suggested that any dose of radiation between the eighth and fifteenth week of gestation could increase the risk of microcephaly and mental retardation by 0.4%/rad and possibly decrease intellectual development (71). Not only was the cohort small, but also the doses of radiation at Hiroshima and Nagasaki that produced these effects came from uncontrolled radiation sources that differed significantly in the two cities (119). Consequently, it cannot be considered readily comparable to the low-LET, filtered radiation used in diagnostic radiology (2). For example, in Hiroshima severe mental retardation was not found in individuals exposed in utero to less than 50 rad, whereas in Nagasaki the risk for central nervous system damage was not increased even at levels of 50–150 rad (120).

It is estimated that the overall risk of malformations and cancer for fetuses exposed in utero during the first 4 months of the pregnancy ranges between 0 and 1 case per 1000 radiated by 1 rad (121). This estimate is reinforced by the U.S. National Council on Radiation Protection, which stated that the risk of malformations at 5 rad or less was negligible when compared to the other risks of pregnancy (122). For stochastic phenomena such as cancer and genetic anomalies, it is estimated that the current practice of radiology in the United States increases spontaneous frequency by less than 1% (123). Performing several radiodiagnostic procedures in a pregnant woman should be avoided, since the radiation dose may accumulate to a hazardous level, especially in the sensitive period of 8–15 weeks postconception.

Table 5 Estimation of the Risks of Radiation in the Human Embryo Based on Human Epidemiological Studies and Mouse and Rat Radiation Embryologic Studies

Embryonic age (days)	Minimal lethal dose (rad)	Approximate LD_{50} (rad)	Minimum dose (rad) for permanent growth retardation in the adult	Increased incidence of mental retardation	Minimum dose for recognized gross anatomical malformation (rad)	Minimum dose for induction of genetic carcinogenic and minimal cell depletion phenomena
1-5	10	<100	No effect in survivors			Unknown
18-28	25-50	140	20-50	20-50 Severe CNS anatomic malformations more likely than mental retardation	20	Unknown
36-50	50	200	25-50	50[a]	50	Unknown
50-150	>50	>100	25-50	50[a]	—[b]	Unknown
To term	>100	Same as	>50	100		Unknown

[a]Information published by Otake and Shull (71) suggest an increased risk at lower exposures.
[b]Anatomical malformations of a severe type cannot be produced this late in gestation except in the genitourinary system and tissue hypoplasia in specific organ systems, such as the brain and testes.
Source: From Ref. 1, used with permission.

Table 6 Estimate of Risks of 1-rad Exposure (Low LET) to the Developing Human Embryo

Age (days)	Mutagenic effect[a-c]	Childhood carcinogenic effect (Stewart)[d]	Maximum childhood carcinogenic effect (ABCC)[b,e]	Gross congenital malformations, death, growth retardation	Permanent cell depletion
1	No data	No data	No data	?[f]	No effect[b]
18–28	10^{-7} per locus	3.2×10^{-4}	5×10^{-6}	Same as controls	?
50		3.2×10^{-4}	5×10^{-6}		
Late fetus to term		3.2×10^{-4}	5×10^{-6}		

[a]Based on an estimated doubling dose for mutagenesis of 100 rad, assuming a linear dose-response curve and no threshold for mutagenic effects.

[b]The mutagenic effects have not been studied in the preimplantation period, or during the perimplantation period, the surviving embryos are not reduced in size even when the dose is very high, although at this stage the embryo is very sensitive to the lethal effects of radiation.

[c]The estimate is assumed to be adult risk because there was no increased carcinogenic effect in the population of exposed fetuses in Hiroshima and Nagasaki.

[d]Stewart's (cited in Ref. 1) data would indicate that the embryo is more sensitive to the carcinogenic effect of radiation than the adult. This is a controversial matter, and others (58,112) feel that this association may be other than a radiation effect.

[e]Atomic Bomb Casualty Commission data on carcinogenesis do not indicate that the embryo and fetus are at increased risk. The risk presented is the same carcinogenic risk attributed to adults, assuming maximal effect at low doses; namely, a linear dose-response curve — and no threshold for carcinogenic effects.

[f]Radiation-induced embryonic death might possibly be a stochastic effect in the first few days of gestation, although the present data involving hundreds of embryos indicate no effect at 5-10 rad.

Source: From Ref. 1, used with permission.

Table 7 Risk of 0.5 rem (Maximum Permissible Exposure for Women Radiation Workers with Reproductive Potential)

Risk	0 rem	Additional risk of 0.5 rem
Spontaneous abortion	$150,000/10^6$	0
Major congenital malformations	$30,000/10^6$	0
Severe mental retardation	$5000/10^6$	0
Childhood malignancy/ 10-year period	$7000/10^6/10$ years	$166/10^6/10$ years or $2.5/10^6/10$ years (ABCC data)[a]
Early- or late-onset genetic disease	$100,000/10^6$	Risk is in next generation
Total risk [using Stewart (cited in Ref. 1)]	$285,700/10^6$	$166/10^6$
Ratio of total risk to additional risk of radiation	1721:1	
Total risk (using ABCC data)[a]	$285,700/10^6$	$2.5/10^6$ (ABCC data)[a]
Ratio of total additional risk of radiation	114,280:1	

[a]Data from Atomic Bomb Casualty Commission.
Source: From Ref. 1, used with permission.

There is general agreement that no woman should be denied a medically justified radiodiagnostic procedure because she is pregnant (74,122). On the other hand, unnecessary use of x-ray procedures is not good medical practice either. The immediate medical care of the mother should take priority over the risks of diagnostic radiation exposure to the embryo. Elective procedures such as employment examinations or follow-up examinations once a diagnosis has been made need not be performed on a pregnant woman even though the risk to the embryo is very small (1). If other procedures can provide adequate information without exposing the embryo to ionizing radiation, they should be used. Examples of such alternative procedures are ultrasound and using a computed tomography (CT) scout view for pelvimetry and excretory urography; with these techniques, radiation doses are significantly lower than with conventional x-ray techniques (124).

The International Commission on Radiological Protection recommended the 10-day rule with regard to the question of when during the menstrual cycle elective x-ray studies should be scheduled (74). They pointed out that it is most improbable that a woman will be pregnant in the 10-day interval following onset of menstruation. This should be regarded as the choice time to perform radiological examinations of the abdomen and pelvis in women of childbearing age (74,122). The pregnancy status of the patient can be determined in several ways:

1. Asking for the date of the last menstrual period and the previous menstrual period, and asking whether the patient possibly could be pregnant.
2. Performing a pregnancy test in cases of uncertainty regarding the pregnancy status.
3. Performing pregnancy tests on all women of reproductive age admitted to the hospital.

Using cost/benefit analysis and simple probability calculations, it was shown that as general public policy, pregnancy tests and elective scheduling procedures are of little value, especially when looking at the current estimates of the morbidity that is associated with low dose radiodiagnostic procedures (3). It is important to discuss with the patient why the diagnostic study is indicated even though she may be pregnant, as well as the possible risks to her offspring. Some authors recommend acquiring written consent before the procedure is initiated (2).

When it has been decided to perform the radiodiagnostic examination, every effort should be made to minimize the expected fetal dose. This can be accomplished by modifying the examination by using only selected views (AP vs. PA), by using efficient collimators, by the deliberate adjustment of maternal bladder volume, and by using lead apron protectors of the pelvic and abdominal areas (3,15,125).

RADIATION DOSE ESTIMATION

Before reviewing the embryonic exposures from various radiodiagnostic procedures, it is important to review the unavoidable radiation the embryo receives (i.e., the background radiation), which includes cosmic rays from outer space, terrestrial radiation from ground and building materials, plus naturally occurring radioisotopes ingested or inhaled (54,126) (Table 8). The total dose to the embryo is less than 100 mrad during the 9 months of pregnancy. This dose will vary in different parts of the world and at different elevations, owing to variation in the terrestrial radiation and cosmic ray radiation. Actually, the embryonic/fetal dose during the pregnancy is less than the maternal because of the higher water content of the embryo (126).

When evaluating the need for a radiodiagnostic procedure during pregnancy, or when counseling a pregnant woman who has been inadvertently exposed to such a procedure, it is important to estimate the embryonic/fetal exposure. Whenever dealing with radiodiagnosis or radiotherapy, it is al-

Table 8 Exposures of a Pregnant Woman to Naturally Occurring Background Radiation During the 9 Months of Pregnancy[a]

| | Exposure (mrad/9 months) | |
Type of radiation	Mother soft tissue	Embryo soft tissue
Potassium-40 (^{40}K)	14–18	10–14[a]
Daughters of radium-226	–	–
Carbon-14 (^{14}C)	0.5–1.3	0.5–1.3
External terrestrial	36	36
Cosmic rays	37	37
Total exposure	90	<86

[a]The dosage to the embryo is less because the embryo has a higher
water content and a higher extracellular volume than the adult. Ossification does not occur in the early stages of pregnancy; therefore,
radium and strontium localization would occur only in the latter portion of gestation.
Source: From Ref. 126, used with permission.

ways recommended to obtain the estimated embryonic/fetal exposure dose
from the radiologist involved in the procedure. This is essential because of
the differences in radiation dose delivered by using different equipment and
techniques, as discussed later.

A few methods are available for estimating organ exposure dose in radiodiagnostic examinations:

1. Thermoluminescent dosimeters (TLD) enable direct measurement of entrance skin doses and doses to superficial organs of interest (127).
2. The Monte Carlo technique is a mathematical method with which entrance doses are converted to organ doses (128). For some organs (thyroid, breast, testes, and lungs) the dose measured with TLD is often higher,
   probably as a result of the limitations of the Monte Carlo method in
   simulating actual irradiation (127).
3. A computerized program is available to enable estimation of output parameters of an x-ray machine from a single test exposure and using the data
   for organ dose estimates (129).
4. Experimentally determined normalized depth-dose curves can be used in
   conjunction with sonographic localization of the embryo/fetus (125).

Methods 1 and 2 are the most frequently used.

Table 9 summarizes the estimated fetal exposure for various radiodiagnostic procedures, as found in several studies (127–131). Fetal exposure is

Table 9 Average Fetal Exposure Dose in Various Radiodiagnostic Procedures (mrad)[a]

Examination	Sweden 1977 (130)	USA 1980 (131)	UK 1986 (128)	Italy 1987 (127)
Head, sinus	<1	<0.01	<1	<1
Full spine		128		227
Cervical spine	<1	<0.01		<1
Dorsal spine	<100	0.6	<1	<1
Lumbar spine	620	408	346	
Lumbosacral region	180	639		385
Shoulder, clavicle, sternum	<1	<0.01		<1
Arm	<1			
Pelvis	190	194	165	238
Hip and femur	370	128		51
Femur (lower two-thirds)	50			
Lower leg, knee	<1			
Lungs, ribs	<3	0.5	<1	
Lung (photofluorography)	<10			<1
Lungs and heart	<5	0.06	<1	<1
Abdomen	200	263	289	233
Upper GI tract	56	48	360	151
Small intestine	180			
Barium enema	700	822	1600	1534
Cholecystography, cholangiography	24	5	60	
Urography (IVP)	880	814	358	505
Retrograde pyelography	800			
Urethrocystography	1500			
Pelvimetry	460			
Obstetrical abdomen	150			
Hysterosalpingography	590			
Cerebral angiography	<10			
Mammography		b		
Dental (single exposure)	0.01			

[a]Fetal dose is considered as equivalent to uterus or ovary dose.
[b]Not computed, but treated as negligible relative to absorbed dose to the female breasts (212–766 mrad).

usually regarded as equivalent to uterine or ovary exposure. The highest dose to the fetus is delivered by barium enema andurethrocystography, whereas the lowest doses are delivered by examinations of remote areas (e.g., skull, thorax). Table 10 shows the estimated fetal dose during CT (132). In another reference, a typical scan study of the abdominal area (several slices) was

Table 10 Fetal Exposure During Computed
Tomography

Examination	Fetal dose (mrad)[a]
Chest	30
Chest/abdomen	450
Abdomen	240
Abdomen/pelvis	640
Pelvis	730

[a]Fetal dose is considered equivalent to ovary dose.
Source: Modified from Ref. 132.

estimated to give an ovarian dose of 0.5–1.1 rad (133). Scattered radiation
to the ovaries during CT scanning of the head measures less than 1 mrad
per single scan (134).

   Fetal dose estimates vary among different studies, as can be readily seen
in Table 9. A few factors influence the fluoroscopic and radiographic radiation exposure (4):

1. Type of x-ray equipment. Exposure may vary by a factor of 2 or more
   with the use of different intensifiers and cameras.
2. Differences in technique used by the radiologist may contribute to the
   variation of exposure by a factor of 1.7 for fluoroscopy and 25 for radiography. Differences in technique may involve variations in fluoroscopic exposure time, number of films taken, beam size, maintenance of
   image quality, and imaging area.
3. Automatic versus manual control of fluoroscopy.
4. Obesity index, which depends on height and weight of the patient.
5. Cooperation of the patient.

MAGNETIC RESONANCE IMAGING

Magnetic resonance imaging (MRI) (interchangeably called nuclear magnetic resonance, NMR) may replace the CT scanner for some diagnostic imaging. With MRI, patients are subjected to very high magnetic fields (static,
rapidly varying, and radiofrequency), but studies thus far have not indicated any potential hazard to the unborn child (135,136). MRI is considered
by some clinicians to be the method of choice for antenatal pelvimetry (137).
Mice exposed to MRI at the magnetic isocenter or at the entrance to the magnetic lumen had a significantly higher rate of eye malformations than controls (138). However, the mouse strain used in this study was genetically prone
to these malformations. Cultured lymphocytes exposed to MRI during growth

and division do not exhibit an increase in chromatid or chromosome lesions (139). The National Radiological Protection Board has indicated that although there is evidence to suggest that the developing embryo is not sensitive to the magnetic field encountered in NMR clinical imaging, more studies are needed to rule out adverse developmental effects. Until more conclusive evidence is available, therefore, it is considered prudent to exclude pregnant women from this procedure during the first trimester, when organ development is taking place (140).

RADIOTHERAPY

Radiotherapy involves large doses of radiation that are likely to affect the fetus deleteriously, especially if given to the abdominal region. If the dose delivered to the embryo during the early organogenetic period is hundreds of rad, the embryo will probably be aborted. During the second and third trimesters there is high chance of irreversible damage to the central nervous system. If the fetus absorbs 50 rad or more at any time during gestation, there is a significant possibility that the fetus may be damaged (1). As mentioned earlier, the fetal exposure dose should be estimated by the radiologist, and the parents should be informed about the real probability of malformations and damage to the central nervous system. In some instances the human fetus has survived and has even appeared normal after exposure to doses exceeding 50 rad (62,141), but this of course should not be regarded as the rule.

OCCUPATIONAL EXPOSURE

Women of childbearing age working regularly with radiation must be monitored (by film or TLD badge) if there is a reasonable possibility of receiving more than a quarter of their maximum quarterly recommended limit of 1.25 rem (142). Few workers, male and female, actually receive an annual dose approaching 5 rem (54). The National Council on Radiation Protection and Measurements recommends a maximum permissible dose equivalent to the embryo and fetus from occupational exposures of the expectant mother of 0.5 rem during the entire pregnancy (143), or 0.05 rem per month (144). If average annual exposure exceeds 3 rem, or if there are peak periods of higher exposure, the worker of childbearing age may receive more than 0.5 rem in the first 2 months of the pregnancy (54). Women radiologists can work without interruption during pregnancy if proper precautions are taken, even with a heavy daily workload (145). The U.S. Nuclear Regulatory Commission suggests that women who are or expect to become pregnant, and whose fetuses could recieve 0.5 rem or more before birth, seek ways to reduce their exposure within their present job or delay having children until they change job locations (146).

PATERNAL IRRADIATION

The effects of radiation on the testes were discussed earlier in this chapter. A study looking at the proportion of malformations in children fathered by testicular cancer patients treated with radiotherapy did not reveal any difference compared to a control group or to the incidence of malformations in the general population (147). The effects of paternal irradiation have been studied in Hiroshima and Nagasaki survivors. No increase in malformations, fetal death rate, or birth weight were found (148,149). Another study showed an association between childhood leukemia and paternal preconception occupational exposure involving radiation (odds ratio, 3.23; 95% CI, 1.36–7.22), as well as with other factors such as wood dust and benzene (150). Ionizing radiation alone gave an odds ratio of 2.35 (95% CI, 0.95–6.22). These results are confounded by small numbers and multiple exposures of some parents.

COSMIC RAYS (AIR TRAVEL)

Exposure to cosmic rays varies with the change in altitude, latitude, and solar activity. The flux of cosmic rays increases by approximately 100% for every 1.5–2.0 km above sea level (2). Assuming that a jet aircraft flies at an average altitude of 8 km, the mean dose rate is 0.84 μGy/h (84 μrad/h) compared to 0.04 μGy/h (3 μrad/h) at sea level. For example, the cosmic ray dose to a person flying from New York to Paris round trip is 31 μGy (3.1 mrem) for subsonic flight and 24 μGy (2.4 mrem) for supersonic flight (subsonic flight is usually at an altitude of approximately 11 km; supersonic flight is at about 19 km) (2). Although supersonic flights take place at high altitudes, the overall absorbed dose is less, since the flight is faster by a factor of 2–3.

The average annual effective dose equivalent from cosmic rays for airline crew members is 0.8 mSv (80 mrem). Astronauts on Apollo space missions and lunar landings have been in the range of 2 mrem/h (2).

COUNSELING THE PREGNANT WOMAN

In all instances of counseling parents concerning the hazards to the embryo/fetus exposed to radiation, biological knowledge is only one facet to be considered. As mentioned earlier, the hazards of exposure to diagnostic radiation (0.02–5.0 rad) present an extremely low risk to the embryo when compared with the "spontaneous" risks. More than 15% of human embryos abort spontaneously. About 3% may have major malformations, 4% have intrauterine growth retardation, and 8–10% have early- or late-onset genetic disease (1). A systematic approach of patient evaluation should be used to obtain the following information:

Stage of pregnancy at time of exposure
Menstrual history
Previous pregnancy history
History of congenital malformations and genetic diseases
Other potentially harmful exposures and environmental factors during the
    pregnancy
Maternal and paternal age
Type of radiation study, dates, and numbers of studies performed
Estimate of the fetal exposure by a radiologist or medical physicist
Status of the pregnancy—wanted or unwanted
Emotional maturity of the family
Religion and ethical values of the family

The applicable abortion laws should also be taken into consideration.

This information should be evaluated with both patient and counselor to arrive at a decision. The information delivered to the patient should be clearly documented in the medical record, including the idea that every pregnancy has a risk of problems. It also should be conveyed that the notion of no increased risk does not mean that the counselor is guaranteeing the outcome of the pregnancy. The physician may consider performing an ultrasound examination to rule out radiation-induced microcephaly or growth retardation.

The maximal theoretical risk attributed to a 1-rad exposure, approximately 0.003%, is thousands of times smaller than the spontaneous risks of malformations, abortions, or genetic diseases (1). Thus, the present maximal permissible occupational exposures of 0.5 rem for pregnant women and 5 rem for medical exposure are extremely conservative. There is no medical justification for terminating pregnancy because of radiation exposure in women exposed to 5 rad or less (1). The specter of radiation hazards should not be invoked to circumvent a social or legal problem.

Although radiodiagnosis involves fetal doses of less than 5 rad, which are not considered to be teratogenic, many pregnant women exposed to it perceive their teratogenic risk as unrealistically high (151). This may be due to the anxiety provoked by the term "radiation" and by misinformation. An effective counseling process in these cases was shown to reduce the perception of teratogenic risk from $25.5 \pm 4.3\%$ to $15.7 \pm 3.0\%$ ($p < 0.05$), thus preventing unnecessary termination of otherwise wanted pregnancies (151).

RADIONUCLIDES

Physics and Biology

An element has a fixed number of protons, which determines it atomic number, but it may have a variable number of neutrons. For instance, ^{12}C, ^{13}C, and ^{14}C, which have six, seven, and eight neutrons, respectively, are referred to as isotopes of carbon, and each of them is a nuclide. Many nuclides have an unstable nucleus, owing to too many or too few neutrons, and they are called radionuclides (radioisotopes). They disintegrate spontaneously and emit various forms of energy, collectively called radiation. The rate of disintegration is measured in units such as the becquerel (Bq) and the curie (Ci); 1 Bq is 1 disintegration per second and 1 Ci is the rate of disintegration of 1 g of pure ^{226}Ra (1 Ci = 3.7×10^{10} Bq). The half-life is the time required for half of a sample of radionuclide to decay. Table 11 shows the halflife and type of radiation of various radionuclides (152).

The heavy alpha particle (positively charged particles; helium nuclei) has a very high LET but penetrates tissue poorly (in contrast to x-rays and gamma rays). Therefore, radionuclides are relatively nonhazardous when used externally, but they can be toxic if ingested. The distribution of absorbed energy is rather uniform in embryos exposed to x-rays and gamma rays. Conversely, radionuclides have a predictable but variable energy distribution in the embryo, depending on placental permeability, fetal distribution, or tissue affinity, and the nature of radiation emitted (alpha particle, beta particle—identical with electrons or positrons, but arising from the nucleus; gamma ray—electromagnetic radiation with wavelength much shorter than that of light or any combination). For example, ^{131}I will be absorbed and incorporated readily into the fetus with the development of the thyroid, as will plutonium and strontium with the development of the skeletal system. Thus, estimating the absorbed dose and hazards of a radionuclide is more complex than estimating externally administered radiation.

The mechanism of action of this form of ionizing radiation as well as its potential to cause congenital malformations, central nervous system damage, growth retardation, or embryonic death was discussed earlier in this chapter.

Types of Radionuclide

The number of agents available in nuclear medicine has expanded rapidly, and 150 substances containing 74 different radionuclides from 36 elements have been in use (153). Over the years, the use of particular radionuclides has changed, the frequency of various procedures in nuclear medicine has increased, several procedures have been introduced, and others have been eliminated (126). For example, placental localization with isotopes (even

Table 11 Physical[a] and Effective[b] Half-Life and Type of Radiation of Various Radioisotopes

Radionuclide	Physical $t_{1/2}$	Effective $t_{1/2}$	Radiation
^{137}Cs	30.1 years	70 days	β^-, e^-, γ
^{47}Ca	4.54 days	4.5 days	β^-, γ
^{14}C	5730 years	12 days	β^-
^{51}Cr	27.7 days	27 days	e^-, γ
^{57}Co	270 days	9 days	e^-, γ
^{58}Co	71 days	8 days	β^+, γ
^{60}Co	5.27 years	10 days	β^-, γ
^{67}Ga	78.26 h		γ
^{198}Au	65 h	62 h	β^-, e^-, γ
^{111}In	67 h		γ
^{113m}In	99.5 min		e^-, γ
^{123}I	13.2 h		γ
^{125}I	60 days	42 days	e^-, γ
^{131}I	8.06 days	8 days	β^-, e^-, γ
^{192}I	74 days		β^-, e^-, γ
^{59}Fe	44.6 days	42 days	β^-, γ
^{197}Hg	64.4 h	55.2 h	e^-, γ
^{203}Hg	46.6 days	11 days	β^-, e^-, γ
^{32}P	14.3 days	14 days	β^-
^{40}K	1.28×10^9 years		e^-, β^-, γ
^{42}K	12.36 h	12 h	β^-, γ
^{75}Se	120 days		e^-, γ
^{22}Na	2.6 years	11 days	β^+, γ
^{24}Na	15.02 h	14 h	β^-, γ
^{85}Sr	64.8 days	64 days	e^-, γ
^{90}Sr	28.5 years	15 years	β^- (DR)[c]
^{35}S	87.4 days	44 days	β^-
^{99m}Tc	6.02 h		e^-, γ
^{201}Tl	73.5 h		γ (DR)
^{204}Tl	3.8 years		β^-, γ
^{224}Ra	3.6 days	3.6 days	β, α (DR)
^{226}Ra	160 years	44 years	α, e^-, γ (DR)
^{3}H	12.35 years	12 days	β^-
^{127}Xe	36.4 days		e^-, γ
^{133}Xe	5.25 days		β^-, e^-, γ
^{90}Y	64.1 days	64 h	β^-

[a]The time required for the activity to decrease by 50%.
[b]The time required for the amount of a particular specimen of a radionuclide in a system to be reduced to half its initial value as a consequence of both radioactive decay and other processes, such as biological elimination.
[c]Daughter radiation (daughter radionuclide is the decay product of a radionuclide).
Source: Modified from Refs. 2 and 152.

with ^{99m}Tc, which delivers a very low dose to the fetus) has been completely replaced by ultrasound.

Radioactive Iodine

The usual forms of iodine are ^{123}I, ^{125}I, and ^{131}I. Isotope ^{125}I is used to label minute doses of hormones for in vivo and in vitro assays. ^{123}I is used for uptake studies. ^{131}I can be given bound to protein or as the inorganic ion. It is used for thyroid uptake scanning and treatment of thyrotoxicosis and thyroid carcinoma, as well as for other medical purposes not related to the thyroid. Inorganic iodides readily cross the placenta, in contrast to protein-bound iodides. Over time, substantial amounts of iodide are released from the protein and then cross the placenta. The fetal thyroid has more affinity to iodides than does the maternal (Table 12), and it begins to absorb and incorporate the iodide by the tenth week of gestation (126). Ablative doses of ^{131}I given to the mother may result in fetal thyroid destruction. So far, the lowest dose reported to destroy the fetal thyroid was 12.2 mCi in a fractionated manner; 9.2 mCi of ^{131}I was given after the seventy-fourth day of gestation (155). There are no reports of immediate deleterious fetal effects from tracer doses of radioactive iodine (126), but there is a theoretical possibility of induction of thyroid carcinoma. The fetal whole-body dose consists mainly of gamma rays, whereas the fetal thyroid dose is a combination of gamma rays and beta particles. This makes the fetal whole-body dose significant compared with the thyroid dose.

Other Radionuclides

Many radionuclides are bound to macroaggregates and macromolecules; they cross the placenta in small amounts, and the radiation dose delivered to the fetus is very small. For example, ^{99m}Tc is used in many diagnostic procedures. Sodium ^{99m}Tc pertechnetate is used for thyroid imaging. The radia-

Table 12 Thyroidal Radioiodine Dose of the Fetus

Gestation period	Fetal/maternal ratio (thyroid gland)	Dose to thyroid (fetus) (rad/μCi)[a]
10–12 weeks	—	0.001 (precursors)
12–13 weeks	1.2	0.7
2nd trimester	1.8	6.0
3rd trimester	7.5	—
Birth imminent	—	8.0

[a]Rad/μCi of ^{131}I ingested by mother.
Source: From Ref. 126 derived from data in Ref. 153, used with permission.

tion dose delivered with this radionuclide is lower than that of iodide because of its short physical half-life and short duration in the thyroid (since little of it is organically bound).

Radioactive phosphorus or gold is used in the treatment of polycythemia or peritoneal malignancies. High dose radioactive phosphorus may result in embryonic abnormality and death in animals; this is also the case for radioactive strontium (156).

Inorganic radioactive potassium, sodium, phosphorus, cesium, thallium, selenium, chromium, iron, and strontium cross the placenta readily, but their use is very limited.

Dose Estimation

The dose to the embryo is dependent on the form of the radionuclide, the site of administration, and the nature of the disease. In any case of exposure to radionuclides during pregnancy, the embryonic dose should be calculated. Often this dose will be less than the maternal dose because the nature of the radionuclide limits its ability to cross the placenta. Methods to estimate the dose to the embryo from radionuclides have been devised (154, 157).

Adult administered activity in various clinical radiopharmaceutical procedures is presented in Table 13 (126,158–160). The estimated embryonic/fetal doses from several radionuclides and nuclear medicine procedures are shown in Tables 14 and 15 (161).

Risk Estimation

Although it has been suggested that background and fallout radiation contribute to spontaneous mutation rate and congenital malformations, most studies have not found a correlation between levels of background radiation and any health hazard, including adverse pregnancy outcome (153, 162–164). It is important to remember these data when considering that many of the exposures from nuclear medicine procedures are within the order of magnitude of background radiation.

The reproductive effects of radionuclides have been less studied and less generalized than those of external radiation. This may be attributed to differences in placental permeability, nonrandom distribution of the radiation, existence of specific target organs, biological differences, or disease states that may affect the metabolism, and the exponential decrease in radiation dose rate over time. In addition, because the amount of energy absorbed over a given length of time (LET) is different for various radiations, 1 Gy aliquots from different radionuclides are not necessarily equally toxic (153).

Table 13 Clinical Radiopharmaceutical Procedures

Radiopharmaceutical	Study	Adult administered activity
^{32}P-sodium phosphate	Therapy, polycythemia vera	2.3 mCi/m^2
^{51}Cr-albumin	GI protein loss	50 μCi IV
^{51}Cr-chromate	Red cell survival	160 μCi IV
^{51}Cr-chromate	Red cell mass	25 μCi IV
^{51}C-chromate	Red cell in vivo	160 μCi IV
^{51}Cr-chromate red blood cells	Spleen imaging	200 μCi IV
^{57}Covitamin B$_{12}$	Vitamin B$_{12}$ absorption	0.5 μCi PO
^{60}Covitamin B$_{12}$	Vitamin B$_{12}$ absorption	0.5 μCi PO
^{59}Fe-citrate	Iron absorption	5 μCi PO (700 μg ferrous ammonium sulfate, 300 mg ascorbic acid)
^{59}Fe-citrate	In vivo counting for effective hematopoiesis	20 μCi IV
^{59}Fe-citrate	Iron plasma clearance and turnover	20 μCi IV
^{59}Fe-citrate	Iron red blood cell uptake	20 μCi IV
^{67}Ga-citrate	Tumor imaging	3–4 mCi IV
^{67}Ga-citrate	Abscess imaging	3–4 mCi IV
^{75}Se-selenomethionine	Pancreas imaging	250 μCi IV or 4 μCi/kg, whichever is less
^{99m}Tc-diphosphonate	Myocardial imaging	15 mCi IV
^{99m}Tc-disphosphonate or pyrophosphate	Bone imaging	15 mCi IV
^{99m}Tc-DTPA	Brain imaging	15–20 mCi IV (no perchlorate)
^{99m}Tc-DTPA	Kidney imaging	15 mCi IV
^{99m}Tc-DTPA iron ascorbate	Kidney imaging	15 mCi IV
^{99m}Tc-human serum albumin	Pericardial imaging	10 mCi IV
^{99m}Tc-human albumin microspheres	Lung perfusion study	3 mCi IV
^{99m}Tc-human serum albumin	Placenta imaging	1–2 mCi IV
^{99m}Tc-macoaggregated albumin	Lung perfusion study	3 mCi IV
^{99m}Tc-macroaggregates	Venous imaging for thrombosis	6 mCi IV
^{99m}Tc-pertechnetate	Vascular flow	20 mCi IV
^{99m}Tc-pertechnetate	Thyroid uptake when uptake is low, organification blocked	1–3 mCi IV

Table 13 Continued

Radiopharmaceutical	Study	Adult administered activity
^{99m}Tc-pertechnetate	Ectopic gastric tissue (e.g., Meckel's diverticulum)	100 μCi/kg
^{99m}Tc-pertechnetate	Brain imaging	15-20 mCi IV (200 mg potassium perchlorate orally prior to exam)
^{99m}Tc-pertechnetate	Carotid or cerebral hemisphere studies	20 mCi IV
^{99m}Tc-sulfur colloid	Bone marrow imaging	10 mCi IV
^{99m}Tc-sulfur colloid	Spleen imaging	3 mCi IV
^{99m}Tc-sulfur colloid	Liver imaging	3 mCi IV
^{111}In-DTPA	Cerebrospinal fluid rhinorrhea	0.5 mCi IT
^{123}I-iodide	Thyroid uptake	100 μCi PO
^{123}I-iodide	TSH thyroid uptake study	100 μCi PO (10 U Thytropar im × 3 days prior to test)
^{123}I-iodide	T_3 suppression thyroid uptake	100 μCi PO (25 μg cytomel t.i.d. × 7 days prior to test)
^{123}I-iodide	Thyroid imaging	100 μCi PO
^{123}I-iodohippurate	Kidney function	1-2 mCi IV
^{123}I-iodohippurate	Kidney imaging	1-2 mCi IV
^{125}I-human serum albumin	Plasma volume	4 μCi IV
^{131}I-fibrinogen	Venous imaging for thrombosis	100 mCi
^{131}I-iodide	Thyroid uptake	10 μCi PO
^{131}I-iodide	TSH uptake study	10 μCi PO (10 U Thytropar IM × 3 days prior to test)
^{131}I-iodide	T_3 suppression	10 μCi PO (25 μg cytomel t.i.d. × 7 days prior to test)
^{131}I-iodide	Thyroid imaging	100 μCi PO
^{131}I-iodide	Thyroid therapy	5-20 mCi PO for thyrotoxicosis; 75-100 mCi Po for thyroid cancer
^{131}I-iodohippurate	Kidney function	3.5 μCi/kg body weight IV not to exceed 300 μCi
^{131}I-iodohippurate	Kidney imaging	200 μCi IV

(continues)

Table 13 Continued

Radiopharmaceutical	Study	Adult administered activity
[131]I-oleic acid	Intestinal fat absorption studies	50 μCi PO
[131]I-rose bengal	Liver imaging	3 mCi IV
[131]I-triolein	Intestinal fat absorption studies	50 μCi PO
[127]Xe gas	Lung ventilation study	15 mCi by inhalation
[133]Xe gas	Lung ventilation study	15 mCi by inhalation
[129]Cs-chloride	Myocardial imaging	5–6 mCi IV
[169]Yb-DTPA	Cerebrospinal fluid rhinorrhea	0.5 mCi IT
[169]Yb-DTPA	Normal pressure hydrocephalus	1 mCi IT
[201]Tl-chloride	Myocardial imaging	3 mCi IV

Source: From Ref. 126, derived from data in Refs. 158–160, used with permission.

Teratogenic, embryonic/fetal, and growth-retarding effects in laboratory animals have been demonstrated for ^{137}Cs, ^{32}P, ^{89}Sr, ^{90}Sr, and [^{3}H]thymidine (165). It is likely that similar effects could be demonstrated for any radionuclide if the exposure could be adjusted to deliver a cytotoxic dose of radiation to the embryo.

Doses to the embryo from standard nuclear medicine procedures are low. This may not be the case for radioactive iodine used for the treatment of thyrotoxicosis and thyroid carcinoma. It is extremely important that a competent expert calculate the fetal dose in any case of fetal or embryonic exposure. If the calculated dose to the embryo is 10 rad or more (about 100 mSv),

Table 14 Dose Estimated to Embryo from Radiopharmaceuticals (131)

Radiopharmaceutical	Embryo dose (rad/mCi administered)
[99m]Tc-human serum albumin	0.018
[99m]Tc-lung aggregate	0.035
[99m]Tc-polyphosphate	0.036
[99m]Tc-sodium pertechnetate	0.037
[99m]Tc-stannous glucoheptonate	0.040
[99m]Tc-sulfur colloid	0.032
[123]I-sodium iodide (15% uptake)	0.032
[131]I-sodium iodide (15% uptake)	0.100
[123]I-rose bengal	0.130
[131]I-rose bengal	0.680

Source: From Ref. 161, derived from data in Ref. 157, used with permission.

Table 15 Fetal Radiation Dose from Various Nuclear Medicine Procedures

Study	Radioisotope	Fetal dose (rad)
Pericardial imaging	^{99m}Tc-human serum albumin	0.18
Placenta imaging	^{99m}Tc-human serum albumin	0.018–0.036
Lung perfusion study	^{99m}Tc-lung aggregate	0.105
Brain imaging	^{99m}Tc-pertechnetate	0.555–0.74
Bone marrow imaging	^{99m}Tc-sulfur colloid	0.32
Spleen imaging	^{99m}Tc-sulfur colloid	0.096
Liver imaging	^{99m}Tc-sulfur colloid	0.096
	^{131}I-rose bengal	2.04
Thyroid uptake (15% uptake)	^{123}I-iodide	0.0032
	^{131}I-iodide	0.001
Thyroid imaging (15% uptake	^{131}I-iodide	0.01
Thyroid therapy	^{131}I-iodide	0.05–2.0 (thyrotoxicosis) 7.5–15.0 (thyroid cancer)

Source: Data derived from Refs. 126 and 161.

the offspring should be considered to have a significant risk of a radiation-induced abnormality (153). The Collaborative Perinatal Project monitored 21 exposures to diagnostic radionuclides (^{131}I, mainly unbound) in the first trimester and found one malformation with standardized relative risk (SRR) of 0.72 (166). For exposures during the whole pregnancy, 3 out of 50 had malformations with SRR of 1.99. It is not mentioned what radionuclides were used in this group, and in addition the numbers were small. However, apart from the well-documented thyroid damage from radioactive iodine, there have been no controlled studies demonstrating an association between nuclear medicine procedures and adverse pregnancy outcome. Nevertheless, it is recommended that pregnant women not undergo nuclear medicine procedures. The use of radioactive iodine should be avoided during pregnancy unless essential for the medical care of the mother and there is no substitute. Even if administered during the first 5–6 weeks of human gestation, when the fetal thyroid has not yet developed, the total fetal dose should be estimated.

In any case of exposure to radionuclides when it is known that the patient is pregnant, or in any case of inadvertent exposure, the guidelines outlined in the section on counseling the pregnant woman should be followed.

The Chernobyl Accident

Accidents in nuclear plants, such as that at Chernobyl in the former Soviet Union, may pose a threat to human reproduction. It seems obvious that lethal radiation levels were reached, and such an exposure can cause fetal damage. Air contamination and radionuclides deposited on the skin or the ground serve as an external source of irradiation, and the inhalation or ingestation of radionuclides in food (especially milk) is considered to be internal exposure. European cities reported doses of radiation of 0.1–1.0 mSv (167), which is equivalent to an extra year of background radiation. Exposure to such levels is unlikely to increase the incidence of gross congenital malformations. An increase in adverse phenomena related to stochastic effects might be expected; for example, increased risk of thyroid carcinoma induced in young children by ^{131}I-contaminated milk (168). In the heavily contaminated southern part of Germany there was a higher rate of trisomy-21 among fetuses conceived during the period of greatest radioactive exposure (169). In Finland there were no differences in the expected/observed rates of congenital malformations, preterm births, and stillbirths (170). In Hungary no measurable germinal mutagenic effect was revealed (171), and in Norway no dose-response associations were observed with perinatal health problems (172). In both countries the rate of live births (171) and the total number of pregnancies (172) somewhat decreased, although there was no increase in the rate of induced or legal abortions. Interestingly, on the other hand, there was an increased rate of termination of pregnancies in Greece and Denmark in the months after the Chernobyl accident, even though the radiation doses measured in these countries were not large enough to induce birth defects (173,174). Thus we see that high levels of anxiety can be invoked even by low amounts of radiation; and in these two countries this anxiety caused more fetal deaths than the radiation itself. The importance of good and reliable counseling in such cases cannot be overemphasized.

RADON

Radon is an odorless, colorless, tasteless, and inert gas. It has several isotopes and radon daughters, all emitting mainly alpha radiation.

Radon in houses comes from building materials, the soil under the house, the water, and the domestic gas. Some building materials such as aerated concrete with alum shale and phosphogypsum from sedimentary ores have higher radium concentrations and cause enhanced radon concentrations indoors. Radon exhalation from walls, floors, and ceilings is dependent on radium concentration, emanation power, diffusion coefficient in the material, and quality and thickness of the applied sealant. Ventilation rate, as determined by meteorological conditions and human activities, has a strong influence on radon levels.

Radon and its daughters, after being attached to environmental airborne dust, stick to bronchial epithelial lining, releasing ionizing radiation (alpha particles), which may induce cancerous transformation.

Increased risk of lung cancer has been clearly documented in uranium miners and certain other miners exposed to radon and its daughters. The level of risk has not been so well quantitated in environmental exposure. There is an additive relationship between radon exposure and cigarette smoking for lung cancer risk.

There are no human or animal data on the effect of maternal exposure to radon during pregnancy. Since radon's main hazard is the ionizing radiation, a small risk cannot be excluded. The main emission consists of alpha particles, which do not penetrate tissues deeply but have high linear energy transfer. A study of 491 males employed at uranium mines revealed in their offspring low birth weight and a decreased male/female ratio (175).

Indoor air concentration of radon should equal outdoor air concentration (0.2–0.7 pCi/L, or 7.4–26 Bq/m^3). Environmental standards for indoor residential air radon are 4–8 pCi/L (148–296 Bq/m^3), as guided by the Environmental Protection Agency and the National Council on Radiation Protection, respectively. These levels may be lowered in the future.

VIDEO DISPLAY TERMINALS

Over the last years, the microprocessor has brought video display terminals (VDTs) into offices and homes, and a massive increase in their use has been observed. It was estimated that in the United States 7 million people were occupationally exposed to VDTs in 1980 (176). The earliest complaints by operators of VDTs were concerned with visual problems and musculoskeletal discomfort (140). Migraine, epilepsy (one case report), and facial dermatitis were also reported (140). The scale of expansion in the use of VDTs has prompted interest in the reproductive effects of radiation from these devices.

Physics

The VDT is a cathode ray tube that directs electrons at a screen coated with a fluorescent target, generally phosphor. The bombardment of the target with electrons causes the fluorescent material to emit light. Television sets operate in the same manner. The energy emitted by VDTs is in the form of electromagnetic radiation. It consists of ionizing radiation (x-ray), the biological effects of which have been discussed earlier in this chapter, and nonionizing radiation (ultraviolet, visible light, infrared, microwave, and electromagnetic fields), some of which can transmit energy to tissues as heat. It is important to remember that electromagnetic radiation decreases in proportion to the square of the distance between a point source and the observer. Therefore, one might expect a rapid decrease in radiation with increasing distance from the screen.

X-rays emitted by the cathode ray tube are entirely absorbed by the glass screen (177). Several studies could not detect measurable ionizing radiation from VDTs (e.g., 0.01–0.05 mrad/h) (177–182).

Ultraviolet and visible light are emitted by the phosphor target of the VDT screen. The amount of ultraviolet radiation measured from VDTs is 2–5 orders of magnitude less than that of the environment (178,180). The amount of heat produced from this type of radiation is estimated to be 1.75 × 10^{-6} cal (183). In addition, the wavelength of ultraviolet radiation emitted from VDTs is not less than 336 nm (180); the harmful range is considered to be higher than 300 nm.

No infrared radiation has been detected from VDTs tested (178,180).

Nonionizing radiation in the form of microwave and extremely low frequency (ELF: 45–60 Hz) and very low frequency (VLF: 15 kHz) electromagnetic fields emitted from VDTs is in the same frequency range given off by most electrical appliances at home (178,184). This amount of radiation is 2 orders of magnitude less than background (180). Some VDTs are equipped with a flyback transformer, responsible for moving the arm of the cathode ray tube back and forth. People coming near the back casing of such a unit may be exposed to lower frequency electromagnetic radiation with powers measured up to 800 mW/cm² (183). The casing can be modified to solve this problem.

Risk Estimation

Over the last years, a few clusters of adverse pregnancy outcomes among women VDT operators were reported (54,140,183). These clusters included spontaneous abortions, prematurity, neonatal respiratory disease, Down's syndrome, and birth defects. The malformations reported, which were different in each affected child, included clubfoot, underdeveloped eye, cleft palate, congenital heart defect, and neural tube defect. None of the reports of abnormal pregnancy presented a distinct or reproducible syndrome.

Current regulations require that x-ray emissions from any cathode ray tube be less than 0.5 mR/h at 5 cm (54). Even at this maximum level, radiation exposure to the uterus (50 cm from the screen) would be minimal. A woman sitting at a VDT console for 30 hours a week would accumulate a maximum uterine dose of 0.006 rem during the first trimester, about one-quarter of the natural background radiation dose she would be receiving at the same time (185). As the fetus grows, it may be physically closer to the terminal, but it would be shielded increasingly by the amniotic fluid.

The amount of nonionizing radiation emitted is very small and consists of frequencies that have not been shown to be harmful. Exposure to an improperly shielded flyback transformer would be associated with absorbing significant low frequency radio waves. Animal studies investigating magnetic field-induced abnormalities in chick embryos are inconclusive (186–188). Epidemiological studies dealing with these issues are fraught with pitfalls. A study reviewing occupations that might entail work with VDTs showed that in pregnancies in which a VDT had not been used, the rate of spontaneous abortions was 5.7%. The rate was 8.2 and 9.3% for women working with VDTs less and more than 15 hours weekly, respectively. In contrast, the rate of spontaneous abortions among women from groups not using VDTs was 7.8% (189). These results were found later on by the authors themselves to be subject to selection bias and recall bias (190). In another study, response bias seemed to be a possible explanation for a suggested association with adverse reproductive effects (191). Comparison of mothers of malformed children and their paired referents found no evidence that exposure to VDTs caused birth defects (192). No mention was made in that report of miscarriages. Schnorr et al. compared a cohort of female telephone operators who used VDTs at work with a cohort of operators who did not use VDTs (184). Operators who used VDTs had higher abdominal exposure to VLF electromagnetic fields (15 kHz), but not to ELF fields (45–60 Hz). VDT operators had no excess risk of spontaneous abortions, and there was no dose-response relation when the women's hours of VDT use per week were examined. In a case control study in Finland, no association was found between cardiovascular malformations and the use of VDTs at work or home among other parameters studied (193).

Based on the current data and the fact that a very large number of women are exposed occupationally to VDTs, it seems likely that the clusters reported were encountered by chance (183). It appears that VDTs offer no known radiation hazard (54). In some countries, pregnant women may request a leave from working with VDTs—and they may be allowed to do so on the grounds of reducing worry (194,195).

MICROWAVES, RADAR, RADIO WAVES, FM, AND DIATHERMY

Physics

Microwave, radar, radio wave, FM, and diathermy radiation sources all involve electromagnetic waves ranging in frequency from 27.5 MHz (diathermy) to 10^4–10^5 MHz (microwave communications) (1). The electromagnetic waves generated by diathermy are highly penetrating and can easily heat the human body. Microwaves of 2450 or 915 MHz produce hyperthermia but are less penetrating. Microwaves exceeding 10,000 MHz produce significant hyperthermia at skin level but are minimally penetrating (1). This type of radiation is incapable of producing ionizations within tissues (14,196).

Biological Studies

Chick embryos exposed to 428 MHz radiofrequency radiation at a power density of 5.5 mW/cm^2 for more than 20 days had higher rates of embryo lethality and teratogenicity (197). A few animal studies using a 27.12 MHz radiofrequency field showed an increased rate of resorption, incomplete cranial ossification, birth defects, reduced fetal weight, prenatal death, and reduced body weight in the exposed dams (198–200). Those effects were related to increased maternal body temperature. In one study, 41.5°C was estimated to be a threshold temperature over which there is an increased incidence of adverse reproductive effects (199). In another study, it appeared possible to ascribe some of the effects to a specific action of the radiofrequency radiation occurring independently of the rise in the temperature (198). When 100 MHz radiofrequency was studied in rats, no increase in maternal colonic temperature or adverse pregnancy outcome was observed (201). This exposure resulted in a specific absorption rate (SAR) of 0.4 W/kg, which corresponds to the maximum permissible level defined in 1982 by the American National Standards Institute. Since the unknowns and uncertainties are potentially significant, it was considered prudent to apply a safety factor of 10, with a resultant SAR limit of 0.04 W/kg (202). Individuals working near FM radio stations, radar, and microwave ovens are not exposed to the maximum permissible levels suggested for occupational and medical exposures (1).

Human studies looking at adverse reproductive effects of radiofrequency radiation are controversial (203). Investigations of human exposures to radiofrequency radiation are confounded by difficulties in determining the type and true extent of exposures, in selecting an appropriate control group for comparisons, in determining the existence and influence of many concomitant environmental factors, and in establishing the presence or measuring the frequency or severity of subjective complaints as well as objective findings in the studied populations (203). In Danish physiotherapists exposed to high frequency electromagnetic radiation, there was a lower rate of male children (23.5%), and these infants also had low birth weight (204), but no increase in congenital malformations (205). In a case control study, maternal exposure to microwave ovens was not found to be associated with cardiovascular malformations (193).

Risk Estimation

There is no way to receive exposure from a microwave oven without bypassing several safety interlocks. In addition, it is easy to shield microwaves with a proper screen or metal foil (1). If there were a door leak, it could theoretically result in a measurable exposure. But it should be remembered that electromagnetic radiation decreases in proportion to the square of the distance, so there should be no consequences several meters away from the microwave oven.

The eye and the embryo are the most vulnerable to the thermal effects of microwave radiation because they cannot dissipate heat efficiently (1). The nonthermal effects have not been clearly demonstrated, but they are still being investigated. There is no indication that this type of electromagnetic radiation can produce malignancy or mutations (1). Microwave ovens properly handled should be regarded as safe.

ULTRASOUND

Ultrasound is a widely used diagnostic modality in obstetrics and other fields. Its use in fetal monitoring and fetal diagnosis is rapidly expanding, and it has replaced obstetrical x-ray examinations. Deep tissue heating with ultrasound is a standard technique in physical therapy.

Physics

Sound is a mechanical energy form in which small particles in a medium are made to oscillate. The oscillation of air molecules at frequencies of 20–20,000 Hz produces sound. Sound waves with a frequency above this range are called *ultrasound*. Medical ultrasound involves frequencies of 1–20 MHz, and the medium is water and tissues instead of air. The intensity of the sound energy, its alteration, and the exposure time determine the amount of energy reaching a given tissue.

In a diagnostic ultrasound examination, a significant proportion of the energy is absorbed and the rest is reflected. The reflection of the sound energy provides the basis for the imaging technique. The fraction of the energy absorbed reduces heat within tissues. It is estimated that ultrasound intensities of 1 W/cm^2 will result in tissue temperature elevation of 0.8°C/min (206). In Doppler fetal heart detectors, intensities are 0.75–75.0 mW/cm^2 (207). Intensities for diagnostic sector scanners may reach peak values of 2–200 mW/cm^2 (208). The theoretical temperature rise 2 cm from an external fetal monitor remains less than 1°C even after prolonged use (206). In addition, further temperature loss occurs owing to removal of heat by circulating blood and by conduction of heat to other tissues.

The nonthermal effects include tissue disruption by the production of cavitation and streaming owing to the movement of particles in the sound field (1). None of these effects occur with the energies utilized in diagnostic ultrasonography (1).

Risk Estimation

In vitro studies have raised the possibility that commonly used ultrasound irradiation causes significant cellular damage (209–213). Detectable biological effects from diagnostic ultrasound were not demonstrated in mammalian studies (208,214,215). The American Institute of Ultrasound in Medicine concluded, in 1982, that there are no independently confirmed significant biological effects of ultrasound in mammals in the low megahertz frequency range and when intensities are below 100 mW/cm². Higher intensities with exposure time less than 500 seconds are not associated with biological effects as long as the product of intensity and exposure time is less than 50 J/cm² (208).

Epidemiological studies did not demonstrate that diagnostic ultrasound has any measurable or significant effects. The fetal anomaly rate was found to be 2.7%, which is comparable to the anomaly rate in the general population (216). No difference was demonstrated in several measurements at birth, in neurological examination, or in developmental testing at 11–15 months of babies exposed antenatally to ultrasound done for amniocentesis (217). Another study also did not find any difference in several birth parameters as well as neurological and cognitive testing at 7–12 years of age (218). In addition, it was concluded that diagnostic ultrasound is safe with regard to the risk of childhood malignancy between birth and the sixth year (219). After this period there appears to be a doubt, but the numbers are very small.

Therapeutic ultrasound involves higher intensity and may produce deep tissue heating. In a study where pregnant rats were exposed to shock-wave lithotriptor, fetuses located nearest the focal area of maximum shock-wave energy showed lower mean weight than controls but no recognizable gross or microscopic fetal damage (220). Because of the potential of hyperthermia to induce birth defects, it is advisable to avoid this form of treatment during pregnancy (208).

Industrial ultrasound also involves very high intensities, and it is unlikely that there will be energy transfer to tissues (208). The only exception is in the case of existence of a satisfactory coupling medium. In addition, standard safety precautions should provide adequate shielding of the ultrasound source.

LASER

Physics

The atomic nucleus is surrounded by electrons in orbits. When an electron is jumped, or excited, from an allowed orbit to a higher level, energy in the form of a photon is absorbed. When the electron returns to a lower energy state, a photon is omitted. This spontaneous emission can be accelerated if the excited state atom is struck by a photon of exactly the same energy as the spontaneously emitted photon. This accelerated process is called *stimulated emission*, and it yields two photons of the same energy level, which leaves the atom in exactly the same direction and phase.

Laser (Light Amplification by Stimulated Emission of Radiation) is an active electron device that uses this process and converts input power into coherent electromagnetic radiation in the range of optic frequencies (ultraviolet, visible, or infrared). Unlike radiation emitted from the usual light sources, the laser produces a very narrow and intense beam of coherent light. The typical laser instrument consists of an energy input source, an active medium (atoms capable of undergoing stimulated emission), feedback mechanisms (totally and partially reflecting mirrors), and standard optical devices to focus the electromagnetic energy. The active medium may be solid (e.g., ruby crystal), liquid (e.g., tunable dyes), gas (e.g., helium-neon, carbon dioxide, argon ion), or a semiconductor. The choice of an active medium depends on the output power and wavelength required for a given application. Output may be delivered in a continuous wave, in a single pulse, or as a series of pulses. Carbon dioxide and excimer lasers produce extremely high output power, up to 10^9 W.

Lasers have various applications in the areas of materials processing, information handling, communication, research, arts and entertainment, and more. Examples of medical applications of lasers include surgery (carbon dioxide laser), various ophthalmological procedures (argon and excimer lasers), vaporization of lung tumors during bronchoscopy (neodymium:yttrium-aluminum-garnet laser), and coronary angioplasties (excimer laser).

The American National Standards Institute classified lasers into four classes (I–IV) in order of increasing risk of hazard (221).

Biological Studies

The effects of laser in biological tissues can be divided into thermal and nonthermal; the latter may include driving chemical reactions, breaking atomic bonds, and creation of shock waves. Skin and eye damage is due mainly to denaturation of proteins resulting from hypothermia. Other hazards may include electrical shock, metal fumes released from processed material, and collateral radiation (e.g., intense light, arc lamps, ultraviolet radiation), which may induce delayed painful photokeratitis (221). The magnitude of damage depends not only on the type of laser involved and its output power, but also on the duration of exposure.

Carbon dioxide laser surgery is used in obstetrics and gynecology via laparoscope for treatment of ectopic pregnancy (222) and intra-abdominally for reproductive pelvic surgical procedures (tubal anastomosis, adhesiolysis, etc.) (223).

Endoscopic fetal surgery by excimer laser (40 and 10 Hz) was studied in premature lambs (224). Laser incisions were associated with smaller zones of devitalization compared to conventional cutting techniques using a scalpel. Albino rat embryos exposed to infrared laser beams (0.89 μm, 300 Hz for 256 and 128 s) had more preimplantation deaths and some disturbances in formation of the osseous skeleton (225). Helium-neon lasers induced an increase in neuritic outgrowths of olfactory bipolar receptor cells in rat fetuses (226).

More studies are needed to evaluate the teratogenic potential of laser and its role in fetal therapy of malformations.

SUMMARY

It is well established that ionizing radiation may have adverse reproductive effects. At present, there is no indication that radiodiagnostic doses of ionizing radiation (< 5 rad) during pregnancy increase the incidence of gross congenital malformations, intrauterine growth retardation, or abortion. The risks of acute exposures involving doses exceeding 5 rad are far below the spontaneous risks of the developing embryo. On the other hand, this does not mean that there are definitely no risks to the embryo exposed to low doses of ionizing radiation. It has not been determined whether there is a linear or exponential dose-response relationship or a threshold exposure for genetic, carcinogenic, cell-depleting, and life-shortening effects. Unnecessary x-ray or nuclear medicine procedures during pregnancy are not good medical practice, whereas medically indicated diagnostic roentgenograms are appropriate for pregnant women. A systematic approach of patient evaluation should be followed in any case of exposure during pregnancy, and not only to consider the biological effects of ionizing radiation.

So far, it has not been proven that exposure to nonionizing radiation (VDT, microwave, ultrasound, etc.) below the maximal permissible level is associated with measurable adverse reproductive outcome. At present, ultrasound not only improves obstetrical care but also reduces the necessity of diagnostic x-ray examinations. Nevertheless, continued surveillance and more studies of potential risks are necessary.

Answer

At 6 weeks of gestation fetal thyroid is not capable of concentrating iodine. Therefore, before 8–10 weeks such risk does not exist. Calculation of fetal dose should be performed as described in this chapter.

REFERENCES

1. Brent RL. The effects of embryonic and fetal exposure to X-ray, microwaves and ultrasound. In Clinics in Perinatology, Teratology, Vol 13 (3) (Brent RL, Beckman DA, ed). Saunders, Philadelphia, 1986, pp 615–648.
2. Mettler FA, Moseley RD. Medical Effects of Ionizing Radiation. Grune & Stratton, New York, 1985, pp 206–209.
3. Mossman KL. Medical radiodiagnosis and pregnancy: Evaluation of options when pregnancy status is uncertain. Health Phys 1985; 48:297–301.
4. Rowley KA, Hill SJ, Watkins RA, Moores BM. An investigation into the levels of radiation exposure in diagnostic examinations involving fluoroscopy. Br J Radiol 1987; 60:167–173.
5. Kendall GM, Darby SC, Harries SV, Rae S. A frequency survey of radiological examinations carried out in National Health Service Hospitals in Great Britain in 1977 for diagnostic purposes, Report No NRPB-R104. HMSO, National Radiological Protection Board, London, 1978.
6. Wall BF, Fisher ES, Shrimpton PC, Rae S. Current levels of gonadal irradiation from a selection of routine diagnostic X-ray examinations in Great Britain, Report No NRPB-R105. HMSO, National Radiological Protection Board, London, 1980.
7. Albert RE, Omran AR, Brauer EW, et al. Follow-up study of patients treated by x-ray for tinea capitis. Am J Public Health 1966; 56:2114–2120.
8. Witherbee WD. Indications for roentgen therapy in chronic tonsillitis and pharyngitis. Am J Roentgenol 1924; 11:331–335.
9. Friedlander A. Status lymphaticus and enlargement of the thymus: With report of a case successfully treated by the x-ray. Arch Pediatr 1907; 24:490–501.
10. Kaplan II. The x-ray treatment of amenorrhea, with a report of 38 cases. Am J Obstet Gynecol 1928; 15:658–661.
11. Lione A. Ionizing radiation and human reproduction. Reprod Toxicol 1987; 1:3–16.
12. Smith H. The detrimental health effects of ionizing radiation. Nuclear Med Commun 1992; 13:4–10.
13. Okada S, Hamilton HB, Egami N, et al. A review of thirty-year study of Hiroshima and Nagasaki atomic bomb survivors. J Radiat Res (Tokyo) 1975; 16 (suppl):1–164.
14. Brent RL. Radiation and other physical agents. In Handbook of Teratology, Vol 1 (Wilson JG, Fraser FC, eds). Plenum, New York, 1977, pp 153–223.
15. Brent RL. The effects of irradiation on the mammalian fetus. Clin Obstet Gynecol 1960; 3:928–950.
16. Lushbaugh CC, Casarett GW. The effects of gonadal irradiation in clinical radiation therapy: A review. Cancer 1976; 37:1111–1120.
17. Heller CG. Effects on germinal cell epithelium. In Radiological Factors in Manned Space Flight, National Radiation Council Publication No 1987 (Langham WH, ed). National Academy of Sciences, NRC, Washington DC, 1967, pp 124–133.

18. Rowley MJ, Leach DR, Warner GA, Heller CG. Effect of graded doses of ionizing radiation on the human testis. Radiat Res 1974; 59:665–678.
19. Lushbaugh CC, Ricks RC. Some cytokinetic and histopathologic considerations of irradiated male and female gonadal tissues. Front Radiat Ther Oncol 1972; 6:229–248.
20. Mandl AM. The radiosensitivity of germ cells. Biol Rev Camb Phil Soc 1964; 39:288–371.
21. Cattanach BM, Barlow JH. Evidence for the re-establishment of a heterogeneity in radiosensitivity among spermatogonial stem cells repopulating the mouse testis following depletion by x-rays. Mutat Res 1984; 127:81–89.
22. Withers HR, Hunter N, Barkley HT, Reid BO. Radiation survival and regeneration characteristics of spermatogenic stem cells of mouse testis. Radiat Res 1974; 57:88–103.
23. Andrews GA, Hubner KF, Fry SA. Report of 21-year medical follow-up of survivors of the Oak Ridge Y-12 accident. In The Medical Basis of Radiation a Accident Preparedness. Elsevier/North Holland, New York, 1980.
24. Searle AG, Beechey CV. Sperm-count, egg-fertilization and dominant lethality after x-irradiation of mice. Mutat Res 1974; 22:63–72.
25. Peters H, Levy E. Effect of irradiation in infancy on the fertility of female mice. Radiat Res 1963; 18:421–428.
26. Oakberg EF. Gamma ray sensitivity of occytes of immature mice. Proc Soc Exp Biol Med 1962; 109:763–767.
27. Baker TG. Radiosensitivity of mammalian oocytes with particular reference to the human female. Am J Obstet Gynecol 1971; 110:746–761.
28. Mandl AM. Superovulation following ovarian x-irradiation. J Reprod Fertil 1964; 8:375–396.
29. Baker TG. The sensitivity in post-natal rhesus monkeys to x-irradiation. J Reprod Fertil 1966; 12:183–192.
30. Parsons DF. An electron microscope study of radiation damage in the mouse oocyte. J Cell Biol 1962; 14:31–48.
31. Sobels FH, ed. Repair from Genetic Radiation Damage and Differential Radiosensitivity of Germ Cells. Pergamon Press, Oxford, 1963.
32. Mandl AM. A quantitative study of the sensitivity of oocytes to x-irradiation. Proc R Soc [Biol] 1959; 150:53–71.
33. Mondorf L, Faber M. The influence of radiation on human fertility. J Reprod Fertil 1968; 15:165–169.
34. Lindop RJ, Sacher GA, eds. Radiation and Aging. Taylor & Francis, London, 1966, p 307.
35. Hahn EW, Morales RL. Superpregnancy following pre-fertilization x-irradiation of the rat. J Reprod Fertil 1964; 7:73–78.
36. Jacox H. Recovery following human ovarian irradiation. Radiology 1939; 32:538–592.
37. Gans B, Bahary C, Levie B. Ovarian regeneration and pregnancy following massive radiotherapy for dysgerminoma. Obstet Gynecol 1966; 22:596–600.
38. Li FP, Gimbrere K, Gelber RD, et al. Outcome of pregnancy in survivors of Wilms' tumor. JAMA 1987; 257:216–219.

39. Lewis EB. Possible genetic consequences of irradiation of tumors in childhood. Radiology 1975; 114:147-153.
40. Schull WJ, Otake M, Neel JV. Genetic effects of the atomic bombs: A reappraisal. Science 1981; 213:1220-1227.
41. Bloomer WD, Hellman S. Normal tissue response to radiation therapy. N Engl J Med 1975; 293:80-83.
42. Riseborough EJ, Grabias SL, Burton RI, Jaffe N. Skeletal alterations following irradiation for Wilms' tumor. J Bone Joint Surg [Am] 1976; 58-A:526-536.
43. Green DM, Jaffe N. Wilms' tumor: Model of a curable pediatric malignant solid tumor. Cancer Treat Res 1978; 5:143-172.
44. Hawkins MM. Is there evidence of a therapy-related increase in germ cell mutation among childhood cancer survivors? J Natl Cancer Inst 1991; 83:1643-1650.
45. Nygaard R, Clausen N, Siimes MA, et al. Reproduction following treatment for childhood leukemia: A population-based prospective cohort study of fertility and offspring. Med Pediatr Oncol 1991; 19:459-466.
46. Desforges JF. Current concepts in genetics. N Engl J Med 1976; 294:393.
47. Advisory Committee on the Biological Effects of Ionizing Radiation. The Effects on Populations of Exposure to Low Levels of Ionizing Radiation. National Research Council, National Academy of Sciences, National Academy Press, Washington, DC, 1980.
48. Russell WL, Russell LB, Kelly EM. Radiation dose rate and mutation frequency. Science 1958; 128:1546-1550.
49. Schull WJ, Otake M, Neel JV. Hiroshima and Nagasaki: A reassessment of the mutagenic effect of exposure to ionizing radiation. In Population and Biological Aspects of Human Mutation. Academic Press, New York, 1981, pp 277-303.
50. Francis J, Snee M. A case-control study of trisomy 21 and maternal pre-conceptional radiography. Clin Radiol 1991; 43:343-346.
51. Freire-Maia A, Krieger H. Human genetic studies in areas of high natural radiation. IX. Effects on mortality, morbidity and sex ratio. Health Phys 1978; 43:61-65.
52. George KP, et al. Investigations on human populations residing in high background radiation areas of Kerala and adjoining regions. In Biological and Environmental Effects and Low-Level Radiation, Vol II. International Atomic Energy Agency, Vienna, 1976, pp 325-329.
53. Ritenour RE. Health effects of low-level radiation: Carcinogenesis, teratogenesis and mutagenesis. Semin Nuclear Med 1986; 16:106-117.
54. Jankowski CB. Radiation and pregnancy: Putting the risks in proportion. Am J Nurs 1986; 86:260-265.
55. Brent RL, Bolden BT. The indirect effect of irradiation on embryonic development. III. The contribution of ovarian irradiation, oviduct irradiation and zygotic irradiation to fetal mortality and growth retardation in the rat. Radiat Res 1967; 30:759-773.
56. Russell LB, Russell WL. The effects of radiation on the preimplantation stages of the mouse embryo. Anat Res 1950; 108:521.
57. Rugh R. Major radiological concepts and ionizing radiation on the embryo and fetus. In Response of the Nervous System to Ionizing Radiation, Vol 3 (Haley TJ, Snider RS, eds). Academic Press, New York, 1962.

58. Russell LB, Russell WL. An analysis of the changing radiation response of the developing mouse embryo. J Cell Comp Physiol 1954; 43:103–149.
59. Brent RL, Gorson RO. Radiation exposure in pregnancy. In Current Problems in Radiology, Vol. 2 (Moseley R, Baker DH, Gorson RO, eds). Year Book, Chicago, 1972, pp 1–48.
60. Moore NW, Adams CE, Rowson LEA. Developmental potential of single blastomeres of the rabbit egg. J Reprod Fertil 1968; 17:527–531.
61. Willadsen SM. A method for culture of micromanipulated sheep embryos and its use to produce monozygotic twins. Nature 1979; 277:298–300.
62. Dekaban AS. Abnormalities in children exposed to x-irradiation during various stages of gestation: Tentative timetable of radiation injury to the human fetus. J Nuclear Med 1968; 9:471–477.
63. Goldstein L, Murphy DP. Microcephalic idiocy following radium therapy for uterine cancer during pregnancy. Am J Obstet Gynecol 1929; 18:189–195, 281–283.
64. Goldstein L, Murphy DP. Etiology of ill health in children born after maternal pelvic irradiation. II. Defective children born after postconceptional maternal irradiation. Am J Roentgenol 1929; 22:322–331.
65. Miller RW. Delayed radiation defects in atomic bomb survivors. Science 1969; 166:569–574.
66. Plummer G. Anomalies occurring in children exposed in utero to the atomic bomb in Hiroshima. Pediatrics 1952; 10:687–692.
67. Wood JW, Johnson KG, Omori Y. In utero exposure to the Hiroshima atomic bomb. An evaluation of head size and mental retardation: Twenty years later. Pediatrics 1967; 39:385–392.
68. Wood JW, Johnson KG, Omori Y, Kawamoto S, Keehn RJ. Mental retardation in children exposed in utero to the atomic bombs in Hiroshima and Nagasaki. Am J Public Health 1967; 57:1381–1389.
69. Zappert J. Über roentgenogene female microcephalie. Monatsschr Kinderheildk 1926; 34:490–493.
70. Blot WJ, MIller RW. Mental retardation following in utero exposure to the atomic bombs of Hiroshima and Nagasaki. Radiology 1973; 106:617–619.
71. Otake M, Schull WJ. In utero exposure to A-bomb radiation and mental retardation: A reassessment. Br J Radiol 1984; 57:409–414.
72. Yoshimaru H, Otake M, Fujikoshi Y, Schull WJ. Effect on school performance of prenatal exposure to the Hiroshima atomic bomb. Nippon Eiseigaku Zasshi 1991; 46:747–754.
73. Otake M, Schull WJ, Yoshimaru H. A review of forty-five years study of Hiroshima and Nagasaki atomic bomb survivors: Brain damage among the prenatally exposed. J Radiat Res (Tokyo) 1991; 32(suppl):249–264.
74. International Commission on Radiological Protection. Developmental Effects of Irradiation on the Brain of the Embryo and Fetus. Annals of the ICRP, vol 16(4). Pergamon Press, Oxford, 1986, p 43.
75. Dobbing J, Sands J. Quantitative growth and development of human brain. Arch Dis Child 1973; 48:757–767.

76. Miller RW, Mulvihill JJ. Small head size after atomic irradiation. Teratology 1976; 14:355–358.
77. D'Amato CJ, Hicks SP. Effects of low levels of ionizing radiation on the developing cerebral cortex of the rat. Neurology 1965; 15:1104–1116.
78. Maroteaux P, Spranger J, Opitz JM, et al. Le syndrome camptomélique. Presse Med 1971; 79:1157–1162.
79. Mole RH. Consequences of pre-natal radiation exposure for post-natal development: A review. Int J Radiat Biol 1982; 42:1–12.
80. Shohoji T, Pasternack B. Adolescent growth patterns in survivors exposed prenatally to the A-bombs in Hiroshima and Nagasaki. Health Phys 1973; 25:17–27.
81. Moriyama IW, Steer A, Hamilton HB. Radiation effects in atomic bomb survivors. Atomic Bomb Casualty Commission Technical Report, 1973, pp 6–73.
82. Kinlen LJ, Acheson FD. Diagnostic irradiation, congenital malformations and spontaneous abortion. Br J Radiol 1968; 41:648–654.
83. Nokkentred K. Effects of Radiation upon the Human Fetus. Munksgaard, Copenhagen, 1968, p 228.
84. Tabuchi A. Fetal disorders due to ionizing radiation. Hiroshima J Med Sci 1964; 13:125–173.
85. Tabuchi A, Nakagawa S, Hirai T, et al. Fetal hazards due to x-ray diagnosis during pregnancy. Hiroshima J Med Sci 1967; 16:49–66.
86. Vilumsen A. Environmental Factors in Congenital Malformations. Foreningen af Danske Laegestuderendes, Copenhagen, 1970.
87. Mossman K, Hill LT. Radiation risks in pregnancy. Obstet Gynecol 1982; 6:237–242.
88. Hammer-Jacobsen E. Therapeutic abortion on account of x-ray examination during pregnancy. Dan Med Bull 1954; 6:113–122.
89. Jacobsen L, Mellemgaard L. Anomalies of the eyes in descendants of women irradiated with small x-ray doses during age of fertility. Acta Ophthalmol (Copenh) 1968; 46:352–354.
90. Brent RL. Irradiation in pregnancy. In Davis' Gynecology and Obstetrics, Vol 2 (Sciarra JJ, ed). Harper & Row, New York, 1972, pp 1–32.
91. Brent RL. The response of the 9.5-day-old rat embryo to variations in dose rate of 150R X-irradiation. Radiat Res 1971; 45:127–136.
92. Brizzee KR, Brannon RB. Cell recovery in foetal brain after ionizing radiation. Int J Radiat Biol 1972; 21:375–378.
93. Bithell JF, Stewart AM. Prenatal irradiation and childhood malignancy: A review of British data from the Oxford Survey. Br J Cancer 1975; 31:271–287.
94. Favus MJ, Schneider AB, Stachura ME, et al. Thyroid cancer occurring as a late consequence of head-and-neck irradiation. N Engl J Med 1976; 294:1019–1025.
95. Einhorn L. Can prenatal irradiation protect the embryo from tumor development? Acta Oncol 1991; 30:291–299.
96. Stewart A, Webb J, Hewitt D. A survey of childhood malignancies. Br Med J 1958; 1:1495–1508.

97. Stewart A, Kneale GW. Changes in the cancer risk associated with obstetric radiography. Lancet 1968; 1:104–107.
98. Mole RH. Antenatal irradiation and childhood cancer: Causation or coincidence? Br J Cancer 1974; 30:199–208.
99. Stewart A. The carcinogenic effects of low-level radiation: A reappraisal of epidemiologists' methods and observations. Health Phys 1973; 24:223–240.
100. Lewis EB. Leukemia and ionizing radiation. Science 1957; 125:965–972.
101. Advisory Committee on the Biological Effects of Ionizing Radiations. The Effects on Populations of Exposure to Low Levels of Ionizing Radiation. National Academy of Sciences, National Research Council, Washington, DC, 1972.
102. Harvey EB, Boice JD, Honeyman M, Flannery JT. Prenatal x-ray exposure and childhood cancer in twins. N Engl J Med 1985; 312:541–545.
103. Jablon S, Kato H. Childhood cancer in relation to prenatal exposure to atomic-bomb radiation. Lancet 1970; 2:1000–1003.
104. United Nations Scientific Committee on the Effects of Atomic Radiation (UNSCEAR). Developmental effects of irradiation in utero. Anex J 1977:655–725.
105. Bithell JF, Stiller CA. A new calculation of the carcinogenic risk of obstetric x-raying. Stat Med 1988; 7:857–864.
106. Mole RH. Fetal dosimetry by UNSCEAR and risk coefficients for childhood cancer following diagnostic radiology in pregnancy. J Radiol Prot 1990; 10: 199–203.
107. Yoshimoto Y, Kato H, Schull WJ. A review of forty-five years study of Hiroshima and Nagasaki atomic bomb survivors: Cancer risk among in utero-exposed survivors. J Radiat Res (Tokyo) 1991; 32(suppl):231–238.
108. Yoshimoto Y, Kato H, Schull WJ. Risk of cancer among children exposed in utero to A-bomb radiations, 1950–84. Lancet 1988; 17:665–669.
109. Lilienfeld AM. Epidemiological studies of the leukemogenic effects of radiation. Yale J Biol Med 1966; 39:143–164.
110. Court Brown WM, Doll R, Bradford Hill A. Incidence of leukemia after exposure to diagnostic radiation in utero. Br Med J 1960; (5212):1539–1545.
111. Burrow GN, Hamilton HB, Hrubec Z. Study of adolescents exposed in utero to the atomic bomb, Nagasaki, Japan. I. General aspects: Clinical and laboratory data. Yale J Biol Med 1964; 36:430–444.
112. Kato H. Mortality in children exposed to the A-bombs while in utero. Am J Epidemiol 1971; 93:435–442.
113. Graham S, Levin MI, Lilienfeld AM. Preconception, intrauterine and postnatal irradiation as related to leukemia. Natl Cancer Inst Monogr 1966; 19: 347–371.
114. Hoshino T, Itoga T, Kato H. Leukemia in the offspring of parents exposed to the atomic bomb at Hiroshima and Nagasaki. Present to the Japanese Association of Hematology, March 28–30, 1965.
115. Rugh R, Duhamel L, Skaredoff L. Relation of the embryonic and fetal x-irradiation to life-time average weights and tumor incidence in mice. Proc Soc Exp Biol Med 1966; 121:714–718.

116. Brent RL, Bolden BT. The long-term effects of low-dosage embryonic irradiation. Radiat Res 1961; 14:453–454.
117. Brent RL, Bolden BT. Indirect effect of x-irradiation on embryonic development. V. Utilization of high doses of maternal irradiation on the first day of gestation. Radiat Res 1968; 36:563–570.
118. Miller RW. Epidemiological conclusions from radiation toxicity studies. In Late Effects of Radiation (Fry RJM, Grahn D, Griem ML, et al., eds). Taylor & Francis, London, 1970.
119. Loewe WE, Mendelson E. Revised dose estimates at Hiroshima and Nagasaki. Health Phys 1981; 41:663–666.
120. Blot WJ. Growth and development following prenatal and childhood exposure to atomic radiation. J Radiat Res (Tokyo) 1975; 16:81–88.
121. Mole RH. Radiation effects on pre-natal development and their radiological significance. Br J Radiol 1979; 52:89–101.
122. National Council on Radiation Protection and Measurements. Medical Radiation Exposure of Pregnant and Potentially Pregnant Women, NCRP Report No 54. Government Printing Office, Washington, DC, 1979, p 320.
123. Hall EJ. Scientific view of low-level radiation risks. Radiographics 1991; 11: 509–518.
124. Friedman WN, Rosenfield AT. Computed tomography in obstetrics and gynecology. J Reprod Med 1992; 37:3–18.
125. Ragozzino MW, Gray JE, Burke TM, Van Lysel MS. Estimation and minimization of fetal absorbed dose: Data from common radiographic examinations. AJR 1981; 137:667–671.
126. Brent RL. Effects and risks of medically administered isotopes to the developing embryo. In Drug and Chemical Action in Pregnancy (Fabro S, Scialli AR, eds). Marcel Dekker, New York, 1986, pp 427–439.
127. Padovani R, Contento G, Fabretto M, Malisan R, Barbina V, Gozzi G. Patient doses and risks from diagnostic radiology in Northeast Italy. Br J Radiol 1987; 60:155–165.
128. Shrimpton PC, Wall BF, Jones DG, et al. Doses to patients from routine diagnostic x-ray examinations in England. Br J Radiol 1986; 59:749–758.
129. McGuire EL, Dickson PA. Exposure and organ dose estimation in diagnostic radiology. Med Phys 1986; 13:913–916.
130. United Nations Scientific Committee on the Effects of Atomic Radiation (UNSCEAR). Sources and Effects of Ionizing Radiation. Report to the General Assembly, 1977, 319.
131. Kereiakes JG, Rosenstein M. Handbook of Radiation Doses in Nuclear Medicine and Diagnostic X-Ray. CRC Press, Boca Raton, FL, 1980, p 211.
132. Murphy F, Heaton B. Patient doses received during whole body scanning using an Elscint 905 CT scanner. Br J Radiol 1985; 58:1197–1201.
133. Schonken P, Marchal G, Coenen Y, Baret AL, Ponette E. Body and gonad doses in computer tomography of the trunk. J Belge Radiol 1978; 61:363–371.
134. McCullough EC, Payne JT. Patient dosage in computed tomography. Radiology 1978; 129:457–463.
135. Budinger TF. Nuclear magnetic resonance (NMR) in vivo studies: Known thresholds for health effects. J Comput Assist Tomogr 1981; 5:800–811.

136. Thomas A, Morris PG. The effects of NMR exposure in living organisms. I. A. Microbial assay. Br J Radiol 1981; 54:615-621.
137. Sigmund G, Bauer M, Henne K, DeGregorio G, Wenz W. A technic of magnetic resonance tomographic pelvimetry in obstetrics. ROFO Fortschr Geb Roentgenstr Nuklearmed 1991; 154:370-374.
138. Tyndall DA, Sulik KK. Effects of magnetic resonance imaging on eye development in the C57BL/6J mouse. Teratology 1991; 43:263-275.
139. Cooke P, Morris PG. The effects of NMR exposure on living organisms. II. A genetic study of human lymphocytes. Br J Radiol 1981; 54:622-625.
140. Lee WR. Working with visual display units. Am J Ophthalmol 1986; 101: 107-111.
141. Ronderos A. Fetal tolerance to radiation. Radiology 1961; 76:454-456.
142. National Council on Radiation Protection and Measurements. Basic Radiation Protection Criteria, NCRP Publication No 39. Government Printing Office, Washington, DC, 1971.
143. Review of NCRP Radiation Dose Limit for Embryo and Fetus in Occupationally Exposed Women, NCRP Publication No 53. Government Printing Office, Washington, DC, 1977, p 3.
144. Edwards M. Development of radiation protection standards. Radiographics 1991; 11:699-712.
145. Wagner LK, Hayman LA. Pregnancy and women radiologists. Radiology 1982; 145:559-562.
146. US Nuclear Regulatory Commission. Instruction concerning prenatal radiation exposure. Reg Guide 1975; 8.13 rev 1:3-4.
147. Senturia YD, Peckham CS, Peckham MJ. Children fathered by men treated for testicular cancer. Lancet 1985; 2:766-769.
148. Schull WJ, Neel JV. Atomic exposure and the pregnancies of biologically related parents. Am J Public Health 1959; 49:1621-1629.
149. Miller RW. Effects of ionizing radiation from the atomic bomb on Japanese children. Pediatrics 1968; 41:257-263.
150. McKinney PA, Alexander FE, Cartwright RA, Parker L. Parental occupations of children with leukaemia in west Cumbria, north Humberside, and Gateshead. Br Med J 1991; 302:681-687.
151. Bentur Y, Horlatsch N, Koren G. Exposure to ionizing radiation during pregnancy: Perception of teratogenic risk and outcome. Teratology 1991; 43:109-112.
152. Reynolds JEF, Prasad AB, eds. Martindale, The Extra Pharmacopeia. Pharmaceutical Press, London, 1982, pp 1386-1400.
153. Fabro S, Brown NA, Scialli AR. Radionuclides in pregnancy. Reprod Toxicol (Med Lett) 1986; 5:17-22.
154. Book SA, Goldman M. Thyroidal radioiodine exposure of the fetus. Health Phys 1975; 29:874-877.
155. Green GH, Gareis FJ, Shepard TH, Kelley VC. Cretinism associated with maternal sodium iodide[131] therapy during pregnancy. Am J Dis Child 1971; 122: 247-249.
156. Sikov MR, Noonan TR. Anomalous development induced in embryonic rat by the maternal administration of radiophosphorus. Am J Anat 1958; 103:137-156.

157. Smith EM, Warner GG. Estimates of radiation dose to the embryo from nuclear medicine procedures. J Nuclear Med 1976; 17:836-839.
158. Saenger EL. Protocol Book of Radioisotope Laboratory. University of Cincinnati Medical Center, Cincinnati, OH, 1976.
159. Kereiakes JG, Feller PA, Ascoi FA, Thomas SR, Gelfand MJ, Saenger EL. pediatric radiopharmaceutical dosimetry. In Radiopharmaceutical Dosimetry Symposium, US Department of Health, Education, and Welfare (Food and Drug Administration) Publication No 76-8044. US DHEW, Bureau of Radiological Health, Rockville, MD, 1976.
160. Roedler HD, Kaul A, Hine GJ. Internal Radiation Dose in Diagnostic Nuclear Medicine. Hoffman, Berlin, 1978.
161. Kereiakes JG, Rosenstein M. Handbook of Radiation Doses in Nuclear Medicine and Diagnostic X-Ray. CRC Press, Boca Raton, FL, 1980, p 170.
162. Brent RL. The prediction of human disease from laboratory and animal tests for teratology, carcinogenicity and mutagenicity. In Controversies in Therapeutics (Lasagna L, ed). Saunders, Philadelphia, 1980, pp 134-150.
163. Brent RL. Cancer risks following diagnostic radiation exposure. Pediatrics 1983; 71:288-289.
164. Brent RL. The Effects of Ionizing Radiation, Microwaves and Ultrasound in the Developing Embryo: Clinical Interpretations and Applications of the Data, Vol 14. Year Book, Chicago, 1984, pp 1-87.
165. Schardein JL, ed. Chemically Induced Birth Defects. Marcel Dekker, New York, 1985, pp 659-668.
166. Heinonen OP, Slone D, Shapiro S. Diagnostic aids, technical aids and rare drugs. In Birth Defects and Drugs in Pregnancy. PSG Publishing, Littleton, MA, 1977, pp 409-415, 444.
167. Webb GAM, Simmonds JR, Wilkins BT. Radiation levels in Eastern Europe. Nature 1986; 321:821-822.
168. Baverstock KF. A preliminary assessment of the consequences for inhabitants of the UK of the Chernobyl accident. Int J Radiat Biol 1986; 50:III-XIII.
169. Sperling K, Pelz J, Wegner RD, Schulzke I, Struck E. Frequency of trisomy 21 in Germany before and after the Chernobyl accident. Biomed Pharmacother 1991; 45:255-262.
170. Harjulehto T, Rahola T, Suomola M, Arvela H, Saxen L. Pregnancy outcome in Finland after the Chernobyl accident. Biomed Pharmacother 1991; 45:263-266.
171. Czeizel AE. Incidence of legal abortions and congenital abnormalities in Hungary. Biomed Pharmacother 1991; 45:249-254.
172. Irgens LM, Lie RT, Ulstein M, et al. Pregnancy outcome in Norway after Chernobyl. Biomed Pharmacother 1991; 45:233-241.
173. Trichopoulos D, Zavitsanos X, Koutis C, Drogari P. The victims of Chernobyl in Greece: Induced abortions after the accident. Br Med J 1987; 295:1100.
174. Knudsen LB. Legally induced abortions in Denmark after Chernobyl. Biomed Pharmacother 1991; 45:229-231.

175. Wiese WH, Skipper BJ. Survey of reproductive outcomes in uranium and potash mine workers: Results of first analysis. Ann Am Conf Govern Ind Hyg 1986; 14:187–192.
176. Bergman T. Eye care health effects of video display terminals. Occup Health Saf 1980; 49:24, 26–28, 53–55.
177. Lazarus MG, Bourke JA. Problems associated with use of video display units by bank clerical staff. Med J Aust 1982; 2:186.
178. Létourneau EG. Are video display terminals safe? Can Med Assoc J 1981; 125:533.
179. Weiss MM, Peterson RC. Electromagnetic radiation emitted from video computer terminals. Am Ind Hyg Assoc J 1979; 40:300–309.
180. Weiss MM. The video display terminals – Is there a radiation hazard? J Occup Med 1983; 25:98–100.
181. US Radiological Health Bureau. An Evaluation of Radiation Emission from Video Display Terminals, US Department of Health and Human Services (Food and Drug Administration) Publication No 81-8153. Government Printing Office, Washington, DC, 1981.
182. Hubar JS, Draus P. Determining the radiation exposure from visual display terminals used in dentistry. J Can Dent Assoc 1991; 57:131–132.
183. Fabro S, Brown NA, Scialli AR. Video display terminals and human reproduction. Reprod Toxicol (Med Lett) 1984; 3:1–4.
184. Schnorr TM, Grajewski BA, Hornung RW, et al. Video display terminals and the risk of spontaneous abortions. N Engl J Med 1991; 324:727–733.
185. Hirning CR, Aitken JH. Cathode-ray tube x-ray emission standard for video display terminals. Health Phys 1982; 43:727–731.
186. Delgado JMR, Leal J, Monteagudo JL, Gracia MG. Embryological changes induced by weak, extremely low frequency electromagnetic fields. J Anat 1981; 134:533–551.
187. Ubeda A, Leal J, Trillo MA, Jimenez MA, Delgado JMR. Pulse shape of magnetic fields influences chick embryogenesis. J Anat 1983; 137:513–536.
188. Maffeo S, Miller MW, Carstensen EL. Lack of effect of weak low frequency electromagnetic fields on check embryogenesis. J Anat 1984; 139:613–618.
189. McDonald AD, Cherry NM, Delorme C, McDonald JC. Work and pregnancy in Montreal – Preliminary findings on work with visual display terminals. In Allegations of Reproductive Hazards from VDUs (Pearce BG, ed). Humane Technology, Loughborough, 1984, pp 161–175.
190. McDonald AD, Chesy NM, Delrome C, McDonald JC. Visual display units and pregnancy: Evidence from the Montreal survey. J Occup Med 1986; 28: 1226–1231.
191. Goldhaber MK, Polen MR, Hiat RA. The risk of miscarriage and birth defects among women who use visual display terminals during pregnancy. Am J Ind Med 1988; 13:695–706.
192. Kurppa K, Holmberg PC, Rantala K, Nurminen T. Birth defects and video display terminals. Lancet 1984; 2:1339.
193. Tikkanen J, Heinonen OP. Maternal exposure to chemical and physical factors during pregnancy and cardiovascular malformations in the offspring. Teratology 1991; 43:591–600.

194. Bergqvist U, Knave B. Video display work and pregnancy—Research in the Nordic countries. In Allegations of Reproductive Hazards from VDUs (Pearce BG, ed). Humane Technology, Loughborough, 1984, pp 49-53.

195. Bayne VJ. Paper outlining a trade union response to the allegations of reproductive hazards from VDUs. In Allegations of Reproductive Hazards from VDUs (Pearce BG, ed). Human Technology, Loughborough, 1984, pp 111-126.

196. Brent RL. X-ray, microwave and ultrasound: The real and unreal hazards. Pediatr Ann 1980; 9:469-473.

197. Saito K, Suzuki K, Motoyoshi S. Lethal and teratogenic effects of long-term low-intensity radio frequency radiation at 428 MHz on developing chick embryo. Teratology 1991; 43:609-614.

198. Tofani S, Agnesod G, Ossola P, Ferrini S, Bussi R. Effects of continuous low level exposure to radiofrequency radiation on intrauterine development in rats. Health Phys 1986; 51:489-499.

199. Lary JM, Conover DL, Johnson PH, Hornung RW. Dose-response relationship between body temperature and birth defects in radiofrequency-irradiated rats. Bioelectromagnetics 1986; 7:141-149.

200. Lary JM, Conover DL, Foley ED, Hanser PL. Teratogenic effects of 27.12 MHz radiofrequency radiation in rats. Teratology 1982; 26:299-309.

201. Lary JM, Conover DL, Johnson PH. Absence of embryotoxic effects from low-level (non-thermal) exposure of rats to 100 MHz radiofrequency radiation. Scand J Work Environ Health 1983; 9:120-127.

202. Cahill DF. A suggested limit for population exposure to radiofrequency radiation. Health Phys 1983; 45:109-126.

203. Roberts NJ Jr, Michaelson SM. Epidemiological studies of human exposure to radiofrequency radiation: A critical review. Int Arch Occup Environ Health 1985; 56:169-178.

204. Larsen AI, Olsen J, Svane O. Gender-specific reproductive outcome and exposure to high-frequency electromagnetic radiation among physiotherapists. Scand J Work Environ Health 1991; 17:324-329.

205. Larsen AI. Congenital malformations and exposure to high-frequency electromagnetic radiation among Danish physiotherapists. Scand J Work Environ Health 1991; 17:318-323.

206. National Council on Radiation Protection and Measurements. NCRP Report No 74, Bethesda, MD, 1983, p 72.

207. World Health Organization, Environmental Health Criteria 22. WHO, Geneva, 1982.

208. Fabro S, Brown NA, Scialli AR. Ultrasound in industry and medicine. Reprod Toxicol (Med Lett) 1984; 3:17-20.

209. Liebeskind D, Bases R, Mendez F, Elequin F, Koenigsberg M. Sister chromatid exchanges in human lymphocytes after exposure to diagnostic ultrasound. Science 1975; 205:1273-1275.

210. Haupt M, Martin AO, Simpson JL, et al. Ultrasonic induction of sister chromatid exchanges in human lymphocytes. Hum Genet 1981; 59:221-226.

211. Siegel E, Goddard J, James AE Jr, Siegel EP. Cellular attachment as a sensitive indicator of the effects of diagnostic ultrasound exposure on cultured human cells. Radiology 1979; 133:175-179.

212. Liebeskind D, Bases R, Elequin F, et al. Diagnostic ultrasound: Effects on DNA and growth patterns of animal cells. Radiology 1979; 131:177-184.
213. Liebeskind D, Bases R, Koenigsberg M, Koss L, Raventos C. Morphological changes in the surface characteristics of cultured cells after exposure to diagnostic ultrasound. Radiology 1981; 138:419-423.
214. Au WW, Obergoenner N, Goldenthal KL, Corry PM, Willingham V. Sister chromatid exchanges in mouse embryos after exposure to ultrasound in utero. Mutat Res 1982; 103:315-320.
215. Wegner RD, Obe G, Meyenburg M. Has diagnostic ultrasound mutagenic effects? Hum Genet 1980; 56:95-98.
216. Hellman LM, Duffus GM, Donald I, Sunden B. Safety of diagnostic ultrasound in obstetrics. Lancet 1970; 11:1133-1135.
217. Scheidt PC, Stanley F, Bryla DA. One year follow-up of infants exposed to ultrasound in utero. Am J Obstet Gynecol 1978; 131:743-748.
218. Stark CR, Orleans M, Haverkamp AD, Murphy J. Short- and long-term risks after exposure to diagnostic ultrasound in utero. Obstet Gynecol 1984; 63:194-200.
219. Wilson MK. Obstetric ultrasound and childhood malignancies. Radiography 1985; 51:319-320.
220. Smith DP, Graham JB, Prystowsky JB, Dalkin BL, Nemcok AA Jr. The effects of ultrasound-guided shock waves during early pregnancy in Sprague-Dawley rats. J Urol 1992; 147:231-234.
221. Krieger GR, Larson J. Lasers. In Hazardous Materials Toxicology: Clinical Principles of Environmental Health (Sullivan JB Jr, Krieger GR, eds). Williams & Wilkins, Baltimore, 1992, pp 1165-1174.
222. Koninckx PR, Witters K, Brosens J, Stemers N, Oosterlynck D, Meuleman C. Conservative laparoscopic treatment of ectopic pregnancies using the CO_2 laser. Br J Obstet Gynaecol 1991; 98:1254-1259.
223. Kelly RW, Diamond MP. Intra-abdominal use of the carbon dioxide laser for microsurgery. Obstet Gynecol Clin North Am 1991; 18:537-544.
224. Schmidt S, Decleer W, Gorissen-Bosselmann S, et al. Endoscopic fetal surgery by excimer laser: An experimental study in premature lambs. J Perinat Med 1991; 19:231-235.
225. Bandazhevskii IuI, Emel'ianchik IuM. Effect of infrared impulse laser irradiation on the development of albino rat embryos. Arkh Anat Gistol Embriol 1991; 100:15-18.
226. Mester AF, Snow JB Jr, Shaman P. Photochemical effects of laser irradiation on neuritic outgrowth of olfactory neuroepithelial explants. Otolaryngol Head Neck Surg 1991; 105:449-456.

Part III

Genetic and Obstetric Considerations

23

Genetic Aspects

Ronald G. Davidson*
McMaster University, Hamilton, Ontario, Canada

Susan Zeesman
Chedoke-McMaster Hospitals, Hamilton, Ontario, Canada

Clinical Case

A pregnant woman with insulin-dependent diabetes mellitus wishes to know the risks for her baby. What is the magnitude of any increased risk, which anomalies are more likely, and what can be done to reduce the risk?

INTRODUCTION

The term congenital anomalies is a broad one used to describe the results of disturbances in the process of prenatal development, and it includes all forms of defects present at birth. These may be structural, functional, or metabolic, and the term provides no causal implications. There is some confusion relating to the interpretation of the word congenital: its meaning is clearly "present at birth." However, inclusion of only anomalies that are visible or detectable at birth is an error that has led to a gross underestimate of the incidence and importance of the problem. On the basis of numerous surveys of variable quality over the past 30 years came the consensus that approximately 3% of newborn children are affected with major congenital malformations. This has led to the widespread quoting of a 2-3% risk for malformations for the general population (1-3), a figure based primarily on defects that are detectable at birth or in the early neonatal period.

---

*Emeritus.

The National Collaborative Perinatal Project (NCPP) of the National Institute of Neurological and Communicative Disorders and Stroke (U.S.) has published the results of its comprehensive prospective study of malformations in children from ages 1–7 (4). The NCPP was a 12-institution study of 53,229 consecutive single deliveries between 1959 and 1965 with known outcome. These include neonatal and fetal deaths for which clinical and autopsy findings were available. It becomes obvious from this study and subsequent others (5,6) that many anomalies, although present in some form at birth, are undetectable at that time, and that these malformations raise the risk of major malformations in childhood from the oft-quoted 3% at birth to 8–9% (4) at age 7 (3547 individuals of the 40,206 examined at 7 years had major malformations).

Examples of malformations that become evident after the neonatal period include pyloric stenosis, abnormalities of the teeth, many cases of craniosynostosis, and tumors of infants and children. Although some would not consider tumors to be malformations, most do fit the definition: for example, retinoblastoma, Wilms' tumor, and neuroblastoma.

TYPES OF CONGENITAL MALFORMATIONS

Malformations have been categorized in a variety of ways, such as by cause, by developmental process (agenesis, hyper- or hypoplasia, etc.), and by specific organ. To use an approach that makes clinical sense, the classification proposed by Spranger et al. (7) is presented.

Malformation: a structural defect of an organ, part of an organ, or larger region of the body resulting from an intrinsically abnormal developmental process. "Intrinsically" implies that the developmental potential is abnormal from the beginning (i.e., at fertilization) and is likely to be genetic, although not necessarily, or even usually, owing to a single mutant gene.

Deformation: an abnormal form, shape, or position of a part of the body caused by mechanical forces. For example, oligohydramnios for any reason can cause clubfoot or increase the likelihood of congenital dislocation of the hip.

Disruption: a structural defect resulting from the extrinsic breakdown of or an interference with, an originally normal developmental process. The anomalies resulting from teratogens fit in here. Although strictly speaking, disruptions cannot be inherited, genes may predispose to and influence the final outcome of the etiological agent.

Dysplasia: an abnormal organization of cells into tissue(s) and its morphological result(s). The connective tissue disorders and many types of short-limbed dwarfs (skeletal dysplasias) fall into this category.

Knowing into which category a defect fits is helpful in determining diagnosis. If type can be ascertained, timing may be determined, and various

Table 1 Malformations in Relation to Timing and Epidemiology

Anatomical site	Malformation	Error	Timing (weeks)	Incidence (at birth)	Recurrence risk (%)	Refs.
Central nervous system	Holoprosencephaly	Failure of the forebrain to divide completely into two vesicles (often associated with a chromosome anomaly, especially trisomy 13)	5th	1/5000	<2 (but rarely can be autosomal recessive)	9
	Neural tube defects (anencephaly, meningomyelocele, etc.)	Anomalous closure of the neural tube	4th	1/400–1/1000	3	10,11
Face	Cleft lip with or without cleft palate	Defective closure of lip fusion of maxillary palatal shelves	10th	1/1000	3–6	12,13
	Isolated cleft palate	Failure of fusion of the lateral palatine processes	9th–12th	1/2000	2	
Cardiovascular	Ventricular septal defect	Defective closure of ventricular septum	6th–7th	1/500	3	14,15
	Atrial septal defect	Defective closure of interatrial septa	Primum-5th, secundum 7th–8th	1/1500	2.5	
	Pulmonary stenosis	Failure of absorption of excess mesenchyme between infundibulum and aortic vestibule	6th–8th	1/1600	2	

(continues)

Table 1 Continued

Anatomical site	Malformation	Error	Timing (weeks)	Incidence (at birth)	Recurrence risk (%)	Refs.
Cardiovascular (continued)	Tetralogy of Fallot	Conal malrotation and mal-septation with narrowing of the infundibilum	5th–8th	1/1800	2.5	
	Coarctation	Constriction of dorsal aorta at the isthmus or between the origin of the left sub-clavian and the ductus, probably due to abnormal blood flow	4th onward	1/2300	2	
	Transposition	Incomplete reduction of the bulboventricular (BV) sulcus and reduced dextro- or levo-torsion of the BV loop	3rd–4th	1/3000	1.5	
	Aortic stenosis	Failure of normal modeling of valves from infundibular and aortic vestibule mesen-chyme	6th–8th	1/2800	2	

System	Malformation	Developmental defect	Critical period	Frequency		Ref.
Gastrointestinal	Omphalocele	Failure of intestines to return to the abdomen during the second stage of rotation of the midgut loop	10th	1/4000	<0.5	16,17
	Diaphragmatic hernia	Incomplete closure of pleuroperitoneal canal	6th	1/2000	0.5	18
Genitourinary	Hypospadias	Incomplete fusion of the urogenital folds and/or lack of normal cannulation of the urethra	8th–14th	1/300 males	9	19
Limbs	Dislocation of the hip	Underdevelopment of the acetabulum, generalized joint laxity, breach delivery	7th onward	1/500 (female preponderance)	4–5	20

Source: Adapted from Ref. 8.

diagnoses can be included or excluded. For example, exposure to medications in the second trimester of pregnancy cannot cause a neural tube defect, since the neural tube is closed by the end of the fourth week. A few of the important embryonic developmental events with their timing and associated malformations are listed in Table 1 (8–20).

ETIOLOGY OF CONGENITAL MALFORMATIONS

Table 2 is an approximation of the etiology of malformations at birth, adapted from Kalter and Warkany (3). For most anomalies, the etiology has yet to be determined.

Table 1 also includes the approximate incidences in the general population of some common congenital anomalies. Sex differences in the incidences of congenital malformations have been well documented, with males being significantly more frequently involved than females for most (21). Racial differences also exist, with blacks having a higher incidence than whites. However, the racial differences are mainly for minor anomalies, most of which are of skin pigmentation (22). The major racial and/or ethnic differences in the incidence of neural tube defects are clearly defined: they are much less common in blacks, Asians, and Ashkenazi Jews, and are particularly frequent in Sikhs, Egyptians, and Irish Catholics (23). It has also been well documented that there is a higher incidence of congenital malformations, in general, among twins (18.33%) (24), especially monozygotic pairs. Neural tube defects, for example, are significantly increased in monozygotic as compared to dizygotic twins (1.6/1000 vs. 1.0/1000), suggesting a possible common etiological factor involved in the process of monozygotic twinning and congenital malformations (25).

Table 2 Causes of Congenital Malformations

	Incidence (%)
Monogenic	8
Chromosomal	10
Multifactorial	25
Environmental	
Maternal infection	2
Maternal illness (noninfectious)	1–2
Drugs and chemicals	2–3
Unknown	50

There is a common misconception that birth defects are on the rise when in actual fact hard data show that this is not the case (23,26–28). Because of a decrease in mortality and morbidity from infectious diseases and other previously important childhood diseases, and improvement in diagnostic and operative techniques, what has occurred is an increased level of relative medical importance and awareness of birth defects (27).

One also begins to feel that the public collectively believes that environmental agents are frequently the cause of birth defects: in fact, the list of proven teratogens is quite short. This overestimation may be partly due to an increase in media coverage of both health and environmental issues, and partly to the litigious nature of our times, with the resultant publicity given to these cases (which are often won by the plaintiff despite scientific evidence in favor of the defendant) (29).

DIABETES MELLITUS

The role of maternal diabetes in causing congenital anomalies warrants special mention for several reasons. Diabetes is a common disease, and it presents a typical example of the complex interaction of genetics and environment in the etiology of malformations. Most important, perhaps, is the recently obtained evidence that the defects may be preventable, although the issue remains controversial (30).

It is now known that the increased risk of congenital malformations in the offspring of women with insulin-dependent diabetes mellitus (IDDM) is due to the metabolic aberrations that occur during pregnancy as a result of the disease rather than to the genes that caused the diabetes. Nevertheless, there is no doubt that diabetes mellitus is primarily a genetically determined group of diseases. One important factor supporting the nongenetic components of etiology of the malformations is the absence of an increased risk when the father has IDDM (31). Furthermore, data from several studies have shown that when the diabetes is meticulously controlled during pregnancy, especially when the careful control is instituted prior to pregnancy, the incidence of malformations drops dramatically and approximates the risk for the general population (30,32). This increased risk does not apply to gestational diabetics, except for those who require insulin during the third trimester. In this group there is an increased risk for major cardiovascular defects among the offspring.

Table 3 lists the malformations most commonly seen in the infants of IDDM mothers (31–33), more or less in order of relative risk. The caudal regression syndrome, for example, has a risk ratio exceeding 200-fold, yet it occurs no more frequently than once in 350 infants born to diabetic mothers. On the other hand, approximately one infant in 40 will have a congenital heart defect (31). It should be noted that the incidence of neural tube defects

Table 3 Malformations Seen Most Often in the Infants of IDDM Mothers

Caudal regression syndrome: from partial agenesis of the sacrum to sirenomelia
Cardiac anomalies: transposition of great vessels, ventricular and atrial septal de-
    fects, coarctation, single ventricle, hypoplastic left ventricle, situs inversus
Renal anomalies: agenesis/dysgenesis, multicystic dysplasia, ureteral duplication
Gastrointestinal defects: anal/rectal atresia, duodenal atresia, small left colon
Neural tube defects: anencephaly, meningocele, myelomeningocele, etc.
Pulmonary hypoplasia

(NTDs) is sufficiently high (2%) to warrant the separation of IDDM women from the rest of the population in screening programs using maternal serum α-fetoprotein for detection of NTDs (34). Some programs use a separately determined median for diabetics, others simply handle these women separately, recommending detailed fetal ultrasonography at 16 weeks and again at 18–19 weeks, often in conjunction with amniocentesis.

THE MULTIFACTORIAL NATURE OF MALFORMATIONS: EXTENDING THE CONCEPT

Understanding the multifactorial concept is crucial to the comprehension of the nature, management, and prevention of congenital malformations (35). Polygenic inheritance, one of the components of multifactorial etiology, indicates an underlying predisposition to some trait, condition, or disease that depends on several genes and typically shows continuous variation: adult height, intelligence, neural tube defects, and congenital heart disease are examples. However, there are very few human characteristics, normal or abnormal, that are determined soley by heredity. Development, both prenatal and postnatal, makes important but as yet poorly understood contributions, exemplified by the frequent and puzzling lack of correlation between cerebral palsy and any detectable causative insult to the fetus during pregnancy, labor, or delivery (36). The third component, of course, is environment, the combination of the individual's changing milieu and life experiences. Just as few traits are purely genetic, few are entirely environmental. The term multifactorial causation covers the vast majority of human characteristics.

With that in mind, if one can now perceive a disease not as an entity, but as a variation or deviation from normal, then the causes of illness are not in themselves necessarily harmful. Rather, they become so when the exceed the adaptive resources of the individual or the whole species. For example, microorganisms inhabit our skin, respiratory mucosa, and gastrointestinal tract at all times; it takes a break in the skin or an alteration in the intestinal flora by an antibiotic before some of us will become ill. Most newborn infants with congenital absence of the thyroid gland will be spared from serious mental retardation as a result of early detection through newborn screening and early institution of thyroid hormone replacement therapy; the defect is still there, but manipulation of the environment has rendered it harmless. Even the bullet would do us no harm if we were wearing an appropriate protective garment, or if, as a species, we were not deficient for the gene or genes that produce the protective shell of the turtle. The strength of this adaptive, more physiologically oriented concept is its flexibility and its emphasis on individuality, variability, and multiplicity of causes. One might conclude, on this basis, that there are no diseases, only sick people. Overemphasis of that notion would lead to a separate diagnosis and a separate treatment for each sick person, and that would of course be impractical. We must accept some categorization of disease so that we can devise workable management schemes and strategies for prevention. Nevertheless, it is extremely important for our patients that those of us who provide care keep firmly in mind that in real life, all phenotypes, normal and abnormal, are multifactorial.

This bears itself out even when the agent at fault is completely external (e.g., rubella, anticonvulsants, alcohol). There are no teratogens, to our knowledge, that cause the same clinical manifestations in every affected individual. Not all infants of alcoholic mothers have the fetal alcohol syndrome. We have no clear-cut experimental data that tell us why, but the adaptive concept would leave us surprised if we did. Surely genetic variability in the sevceral enzymes that metabolize alcohol in both the mother and the fetus are important, and there are undoubtedly critical periods in embryonic and fetal development when specific organs or tissues are particularly susceptible to damage from alcohol and/or its breakdown products. The nutritional status of the mother may also play a role, and there may be a host of further genetic, developmental, and environmental factors about which we know nothing. In other words, although the direct cause may be environmental, the manifestation of the insult (i.e., the phenotype) depends on the genetic background, the developmental timing, and the environment.

In summary, as Barton Childs, who has written extensively on this issue so aptly put it, "in this personal evolution the genes set the limits of homeostatic capacity: the genes propose, the environments dispose, and if those limits are exceeded the result is illness or death" (37).

GENETIC ASESSMENT

A genetic assessment is a crucial component of a teratology workup. The most central and critical aspect of a proper genetic assessment is the formulation of a correct diagnosis, be it in assessing a dysmorphic child or responding

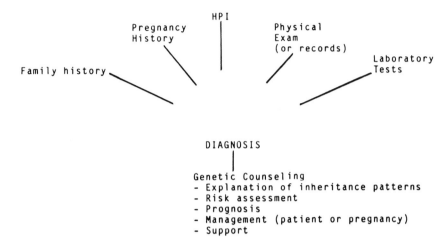

Figure 1   Elements of a genetic assessment (HPI = history of the patient's illness).

to a periconceptual inquiry. Lack of diagnosis diminishes the ability to prognosticate, to predict recurrence risk, and to anticipate the development of complications that may be preventable if detected early enough (e.g., the hypoglycemia that could cause mental retardation in patients with Beckwith-Wiedemann syndrome). Uncertainty may also make it more difficult for families to accept what has occurred, resulting in a decreased ability to move through the grieving process. Obviously, an incorrect diagnosis may lead not only to improper management and prognosis, but also to incorrect assignment of recurrence risks.

The components of the genetic assessment (Fig. 1) are discussed in the following sections.

Family History

Asking for the presence of genetic, or even inherited, diseases is not useful, since it presumes that the consultand understands the principles of heredity; additionally, it puts the burden of diagnosis on the consultand.*

More specific questions must be asked, as outlined in Table 4. A positive response to any of these questions may be an indicator of genetic, chromosomal, or teratogenic factors acting in the family. If a positive response is

---

*The neologism, *consultand*, was coined by geneticists to represent the individual being counseled: often it is neither the affected patient nor the proband (the individual through whom the family came to medical attention), but a relative who may or may not be at risk.

Table 4 Family History Screening Questions

Two or more spontaneous abortions?
Stillbirth?
Neonatal death?
Infertility?
Malformations/birth defects?
Mental retardation?
Familial conditions?
Maternal and paternal age?
Early deaths and/or unexplained infant deaths?
Consanguinity?
Ethnic origin?
Other medical problems (define)?

elicited, the consultand's relationship to the affected individual must be established by drawing the family tree. A three-generation family history is usually sufficient and can be elicited quite rapidly.

The clinician must beware of the medical diagnoses supplied by family members. In the past, particularly, many different forms of mental retardation were labeled mongolism. The term spina bifida may be erroneously applied to cases of isolated hydrocephalus and to the apparently unrelated and very common minor defect(s) in the bony arch of the spinal column, spina bifida occulta, which can be found, if one looks hard enough at x-rays, in up to 50% of the population (38). Medical records should be obtained if possible on any relatives whose history may be relevant to your patient. Family members frequently know only part of the story and may be aware of only one malformation in a person who has many, or they may be unaware that a tentative diagnosis was never confirmed.

Consanguinity

The risk of both autosomal recessive and multifactorial conditions increases when parents are consanguineous. For incestuous matings (brother/sister, parent/child), no accurate data have ever been collected, but estimates indicate that greater than 20% of such offspring have major genetically caused problems (39). For second-degree relatives (uncles/aunts, nieces/nephews), the risk is about double the general population incidence for multifactorial and autosomal recessive conditions (about 6%); and for first cousins, the risk is less than is commonly perceived, probably about 1% over the population risk of 2–3% when the family history is negative and carrier status for "ethnic" conditions ruled out (40,41).

It is tempting to implicate consanguinity when a child is born with a malformation. However, full investigations must be done to ascertain what has really gone awry. A good example is hemophilia A in the royal families of Europe (42). You will still read in the lay literature that this condition was caused by inbreeding, which of course is not true, since the condition is X-linked. Although its *presence* in the various royal houses of Europe was a direct consequence of the fact that the families were related, the hemophilia itself did not persist in these families because of individual consanguineous matings. This distinction is important, but not commonly understood.

Ethnic Origin

National and ethnic origins must be obtained. Inbreeding is common in Middle Eastern countries and certain ethnic groups. The Amish, for example, may have an almost total monopoly on one genetically determined syndrome, cartilage-hair hypoplasia or metaphysieal chondrodysplasia (43). The carrier frequency for Tay-Sachs disease is about 1 in 30 Ashkenazi Jews (Jews of eastern European origins). Up to 10% of Italians and other peoples from the Mediterranean areas are carriers of one of the many mutations for β-thalassemia. Approximately 8% of North American blacks are carriers of the sickle gene, and many are carriers of the β-thalassemia mutants. The immigration of large numbers of Asians to Canada and the United States has brought α-thalassemia to the fore (44). It is clearly the responsibility of every practising physician to determine the ethnic and national origins of couples planning to have children in order to inform special groups of their unique genetic risks and to ensure that they are aware of the available carrier tests and of prenatal diagnosis.

Maternal and Paternal Age Effect

Table 5 presents the increasing risk of chromosome anomalies with advancing maternal age. The most common anomaly by far is trisomy 21, and it

Table 5 Risk of Chromosomal Anomalies with Advancing Maternal Age

Maternal age at delivery	Down's syndrome (trisomy 21)	Klinefelter syndrome (47,XXY)	Male 47,XYY	Total
20	1/2000	1/2500	1/2000	1/530
30	1/1000	1/2000	1/2000	1/390
35	1/350	1/1100	1/2000	1/180
37	1/200	1/900	1/2000	1/125
40	1/100	1/550	1/2000	1/80
45	1/30	1/200	1/2000	1/19

shows the most striking age effect. Trisomies 13 and 18 also show some maternal age effect, but even by age 40 the risk only rises to 1/1000–1/2000 from around 1/10,000 at age 20 (45). There is a paternal age effect (46), but it is barely significant (47); for example, it has been calculated that to advance a woman at age 34 to the risk category of a woman at age 35 on the basis of paternal age, the father would have to be over 55 (46).

A paternal age effect has been observed in some autosomal dominant conditions (48). The best documented example is achondroplasia. In this autosomal dominant condition, approximately 80% of affected individuals are born to nondwarf parents. The vast majority of these cases are a result of a spontaneous mutation in a parental germ cell, and there is a statistically significant increase in the age of the father in these families.

Pregnancy History—Past and Present

Pregnancy history is dealt with in other chapters, but a few points warrant emphasis. Medications are easily forgotten, but patients may recall them when they recall an illness during the pregnancy. Chronic diseases sometimes become such a part of daily living that they are unmentioned (e.g., the epileptic mother who has been seizure-free for years but still takes her daily phenytoin). Multiple spontaneous abortions, especially if they occur in more than one couple in a family, may be due to inherited chromosomal rearrangements.

The amount of amniotic fluid may provide clues to diagnosis. Throughout the latter half of pregnancy much of the amniotic fluid is fetal urine, and homeostasis depends on intact fetal gastrointestinal and urinary tracts as well as a functional brain to control normal fetal swallowing. If the fetus cannot swallow, or if the gut is not fully patent, polyhydramnios will occur; if the kidneys are dysplastic, severely cystic or absent, or if the outflow tract is obstructed, oligohydramnios results and the infant will show some or all of the deformations of Potter syndrome.

History of the Patient's Illness

It may sound odd to include a history of the patient's illness as part of the assessment because, by definition, congenital malformations are present at birth. However, as pointed out earlier in this chapter, many malformations, even though present at birth, may not be detectable by even the most skilled examiners. One of the most important points about, for example, developmental delay (motor, physical, or intellectual) is the timing. A period of well-documented normal motor and intellectual development for weeks or months, followed by deterioration, almost by definition puts the patient into the neurodegenerative group of diseases rather than cerebral palsy or a developmental brain anomaly, such as holoprosencephaly or porencephaly. The family album may be helpful. Photographs of an infant doing things at 6 months that are clearly not achievable 6 months later are better than hundreds of words of description.

The Syndrome-Oriented Physical Examination

When examining a child or a child's medical records, keep in mind the cliché, if you find one malformation, look for others. An important point is that many "malformations" are subtle—mere variations from what is normal or perhaps most usual—and often of no functional importance in and of themselves. However, it is the constellation of minor variations and major anomalies that constitute a syndrome, and the physician who is unable to recognize the minor anomalies or to link the various findings will have difficulty in arriving at the correct diagnosis. Several associations of congenital anomalies occur, and many are obvious ones. These include abnormal external ears and hearing problems; concurrent anomalies of genital, lower renal, and lower bowel segments; and cleft palate, micrognathia, glossoptosis, and difficulty breathing [the Pierre Robin complex (49)]. Less obvious associations are hearing loss and kidney disease, and vertebral, anal, cardiac tracheoesophageal, renal, and limb (VACTERL) anomalies (50). Cleft lip and cleft palate serve as good examples of common malformations that occur not only as isolated defects, but also in association with over 250 recognized syndromes (51).

Examination of both the parents and the siblings, if any, is often important. Again, human variability is extensive, and all too often the "dysmorphic" infant is a near replica of one of the parents. On occasion, a parent or sibling may have a mild and undiagnosed form of the same condition: neurofibromatosis and myotonic dystrophy are examples of conditions that come up frequently. Unavailable relatives can usually be "examined" via photographs. The family album is one of the most useful and most underutilized diagnostic tools.

In addition, when a dysmorphic child is being examined, one must be wary of phenocopies: that is, environmentally induced conditions that mimic genetic diseases. For example, the teratogenic effects of thalidomide may be indistinguishable from the physical signs of the cardiac limb, or Holt-Oram syndrome, inherited as an autosomal dominant trait. The limb reduction defects and stippling of the epiphyses of long bones and vertebrae seen in the warfarin embryopathy may be indistinguishable from the defects of the Conradi-Hunnermann, or chondrodystrophia calcificans syndrome, inherited as an autosomal recessive trait. It should be appreciated that occasionally environmentally induced disorders occur repetitively in families. We recently saw a child with the fetal alcohol syndrome who bore a striking resemblance, physically and mentally, to her mother—further history revealed that the grandmother had been a heavy drinker, as was the child's mother. Similarly, nearly all the offspring of a woman with classic phenylketonuria (PKU) (maternal PKU) who is untreated during pregnancy will be mentally retarded and will frequently have a variety of malformations, with microcephaly being the most common (52). None is likely to be homozygous for the gene that causes PKU—they are usually heterozygotes, damaged in utero by high blood levels of phenylalanine and its metabolites that cross the placenta to the fetus.

In attempting to elicit easy-to-miss physical signs, special attention should be paid to the following areas.

Head: The head and face should be viewed from several angles for asymmetries.

Limbs: Lack of movement of the limbs may mean severe hypotonia, nerve palsy, or underlying fracture. Assymetrical limbs are also easy to miss.

Eyes: The lids of a neonate are often swollen, but failure to open them will result in missing a coloboma, a white pupil (retinoblastoma or severe corneal clouding), or congenital microphthalmia/anophthalmia.

Ears: It is important to document abnormal folds of the helix, absence of the posterior crura of the antihelix, ear lobe creases, presence of skin tags or sinuses, and overall size [there are tables of ear sizes (9)]. Recognizing low set ears is not difficult. A major clue comes from embryology. The external ears originate from outgrowths of the first and second branchial arches; the cleft between the arches contributes to the ear canal and the eustachian tube. The developing ear has to migrate up and forward from the side of the neck. Therefore, if the ear appears low and is also tilted posteriorly, it probably really is low set. If one uses the *medial* canthus of the eye as the fixed point and draws an imaginary line backward parallel to the floor, it should pass within a centimeter or two of the external auditory meatus. (If you make the common error of using the lateral canthus as your reference point, you will overdiagnose low set ears.) If in doubt about low set ears, disregard this feature because it is probably not significant.

Mouth: It is surprisingly easy to miss a cleft palate, abnormalities of the tongue, or alveolar hyperplasia. Presence or absence of teeth should be ascertained as well as their arrangement, size, structure, and color.

Neck: Masses are routinely sought, but also check for low hair line, webbing, redundant skin folds, and short neck.

Chest: If the nipples are in the anterior axillary line, they are wide set. If in doubt, there are tables (9). Note pectus, if present, or a bell-shaped small chest cavity, and watch for asymmetries that might indicate absence of underlying muscles, which occurs in Poland syndrome and the cardiac-limb syndrome.

Extremities: A short little finger with a single crease, with or without clinodactyly (bent finger), is the commonest physical sign associated with chromosomal disorders. The single palmar crease, in contrast, is present in close to 5% of the general population. Look carefully for extra digits. Even a tiny "nubbin" on the thumb (preaxial polydactyly) or little finger (post-axial polydactyly) counts. It is surprisingly easy to miss short limbs: The fingertips, even in a newborn infant, should reach down to the upper thigh if the upper limbs are of normal length. Hypoplasia of the finger- or toenails may be a subtle sign of a limb reduction defect, as seen in the fetal hydantoin syndrome.

Genitalia: Hypoplasia of the external genitalia occurs in females as well as in males with conditions such as Prader-Willi and Laurence-Moon-Biedl syndromes; the manifestations just are not as obvious as a micropenis and underdeveloped scrotum. Look for poorly developed or even nearly absent labia minora as well as for a very small clitoris. If the genitalia are ambiguous, check carefully for inguinal mases. If you can find a palpable gonad, it will nearly always be a testicle and the infant is a biological male. In addition, if the urethral opening is at or near the tip of a penile/clitoral structure, it is more likely to be a penis.

Skin and hair: One rarely sees café-au-lait spots in a newborn with neuro-fibromatosis, but areas of depigmentation may be a diagnostic clue for tuberous sclerosis and other neurocutaneous syndromes. It is worth noting that anomalies of the hair are among the relatively rare "malformations" that occur in inherited metabolic diseases: the kinky hair of Menkes syndrome, the decrease of pigment in untreated PKU and in albinism, the coarse hair of patients with mucopolysaccharidoses or hypothyroidism.

Laboratory Testing

Since inherited metabolic diseases are so rarely associated with malformations, expensive laboratory assays are rarely necessary. However, some key tests repeatedly yield helpful results.

1. *Karyotype*: Indicated whenever there are combinations of malformations with or without mental retardation and the diagnosis is not established. Sometimes a prenatal karyotype is important when malformations are detected by ultrasound — even if it is too late in the pregnancy to consider termination. Knowing the specific chromosome anomaly prior to delivery of an infant with trisomy 13, for example, might have a major influence on the management of the newborn infant.
2. *X-rays and ultrasound*: It is often said that the radiologist is the dysmorphologist's best friend. Total body x-rays may reveal major and even pathognomonic anomalies that would be otherwise missed. Ultrasound may be extremely helpful in detecting a variety of internal organ anomalies, especially those of the brain and kidneys.

3. *CBC*: Combinations of anemia and thrombocytopenia occur in some syndromes in association with such malformations as aplastic anemia and absent thumbs in Fanconi's anemia and low platelet counts and absence of the radii in the TAR (*t*hrombocytopenia-*a*bsent-*r*adius) syndrome.
4. *Testing for infections*: Multiple congenital malformations can be caused by viruses, bacteria, and other infectious agents. Important clues are hydro- or microcephalus, chlorioretinitis, and intracranial calcifications. The TORCH (*to*xoplasmosis, *r*ubella, *c*ytomegalovirus, and *h*erpes) screen and VDRL (*v*enereal *d*isease *r*esearch *l*aboratory) are old but still important procedures.

The autopsy, although hardly a routine laboratory procedure, is extremely important when a malformation syndrome or genetic disease is suspected in a stillborn infant (53) or neonatal death (54) even as an outside possibility. The following checklist of procedures provides the maximum opportunity to come up with a diagnosis, which is often crucial for genetic counseling.

1. *Photographs (before and during the autopsy)*: If not obtained during life or if the newborn photographs are distorted by tubes, intravenous lines, and monitors.
2. *X-rays (total body) and ultrasound of head*: Postmortem autolysis may obscure significant intracranial malformations, especially if there is any delay in obtaining consent for autopsy.
3. *Tissue for karyotype*: Heart blood should be obtained as soon as possible after death, but may yield viable lymphocytes for culture even 2–3 days later. Skin and pleura also serve as good sources of viable cells. If chromosome culture medium is not available, tissues should be placed between sterile gauze pads kept moist with sterile saline. For stillbirths and neonatal deaths, tissue from the fetal surface of the placenta and a small section of the umbilical cord should be added to the above. Occasionally a chromosomal diagnosis can be obtained from the placenta or cord when the fetus is too macerated for either autopsy or for the obtaining of viable cells for culture.
4. *Tissues for cell culture (skin, pleura, etc., as above)*: Should be obtained if there is any suggestion that the condition might be an inherited metabolic disease. In addition, the following samples should be obtained for storage in the deep-freezer: serum and urine for amino and organic acids, and liver for possible future enzyme or molecular analysis.

Making a Diagnosis

At this point the physician should have a complete list of historical, physical, and laboratory findings, which do not necessarily add up to a syndrome that can be recalled. The following are the sequential steps to take.

1. *Consultation.* Medical geneticists and pediatricians generally have the most experience with syndrome diagnosis. Nearly every medical school in North America provides a clinical genetics service. A complete listing of centers, including staff and service areas covered, can be obtained through the Canadian College of Medical Geneticists or the American Society of Human Genetics. Many states and provinces also provide outreach or satellite genetics clinics on a regular basis. Genetic services include diagnostic tests, family studies when indicated, genetic counseling, prenatal diagnosis, and follow-up, if the physician and/or family wish it. Genetics centers also serve as sources of up-to-date information for referring physicians who may wish to do their own investigative work-up and counseling.

2. *The malformation atlas.* The book *Recognizable Patterns of Human Malformations* (9) is one of the best because it contains several tables of measurements of many parts of the body as well as the extremely useful tables of individual anomalies. The latter allow the physician to select one or two of the most significant anomalies seen in the patient and then obtain a relatively short list of the syndromes wherein that anomaly is found.

3. *Computer-assisted diagnosis programs.* Several are now in existence and soon will be available, directly or through genetics centers, to all physicians. The data are now on laser or compact discs that provide printed, audio, and pictorial output. The operator simply enters the patient's clinical and laboratory data, and the machine matches the patient to the syndromes that best fit. The best programs provide brief descriptions of any of the listed conditions and appropriate references upon request, along with photoimages of patients with that diagnosis on a video screen. The computer has one major advantage over the physician—it will not forget anything that has been entered into its memory bank. But it cannot do a physical examination or take a history. Missed signs and omitted data diminish the machine's diagnostic accuracy, although some programs will ask if certain physical signs were elicited or recommend specific investigations. Sometimes geneticists will send photographs, x-rays, sonograms, and/or pathological specimens to experts in other genetics centers for an opinion.

4. *Follow-up examinations.* Review and reexamination of an undiagnosed infant or child 4–6 months later may be very helpful because fetures can change quite quickly and dramatically. The facial features of the Cornelia de Lange syndrome (55), for example, have been documented as becoming much more obvious over the latter part of the first year of life, and the obesity of the Prader-Willi and Laurence-Moon-Biedl syndromes may not become obvious for months.

GENETIC COUNSELING

Genetic counseling has been defined as a communication process which deals with the human problems associated with the occurrence, or risk of occurrence, of a genetic disorder in a family. This process involves an attempt by one or more appropriately trained persons to help the individual or the family to (1) comprehend the medical facts, including the diagnosis, the probable course of the disorder and the available management; (2) appreciate the way heredity contributes to the disorder and the risk of recurrence in specified relatives; (3) understand the options for dealing with the risk of recurrence; (4) choose the course of action which seems appropriate to them in view of their risk and their family goals and act in accordance with that decision; and (5) make the best possible adjustment to the disorder in the affected family member and/or to the risk of recurrence of that disorder (56). The counseling is usually done by a medical geneticist or genetic counselor, but the follow-up is often the responsibility of the referring physician. In either case, reinforcement is essential, since few individuals or families absorb all the genetic data the first time they are presented. A letter to the family describing the condition and the genetics involved is often helpful. An unresolved problem is the physician's responsibility toward other relatives at risk, some of whom may reside in distant communities or even other countries—the issues of confidentiality versus an individual's right to knowledge may be in conflict.

Risk Assessment

The assignment of an accurate recurrence risk depends on arriving at a correct diagnosis, as described above, determining the mode of inheritance, and noting the relationship of the consultand to the affected individual or proband. Qualitative descriptions of risks should be avoided. No malformation is as rare as "one in a million," and even experienced physicians have been shown to differ widely in their interpretation of such terms as rare, uncommon, and unlikely (57).

Many people have difficulty comprehending probabilities, especially when applied to their personal situation. The 50:50 risk of autosomal dominant inheritance can be misconstrued as meaning that if the first offspring is affected, the next one will be normal. The coin toss analogy is helpful there, as is the relationship between drawing playing cards out of a deck for autosomal recessive inheritance. In the latter, you know you have made your point when the consultand adds that you have to replace the drawn card each time. Clinical experience leads us to conclude that many people have a clearer conception of ratios than percentages; that is, stating the risk as one out of every 30 babies born is better understood than 2–3%.

Couples concerned about teratogenic effects of medication, radiation, or other environmental toxic exposures in a pregnancy should understand the background risk for the general population as well as their personal risk for malformations (maternal or paternal age, ethnic diseases, familial genetic problems) so that an abnormal outcome is not automatically attributed to the environmental agent.

When the strategies above fail to determine either a specific cause for the condition or a specific diagnosis, the family still needs some indication of at least the range of risk. It is rarely if ever zero, but may be almost that low if infection or other correctable environmental factor were the cause. The empiric or observed recurrence risk for multiple congenital malformations of unknown cause is 4–6% (58), and this is an often presented figure for parents of such a child. It is important to mention to parents that sometimes, even without consanguinity, the mode of inheritance could be autosomal recessive, in which case the recurrence risk would be 25%. With increasing frequency, considerable reassurance during future pregnancies can be provided by detailed ultrasound examinations looking specifically for whatever malformations are present in the proband. Any "open" defects (neural tube defects, extrophy of the bladder, omphalocele, etc.) ought to cause an increase in amniotic fluid and maternal serum α-fetoprotein (59).

Management

Carrier detection for autosomal recessive and X-linked conditions, and presymptomatic detection of late-onset autosomal dominant conditions are rapidly expanding components of genetic counseling, mainly as a result of the establishment of molecular genetics diagnostic services. Thus, intrafamilial screening for the detection of at-risk relatives is now an established component of the activities of genetics centers. It is important to have such procedures done before a pregnancy is under way to avoid rushing sometimes complex tests and creating anxiety for both the couple and the laboratory personnel. Detection of a carrier often leads to studies of the spouse and preparation for prenatal diagnosis.

Many couples go on to therapeutic abortion when an affected fetus is diagnosed. Those who decide to continue the pregnancy, however, value the time that prenatal diagnosis provides to prepare for the predicted problems. Knowing about problems in advance can be important in managing the delivery. The mother might benefit from being transferred to a major medical center prior to delivery so that facilities for early treatment will be immediately available if required.

Prenatal diagnosis is not, however, the only approach to reduction or elimination of risk for genetic/chromosomal anomalies. In some social and ethnic groups where abortion is unacceptable and marriages are still arranged, premarital testing of couples is already occurring: In some Orthodox Jewish communities, for example, prospective spouses are routinely screened for carrier status for Tay-Sachs disease (TSD) – if both are carriers of the TSD gene, new partners are chosen.

Artificial insemination by donor (AID), now referred to as therapeutic donor insemination (TDI), has been available for decades to couples facing the 1 in 4 risk of an autosomal recessive condition, or a 50% risk in the case of a male with an autosomal dominant disease, but few have availed themselves of this option. This reluctance is diminishing, and requests for donor insemination for genetic reasons are rising in North America (60). In vitro fertilization of donor eggs by the husband's sperm when the wife has an autosomal dominant condition is now technically feasible, as is preimplantation genetic diagnosis. The latter involves in vitro fertilization, removal of a single cell from the preembryo by micromanipulation and molecular analysis of amplified DNA extracted from that single cell (61).

Patients are frequently referred for, or themselves request, amniocentesis or chorionic villus sampling after exposure to a real or potential teratogen. Unfortunately, these procedures rarely provide relevant information. Assessment of chromosomal breakage after fetal exposure to x-rays or hallucinogenic drugs is of no value because of marked variability in the unexposed fetal population. A detailed ultrasound examination may help allay anxiety, but great care must be taken to ensure that the parents realize that a normal fetal sonogram does not in any way guarantee a normal newborn.

Support

Today there are a large number of disease-oriented patient, parent, and family support groups, even for conditions as rare as Williams syndrome and epidermolysis bullosa. Many find these groups extremely helpful, primarily because it puts them in contact with other families who have faced the same problems and managed to cope. Libraries may provide little if any understandable information on malformations for parents and often, sad to say, descriptions in texts are out of date, wrong, and/or misleading. The classic presentation of the Klinefelter male – a tall, eunuchoid, sexually underdeveloped, and mentally retarded person – is, in fact, seen only rarely: most 47,XXY males are normal except for small testes and azospermia.

The support groups tend to organize meetings, produce readable descriptions of genetic conditions, publish periodic newsletters, and provide someone to talk to when the parents are in need of advice from other individuals or families who have had the same problems. Information on diseases and syndrome-oriented groups is available from most genetics centers.

SUMMARY

We have documented the high incidence and importance of malformations in human populations, and the complexity of their causes. Emphasis has been placed on the assessment of the dysmorphic patient, including historical, physical, and laboratory aspects. The availability of services and organizations that may be helpful to the clinician in making accurate diagnoses and providing optimal management strategies has been noted. Prevention of birth defects is already part of the practice of medicine, but it must be orchestrated with extreme care. Newborn screening for PKU and congenital hypothyroidism is now of proven value and relatively free of controversy, but the maternal serum screening programs for prenatal detection of NTDs and Down's syndrome are very different. They require administration that must include well-informed consent and must remain voluntary: some couples do not desire prenatal detection for moral and ethical reasons. Great care must be taken in all prenatal diagnostic testing to ensure that the patient understands the risk of the procedure, its specificity and sensitivity, and the fact that normal results do not guarantee that the infant will be normal. The discovery of a congenital anomaly or a chromosome aberration in a fetus often puts the geneticist and/or the referring physician into the most challenging position likely to be faced vis-à-vis maintaining the stance of nondirective counseling. One's own biases may easily get in the way of allowing a couple to make a decision based on the known facts and figures and their own ethical values.

Finally, it is important and exciting to look to the future. Realistically, correcting genetic errors through gene replacement or other forms of direct genetic engineering remains in the research area. However, new techniques for diagnosis, both pre- and postnatal, are here, and their benefits are growing. Many of our house officers become frustrated with the difficulty of remembering the features of so many syndromes. Newer and better atlases and computer-assisted diagnosis have been of great help, but now the molecular geneticists are also coming to the rescue. Hardly a week goes by without a report on the identification, cloning, and characterization of yet another disease- or malformation-causing mutant gene. Obviously, these discoveries are a great help in distinguishing between genetically determined syndromes and those due primarily to environmental teratogens. Apparent exceptions to Mendel's laws, such as genetic "anticipation" (the apparent worsening of the deleterious effects of a gene as it passes down from generation to generation in a family — myotonic dystrophy and the fragile-X syndrome being prime examples) (62) and imprinting (the difference in expression of a mutation depending on its parental origin, as in the Prader-Willi and Angelman syndromes) (63) are beginning to be understood through molecular genetics research. Perhaps most relevant to genetic aspects of maternal–fetal toxicology is the emerging proof of the existence of modification of expression of major genes by either alleles or by genes at other loci. A recent example is the variation in age of onset in Huntington's disease (64) and the existence of two distinct phenotypes, fatal familial insomnia and familial Creutzfeldt-Jakob disease, both due to the same mutation but with expression determined by a common polymorphism (65). It is surprising that at least some of the variation in phenotypes due to teratogens is the result of genetic susceptibilities and modifications by a variety of genes. Should it become possible to identify specific predisposing or modifying genes, assignment of risks for parents on drug treatment would become more accurate and more specific.

We conclude by harking back to the quotation by Childs in the section on the multifactorial nature of malformations. As we shed more and more light on the genes that propose, we may mitigate the ways that the environments dispose. The beneficiaries will be our patients who require medications during pregnancy and who wish to become parents with the maximum of safety for their unborn children.

Answer

A two- to threefold increase in the incidence of congenital anomalies over the general population risk. Caudal regression syndrome, congenital heart defects, neural tube defects, macrosomia, and neonatal hypoglycemia are major problems. Meticulous control of the diabetes prior to and during pregnancy significantly reduces the risk.

REFERENCES

1. Holmes LB. Current concepts in genetics. Congenital malformations. N Engl J Med 1976; 295:204–207.
2. Van Regemorter N, Dodion J, Druart C, Hayez F, Vamos E, Flament-Dorand J, Perlmutter-Cremer N, Rodesch F. Congenital malformations in 10,000 consecutive births in a university hospital: Need for genetic counseling and prenatal diagnosis. J Pediatr 1984; 104(3):386–390.
3. Kalter H, Warkany J. Congenital malformations. Etiologic factors and their role in prevention. New Engl J Med 1983; 308:424–431, 491–497.
4. Myrianthopoulos NC. Malformations in children from one to seven years. A report from the collaborative perinatal project. Alan R Liss, New York, 1985.
5. Christianson RE, Van Den Berg BJ, Milkovich L, Oechsli FW. Incidence of congenital anomalies among white and black live births with long-term follow-up. Am J Public Health 1981; 71(12):1333–1341.
6. Baird PA, Anderson TW, Newcombe HB, Lowry RB. Genetic disorders in children and young adults: A population study. Am J Hum Genet 1988; 42:677–693.
7. Spranger J, Benirschke K, Hall JG, Lenz W, Lowry RB, Opitz M, Pinsky L, Schwarzacher HG, Smith DW. Errors of morphogenesis: Concepts and terms. J Pediatr 1982; 100:160–165.
8. Moore KL. The Developing Human, 2nd ed. Saunders, Philadelphia, 1977.

9. Jones D. Recognizable Patterns of Human Malformation. Genetic, Embryologic and Clinical Aspects, 4th ed. Saunders, Philadelphia, 1988.

10. Winsor EJT, Brown BSJ. Prevalence and prenatal diagnosis of neural tube defects in Nova Scotia in 1980-84. Can Med Assoc J 1986; 135:1269-1273.

11. Keena B, Sodovnick AD, Baird PA, Hall JG. Risk to sibs of probands with neural tube defects: Data for clinic populations in British Columbia. Am J Med Genet 1986; 25:563-573.

12. Malnick M, Bixler D, Fogh-Andersen P, Conneally PM. Cleft lip + cleft palate: An overview of the literature and an analysis of Danish cases born between 1941 and 1968. Am J Med Genet 1980; 6:83-97.

13. Welch J, Hunter AGW. An epidemiological study of facial clefting in Manitoba. J Med Genet 1980; 17:127-132.

14. Keith JK, Rowe RD, Vlad P. Heart Disease in Infancy and Childhood, 3rd ed. Collier Macmillan Canada, Toronto, 1978.

15. Nora JJ, Nora AH. Update on counseling the family with a first-degree relative with a congenital heart defect. Am J Med Genet 1988; 29:137-142.

16. Baird PA, MacDonald EC. An epidemiologic study of congenital malformations of the anterior abdominal wall in more than half a million consecutive live births. Am J Hum Genet 1981; 33:470-478.

17. Lowry RB, Baird PA. Familial gastroschisis and omphalocele. Am J Hum Genet 1982; 34:517-518.

18. Wolff G. Familial congenital diaphragmatic hernia: Review and conclusions. Hum Genet 1980; 54:1-5.

19. Calzolari E, Contiero MR, Roncarati E, Mattiuz PL, Volpato S. Aetiological factors in hypospadias. J Med Genet 1986; 23:333-337.

20. Artz TD, Levine DB, Lim WN, Salvati EA, Wilson PD Jr. Neonatal diagnosis, treatment and related factors of congenital dislocation of the hip. Clin Orthoped 1975; 110:112-135.

21. Myrianthopoulos NC. Sex differences. In Malformations in Children from One to Seven Years. A Report from the Collaborative Perinatal Project. Alan R Liss, New York, 1985, pp 45-53.

22. Myrianthopoulos NC. Racial differences. In Malformations in Children from One to Seven Years. A Report from the Collaborative Perinatal Project. Alan R Liss, New York, 1985, pp 55-64.

23. Mortimer EA Jr. The puzzling epidemiology of neural tube defects. Commentaries. Pediatrics 1980; 65:636-638.

24. Myrianthopoulos NC. Congenital malformations in twins. Epidemiologic survey. Birth Defects Orig Article Ser 1975; 11:1-39.

25. Windham GC, Bjerkedal T, Sever LE. The association of twinning and neural tube defects. Acta Genet Med Gemellol (Roma) 1982; 31:165-172.

26. Persaud TVN. Classification and epidemiology of developmental defects. In Basic Concepts in Teratology (Persaud TVN, Chudley AD, Skalko RG, eds). Alan R Liss, New York, 1985, pp 13-21.

27. Chudley AE. Genetic contributions to human malformations. In Basic Concepts in Teratology (Persaud TVN, Chudley AD, Skalko RG, eds). Alan R Liss, New York, 1985, pp 31-68.

28. Windham GC, Edmonds LC. Current trends in the incidence of neural tube defects. Pediatrics 1982; 70:333–337.
29. Mills JL, Alexander D. Teratogens and litogens. N Engl J Med 1986; 315(19): 1234–1236.
30. Mills JL, Knopp RH, Simpson JL, Jovanovic-Peterson L, Metzger BE, Holmes LB, Aarons JH, Brown Z, Reed GF, Bieber RF, Van Allen M, Holzman I, Ober C, Peterson CM, Withiam MJ, Duckles A, Mueller-Heubach E, Polk BF, and National Institute of Child Health and Human Development Diabetes in Early Pregnancy Study. Lack of relation of increased malformation rates in infants of diabetic mothers to glycemic control during organogenesis. N Engl J Med 1988; 318:671–676.
31. Becarra JE, Khoury MJ, Cordero JF, Erickson JD. Diabetes mellitus during pregnancy and the risks for specific birth defects: a population-based case-control study. Pediat 1990; 85:1–9.
32. Cousins L. Congenital anomalies among infants of diabetic mothers. Etiology, prevention, prenatal diagnosis. Am J Obstet Gynecol 1983; 147(3):333–337.
33. Steel JM, Johnstone FD, Hepburn DA, Smith AF. Can prepregnancy care of diabetic women reduce the risk of abnormal babies? British Med J 1990; 301: 1070–1074.
34. Milunsky A, Alport E, Kitzmiller JL, Younger MD, Neff RK. Prenatal diagnosis of neural tube defects: VIII. The importance of serum α-fetoprotein screening in diabetic pregnant women. Am J Obstet Gynecol 1984; 142:1030–1032.
35. Fraser FC, Nora JJ. Multifactorial inheritance. In Genetics of Man, 2nd ed. Lea & Febiger, Philadelphia, 1986, pp 173–183.
36. Nelson KB. What proportion of cerebral palsy is related to birth asphyxia? J Pediatr 1988; 112:572–573.
37. Childs B. Genetic factors in human disease. In Genetic Issues in Pediatric and Obstetric Practice (Kaback M, ed). Year Book, Chicago, 1980, pp 3–16.
38. Warkany J. Spina bifida. In Congenital Malformations. Notes and Comments. Year Book, Chicago, 1971, pp 272–291.
39. Baird PA, McGillivray B. Children of incest. J Pediatr 1982; 101:854–857.
40. Fried K, Davies AM. Some effects on the offspring of uncle-niece marriage in the Moroccan Jewish community in Jerusalem. Am J Hum Genet 1974; 26: 65–72.
41. Fraser FC, Biddle CJ. Estimating the risks for offspring of first-cousin matings: An approach. Am J Hum Genet 1976; 28:522–526.
42. Levitan M. Relationship and consanguinity. In Textbook of Human Genetics, 3rd ed. Oxford University Press, New York, 1988, p 247.
43. McKusick VA, Eldridge R, Hostetler JA, Ruargwit U, Egeland JA. Dwarfism in the Amish. II. Cartilage-hair hypoplasia. Bull Johns Hopkins Hosp 1965; 116:285–326.
44. McKusick VA. The ethnic distribution of disease in the United States. In Mendelian Inheritance in Man. Catalogs of Autosomal Dominant, Autosomal Recessive and X-Linked Phenotypes (Foreword), 5th ed. Johns Hopkins University Press, Baltimore, 1978, pp 59–61.
45. Hook EB. Rates of chromosome abnormalities at different maternal ages. Obstet Gynecol 1981; 58:282–285.

46. Stene J, Stene E, Stengel-Rutowski S, Murken J. Paternal age and Down's syndrome. Data from prenatal diagnoses. Hum Genet 1981; 59:119–124.
47. Hook EB, Cross PK. Paternal age and Down syndrome genotypes diagnosed prenatally: No association in New York State data. Hum Genet 1982; 62:167–174.
48. Friedman JM. Genetic diseases in the offspring of old fathers. Obstet Gynecol 1981; 57:745–749.
49. Sheffield LJ, Reiss JA, Strohm K, Gilding M. A genetic follow-up study of 64 patients with the Pierre Robin complex. Am J Med Genet 1987; 28:25–36.
50. Khoury MJ, Cordero JF, Greenberg F, James LM, Erikson JD. A population study of the VACTERL association: Evidence for its etiologic heterogeneity. Pediatrics 1983; 71:815–820.
51. Shprintzen RJ, Siegel-Sadewitz VL, Amato J, Goldberg RB. Anomalies associated with cleft lip, cleft palate, or both. Am J Med Genet 1985; 20:585–595.
52. Levy HI, Waisbren SE. Effects of untreated maternal phenylketonuria and hyperphenylalaninemia on the fetus. N Engl J Med 1983; 309:1269–1274.
53. Mueller RF, Sybert VP, Johnson J, Brown ZA, Chen W. Evaluation of a protocol for post-mortem examination of stillbirths. N Engl J Med 1983; 309:586–590.
54. Kronick JB, Goodyer PR, Kaplan PB. A perimortem protocol for suspected genetic disease. Pediatrics 1983; 71:960–963.
55. Passarge E, Mecke S, Altrogge HC. Cornelia de Lange syndrome: Evolution of the phenotype. Pediatrics 1971; 48:833–836.
56. Fraser FC. Genetic counseling. Am J Hum Genet 1974; 26:636–659.
57. Bryant GD, Norman GR. Expressions of probability: Words and numbers. N Engl J Med 1980; 302:411.
58. Czeizel A, Metreki J. Empirical recurrence risk after unidentified multiple congenital abnormalities. J Med Genet 1983; 20:367–371.
59. Nelson LH, Bensen J, Burton BK. Outcomes in pregnancy with unusually high maternal serum α-fetoprotein levels. Am J Obstet Gynecol 1987; 157:572–576.
60. Curie-Cohen M, Luttrell L, Shapiro S. Current practice of artificial insemination by donor in the United States. N Engl J Med 1979; 300:585–590.
61. Verlinsky Y, Kuliev A. Preimplantation genetic diagnosis. In Genetic Diagnosis and the Fetus: Diagnosis, Prevention and Treatment, 3rd ed. (Milunsky A, ed). Johns Hopkins University Press, Baltimore, 1992, pp. 745–758.
62. Sutherland GR and Richards RI. Invited editorial: Anticipation legitimized: Unstable DNA to the rescue. Am J Hum Genet 1992; 51:7–9.
63. Hall JG. Genomic Imprinting: Review and relevance to human diseases. Am J Hum Genet 1990; 46:857–873.
64. Farrer LA, Cupples LA, Wiater P, Conneally PM, Gusella JF, and Myers H. The Normal Huntington Disease (HD) Allele, or a closely linked gene, influences age at onset of HD. Am J Hum Genet 1993; 53:125–130.
65. Goldfarb LG, Petersen RB, Tabaton M, Brown P, LeBlanc AC, Montagna P, Cortelli P, Julien J, Vital C, Pendelbuy WW, Haltia Autilio-Gambetti L, Gajdusek DC, Lugarsi E, and Gambetti P. Fatal familial insomnia and familial Creutzfeldt-Jakob disease: Disease phenotype determined by a DNA polymorphism. Science 1992; 258:806–808.

24

Prenatal Diagnosis in Clinical Practice

David Chitayat
The Hospital for Sick Children, Toronto, Ontario, Canada

Kathy A. Hodgkinson
The Toronto Hospitals, Toronto, Ontario, Canada

Philip R. Wyatt
*North York General Hospital and Children's Centre,
Toronto, Ontario, Canada*

Clinical Case

*A 45-year-old G1 P0 patient hesitates about undergoing amniocentesis. She
has heard that the risk of the procedure is substantial, and she does not wish
to jeopardize this long awaited pregnancy.*

INTRODUCTION

The prenatal diagnosis and treatment of both inherited and noninherited
congenital disorders has undergone significant change over the last decade.
The ability to detect developmental defects before birth allows informed
choices prior to and during a pregnancy, as well as the luxury of qualified
reassurance with negative results (especially for those at high genetic risk)
and the possibility of early treatment, either prenatally or at birth. The delivery of these services is multidisciplinary, entailing many clinical and laboratory services.

Every pregnancy has at least a 2–3% risk of producing a child with a congenital disorder. Of this group, 20% will have multiple abnormalities, of which
only 40% will have a known cause. Chromosome abnormalities account for
6%, single gene disorders, 7.5%, teratogenic exposure during pregnancy or

maternal disease, 6.5%, with the remainder considered to be multifactorial, that is, a mixture of genetic and environmental factors. The overall risk for any form of congenital disorder in any pregnancy, however, is low. To detect the majority of these disorders, invasive and noninvasive diagnostic methods have been developed. The latter include a detailed assessment of family, medical, and obstetric history, plus fetal imaging techniques (mainly ultrasound). More recently maternal serum biochemical screening has become available. Invasive techniques involve direct fetal sampling and include amniocentesis, transcervical and transabdominal chorionic villus sampling (CVS), percutaneous umbilical blood sampling (PUBS), and other fetal biopsy methods. The cells obtained are used for cytogenetic, molecular genetic, and biochemical investigations. Future avenues include preimplantation diagnosis and analysis of nucleated fetal cells in maternal blood. This chapter is an overview of the subject and briefly describes the methods used in prenatal diagnosis, the indications for each procedure, and the associated risks.

INVASIVE PRENATAL
DIAGNOSTIC PROCEDURES

The invasive testing procedures, with their associated fetal morbidity and mortality, are not clinically applicable for most pregnant women. The indications for their use are outlined in Table 1.

Increased Risk for Fetal Chromosome
Abnormality or Single Gene Disorders
Diagnosable Cytogenetically

This is the most common indication for prenatal testing. The procedures used to obtain fetal cells are amniocentesis, CVS, and PUBS. Cells obtained through the latter method are stimulated by phytohemoglutinin and cultured for 48–72 hours. All other methods use cell culture techniques; that is, cells are cultured in flasks or on coverslips in appropriate growth media until a sufficient amount of material is available to harvest. Routine cytogenetic techniques are then applied, and a fetal karyotype is obtained (1). More recently the detection of chromosomal aneuploidy in interphase cells using fluorescent in situ hybridization techniques (with cloned DNA from flow-sorted human chromosomes as a probe) has become routine in some centers (2).

The association of fetal chromosome aneuploidy, specifically Down's syndrome, and advanced maternal age is well established (3) (Tables 2 and 3). Since most pregnancies occur in younger women (in their second and third

Table 1 Indications for Invasive Prenatal Diagnosis

1. *Cytogenetic analysis*
Techniques: CVS, amniocentesis, PUBS, rarely direct biopsy
Considerations
  Maternal age
  Abnormal maternal serum markers (AFP, hCG, uE3)
  Previous child with a chromosome abnormality
  Parental chromosome rearrangement
  Ultrasound abnormality
  Single gene disorder with an identifiable chromosome abnormality
  Sex determination in X-linked disorders
  Parental exposure to therapeutic irradiation
2. *DNA analysis* (direct gene analysis or linked markers)
Techniques: CVS, amniocentesis, rarely PUBS
Considerations
  Autosomal recessive conditions
  Autosomal dominant conditions
  Sex-linked conditions
3. *Biochemical/histopathological analysis*
Techniques: CVS, amniocentesis, direct fetal biopsy
For single gene disorders
4. *As a result of biochemical screening*
Techniques: amniocentesis, PUBS
Considerations
  Raised MSAFP maternal serum α-fetoprotein
  Low maternal serum α-fetoprotein
  Abnormal triple screen

Table 2 Comparison of CVS and Amniocentesis

	CVS	Amniocentesis
Total risk of miscarriage	Approx. 5% (after 10 weeks)	Approx. 3% (after 16 weeks)
Risk of miscarriage due to procedure	approx. 1%	Approx. 0.5%
Chance of obtaining result	96%	99%
Time for chromosome result	3–4 weeks	3–4 weeks
Accuracy of chromosome diagnosis	Highly accurate	Highly accurate
Detection of spina bifida	No	Yes

Table 3   Risks of Down's Syndrome and All Chromosome Abnormalities with Maternal Age

Maternal age at delivery	Risk of Down's syndrome	Risk of all chromosome abnormalities
25	1/1270	1/480
30	1/970	1/390
35	1/330	1/180
36	1/255	1/150
37	1/205	1/125
38	1/155	1/100
39	1/125	1/80
40	1/95	1/65
41	1/73	1/50
42	1/55	1/40
43	1/45	1/30
44	1/35	1/24
45	1/28	1/19

decades) only 30% of all chromosomally abnormal babies are born to women above the age of 35. To detect all cases, invasive procedures would have to be offered to all pregnant women. Because these diagnostic measures are expensive and have an element of risk, however, they are usually offered to women with a risk of having a chromosomally abnormal fetus greater than 1/200. Generally this applies to women of 35 and above, although the newer screening methods may change this.

Prenatal diagnosis is offered to mothers who have had a child (live born or stillborn) with a chromosomal aneuploidy. For women under 30 the risk of a second event is about 1 in 100. The same risk probably applies to women between 31 and 35 years old. For women above the age of 35, the risk remains at their age-related risk. When the aneuploidy involves the sex chromosomes, the recurrence risk is considered to be negligible (4). It is interesting to note that an aneuploid spontaneous abortion (miscarriage) is not associated with an increased risk (5). Since about half of all recognized losses in the first trimester of pregnancy are chromosomally abnormal (6), this is an important consideration.

Couples in which one member is a carrier of a significant chromosome rearrangement are at high risk of having a chromosomally unbalanced child. The actual risk depends on the chromosomes involved, the type of rearrangement, whether it is maternally or paternally carried, and the mode of ascertainment of the family (7).

When fetal anomalies are detected by ultrasound, chromosome analysis is often indicated (8). Single abnormalities have an association with specific chromosome abnormalities, such as cystic hygroma (Turner's syndrome; 45,X), duodenal atresia, nuchal thickening (Down's syndrome, trisomy 21), holoprosencephaly (Patau's syndrome, trisomy 13), although none are considered to be pathognomonic. The incidence of chromosome abnormalities in fetuses with two or more defects is 10–20% (9,10).

Chromosome analysis is indicated for those at risk of having children with single gene disorders associated with increased chromosome breakage or other cytogenetic markers, including Fanconi's anemia (11), Bloom's syndrome, ataxia telangiectasia (12), xeroderma pigmentosum, and Roberts' syndrome (13).

Sex determination for X-linked conditions not diagnosable by molecular techniques may still occur, although for many of these, the gene responsible is cloned, and direct DNA analysis available.

When either member of a couple has had therapeutic levels of radiation or cytotoxic drugs in the months prior to conception, amniocentesis may be warranted.

Increased Risk for Single Gene Disorders Diagnosable by DNA Analysis

Any fetal sampling technique may be used. Many dominant, recessive, and X-linked disorders can now be prenatally diagnosed using either linked DNA markers, intragenic probes, or direct gene analysis. Historically, individuals from such families had to accept their a priori risk of transmission of a disorder, although sex determination by chromosome analysis for families with X-linked conditions has been available for some time. Often family studies are required for ascertainment of phase of the disease with linked markers, and in such cases the accuracy of diagnosis is limited. The fetus is placed at either high or low risk of having inherited the "at-risk" chromosome. Increasingly the genes themselves are cloned and the mutations identified, which allows for direct gene analysis with no necessity for family studies and linked markers. In some instances the result can provide prognostic information (14), while in other cases the prognostic indications are of value within families rather than between families (15). For those with an a priori pedigree risk of between 25 and 50%, the advent of this technology has meant the possibility of having disease-free children. In all cases however, the sequela to a positive result is for the pregnancy to be terminated (if desired by the parents), and recent impetus has been toward preimplantation diagnosis (16). This technique uses a single cell obtained by biopsy of a fertilized egg, obtained through in vitro fertilization (IVF) at the eight-cell stage. The DNA contained within the cell is amplified using polymerase chain reaction (PCR) (17). Both sex determination and the successful diagnosis of cystic fibrosis have been reported (18,19).

Increased Risk for Single Gene Disorders Not Diagnosable by DNA Analysis

The diagnosis of many inborn errors of metabolism relies on biochemical studies of the cell-free amniotic fluid or of the cells themselves. Tay-Sachs disease and mucopolysaccharidosis are two conditions diagnosable in this way (20). Prior to the advent of DNA analysis for cystic fibrosis, microvillar intestinal enzymes were measured in the amniotic fluid (21). Histopathological studies of amniocytes can also be used in the diagnosis of neuronal ceroid lipofuscinosis (22) and mucolipidosis IV (23).

Increased Risk for Fetal Abnormalities Associated with Maternal Serum Screening

In cases of high maternal serum α-fetoprotein (MSAFP), the increased risk of having a child with a neural tube defect (NTD), ventral wall defect (VWD), Finnish-type congenital nephrosis (24,25), or other problem warrants further investigation. Both ultrasonography and analysis of acetylcholinesterase in amniotic fluid refine the risk. For low MSAFP, the risk of Down's syndrome increases. This risk is refined further by other biochemical markers. (See "Biochemical Screening for Down's Syndrome.")

METHODS OF PRENATAL DIAGNOSIS

Amniocentesis

The aspiration of amniotic fluid from the amniotic cavity continues to be the most widely used procedure in prenatal diagnosis. It was performed as a technique for the management of oligohydramnios as long ago as the eighteenth century (26,27) but did not gain wide acceptance until the mid-19th century when it was successfully used in the management of erythroblastosis fetalis (28). The diagnosis of metabolic disorders became possible (29, 30), and in 1966 Steele and Berg (31) successfully cultured and karyotyped amniotic fluid cells, leading to the first antenatal diagnosis of Down's syndrome (32).

Midtrimester Amniocentesis

Midtrimester amniocentesis is carried out at 15–17 weeks gestation. Gestational age is confirmed by ultrasound (measuring the fetal biparietal diameter and femur length), which also determines zygosity, placental position, cardiac activity, structural normality of the fetus, and the optimal position for needle insertion. Once determined, a 20 gage (or smaller) spinal needle is inserted transabdominally into the uterine cavity, through which a 10–20 mL sample of amniotic fluid is drawn (Fig. 1). Some centers infiltrate the subcutaneous area with lidocaine prior to needle insertion, although this is not considered necessary. The first few milliliters of the sample are discarded to minimize maternal cell contamination, after which the greater part of the sample is used for cell culture. A small amount of cell-free amniotic fluid is used to determine the α-fetoprotein (AFP) levels, and when indicated acetyl-cholinesterase (AChE) is assayed. Failure to obtain amniotic fluid rarely occurs, although historically, before the availability of ultrasound, it was common (33).

Amniotic fluid cells are heterogeneous and derive from fetal skin, the inner epithelial surfaces of the respiratory and genitourinary tracts, and the uterine membranes. They can be used for biochemical and molecular genetic studies in addition to the more usual cytogenetic studies. Culture time varies considerably, depending on the type and number of viable cells and other less easily classifiable variables. Most centers have results in less than 4 weeks. Culture failure is rare, and maternal cell contamination is considered to be less than 0.5% (34).

As with all invasive prenatal testing, there is compromise between obtaining accurate information and possibly harming an otherwise normal fetus. The impetus over the last three decades has been to assess the possible disadvantages

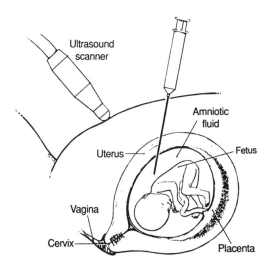

Figure 1 Amniocentesis.

of each method to both the fetus and the mother. There is still uncertainty about the exact fetal loss rate due to amniocentesis. The background rate, however, is well established (35); it bears some relation to the number of needle insertions (36), with two attempts to obtain fluid at any one procedure being the recommended maximum. Although the figure quoted for fetal loss above the background rate is 1 in 200 (0.5%) (36,37), the actual risk is difficult to ascertain and may be lower (38). Fetal trauma is rare, and maternal risks are negligible.

The timing of the procedure and the cell culture requirements mean that chromosome results are not available much before 19 weeks of pregnancy. For a couple found to have an abnormal fetus, the emotional burden is large. In addition, there is an increase in morbidity and mortality associated with later pregnancy termination. The need for earlier prenatal diagnosis led to the development of CVS and early amniocentesis as alternative methods. Both procedures became possible as fetal imaging technology improved.

Early Amniocentesis

The smaller volume of amniotic fluid found in earlier pregnancy was thought to contraindicate this type of sampling. At 10-11 weeks there is 30-40 mL, which increases to 50-100 mL between weeks 12 and 14, with a volume of approximately 200 mL at 16 weeks (39). Since 1987, however, some centers have been offering amniocentesis prior to 15 weeks gestation (40,41). The procedure is the same as described for midtrimester amniocentesis, although less amniotic fluid is drawn. About 1 mL of fluid per week of gestation is considered a rule of thumb. Culture success rate is high (42), and fetal loss rate is similar in magnitude to other procedures at the same gestational age. Concern exists regarding the proportion of amniotic fluid removed in early gestation as a function of the total volume; concerns regarding possible positional, neurodevelopmental, or respiratory effects previously raised with midtrimester amniocentesis (43) are unresolved. So far there has been no reported randomized study comparing early amniocentesis to midtrimester amniocentesis and CVS in terms of fetal loss and morbidity.

Chorionic Villus Sampling (CVS)

Chorionic villus sampling [the removal of a sample of chorionic (placental) tissue as a source of fetal cells] developed in response to the limitations of midtrimester amniocentesis. First suggested in the late 1960s (44), this technique was overshadowed in the 1970s by amniocentesis. With the advent of molecular genetic technology, and the possibility of prenatally diagnosing genetic disorders with small amounts of tissue, interest in CVS resurfaced, and in the early 1980s the technique was refined and came into more general usage (45,46).

The technique relies on the biopsy of rapidly dividing cells in the first trimester. At 7–10 weeks postconception (9–12 weeks from the last menstrual period) the gestational sac does not yet fill the uterine cavity. The chorion surrounding the gestational sac is differentiated into the chorion laeve (smooth), which faces the uterine cavity and later degenerates and attaches to the uterine wall, and the chorion frondosum, which is attached to the uterine wall that forms the future placenta and contains rapidly dividing cells.

The transcervical method uses the space within the uterine cavity that is not filled by the gestational sac and is accessible by catheterization through the cervix into the chorion frondosum (Fig. 2). Before sampling, the positions of the gestational sac and the placenta are determined by ultrasonography. Gestational age is assessed and if necessary the procedure rescheduled. In older mothers especially, a discrepancy between dates and scan measurements may indicate an impending miscarriage. Once the chorion frondosum has been recognized, a flexible catheter with a metal obturator is inserted under continuous ultrasound guidance. The metal obturator is removed, and a 20 mL syringe containing media is attached. A negative suction is applied together with to and fro movements of the catheter, followed by withdrawal. The tissue is immediately assessed microscopically; usually 10–25 mg is obtained. If the first attempt fails to obtain sufficient tissue, up to three attempts (each with a new catheter) may be performed, although the

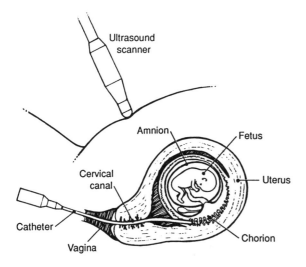

Figure 2 Transcervical chorionic villus sampling.

risk of miscarriage appears to increase proportionally with each attempt after the first (47). Often the choice of method is determined as much by practitioner preference as by clinical necessity. However, genital herpes, cervical polyps, infection, uterine abnormalities, or a pregnancy greater than 12 weeks gestation will render the transabdominal approach the one of choice. As with all methods described, ultrasound evaluation is required before and during the procedure. The transabdominal procedure most commonly used follows that of Brambati and colleagues (48) in which an 18–20 gage needle is introduced through the maternal abdomen and uterine wall into the placenta. Negative suction is applied to the syringe with simultaneous movement of the needle tip. The advantage of this method over the one described earlier is that it can be performed at any stage of pregnancy if the placenta is in an accessible position. When obtaining fetal cells by any other method is difficult, this may be an option.

Complications related to the procedure are reported. Vaginal bleeding occurs in 15–20% of women after transcervical CVS, while this finding is rare (< 1%) in transabdominal CVS. The report of two life-threatening infections after transcervical CVS (49,50) led to the recommendation that a new catheter be used for each insertion. The overall incidence of chorioamnionitis after transcervical CVS, however, is 0.2% or less (51). Rupture of the membranes is a rare complication with an incidence of 0.3% (52). The realization that MSAFP was elevated in the majority of women post-CVS (regardless of method) led to the recommendation that every nonsensitized Rh-negative woman undergoing CVS (and every invasive prenatal procedure) be given anti-D immunoglobulin. CVS in Rh-negative sensitized women is contraindicated (53).

Chorionic villi contain a mesenchymal core, a cytotrophoblast layer, and an outer single-layer syncytiotrophoblast. Cells from all layers are used for extraction of DNA for molecular analysis, whereas cytogenetics uses cells from the cytotrophoblast and the mesenchymal core. The cytotrophoblast contains dividing cells, which are used for direct analysis; the results usually are available within days. The mesenchymal core cells are cultured, with results usually available within 2–3 weeks.

Initial concern with CVS focused on maternal cell contamination. The acquisition of experience in dissociating maternal tissue from fetal tissue has lessened this problem; other problems, however, became apparent. Obtaining earlier results was an advance over amniocentesis, but discrepancies were noted between results obtained through direct analysis and those obtained through long-term CVS culture, or amniocentesis or after birth. This, in addition to the poorer quality of direct preparations, led many centers to stop direct analysis. This approach should be considered, however, if a chromosome aneuploidy is suspected on the basis of fetal ultrasound findings.

Mosaicism (i.e., the presence of two or more cell lines in the same tissue) has been reported in most large CVS studies. It is found twice as frequently in direct versus cultured preparations and is considered to have an incidence of between 0.6% and 1.0%. In about 75% of the cases the mosaicism is confined to the placenta (47,54). Confined placental mosaicism is associated with intrauterine growth retardation and perinatal complications (55,56), probably as a result of placental dysfunction. When mosaicism is found at CVS, a follow-up amniocentesis is usually recommended. The addition of this second invasive procedure is not thought to increase the risk of fetal loss (57). If the mosaicism involves a chromosome complement not known to result in a live-born child, a detailed fetal ultrasound examination may be sufficient. In all cases the possibility of failure to detect uniparental disomy (a rare but reported complication) during follow-up screening should be considered (58).

Whether CVS places the fetus at higher risk than other sampling methods has been the subject of much debate. Randomized multicenter trials comparing CVS with midtrimester amniocentesis found little difference with a figure from the Canadian study of 0.8% higher fetal loss rate after transcervical CVS than after amniocentesis (54). The Medical Research Council (MRC) European study (59) projected a grimmer prognosis, but the study was confounded. More recent controversy surrounds the issue of fetal damage with the report from the Oxford group (60) of an association between limb reduction defects and early (< 10 weeks gestation) CVS. Subsequent reports (61,62) seemed to confirm the finding. However the World Health Organization (63) concluded that in centers with extensive experience, the rate of limb reduction defects following CVS was similar to that in the general population (6.0/10,000 vs. 5.4/10,000, respectively). Most cases so far reported have been with CVS performed before 9 weeks gestation. Mentioned in discussions of the possible etiology of the association have been vascular disruption, poor technique, and premature sampling, and it has been recommended that CVS be performed after 10 weeks gestation. Further studies are required to determine accurate risks to the fetus.

Percutaneous Umbilical Blood Sampling (PUBS)

Fetal blood sampling is used for both diagnostic and therapeutic purposes. Initially the procedure was performed by fetoscopy and the fetal loss reported as 3–7% (64). Fetoscopy, however, has been replaced by the safer ultrasound-guided transabdominal needle puncture of the cord insertion known as cordocentesis or PUBS. Other sources of fetal blood include the heart (cardiac ventricles) and intrahepatic veins (65). As with all sampling techniques, an ultrasound evaluation of the fetus and uterus is a mandatory prelude to the invasive act.

The procedure is performed by the insertion of a 20–25 gage spinal needle through the maternal abdominal wall, and the uterine wall, and into the umbilical artery, 2–3 cm from the placental insertion site; 1–5 mL of blood is removed. Other sites are directly sampled. It is important to always confirm that fetal blood has been aspirated (66).

Unlike amniotic fluid cells, stimulated cultured lymphocytes can provide chromosome results within days. PUBS is indicated therefore when abnormalities detected by ultrasonography indicate a possible chromosome problem, both when termination is still an option and prior to delivery, for obstetric guidance regarding the management. It may also be indicated when mosaicism or pseudomosaicism is detected by amniocentesis or CVS.

Intrauterine infections (such as toxoplasmosis and rubella) have been diagnosed using fetal blood (67,68), as have several hematological disorders, including the hemoglobinopathies, hemophilia, and familial combined immune deficiency disorders (69). Many are now amenable to DNA diagnosis using other sampling methods. The diagnosis of Rhesus disease and the measurement of acid-base balance in cases with symmetric intrauterine growth retardation (70) are clinical indications for the use of PUBS.

Although PUBS is considered to be a higher risk procedure than other methods at gestations under 20 weeks, with a fetal loss rate of 5% at 12–18 weeks gestation versus 2.5% at 19–21 weeks (71), the risks compared to the benefits are considered to be low.

Other Fetal Tissue Sampling Techniques

Skin biopsies are indicated for the prenatal diagnosis of inherited congenital skin disorders, which include epidermolysis bullosa lethalis (72), epidermolysis bullosa dystrophica (73), epidermolytic hyperkeratosis (74), and harloquin ichthyosis (75). Liver biopsies can diagnose rare inherited metabolic disorders in which the enzyme is formed only in the liver, including ornithine carbamyl transferase deficiency, carbamyl phosphate synthetase deficiency, and glucose-6-phosphatase and alanine glyoxalate aminotransferase deficiency (76). Biopsies of samples from other organs, such as lungs, kidneys, and muscle (77), have been performed for prenatal diagnosis of disorders detectable histopathologically.

NONINVASIVE PRENATAL TECHNIQUES

The most widely used technique for assessing fetal well-being for most pregnant women is ultrasound examination. Other techniques for visualizing fetal structure are x-rays, magnetic resonance imaging (MRI), and echoplanar imaging (EPI).

Fetal Ultrasonography

Obstetric ultrasound imaging involves transmitting sound waves with a frequency between 2 and 7.5 MHz into the pregnant abdomen and recording the echoes from the tissues in the path of the beam. This allows analysis of fetal structure. The lower frequencies have greater penetration, whereas the higher frequencies allow for better resolution of the image.

Ultrasound has been used as a technique in obstetrics since the early 1960s. Initially the pictures were static and fuzzy, but the development of grayscale ultrasonography and real-time imaging in the last 20 years has markedly increased our ability to identify fetal abnormalities. An ultrasound examination may be performed at any point in gestation. In the first trimester it is used to assess viability of the pregnancy and to determine gestational age (by measuring crown-rump length). Later in pregnancy fetal structure may be examined more closely. The American College of Obstetrics and Gynecology, therefore, has addressed the issue of different levels of fetal ultrasound examination (78) and suggested a basic and a targeted level, as well as minimal requirements for each. The basic examination, which is considered to be appropriate for routine obstetric patients, includes determination of gestational age (using at least two parameters), zygosity, viability and presentation, placental localization, and amniotic fluid volume. The fetal head and spine, four-chamber heart, gastrointestinal tract, kidney and bladder, umbilical cord insertion, extremities, and genitalia should be adequately visualized and assessed. The delineation of abnormalities detected on a basic ultrasound resembles the post-natal physical examination; most are unexpected. Once an abnormality has been detected, however, a targeted fetal ultrasound examination is recommended. Other indications (among many) include maternal diabetes mellitus [with an increased risk of NTD, congenital heart defect (CHD), and sacral agenesis], maternal systemic lupus erythematosus (congenital heart block), and maternal myasthenia gravis (arthrogryposis). Exposure to potential teratogens such as antiepileptic medications (an increased risk for NTD) or vitamin A congeners (hydrocephaly, microcephaly, and cardiac defect) would warrant further investigation. In all cases a detailed family and pregnancy history is invaluable in determining pertinent risks.

The technique is not perfect. Even with modern high resolution equipment and experienced operators, abnormalities may be missed. Technical difficulties such as maternal obesity or oligohydramnios may hamper diagnostic ability. In addition, variations in structure may be seen about which little is known, and both diagnostic and prognostic information will be difficult to assess.

The ability to detect subtle findings on fetal ultrasound (79) coupled with the fact that most women have at least one such examination during a pregnancy led to the suggestion of using ultrasound as a screening test for Down's syndrome. A relationship between shortened femurs and Down's syndrome is known (80–82). Other features include nuchal folds, hypoplastic middle phalanx of the fifth digit, cardiac defects (83), mild dilatation of the cerebral ventricles, and hyperechogenic bowel (84). Detection of up to 75% of fetuses with Down's syndrome may be possible (85).

Ultrasound is both a diagnostic and a screening test; in the latter mode, it detects individuals in an otherwise normal population who are at higher risk, hence are then offered further investigations. In the former it diagnoses fetal abnormality directly.

SCREENING METHODS IN PRENATAL DIAGNOSIS

Screening for Neural Tube Defects (NTDs)

Biochemical screening for open neural tube defects (ONTDs) between 16 and 18 weeks of gestation has been available since the 1970s. The screening test ascertains the level of AFP in the maternal serum. With improvements in ultrasonography, severe ONTDs are often diagnosed directly, with anencephaly almost always diagnosed before 16 weeks.

AFP is a glycoprotein found in high concentrations in fetal serum and consequently in amniotic fluid through fetal urination. It is synthesized initially by the yolk sac, then by the fetal liver and gastrointestinal tract. Peak concentrations of amniotic fluid AFP (AFAFP) occur at 12–14 weeks gestation, then steadily decline. Levels of AFP in maternal serum are an order of magnitude lower. The interchange between mother and fetus probably occurs directly via the placenta, and indirectly via the amniotic fluid and the fetal membranes.

The association between raised AFAFP and NTDs was reported in the early 1970s (86) when stored amniotic fluid samples from NTD pregnancies were retrospectively studied and found to have levels of AFP far in excess of normal levels. The increase is assumed to be due to leakage of AFP from fetal sera or cerebrospinal fluid. Since leakage will occur from other anatomical defects, AFP levels are not specific for NTDs. The introduction in the late 1970s of both a quantitative and a qualitative assay for acetylcholinesterase (AchE), an enzyme synthesized in the central nervous system (CNS) and present in the cerebrospinal fluid (CSF), was an improvement (87,88). The leakage of CSF into the amniotic fluid when there is an ONTD results in a marked rise in AChE levels. The assessment of AChE uses the qualitative method of polyacrylomide gel electrophoresis (PAGE), where fluid from unaffected pregnancies produces a single band of pseudocholinesterase, whereas ONTDs have a faster second band of AChE. A second band is not specific for NTDs and can also be present with ventral wall defects. AChE is not present in cases of high AFP related to congenital nephrosis, an autosomal recessive condition prevalent in the Finnish population. False positives can occur with either assay if fetal blood is present in the sample. If in doubt, a Kleihauer-Betke test should be applied.

The detection of open NTDs by measuring AFP and AChE in amniotic fluid was an improvement; it related, however, to a small subsection of the population undergoing amniocentesis. The use of MSAFP allowed for all pregnant women to be screened. However, unlike AFAFP there is considerable overlap between normal and abnormal pregnancies; at between 16 and 18 weeks the separation of the two distributions is most distinct, although the remaining overlap makes optimum cutoff levels difficult to ascertain. The final value is ultimately a compromise between ascertaining all abnormals and subjecting too many women to invasive tests, with consequent risks, as well as costs to the care providers. A cutoff level of 2.5 multiples of the median (MoMs) of MSAFP is used, which is considered to have a pickup rate of approximately 75% of ONTDs and about 3% false positives (89). It will not pick up all ONTDs or ventral wall defects, since by definition it is a screening test.

Causes other than an anatomical defect resulting in leakage of AFP into the amniotic fluid are known to cause a rise in MSAFP. These include incorrect gestation at the time of sampling (as the normal values are gestation based), multiple pregnancy, conditions that cause oligohydramnios (renal agenesis and urethral obstruction), conditions that interfere with kidney resorption [congenital nephrosis (24,90), polycystic kidneys], and fetal death, with its consequent autolysis of tissues. If the MSAFP is raised for no apparent reason, there is an associated high risk of fetal death, intrauterine growth retardation (IUGR), and prematurity (91). Syndromes associated with NTDs or VWDs may be detected, and it is thought that the risk of having a significant chromosome abnormality following a raised MSAFP in the second trimester is in the region of 1% (92,93). The high concentration gradient between amniotic fluid and maternal serum means that any placental abnormalities (e.g., an intrauterine infection or maternal lupus anticoagulant) may result in a rise in MSAFP (94). Other findings linked to raised MSAFP include fetal cardiovascular defects (95), maternal hepatic tumor, ovarian cysts, and prior fetal reduction. Whatever the cause, a raised MSAFP should prompt further investigation. If no obvious cause is ascertained, regular surveillance of the pregnancy should occur, and amniocentesis should be considered.

Screening for Down's Syndrome

Prior to the possibility of screening for defects by ultrasound, the only marker for Down's syndrome was maternal age. The majority of Down's syndrome babies therefore remained undetected, and a large number of invasive tests were performed unnecessarily. With the introduction of midtrimester MSAFP screening for NTDs came the unexpected correlation between low levels of AFP and Down's syndrome pregnancies (96). Subsequently other maternal serum markers were found to be associated with an increased risk for Down's syndrome. These include human chorionic gonadotrophin (97), unconjugated estriol (98), pregnancy-specific β_1-glycoprotein (99), and urea-resistant neutrophil alkaline phosphatase (100). The latter, which is considered to be the single most effective marker for the detection of Down's syndrome, assesses the staining of cytoplasmic granules in neutrophils. The technique is both labor intensive and subjective, and it was not used as a routine screening test at the time of writing. The four principal markers used in most screening programs are maternal age, α-fetoprotein (AFP), unconjugated estriol (uE3), and human chorionic gonadotropin (hCG).

Pilot studies using MSAFP alone for the detection of Down's syndrome among women younger than 35 years of age revealed that 26% of the incidences of Down's syndrome expected were detected, compared to 10–20% detected by fetal karyotyping in women 35 years or older (101). In a Canadian study the mean second-trimester MSAFP level found in pregnancies that resulted in a Down's syndrome baby was 0.79 MoM.

Estriol is a steroid hormone, produced by the syncytiotrophoblast from fetal precursors. The fetal liver produces dehydroepiandrosteronesulfate (DHEAS), which is converted to 16α-OH-DHEAS. The sulfate is deconjugated by sulfatase in the placenta and forms unconjugated estriol. The presence of estriol in the maternal serum was found to be discriminatory for Down's syndrome, with a geometric mean for affected pregnancies of 0.73 MoM, a concentration 25% lower than normal.

Human chorionic gonadotropin is a glycoprotein hormone consisting of an α and a β subunit. The α subunit is identical to the α subunit of lutinizing hormone, follicle stimulating hormone, and thyrotropin stimulating hormone; its specificity is determined by its unique β subunit. Excreted by the syncytiotrophoblast, hCG appears in the maternal circulation shortly after implantation. It rises rapidly to a peak at 9–10 weeks gestation, after which it declines steadily to a plateau at 18 weeks, where it remains until delivery. Both retrospective and prospective studies have shown a strong correlation between elevated midtrimester hCG and Down's syndrome. Median hCG maternal serum values from Down's syndrome pregnancies between 15 and 19 weeks gestation were above the 95th percentile compared to unaffected pregnancies. In a retrospective study, 64% of Down's syndrome pregnancies were detected on the basis of a single hCG assay (97). Prospective studies confirmed results and showed that the average maternal serum concentration of hCG was at least twice that of normal pregnancies (102). Interestingly, a low midtrimester MS-hCG was found to be associated with trisomy 18 pregnancies (103) and was used in the detection of this anomaly (104).

In a prospective study using all three maternal serum markers in combination with maternal age, more than 60% of Down's syndrome fetuses were detected with a false-positive rate of 5% (102). When all three biochemical markers were low, the detection of fetuses with trisomy 18 was as high as 80%. Confounders exist that render the test less efficient. An inaccurate gestational age will skew the results, for example, because the normal levels are gestation based. Maternal obesity decreases the concentration of all three serum markers, as does insulin-dependent diabetes mellitus, whereas twin pregnancies increase the levels. A correction factor exists for the latter two scenarios (105,106). Smoking in pregnancy increases MSAFP levels, while reducing both hCG and uE3 (107). An adjustment factor is not considered necessary.

Many say that serum screening for Down's syndrome should be carried out on women regardless of age and believe that the automatic offer of invasive procedures to all women above the age of 35 should be rescinded. Thus women previously assigned high risk might avoid invasive testing and its inherent risks. Meanwhile the refining of screening tests continues.

The possibility of isolating fetal cells from the maternal serum and using them as a source of tissue for prenatal testing was first suggested in 1969 (108), when lymphocytes in the maternal serum were detected containing a Y chromosome from a male fetus. Subsequent reports however failed to consolidate the findings (109,110). The PCR technique revived interest in the possibility of assessing small amounts of fetal cells in maternal blood and has been used successfully in the detection of fetal sex (111). The amount of fetal blood that must be present in the maternal circulation to permit detection, the type of fetal cells, and the optimum time of gestation for testing are questions that have been addressed by several authors (112,113).

SUMMARY

This chapter has focused on techniques and methods used in prenatal diagnosis; other facets (such as sequelae to an abnormal result, fetal therapy, and legal and ethical aspects) are covered by cited references in the bibliography. The discpline itself is relatively new in medicine, and the issues increase in complexity as more tests become available. Concerns exist regarding the provision of services and the availability of accurate counseling. The techniques alone cannot replace accurate risk estimation based on family history and ethnic background, nor can they deal with the complexity of the decision-making process in which couples are often involved.

The Royal College of Physicians in London in 1989 attempted to address the issues and recommended that both genetic screening and prenatal diagnosis be recognized as intrinsic components of maternal and child health services. The report stated:

> While prenatal tests should not be pressed upon everyone, they should be made available, even to women who are completely opposed to abortion, since testing may provide welcome reassurance, or an informed choice to care for a child with a known handicap, or allow the option of abortion to be reconsidered on the basis of known facts (114).

Whatever the future holds, the push for earlier and safer noninvasive methods of prenatal diagnosis, and the debate surrounding the efficient assessment of the unborn, will continue.

Answer

At age 45 the risk for Down's syndrome is around 4%. The risk for loss of pregnancy is less than 0.5%. Among other points, you may choose to discuss whether the patient wishes to continue her pregnancy if Down's syndrome is detected.

REFERENCES

1. Barch MJ, ed. ACT Cytogenetics Laboratory Manual, 2nd ed. Rowan Press, New York, 1991.
2. Jauch A, Daumer C, Lichter P, Murken J, Schroeder-Kurth TM, Cremer T. Chromosomal in situ suppression hybridization of human gonosomes and autosomes in its use in clinical cytogenetics. Hum Genet 1990; 85:145–150.
3. Hook EB. Rates of chromosome abnormalities at different maternal ages. Obstet Gynaecol 1981; 58:282–285.
4. Harper PS. Practical Genetic Counselling, 3rd ed. Butterworth and Heinemann, London, 1988.
5. Warburton D, Kline J, Stein Z, Hutzler M, Chin A, Hassold T. Does the karyotype of a spontaneous abortion predict the karyotype of a subsequent abortion? Evidence from 273 women with two karyotyped spontaneous abortions. Am J Hum Genet 1987; 41:465–483.
6. Carr DH, Gedeon M. Population cytogenetics of human abortuses. In Population Cytogenetics. Studies in Human Reproduction (Hook EB, Porter IH, eds). Academic Press, New York, 1977.
7. Daniel A, Hook EB, Wolf G. Risks of unbalanced progeny at amniocentesis to carriers to chromosome rearrangements: Data from United States and Canadian laboratories. Am J Med Genet 1989; 33:14–53.
8. Eydoux P, Choiset A, Le Porrier N, Thepot F, Szpiro-Tapia S, Alliet J, Ramond S, Viel JF, Gautier E, Morichon U, et al. Chromosomal prenatal diagnosis: Study of 936 cases of intrauterine abnormalities after ultrasound assessment. Prenatal Diagn 1989; 9:255–268.

9. Hentemann M, Rauskolb R, Ulbrich R, Bartels I. Abnormal pregnancy sonogram and chromosomal anomalies: Four years' experience with rapid karyotyping. Prenatal Diagn 1989; 9:605–612.
10. Wilson RD, Kendrick V, Wittman BK, McGillvray BC. Spontaneous abortion and pregnancy outcome after normal first-trimester ultrasound examination. Obstet Gynecol 1985; 67(suppl):352–355.
11. Auerbach AD, Sagi M, Adler BA. Fanconi anemia: Prenatal diagnosis in 30 fetuses at risk. Pediatrics 1985; 76:794–800.
12. Shaham M, Voss R, Becker Y, Yarkoni S, Ornoy A, Kohn G. Prenatal diagnosis of ataxia telangiectasia. J Pediatr 1982; 100:134–137.
13. Stanley WS, Pai GS, Horger EO III, Yan YS, McNeal KS. Incidental detection of premature centromere separation in amniocytes associated with a mild form of Roberts syndrome. Prenatal Diagn 1988; 8:565–569.
14. Sutherland GR, Richards RI. Fragile-X syndrome. In Prenatal Diagnosis and Screening (Brock DJH, Rodeck CH, Ferguson-Smith MA, eds). Churchill & Livingstone, New York, 1992, pp 393–403.
15. Hunter A, Tsilfidis C, Mettler G, Jacob P, Mahadervan M, Surh L, Korneluk R. The correlation of age of onset with CTG trinucleotide repeat amplification in myotonic dystrophy. J Med Genet 1993; 29:774–779.
16. Monk M. Preimplantation diagnosis – A comprehensive review. In Prenatal Diagnosis and Screening (Brock DJH, Rodeck CH, Ferguson-Smith MA, eds). Churchill & Livingstone, New York, 1992, pp 627–638.
17. Childs B, Holtzman NA, Kazazian HH, Valle DL, eds. Molecular Genetics in Medicine: Progress in Medical Genetics, new series, Vol 7. Elsevier, New York, 1988.
18. Handyside AH, Kontogianni EH, Hardy K, Winston RML. Pregnancies from biopsied human preimplantation embryos sexed by Y-specific DNA amplification. Nature 1990; 344:768–770.
19. Handyside AH, Lesko JG, Tarin JJ, Winston RML, Hughes MR. Birth of a normal girl after in vitro fertilization and preimplantation diagnostic testing for cystic fibrosis. N Engl J Med 1992; 327:905–909.
20. Weaver DD. Catalog of Prenatally Diagnosed Conditions, 2nd ed. Johns Hopkins University Press, Baltimore, 1992.
21. Brock DJH. A comparative study of microvillar enzyme activities in the prenatal diagnosis of cystic fibrosis. Prenatal Diagn 1985; 5:129–134.
22. Conradi NG, Uvebrant P, Hokegard K-H, Wahlstrom J, Mellqvist L. First trimester diagnosis of juvenile neuronal ceroid lipofuscinosis by demonstration of fingerprint inclusions in chorionic villi. Prenatal Diagn 1989; 9:283–287.
23. Ornoy A, Arnon J, Grebner EE, Jackson LG, Bach G. Early prenatal diagnosis of mucolipidosis IV (letter). Am J Med Genet 1987; 27:983–985.
24. Seppala M, Rapola J, Karjalainen O, Huttunen MP, Ruoslahti E. Congenital nephrotic syndrome: Prenatal diagnosis and genetic counselling by estimation of amniotic fluid and maternal serum a-fetoprotein. Lancet 1976; 2:123–124.
25. Thomas RL, Blakemore KJ. Evaluation of elevations in maternal serum a-fetoprotein: A review. Obstet Gynecol Rev 1990; 45:269–283.
26. Lambl D. Ein seltener Fall von Hydramnios. Centralbl Gynekol 1881; 5:329–353.

27. Prochownick L. Beitrage zur Lehre vom Fruchtwasser und seiner Entstellung. Arch Gynekol 1877; 11:305-345.
28. Liley AW. The use of amniocentesis and fetal transfusion in erythroblastosis fetalis. Pediatrics 1965; 35:836-847.
29. Jeffcoate TNA, Fleigner JRN, Russel SN, Davis JC, Wade AP. Diagnosis of adrenogenital syndrome before birth. Lancet 1965; 2:553-555.
30. Nadler HL. Antenatal detection of hereditary disorders. Pediatrics 1968; 42: 912-918.
31. Steele MW and Berg WT. Chromosome analysis of human amniotic fluid cells. Lancet 1966; 1:383-385.
32. Valenti C, Schutta EJ, Kehaty T. Prenatal diagnosis of Down syndrome. Lancet 1968; 2:220.
33. Crandon AJ, Peel KR. Amniocentesis with and without ultrasound guidance. Br J Obstet Gynaecol 1979; 86:1-3.
34. Benn PA, Hsu LYF. Maternal cell contamination of amniotic fluid cell cultures. Results of a nationwide survey. Am J Med Genet 1983; 14:361-365.
35. MacKenzie WG, Holmes DS, Newton JR. Spontaneous abortion rate in ultrasonographically viable pregnancies. Obstet Gynaecol 1988; 71:81-83.
36. Simpson NE, Dallaire L, Miller JR, Siminovich L, Hamerton JL, Miller J, McKeen C. Prenatal diagnosis of genetic disease in Canada: Report of a collaborative study. Can Med Assoc J 1976; 115:739-748.
37. Hunter AGW, Thompson D, Speevak M. Midtrimester genetic amniocentesis in Eastern Ontario: A review from 1970 to 1985. J Med Genet 1987; 24:335-343.
38. Halliday JL, Lumley J, Sheffield LJ, Robinson HP, Renou P, Carlin JB. Importance of complete follow-up of spontaneous fetal loss after amniocentesis and chorion villus sampling. Lancet 1992; 340:886-890.
39. Abramovich DR. The volume of amniotic fluid and its regulating factors. In Amniotic Fluid — Research and Clinical Application, 2nd ed (Fairweather DVI, Eskes TKAB, eds). Excerpta Medica, Amsterdam, pp 31-49.
40. Chadefaux B, Rabier D, Dumez Y, Oury JF, Kamoun P. Eleventh week amniocentesis for prenatal diagnosis of metabolic diseases (letter). Lancet 1989; 1:849.
41. Rooney D, MacLachlan N, Smith J, Rebello MT, Loeffler FE, Beard RW, Rodeck CH, Coleman DV. Early amniocentesis: A cytogenetic evaluation. Br Med J 1989; 299:25.
42. Nevin J, Nevin NC, Dornan JC, Sim D, Armstrong MJ. Early amniocentesis: Experience of 222 consecutive patients, 1987-1988. Prenatal Diagn 1990; 10: 79-83.
43. Gilberg C, Ramussen P, Wahlstrom J. Long-term follow-up of children born after amniocentesis. Clin Genet 1982; 21:69-73.
44. Mohr J. Foetal genetic diagnosis: Development of techniques for early sampling of foetal cells. Acta Pathol Microbiol Scand 1968; 73:7377.
45. Old JM, Ward RHT, Karaguzlu F, Petru M, Modell B, Weatherall DJ. First trimester fetal diagnosis for haemoglobinopathies: Three cases. Lancet 1982; 2: 1413-1416.

46. Ward RHT, Modell B, Petrou M, Karaguzlu F, Douratsos E. Method of sampling chorionic villi in first trimester of pregnancy under guidance of real-time ultrasound. Br Med J 1986; 286:1542–1544.
47. Rhoads GG, Jackson LG, Schlesselman SE, de la Cruz FF, Desnick RJ, Golbus MS, Ledbetter DH, Lubs HA, Mahoney MJ, Pergament E, et al. The safety and efficiency of chorionic villus sampling for early prenatal diagnosis of cytogenetic abnormalities. N Engl J Med 1989; 320:609–617.
48. Brambati B, Oldrini A, Lanzani A. Transabdominal chorionic villus sampling: A freehand ultrasound-guided technique. Am J Obstet Gynecol 1987a; 157: 134–137.
49. Blakemore KJ, Mahoney MJ, Hobbins JC. Infection and chorionic villus sampling. Lancet 1985; 2:339.
50. Barela A, Kleinman GE, Golditch IM, Menke DJ, Hogge WA, Golbus MS. Septic shock with renal failure after chorionic villus sampling. Am J Obstet Gynecol 1986; 154:1100–1102.
51. Brambati B, Oldrini A, Ferrazzi E, Lanzani A. Chorionic villus biopsy: An analysis of the obstetric experience of 1000 cases. Prenatal Diagn 1987; 7:157–169.
52. Hogge WA, Schoberg SA, Golbus MS. Chorionic villus sampling: Experience of the first 1000 cases. Am J Obstet Gynecol 1986; 154:1249–1252.
53. Moise KJ, Carpenter RJ, Wapner RJ, Shah DM, Boehm FM. Increased severity of fetal hemolytic disease with known Rhesus alloimmunization after first trimester transcervical chorionic villus biopsy. Fetal Diagn Ther 1990; 5:76–78.
54. Canadian Collaborative CVS-Amniocentesis Clinical Trial Group. Multicentre randomized clinical trial of chorion villus sampling and amniocentesis. Lancet 1989; 1:1–6.
55. Kalousek D, Dill F. Chromosomal mosaicism confined to the placenta in human conceptions. Science 1983; 221:665–667.
56. Johnson A, Wapner RJ, Davis GH, Jackson LG. Mosaicism in chroionic villus sampling: An association with poor perinatal outcome. Obstet Gynecol 1990; 75:573–577.
57. Brandenburg H, Jahoda MGJ, Pijpers L, Reuss A, Kleyer WJ, Wladimiroff JW. Fetal loss rate after chorionic villus sampling and subsequent amniocentesis. Am J Med Genet 1990; 35:178–180.
58. Cassidy SB, Li-Wen L, Erickson RP, Magnuson L, Thomas E, Gendron R, Herrmann J. Trisomy 15 with loss of the paternal 15 as a cause of Prader-Willi syndrome due to maternal disomy. Am J Hum Genet 1992; 51:701–708.
59. MRC European Trial of Chorionic Villus Sampling. Lancet 1991; 337:1491–1496.
60. Firth HV, Boyd PA, Chamberlain P, MacKenzie IZ, Lindenbaum RH, Husan SM. Severe limb abnormalities after chorion villus sampling at 56–66 days gestation. Lancet 1991; 337:726–763.
61. Mastroiacovo P, Cavalcanti DP. Limb-reduction defects in chorionic villus sampling. Lancet 1991; 337:1091.
62. Burton BK, Schultz CJ, Burd LI. Limb anomalies associated with chorionic villus sampling. Obstet Gynecol 1992; 79:726–730.

63. World Health Organization. Risk Evaluation of CVS. Copenhagen, WHO/ EURO, 1992.
64. Special report. The status of fetoscopy and fetal tissue sampling. Prenatal Diagn 1984; 5:93–105.
65. Nicolini U, Nicolaidis P, Fisk NM, Tannirandorn Y, Rodeck CH. Fetal blood sampling from the intrahepatic vein: Analysis of safety and clinical experience with 214 procedures. Obstet Gynecol 1990b; 76:47–53.
66. Forestier F, Cox WL, Daffos F, Rainaut M. The assessment of fetal blood samples. Am J Obstet Gynecol 1988; 158:1184–1188.
67. Daffos F, Forestier F, Capella-Pavlovsky M, Thulliez P, Aufrant C, Valenti D, Cox WZ. Prenatal management of 746 pregnancies at risk for congenital toxoplasmosis. N Engl J Med 1988; 318:271–275.
68. Lange I, Rodeck CH, Morgan-Capner P, Simmons A, Kangro HO. Prenatal serological diagnosis of intrauterine cytomegalovirus infection. Br Med J 1982; 284:1673–1674.
69. Levinsky RJ. Prenatal diagnosis of severe combined immunodeficiency. In Prenatal Diagnosis. Proceedings of the Eleventh Study Group of the Royal College of Obstetricians and Gynecologists (Rodeck CH, Nicolaides KH, eds). RCOG, London, 1984, pp 137–146.
70. Nicolini U, Nicolaidis P, Risk NM, Vaughan JI, Fusi L, Gleeson R, Rodeck CH. Limited role of fetal blood sampling in prediction of outcome in intrauterine growth retardation. Lancet 1990; 336:768–772.
71. Orlandi F, Damiani G, Jakil C, Lauricella S, Bertolino O, Maggio A. The risks of early cordocentesis (12–21 weeks): Analysis of 500 procedures. Prenatal Diagn 1990; 10:425–428.
72. Nazzaro V, Nicolini U, De Luca L, Berti E, Caputo R. Prenatal diagnosis of junctional epidermolysis bullosa associated with pyloric stenosis. J Med Genet 1990; 27:244–248.
73. Anton-Lamprecht I, Rauskolb R, Jovanovich V, Kern B, Arnold ML, Schenck W. Prenatal diagnosis of epidermolysis bullosa dystrophica Hallopeau Siemens with electron microscopy of fetal skin. Lancet 1981; 1077–1079.
74. Golbus MS, Sagebiel RW, Filly RA, Gindhart TD, Hall JG. Prenatal diagnosis of bullous ichthyosiform erythroderma (epidermolytic hyperkeratosis) by fetal skin biopsy. N Engl J Med 1980; 302:93–95.
75. Elias J, Mazur M, Sabbagha R, Esterly J, Simpson JL. Prenatal diagnosis of harloquin ichthyosis. Clin Genet 1980; 17:275–279.
76. Golbus MS, McGonigle KF, Goldberg JD, Filly RA, Callen PW, Anderson RL. Fetal tissue sampling. The San Francisco experience with 190 pregnancies. West J Med 1989; 150:423–430.
77. Evans MI, Greb A, Kunkel LM, Sacks AJ, Johnson MP, Boehm C, Kazazian HH Jr, Hoffman EP. In utero fetal muscle biopsy for the diagnosis ofr Duchenne muscular dystrophy. Am J Obstet Gynecol 1991; 165:728–732.
78. American College of Obstetrics and Gynecology. Ultrasound in pregnancy. Technical Bulletin No 116. ACOG, 1988.
79. Whittle MJ, Gilmore DH, McNay MB. Obstetric aspects of prenatal diagnosis methods. J Inherited Metab Dis 1989; 12(suppl I):97–104.

80. Benacerraf BR, Neuberg D, Frigoletto FD. Humeral shortening in second-trimester fetuses with Down syndrome. Obstet Gynecol 1991; 77:223–227.
81. Lockwood C, Benacerraf B, Krinsky A, Blakemore K, Belanger K, Mahoney M, Hobbins J. A sonographic screening method for Down syndrome. Am J Obstet Gynecol 1987; 157:803–808.
82. Grist TM, Fuller RW, Albiez KL, Bowie JD. Femur length in the US: Prediction of trisomy 21 and other chromosomal abnormalities. Radiology 1990; 174: 837–839.
83. Fitzsimmons J, Droste S, Shepard TH, Pascoe-Mason J, Chinn A, Mack LA. Long-bone growth in fetuses with Down syndrome. Am J Obstet Gynecol 1989; 161:1174–1177.
84. Nyberg DA, Resta RG, Luthy DA, Hickok DE, Mahony BS, Hirsch JH. Prenatal sonographic findings of Down syndrome: Review of 94 cases. Obstet Gynecol 1990; 76:370–377.
85. Benacerraf BR, Gelman R, Frigoletto FD. Sonographic identification of second-trimester fetuses with Down's syndrome. N Engl J Med 1987; 317:1371–1376.
86. Brock DJH, Sutcliffe RG. Alphafetoproteins in the antenatal diagnosis of anencephaly and spina bifida. Lancet 1972; 2:197–199.
87. Chubb IW, Pilowsky PM, Springwell HJ, Pollard AC. Acetylcholinesterase in human amniotic fluid: An index of fetal neural development. Lancet 1979; 1: 688–690.
88. Smith AD, Wald NJ, Cuckle HS, Stirrat JM, Bobrow M, Lagercrantz H. Amniotic fluid acetylcholinesterase as a possible diagnostic test for neural tube defects in early pregnancy. Lancet 1979; 2:685–688.
89. Wald NJ, Cuckle HS. Biochemical screening. In Prenatal Diagnosis and Screening (Brock DJH, Rodeck CH, Ferguson-Smith MA, eds). Churchill & Livingstone, New York, 1992, pp 569ff.
90. Albright SG, Warner AA, Seeds JW, Burton BK. Congenital nephrosis as a cause of elevated α-fetoprotein. Obstet Gynaecol 1990; 76:969–971.
91. Waller DK, Lustig LS, Cunningham GC, Golbus MS, Hook EB. Second trimester maternal serum α-fetoprotein levels and the risk of subsequent fetal death. New Engl J Med 1991; 1:6–10.
92. Bixenman HA, Wagner RM, Slotnick N, Macdonald ML. Increased risk for cytogenetic abnormality in patients with elevated maternal serum α-fetoprotein, independent of open neural tube or ventral wall defects. Am J Hum Genet 1991; 49:211 (abstr).
93. King DA, Fallon L, Dorfman A, Jones SL, McCorkle RD, Schulman JD. Amniocentesis after elevated maternal serum α-fetoprotein (AFP) concentrations: Cytogenetic considerations in women under age 35. Am J Hum Genet 1991; 49: 221 (abstr).
94. Fleischer AC, Kurtz AB, Wapner RJ, Ruch D, Sachs GA, Jeanty P, Shah DM, Boehm FH. Elevated α-fetoprotein and a normal fetal sonogram: Association with placental abnormalities. AJR 1988; 150:881–883.
95. Oman-Ganes LA, Shapiro LR, Cummings KR, Lorsung EM, Fish B, Gewitz MH. Elevated maternal serum α-fetoprotein due to fetal cardiac disease. Am J Human Genet 1991; 49:227 (abstr).

96. Merkatz IR, Nitowsky HM, Macri JN, Johnson WE. An association between low maternal serum α-fetoprotein and fetal chromosome abnormalities. Am J Obstet Gynecol 1984; 148:886–894.

97. Bogart MH, Pandia MR, Jones CW. Abnormal maternal serum chorionic gonadotrophin levels in pregnancies with fetal chromosome abnormalities. Prenatal Diagn 1987; 7:623–630.

98. Canick JA, Knight GJ, Palomaki GE, Haddow JE, Cuckle HS, Wald JH. Low second trimester maternal serum unconjugated oestriol in pregnancies with Down syndrome. Br J Obstet Gynaecol 1988; 95:330–333.

99. Bartels I, Lindemann A. Maternal levels of pregnancy-specific β_1-glycoprotein (SP-1) are elevated in pregnancies affected by Down's syndrome. Hum Genet 1988; 80:46–48.

100. Cuckle HS, Wald NJ, Goodburn SF, Sneddon J, Ames JAL, Dunn SC. Measurement of activity of urea-resistant neutrophil alkaline phosphatase as an antenatal screening test for Down's syndrome. Br Med J 1990; 301:1024–1026.

101. DiMaio MS, Baumgarten A, Greenstein RM, Saal HM, Mahoney MJ. Screening for fetal Down's syndrome in pregnancy by measuring serum α-fetoprotein levels. N Engl J Med 1987; 317:342–346.

102. Muller F, Boue A. A single chorionic gonadotropin assay of maternal screening for Down's syndrome. Prenatal Diagn 1990; 10:389–398.

103. Barkai G, Chaki R, Sochat M, Goldman B. Human chorionic gonadotropin and trisomy 18. Am J Med Genet 1991; 41:52–53.

104. Haddow JE, Palomaki GE, Knight GJ, Williams J, Pulkkinen A, Canick JA, Saller DN Jr, Bowers GB. Prenatal screening for Down's syndrome with use of maternal serum markers. N Engl J Med 1992; 327:588–593.

105. Wald NJ, Cuckle HS, Wu T, George L. Maternal serum unconjugated oestriol and human gonadotrophin levels in twin pregnancies; implications for screening for Down's syndrome. Br J Obstet Gynaecol 1991; 98:905–908.

106. Wald NJ, Cuckle HS, Densem JW, Stone RW. Maternal serum unconjugated oestriol and human chorionic gonadotropin in pregnancies with insulin-dependent diabetes: Implications for Down's syndrome screening. Br J Obstet Gynaecol 1992; 99:51–53.

107. Bernstein L, Pike MC, Lobo RA, Depue RH, Ross RK, Henderson BE. Cigarette smoking in pregnancy results in marked decrease in maternal hCG and oestradiol levels. Br J Obstet Gynaecol 1989; 96:92–96.

108. Wlaknowska J, Conte FA, Grumbach MM. Practical and theoretical implications of fetal/maternal lymphocyte transfer. Lancet 1969; 1:1119–1122.

109. Zilliacus R, de la Chapelle A, Schroder J, Tilikainen A, Kohue E, Kleihauer E. Transplacental passage of foetal blood cells. Scand J Haematol 1975; 15: 333–338.

110. Schroder J, Schroder E, Cann HM. Lack of response of fetal cells in maternal blood to mitogens and mixed leukocyte culture. Hum Genet 1977; 38:91–97.

111. Muller UW, Hawdes CS, Wright AE, Petropoulos A, DeBoni E, Firgairia FA, Morley AA, Turner DR, Jones WR. Isolation of fetal trophoblast cells from peripheral blood of pregnant women. Lancet 1990; 2:197–200.

112. Adinolfi M, Camporese C, Carr T. Gene amplification to detect fetal nucleated cells in pregnant women. Lancet 1989; 2:328–329.
113. Covone A, Kozma R, Johnson PM, Latt SA, Adinolfi M. Analysis of peripheral maternal blood samples for the presence of placenta-derived cells using Y-specific probes and McAb H315. Prenatal Diagn 1988; 8:591–607.
114. Royal College of Physicians. Prenatal diagnosis and genetic screening: Community and service implications. Summary and recommendations of a report of the Royal College of Physicians. J R Coll Physicians Lond 1989; 23:215–220.

25

Fetal Malformations Associated with Drugs and Chemicals

Visualization by Sonography

Gideon Koren and Irena Nulman
The Hospital for Sick Children, Toronto, Ontario, Canada

Clinical Case

You are following the pregnancy of a woman who is being treated with carbamazepine for neuralgia. Attempts to discontinue the drug have resulted in reappearance of severe pain. The woman wants to know whether an ultrasound examination will help to decrease her risks of resuming carbamazepine therapy by detecting malformations.

INTRODUCTION

The ability to detect fetal malformation antenatally is important both in order to allow families to terminate such pregnancies if they so wish and to plan for optimal fetal and/or neonatal management if pregnancy continues.

Since the thalidomide disaster in the 1950s, an increasing number of drugs and chemicals have been incriminated as causing teratogenicity or fetal toxicity. As the majority of pregnant women are exposed to at least one medication during pregnancy, either before or after realizing that they are pregnant (1), the need to determine the relative risk that a certain agent will cause malformations is of utmost importance.

Data on chemically induced teratogenic risk are derived from animal studies, human case reports, or epidemiological studies. While such information is essential for assigning a relative risk to a potential teratogen, it may be of little help for medication in a specific case. Sonography has emerged as a

Table 1 Common Drugs

Drug	Central nervous system	Cardiovascular	Skeleton
Acetaminophen (overdose)			Clubfoot
Acetazolamide			Sacrococcygeal teratoma
Acetylsalicyclic acid	Intracranial hemorrhage		
Albuteral		Fetal tachycardia	
Alcohol	Microcephaly	Heart malformations	Short nose, hypoplastic maxilla, small mandible, poorly formed orbits, incomplete skull ossification
Amantadine		Single ventricle with pulmonary atresia	
Aminopterin[b]	Meningoencephalocele, incomplete skull ossification, brachycephaly, anencephaly		Hypopolasia of thumb and fibula, clubfoot, syndactyly, cranial anomalies, small mandible
Amitriptyline	Hydrocephalus		Small mandible
Amobarbital	Anencephaly	Heart malformations	
Antithyroid drugs			Scalp and finger-toe abnormalities
Azathioprine[b]	Cerebral hemorrhage, plagiocephaly	Atrial septal defects, pulmonary valvular stenosis	
Betamethasone	Reduced head circumference		
Bromides	Microcephaly	Heart malformations	
Busulfan			
Caffeine			Musculoskeletal defects
Captopril			
Carbon monoxide[b]	Cerebral atrophy, hydrocephalus, microcephaly	Fetal bradycardia	

Extremities	Gastrointestinal	Genitourinary	Miscellaneous	Source[a]
Dislocation of the hip			Polyhydramnios	CR
Oral cleft			Growth retardation	CR PS CR PS
	Cleft lip/palate, diaphragmatic hernia	Renal defects, hypospadias, labial hypoplasia	Growth retardation, microphthalmia	CR PS
				CR
Abnormal position of extremities, short forearms, talipes, clubfoot		Cleft lip/palate	Low set ears	CR
Limb reduction, swelling of hands and feet		Urinary retention, hypospadias		CR
Severe limb deformities, hip dislocation, polydactyly, clubfoot	Oral cleft	Intersex, hypospadias, hydrocele	Soft tissue deformity of neck, accessory auricle, inguinal hernia	PS CR
			Goiter, aplasia cutis	CR
Limb reduction, preaxial polydactyly (thumb polydactyly type)		Hypospadias	Growth retardation	RS CR
			Premature babies	PS
Polydactyly, clubfoot, dislocation of hip	Gastrointestinal anomalies		Growth retardation	CR
	Pyloric stenosis, cleft palate, bipolar spleen, hepatic subcapsular calcification	Hydronephrosis, kidney/ureter anomalies	Microphthalmia, growth retardation	CR
Leg reduction		Hydronephrosis		PS
	Renal defects, renal insufficiency		Stillbirth	CR CR
			Stillbirth	CR PS

(continues)

Table 1   Continued

Drug	Central nervous system	Cardiovascular	Skeleton
Carbamazepine	Meningomyelocele, spina bifida, decreased head circumference	Atrial septal defect, patent ductus arteriosus	Nose hypoplasia, hypertelorism
Chlordiazepoxide	Microcephaly	Heart malformations	
Chloroquine	Tetralogy of Fallot		
Chlorpheniramine	Hydrocephalus		
Chlorpropamide	Microcephaly, anencephaly	Atrial septal defect	Vertebral anomalis
Clomiphene	Meningomyelocele, hydrocephalus, microcephaly, anencephaly, neural tube defect		
Codeine	Hydrocephalus	Heart malformations	Musculoskeletal malformations
Cortisone	Hydrocephalus, cyclopia	Ventricular septal defect, coarctation of aorta	
Coumadin[b]	Encephalocele, anencephaly, spina bifida, agenesis of corpus callosum, Dandy-Walker malformation	Heart malformations	Nasal hypoplasia, scoliosis, skeletal deformities, absence of clavicles
Cyclophosphamide[b]	Microcephaly	Tetralogy of Fallot	Dysmorphic facies, flattened nasal bridge
Cytarabine	Anencephaly	Tetralogy of Fallot	
Daunorubicin[b]	Anencephaly	Tetralogy of Fallot	
Dextroamphetamine	Exencephaly, hydrocephalus, microcephaly	Heart malformations, atrial septal defect	
Diazepam	Spina bifida	Heart malformations	Hypertelorism
Diphenhydramine		Ventricular-spetal defects	

Extremities	Gastrointestinal	Genitourinary	Miscellaneous	Source[a]
Polydactylia, talipes, hip dislocation	Anal atresia, cleft	Ambiguous genitalia	Inguinal hernia	PS CR
	Duodenal atresia, Meckel's diverticulum			RS
			Wilms' tumor, hemyhypertrophy	CR
Polydactyly, dislocation of hip	Gastrointestinal defects		Eye and ear defects, inguinal hernia	PS
Dysmorphic hand and fingers	Stricture of lower ileum, cleft palate		Preauricular sinus, ear tags, perinatal death	CR
Syndactyly, clubfoot, polydactyly	Esophageal atresia, cleft lip/palate	Hypospadias, ovarian dysplasia	Hemangiomas	CR RS
Dislocated hip	Pyloric stenosis, oral cleft, umbilical and inguinal hernia	Genitourinary abnormality	Respiratory pathway malformations	PS RS
Clubfoot	Cleft lip, gastroschisis			CR
Stippled epiphysis, chondroplasia punctata, short phalanges, toe defects	Incomplete rotation of gut, asplenia, cleft palate	Single kidney	Growth retardation, bleeding, microphthalmia	CR RS
Four toes on each foot, hypoplastic mid-phalanx, syndactyly, absence of nails/thumbs	Inguinal and/or umbilical hernia, imperforate anus, rectovaginal fistula		Hemangiomas, growth retardation, microphthalmia	CR
Lobster claw malformations, missing toes, syndactyly			Growth retardation, atresia of external auditory canal	CR
Syndactyly			Growth retardation	CR
Dislocation of hip, absence of arm, syndactyly, absence of thumbs	Biliary atresia, cleft lip/palate	Urogenital defects	Growth retardation	CR RS
Clubfoot	Cleft palate/lip, inguinal hernia	Renal defects	Hemangiomas, growth retardation	PS CR
	Cleft palate, inguinal hernia	Hypospadias, genitourinary malformations other than hypospadias		PS CR

(continues)

Table 1   Continued

Drug	Central nervous system	Cardiovascular	Skeleton
Disulfiram			Vertebral fusion
Diuretics			
Estrogens		Heart malformations	
Ethanol[b]	Microcephaly	Ventricular septal defect, atrial septal defect, double outlet of right ventricle, pulmonary atresia, dextrocardia, patent ductus arteriosus, tetralogy of Fallot	Short nose, hypoplastic philtrum, micrognathia, pectus excavatum, radioulnar synostosis, bifid xyphoid, scoliosis
Ethosuximide	Hydrocephalus, microcephaly		Short neck
Fluorouracil	Hydrocephalus, anencephaly	Hypoplasia of aorta, lung	
Folic acid (absence)	Neural tube defect		
Fluphenazine			Poor ossification of frontal bone, ocular hypertelorism
Haloperidol		Aortic valve defect	
Heparin[b]			
Hormones, progestogenic	Anencephaly, hydrocephalus	Tetralogy of Fallot, truncus arteriosus, ventricular septal defect	Spina bifida
Imipramine	Exencephaly		
Indomethacin		Premature closure of ductus arteriosus, tricuspid regurgitation	
Isoniazid	Meningomyelocele		Spina bifida

Extremities	Gastrointestinal	Genitourinary	Miscellaneous	Source[a]
Clubfoot, radial aplasia, phocomelia	Tracheoesophageal fistula			CR PS
Limb reduction				CR PS
Wormian bones, dislocated hips, absent tibia, polydactyly	Cleft palate	V — vertebral A — anal C — cardiac T — tracheal E — esophageal R — renal or radial L — limb	Eye and ear anomalies	PS CR
	Oral cleft, diaphragmatic hernia	Renal defects, hypospadias, labial hypoplasia	Growth retardation	CR RS PS
	Oral cleft			CR
Radial aplasia, absence of thumbs and fingers	Aplasia of esophagus, duodenum; absence of appendix; imperforate anus/cloaca; hypoplasia of duodenum, bile duct	Hypoplasia of uterus	Hypoplasia of thymus	CR
				CR PS RS
	Oral cleft, imperforate anus	Retrourethral fistula, hypospadias		PS CR
Limb deformities				RS
			Bleeding	RS
Absence of thumbs	Inguinal hernia	Hypospadias, ambiguous genitalia		RS CR
Limb reduction	Cleft palate, diaphragmatic hernia	Renal cystic degeneration	Adrenal hypoplasia, defective abdominal muscles	CR
Phocomelia	Intestinal perforation and bleeding	Reduced fetal urine output, oliguria	Stillbirth, hemorrhage, oligohydramnion	CR
Talipes				PS

(continues)

Table 1   Continued

Drug	Central nervous system	Cardiovascular	Skeleton
Lithium	Hydrocephalus, meningomyelocele	Ventricular septal defect, Ebstein's anomaly, mitral atresia, patent ductus arteriosus, dextrocardia	Spina bifida
Lysergic acid diethylamide	Hydrocephalus, encephalocele, meningomyelocele	Tetralogy of Fallot	Spina bifida occulta
Meclizine	Meningocele, hydrocephalus, spina bifida	Hypoplasia cardis, hypoplastic left heart	
Meprobamate		Heart malformations	
Methotrexate[b]	Anencephaly, oxycephaly, absence of frontal bone, large fontanelles	Dextrocardia	Hypoplastic mandible, hypertelorism
Methyl mercury[b]	Microcephaly, asymmetric head		
Metronidazole	Brain defects, holotelencephaly		Midline facial defects
Nortriptyline			
Oral contraceptives	Meningomyelocele, hydrocephalus, anencephaly	Heart malformations	Vertebral malformations
Paramethadione	Tetralogy of Fallot		
Penicillamine	Hydrocephalus, intraventricular hemorrhage	Ventricular septal defect	Small mandible
Phenobarbital	Hydrocephalus, meningomyelocele		
Phenothiazine	Microcephaly		
Phenylephrine			
Phenylpropanolamine			Pectus excavatum
Phenytoin[b]	Microcephaly	Heart malformations	Rib-sternal abnormalities; wide fontanelle; broad alveolar ridge; short neck; hypertelorism; spotted calcification in skull, fontanelle, and sagittal suture; webbed neck, small mandible; short nose; broad nasal bridge

Extremities	Gastrointestinal	Genitourinary	Miscellaneous	Source[a]
Clubfoot, dislocated			Stillbirth	CR
hip				RS
				PS
Limb deficiencies,			Neuroblastoma	PS
bilateral defects of				CR
limbs				
	Imperforate anus	Renal hypoplasia	Respiratory pathway	PS
	pyloric stenosis		defects, eye and ear	CR
			defects, inguinal	
			hernia	
Dysplastic hips			Abdominal wall	CR
			defect	PS
Long webbed fingers,			Growth retardation,	CR
absence of digits,			low set ears	
abnormal ribs				
				CR
Dislocated hip, limb	Oral cleft	Genital defects,		CR
abnormalities		hydrocele		PS
Limb reduction				CR
Limb reduction	Tracheoesophageal	Renal malformations	Growth retardation	RS
	+ anal malforma-			CR
	tions			
			Growth retardation	PS
Dislocated hip, bilat-	Pyloric stenosis,		Growth retardation,	CR
eral clubfoot, limb	perforated bowel		stillbirth, inguinal	
deformations			hernia, low set ears	
Digital anomalies	Cleft palate, ileal		Growth retardation,	CR
	atresia		pulmonary hypo-	
			plasia	
Syndactyly, clubfoot	Omphalocele, ab-			CR
	dominal distension			PS
Syndactyly, clubfoot,	Umbilical hernia	Eye and ear abnor-		PS
dislocation of hip		malities		
Polydactyly, disloca-		Hypospadias		PS
tion of hip				
Hypoplastic distal,	Cleft palate/lip,		Growth retardation,	CR
phalanges and nails,	diaphragmatic		Neurotumors	PS
digitalized thumb,	hernia		Low set ears	RS
dislocated hip				

(continues)

Table 1   Continued

Drug	Central nervous system	Cardiovascular	Skeleton
Polychlorinated biphenyl[b]	Smaller head sizes		
Procarbazine[b]	Cerebral hemorrhage	Ventricular septal defect	Oligodactyly and other finger and limb abnormalities
Quinine	Hydrocephalus	Heart malformations	Facial defects, vertebral anomalies
Retinoic acid[b]	Hydrocephalus, microcephaly	Heart malformations	Malformations of cranium, ear, face, ribs, micrognatia
Spermicides			
Sulfonamide			
Tetracycline			Clubfoot
Thalidomide[b]		Heart malformations	Spine malformation
Thioguanine		Tetralogy of Fallot	
Tobacco			
Tolbutamide		Heart malformations	
Trifluoperazine		Transposition of great arteries	
Trimethadione[b]	Microcephaly	Atrial septal defect, ventricular septal defect	Low set ears, broad bridge
Valproic acid[b]	Lumbosacral meningomyelocele, microcephaly, wide fontanelle	Tetralogy of Fallot, ventricular septal defect, valvular aortic stenosis	Depressed nasal bridge, hypoplastic nose, low set ears, small mandibles

Extremities	Gastrointestinal	Genitourinary	Miscellaneous	Source[a]
			Stillbirth, growth retardation	PS
		Malformed kidneys	Growth retardation, multiple hemangiomas	CR
Dysmelias, limb deformities	Gastrointestinal abnormalities	Urogenital abnormalities	Hernias	CR
			Stillbirth, thymic defects, microphthalmia	RS
				PS
Limb reduction, hypoplasia of limb or part of it, foot defects		Hypospadias		PS
				CR
				RS
Hypoplasia of limb or part of it, clubfoot		Urethral obstructions	Adrenal atrophy, benign tumors	PS
				CR
Limb reduction (amelia, phocomelia), hypoplasia	Duodenal stenosis or atresia, pyloric stenosis	Hypospadias	Inguinal hernia	PS
				CR
Missing digits			Microtia	CR
Limb and digit abnormalities			Fetal death, growth retardation	CR
			Growth retardation	PS
Finger-toe syndactyly, absent toes, accessory thumb	Cleft palate, tracheoesophageal fistula	Renal anomalies	Stillbirth	RS
Phocomelia				CR
Malformed hands, clubfoot	Esophageal atresia, imperforate anus, oral cleft	Hypospadias, kidney and ureter abnormalities, ambiguous genitalia	Growth retardation, inguineal hernia	CR
				PS
Limb, finger, toe, nail abnormalities	Oral cleft, duodenal atresia, inguinal hernia		Growth retardation, umbilical hernia	CR

---

[a]Since only malformations that can be visualized by current ultrasonographic techniques are listed, the guide cannot be used as a complete list of drug-induced teratogenicity. CR, case reports; RS, retrospective studies; PS, prospective studies; AS, animal studies.

[b]Proved to be teratogenic.

Source: Koren et al. (Am J Obstet Gynecol 1987; 156:79–85), with permission of CV Mosby Company.

powerful tool for antenatal detection of fetal anomalies. It is conceivable therefore that more and more pregnant women exposed to drugs and chemicals will be referred for diagnosis of or to rule out malformations associated with these agents. Currently, pregnant women who attend the Motherisk Clinic for antenatal counseling of drug-chemical exposure are scheduled for a level 2 sonographic evaluation in 17–18 weeks of gestation if there is an increased risk for malformations or when gestational age is not known.

This guide aims at providing the sonographer with a practical list of malformations that have been described in association with specific drugs or chemicals. It is an updated version of our original publication several years ago (1).

METHODOLOGICAL CONSIDERATIONS

Two groups of agents are included (1). Common drugs and chemicals that have been associated with the malformations are listed. In many cases the incriminating data are controversial; hence the inclusion of a certain malformation in this guide by no means suggests that we are convinced that the agent is a teratogen. Because of the heterogeneity of the data, the source of information is mentioned (for instance, case reports, retrospective or prospective studies) (2). Drugs and chemicals that have been proved beyond doubt as teratogens are marked (see Table 1).

Table 1 includes only malformations that can be visualized by current ultrasonographic techniques and cannot be used as a complete list of drug-induced teratogenicity. The data in this guide have been extracted from currently available literature (2–9).

Certain points with respect to the ultrasound examination itself should be stressed. It is probably best carried out by a physician ultrasonographer who has had significant experience in looking at fetuses. A very meticulous technique and high resolution, real-time equipment should be used. The examination is best recorded on videotape so that it can be reviewed as needed. A great deal of patience is required in this type of study, especially when one is examining the face, digits, and heart. At the outset of the examination it should be explained to the patient that the examination may take some time to complete and that more than one sitting may be required.

Answer

It is estimated that about 1% of carbamazepine users will have babies with neural tube defects (a relative risk of around 10 compared to the general population). Detailed ultrasound examination can detect most cases of neural tube defects. However, α-fetoproteins in blood and/or amniotic fluids should also be examined.

REFERENCES

1. Koren G, Brill Edwards M, Miskin M. Fetal malformations associated with drugs and chemicals: Visualization by sonography. In Maternal-Fetal Toxicology, 1st ed (Koren G, ed). Marcel Dekker, New York, 1990, pp 297–307.
2. Schardein J. Chemically Induced Birth Defects. Marcel Dekker, New York, 1985.
3. Fabro S. Reproductive Toxicology. A Medical Letter. Reproductive Toxicology Center, Washington, DC, 1984.
4. Mattison DR. Reproductive Toxicology. Alan R Liss, New York, 1983.
5. Briggs GG, Bodendorfer TW, Freeman RK, Yaffe SJ. Drugs in Pregnancy and Lactation, 3rd ed. Williams & Wilkins, Baltimore, 1990.
6. Heinonen OP, Slone D, Shapiro S, Birth Defects and Drugs in Pregnancy. PSG Publishing, Littleton, MA, 1977.
7. Shepard TH. Catalog of Teratogenic Agents, 6th ed. John Hopkins University Press, Baltimore, 1989.
8. Onnis A, Grella P. The Biochemical Effects of Drugs in Pregnancy. Ellis Horwood, Chichester, 1984.
9. Berglund F, et al. Drug use during pregnancy and breast-feeding. A classification system for drug information. Acta Obstet Gynecol Scand Suppl 1984; A medical letter "Ultrasound in Industry and Medicine" 126:1–55.

26

Maternal Disorders Leading to Increased Reproductive Risks

Ron Gonen
B'nai Zion Medical Center, Technion, Haifa, Israel

Kathleen Shilalukey, Laura Magee, and Gideon Koren
The Hospital for Sick Children, Toronto, Ontario, Canada

Jerry Shime
Women's College Hospital, Toronto, Ontario, Canada

Clinical Case

A young Type I diabetic woman, known to your clinic for many years, is in the first trimester of her first pregnancy. She is concerned that her daily injections of insulin may adversely affect the baby.

INTRODUCTION

When pregnancy and maternal medical disease coexist, there may be serious consequences for mother, fetus, and child. For example, maternal risks include preeclampsia in the hypertensive woman, increased vaso-occlusive crises in the presence of sickle cell disease, and functional deterioration in cardiac patients. The fetus or neonate is predisposed to congenital anomalies if the mother has diabetes, to hemorrhage if she suffers from autoimmune thrombocytopenia, and to heart block in the presence of maternal lupus. In later years, the child may exhibit manifestations of genetic transmission, as with thalassemia or Marfan's syndrome, and in addition is subject to the potential repercussions from growing up in an environment rendered less secure by the mother's medical condition.

Aside from events that relate directly to the interaction between maternal health and pregnancy, there are risks arising from the treatment of several underlying medical disorders. For example, warfarin (in the woman with a prosthetic heart valve) and valproic acid (in the treatment of seizure disorders) are known teratogens. Propylthiouracil, used in the management of hyperthyroidism, can result in fetal goiter and hypothyroidism. Other drugs such as the anticancer chemotherapeutic agents and posttransplant immunosuppressants are potentially dangerous and require further evaluations.

Finally, certain maternal factors that relate primarily to lifestyle carry increased reproductive risks. Aside from the obvious disadvantages to maternal health brought on by alcohol, drug abuse, and dietary extremes, there are recognized corresponding fetal and neonatal hazards such as fetal alcohol syndrome, placental abruption, and stillbirth.

During the past three decades, we have witnessed an explosion of activity directed toward the identification of the fetus at risk, the management of preterm labor, and the intensive care of the prematurely born neonate. These efforts have been accompanied by significant reductions in perinatal mortality and morbidity. More recently, the component of high risk pregnancy arising from compromised maternal health has acquired a growing, if not novel importance, as evidenced by a proliferation of scientific articles as well as new and revised editions of textbooks addressing this theme (1–43).

There are several good reasons for intensified interest in the influence of maternal factors on reproductive risks.

First, advances in medical and surgical care have made pregnancy feasible in a variety of conditions in which previously the mother's life was seriously threatened and perinatal results were disastrous. Examples include surgical correction of congenital heart disease, renal transplantation, and the medical management of systemic lupus erythematosus.

Second, societal factors are altering the composition of the population at risk. For example, growing immigration from the Orient has resulted in an increase in the incidence of hepatitis and some of the hemoglobinopathies. In the adolescent population, intravenous drug abuse has become more prevalent, and there are already many documented cases of pregnant women with autoimmune deficiency syndrome (AIDS) and vertical transmission to the neonate. With the advent of in vitro fertilization and the expansion of career options for women, many have delayed childbearing (comforted by the availability of prenatal diagnosis for advanced maternal age); thus, it is likely that we will increasingly see during pregnancy certain conditions that occur with aging, such as hypertension and diabetes.

Third, with the heightened awareness by members of the medical profession, as well as legislators and consumers, of the importance of preventive medicine and quality of life, it is no longer sufficient merely to see a woman

Table 1 Maternal Disease and Pregnancy Outcome

Condition	Epidemiology/ incidence	Effects of the disease on pregnancy	Effects of pregnancy on the disease	Practice points
AIDS (1–4)	Current seroprevalence of HIV infection is 0.15% among America women of childbearing age, but as high as 8% in urban areas. In parts of Central Africa and Haiti it may be 5–30%. High risk women: prostitutes, IV drug abusers, chronic recipients of blood products (especially before screening), bisexual spouses	Current vertical transmission averages 25–30%, but may be as low as 12.9% or as high as 45%. Vertical transmission may result in: Intrauterine growth retardation Increased risk of premature rupture of membranes Increased cesarean delivery rate Neonatal AIDS	May become fulminant even for previously asymptomatic women.	Women who are seropositive or whose partners are seropositive should avoid pregnancy. Avoid monitoring fetus by cordocentesis or scalp electrode. Staff should not use DeLees suction catheters. HIV-1 infection may be transmitted through breast milk; women should refrain from breastfeeding. HIV-infected women with pelvic inflammatory disease are more prone to tubo-ovarian abscesses, requiring more surgical intervention. HIV disease appears to increase the rate of progression and the severity of cervical neoplastic lesions.

(continues)

Table 1 Continued

Condition	Epidemiology/ incidence	Effects of the disease on pregnancy	Effects of pregnancy on the disease	Practice points
Anemia (1,5,6)	Most frequent maternal complication diagnosed during pregnancy; using WHO definition of hemoglobin (Hb) ≤ 13.0 g/dL (130 g/L), 50% of all US gestations are complicated by anemia. However Hb ≤ 11.0 g/L (110 g/L) is the usual clinical definition of anemia.	Refer to specific type of anemia.	Significant maternal complications with Hb < 6 g/dL (60 g/L).	
Asthma (7)	Common, occurring in 0.4–1.3% pregnant women.	Increased frequency of maternal complications (hyperemesis, vaginal hemorrhage, pre-eclampsia, and complicated labor). Significant relationship exists between level of chronic asthma control and infant gestational age, intrauterine growth retardation, and perinatal mortality.	Course unpredictable for first pregnancy, but more severe asthma often associated with worsening during pregnancy; exacerbation usually between 28 and 36 weeks. Asthma course similar in subsequent pregnancies.	Therapy should be guided by *objective* measures of airway obstruction, as subjective complaints are unreliable. Considered *safe* in pregnancy: inhaled β_2-selective agents, steroids, disodium chromoglycate, ipratropium; when required, IV/PO steroids.

			Ripening of cervix with Prostin Gel (PGE2) not contraindicated. Use inhaled β_2 agonists sparingly near labor, as they suppress uterine contractions.
B_{12} vitamin deficiency (1,5,6)	1/6000–1/8000 pregnancies.	Pernicious anemia associated with infertility. Maternal levels of vitamin B_{12} fall progressively during gestation to intermediate levels (80–120 g/mL). Fetus is protected from deficiency because of efficient placental transfer except in transcobolamin 2 deficiency. Breast-fed neonates whose mothers have maternal B_{12} deficiency may develop severe deficiency 4–12 months after birth.	No effect of pregnancy on vitamin B_{12} deficiency.	Therapy necessary for vitamin B_{12} < 50 pg/mL. Breastfeeding not recommended until deficiency corrected.
Cancer				
Acute leukemias (1,5,6)	1/75,000 pregnancies (approximately 400 cases have been reported in the literature thus far).	Increased risk of spontaneous abortions, premature births, stillbirths.	Pregnancy does not affect course or prognosis adversely. Overall, complete remission rate for stan-	Once the diagnosis of acute leukemia has been made, treatment should not be delayed.

(continues)

Table 1 Continued

Condition	Epidemiology/ incidence	Effects of the disease on pregnancy	Effects of pregnancy on the disease	Practice points
Cancer				
acute leukemias (continued)		Increased risk of maternal bleeding and infection if peripheral blood counts are suppressed by chemotherapy. Chemotherapy increases risk of fetal abnormalities; congenital malformations occur in < 10–15% of cases.	dard induction chemotherapy is comparable to that in general population (50–80%). Suboptimal treatment and delay of treatment in an attempt to protect the fetus may adversely affect chances of remission/cure.	Therapeutic abortion is recommended if diagnosed in first half of pregnancy because of poor maternal prognosis and the effects of multidrug chemotherapy on the fetus. If chemotherapy is administered close to time of delivery, neonatal hematological status should be assessed.
breast cancer (1,5,6,8)	1–3% of breast cancers occur during pregnancy or lactation. More likely to be invasive ductal carcinoma.	Breast cancer is not transmitted from mother to fetus.	Stage-for-stage survivals similar in pregnant and nonpregnant women, but diagnosis may be delayed by pregnancy, thus worsening the prognosis. Pregnancy may affect the course of breast cancer by altering the incidence, altering the ability to diagnose, limiting therapeutic	During the first trimester, termination of pregnancy may be necessary to initiate chemotherapy for metastatic disease. Chemotherapy causes a malformation rate of 11.6% in the first trimester, with no reported malformations when given in the second or third trimester.

The effect of gestational exposure to chemotherapy on female fetuses is of concern because eggs are formed during gestation. Mutations/chromosomal abnormalities produced in such gametes could result in embryopathology in the next generation; recessive mutations might not become manifest until subsequent generations.

options, or altering cure rates.
A first pregnancy after 30 years is associated with increases in the likelihood of developing breast cancer.

	Incidence	Effect on fetus	Comments
cervical cancer (1,5,6)	In situ: 0.13% (1 in 770) of pregnancies. Invasive: 0.05% (1 in 2205) of pregnancies.	Fetus is not affected.	Survival not influenced by pregnancy. Mode of delivery does not affect prognosis. Treatment of invasive cervical cancer in pregnancy depends on the stage of disease at diagnosis. Cervical cancer invasive to less than 3 mm (as diagnosed by cone biopsy) may be deferred until fetal maturity, when cesarean section and hysterectomy are performed. Pregnancy termination may be advisable with more advanced stages.

647

Table 1 Continued

Condition	Epidemiology/ incidence	Effects of the disease on pregnancy	Effects of pregnancy on the disease	Practice points
Cancer				
Hodgkin's disease (1,9)	Not rare in pregnancy. 7500 cases of Hodgkin's are diagnosed/year in United States. 50% of cases occur in women between ages 30 and 40.	Disease does not affect pregnancy outcome; however during the first trimester diagnostic and/or therapeutic radiological procedures may be hazardous to to the fetus.	Pregnancy does not affect course or prog-	Pregnancies < 16 weeks of gestation may warrant therapeutic abortion because of chemotherapy, irradiation, or aggressive/advanced disease. Pregnancies > 16 weeks, if asymptomatic, can be followed until early delivery is carried out. Radiation doses to the pelvis > 10 rad, or full doses of chemotherapy during the first trimester, can be deleterious to fetal health.
melanoma (1,5,6,9)	Presently 1/128 in United States. Death rates increasing by 5% per year in United States. Overall, incidence of metastatic/recurrent disease may be increased by 10% in pregnant patients.	Generally, no adverse effects. Metastases of maternal cancers to fetus and placenta are extremely rare, but several cases of neonatal melanomas have been reported.	Conflicting data concerning the influence of pregnancy on survival or growth rates of malignancy. This confusion results from studies in which groups evaluated were not homogeneous.	Primary lesions should be treated surgically as soon as discovered.

ovarian cancer (1,5,6,9)	1/23,000 deliveries. 3.5% of pregnant patients undergoing surgery for an adnexal mass.	Fetus usually not affected. In advanced malignancy: fetal growth retardation may occur. Possible virilization of fetus due to androgens produced by ovarian stromal tumors	Pregnancy does not promote/predispose to ovarian cancer, but rather is considered protective to subsequent ovarian cancer.	Exploratory laparotomy to evaluate an adnexal mass detected in early pregnancy should not be delayed beyond 16 weeks gestation. 12% of ovarian masses may present as an acute surgical abdomen not allowing for planned surgery. Postoperative therapy for ovarian cancer should be given in nearly all instances. Serum markers should be followed as they indicate tumor status (e.g., α-fetoprotein human chorionic gonadotropin, lactase dehydrogenase, Ca-125).
Chlamydia trachomatis infections (1,5,6)	Prevalent in young women of lower socioeconomic status. Cultured from 5–30% of women attending prenatal clinics, many of whom are asymptomatic.	In infants of untreated mothers, ophthalmia neonatorum occurs in 40–50% and 10–20% develop pneumonia. May increase risk of premature labor and perinatal death. Risk of intrapartum fever and postpartum endometritis increased.	Pregnancy does not alter the course of the disease.	Topical erythromycin soon after delivery protects neonate against chlamydial conjunctivitis.

(continues)

Table 1 Continued

Condition	Epidemiology/ incidence	Effects of the disease on pregnancy	Effects of pregnancy on the disease	Practice points
Cytomegalovirus (CMV) infection (1)	Congenital infection in 1–3% pregnancies. Most important cause of infectious mental retardation and congenital deafness in United States. Seropositivity more prevalent in lower socioeconomic class (90% vs. 50% in mid-upper class) age >30 years non-Caucasian background	50% of primary infections and almost all recurrent infections are asymptomatic. Congenital transmission after CMV infection during pregnancy occurs in 2–3% of seropositive women (either reinfection or reactivation) and 25–50% of seronegative women (primary infection). Infection in the latter group associated with more severe disease, with risk of a severely affected infant of ≤5%. However, sequelae can occur with infection at *any* stage of gestation, and abnormalities are *progressive*.	No change in incidence/ severity of maternal disease.	Consider screening women in *high risk* situations. Culture of amniotic fluid by amniocentesis not 100% sensitive. Prophylactic cesarean section not necessary. Breastfeeding not contraindicated.
Diabetes mellitus (10,11)	Type I DM: 1% pregnancies.	*Maternal* Increased in frequency: chronic hypertension,	Insulin requirements increase progressively during pregnancy.	Excellent preconceptional control and in early pregnancy may reduce

(continues)

Gestational diabetes (GDM): 3% pregnancies.

probably pregnancy-induced hypertension in Type I DM, polyhydramnios, maternal mortality (≤ 0.11%).

Fetal/neonatal

Type I DM; rate of congenital malformations increased 2-6-fold (7.5–12.9%).

Preconceptional counseling recommended, as preconception hemoglobin A1C (glycosilated hemoglobin) within 1% of upper limits of normal (6–7%) has decreased rate of malformations almost to levels seen in nondiabetic patients (2–3%)

Cardiac and *neural tube* defects most common, followed by skeletal, GI, urinary tract abnormalities. Increased perinatal mortality and morbidity (macrosomia,

Type I DM: *diabetic retinopathy:* nonproliferative usually does not progress; proliferation may progress during pregnancy.

Diabetic nephropathy: proteinuria usually *increases* during pregnancy, whereas creatinine clearance may *decrease* in up to one-third of patients.

However, *most* values return to normal postpartum, following same rate of progression thereafter as in men.

risk of fetal malformations.

Diabetic diet should be reviewed with a dietitian.

Type I DM should be managed by an endocrinologist for intensive insulin therapy and monitoring; have basic ophthalmologic assessment, and 24-hour urine collection for protein and creatinine clearance (the latter to be repeated every trimester.

Level II ultrasound and serum α-fetoprotein recommended in mid-second trimester.

Cesarean delivery for obstetrical indications only.

Table 1 Continued

Condition	Epidemiology/ incidence	Effects of the disease on pregnancy	Effects of pregnancy on the disease	Practice points
Diabetes mellitus (continued)		cesarean delivery, birth trauma, respiratory distress syndrome, hypoglycemia, hypocalcemia, hyperbilirubinemia, polycythemia) that *may* be decreased by good glycemic control.		
Epilepsy (1,5,6,9)	0.3–0.5% of pregnancies.	Two- to threefold increase in fetal malformations, especially facial clefts and cardiac problems (baseline risk 1–3%). Increased risk of preterm birth and intrauterine growth retardation with trauma due to fall, with poor control of generalized seizures.	Variable effect of pregnancy on seizure frequency; increased in 45%, unchanged in 50%, decreased in 5%.	Serum concentrations of antiepileptic medications tend to decline as pregnancy progresses but free levels increase; blood levels should be measured at regular intervals. Seizure control first priority. Carbamazepine, drug of choice for grand mal seizures; 1% risk of neural tube defect (NTD). 4 mg/day folate decreases risk of NTD; start taking it when trying to conceive.

| Folic acid deficiency (1,5,6) | Frank megaloblastic anemia in 1/70–1/250 pregnancies. WHO report 1 in 3 women worldwide suffer from folic acid deficiency. 30–69% U.S. women in low socioeconomic classes have this deficiency. | Prospective human studies show a cause-and-effect relationship between folate deficiency and increased risk for neural tube defects (both in normal population and high risk families). | Pregnancy aggravates folic acid depletion. | 0.5 mg supplemental folate adequate for prophylaxis and overt maternal folate deficiency. Folate supplementation periconceptually and prenatally has been reported to reduce neural tube defects. |
| Gonorrhea (1,5,9) | 2–5% of prenatal patients in North America have endocervical gonorrhea; 75–90% are asymptomatic. | Vertical transmission occurs by ascending in presence of premature rupture of membranes or by delivery through an infected birth canal. Higher incidence of premature rupture of membranes, preterm labor, intrauterine growth retardation, and chorioamnionitis in untreated cases. Newborn infections may involve eye, ear canal, oropharynx, stomach, anorectal mucosa, or hematogenous dissemination. | Risk of disseminated infection increases in pregnancy. | Since most women are asymptomatic, routine endocervical cultures are essential in early pregnancy. Treatment of the mother with penicillin or ceftriaxone, and topical application of 1% silver nitrate or erythromycin to the newborn's eyes dramatically decrease neonatal infection and ophthalmia neonatorum. |

(continues)

Table 1 Continued

Condition	Epidemiology/ incidence	Effects of the disease on pregnancy	Effects of pregnancy on the disease	Practice points
Heart disease (12)	Heart disease complicates 1–4% of all pregnancies, has remained stable over time. Rheumatic and congenital etiologies most common.	Poor cardiovascular status associated with spontaneous abortions, intrauterine growth retardation, and premature labor. Women with congenital heart disease (CHD) have a 3–4% risk of having a baby with CHD, especially in the presence of obstruction to left ventricular outflow. Critical period of exposure for causing fetal warfarin syndrome is between 6–12 weeks, when one-third of babies are affected. Exposure to warfarin *after* the first trimester *may* present a risk of CNS damage and stillbirth due to hemorrhage; however, degree of risk unclear	Cardiac output increases by 40%, peaking by end of second trimester. Vast majority of patients can be safely managed to term. Maternal mortality is 0.4% with New York Heart Association (NYHA) Class I or II, but increases to 6.8% with Class III or IV. Pregnancy not recommended with high risk cardiac lesions: any cardiac disease with Class III or IV symptoms, unrepaired cyanotic CHD, critical aortic stenosis, primary pulmonary hypertension, Eisenmenger's syndrome, Marfan's syndrome, or peripartum cardiomyopathy with persistent cardiomegaly.	Management in high risk obstetrics center recommended. Rest, reassurance, and monthly examinations are mainstay of treatment. Coumadin should be changed to SC heparin either prior to conception or certainly before 6 weeks gestation. Digoxin, β-adrenergic blockers, heparin are *not* teratogenic. Fetal echocardiography recommended at 18–20 weeks gestation to rule out CHD. Method of delivery dictated by obstetrical considerations; deterioration can occur in labor and especially postpartum period. American Heart Association does *not* rec-

	and must be balanced against risks to the mother (e.g., of stroke in the case of mechanical heart valves).	Maternal complications include congestive heart failure and risk of aortic rupture in Marfan's syndrome or coarctation of aorta (even repaired).	ommend antibiotic prophylaxis for vaginal delivery.
Hepatitis (viral) (13–17)	0.2% of pregnant women, however, 1–5% of adults may develop chronic infection and peristent viremia, depending on the etiological agent.	No vertical transmission of hepatitis A (HA). Significant risk of vertical transmission of hepatitis B (HB) from mother with acute or chronic hepatitis and asymptomatic carriers. If maternal HBe antibody positive or HBe antigen negative, there is a 10–20% risk of perinatal infection. If maternal HBe antigen positive, the risk is 80–90% for either infant hepatitis or carrier state. Prematurity 2–3 times higher with maternal viral hepatitis. In fulminant hepatitis, fetal wastage > 70%. Disease unaltered by pregnancy; thus risk of fulminant hepatitis is well below 2%.	Pregnant women in contact with HAV infective cases should receive immunoglobin (0.02 mL/kg) as soon as possible. Pregnant women exposed to HBV should receive HBIg (0.04–0.07 mL/kg), first of 3 1 mL HBV vaccines as soon as possible, the second and third vaccines given 1 and 6 months later. Prevention of HBV transmission currently dependent on identification of HB surface antigen (HBsAg) and HBeAg carriers among pregnant women and recognizing acute HBV

(continues)

Table 1 Continued

Condition	Epidemiology/ incidence	Effects of the disease on pregnancy	Effects of pregnancy on the disease	Practice points
Hepatitis (viral) (continued)				infection in the latter half of pregnancy/postpartum period. Newborns of HBsAg-positive women should receive HBIg (0.5 mL within 1 hour and 0.5 mL HBV within a week of birth). Test infants for HBsAg and anti-HBc at 1 year to determine treatment success. The presence of HBsAg ± IgM anti-HBc indicates treatment failure, since infant is actively infected. Anti-HBs alone suggests that vaccine-induced immunity can last ≈ 5 years. Boosters needed every 5 years for continued protection.

| Herpes simplex (18,19) | 20–50% of primary infections are due to herpes simplex virus 1 (HSV-1), but > 80% of recurrent infections are due to HSV-2.
HSV can be isolated from 0.2–4.0% of pregnant women at delivery. Women may shed virus in absence of clinical history of HSV infection. | True congenital infections with HSV rare and are invariably associated with *primary* maternal infection during pregnancy.
Primary infections that occur in first trimester are not indications for therapeutic abortion, since malformations usually not consistent with life; later infections may cause intrauterine growth retardation, major multiorgan sequelae, significant fetal mortality, or prematurity.
Recurrent infections during pregnancy are reservoir for neonatal infectins but do not contribute significantly to fetal morbidity/mortality.
Perinatally acquired infections occur in | Primary maternal infection during pregnancy associated with greater risk of recurrence and viral excretion during labor.
Recurrences tend to increase in frequency as pregnancy progresses. Overriding concern is transmission to baby, since maternal infection usually follows self-limited course. | Consideration can be given to oral acyclovir treatment for frequent recurrences of HSV, since reported use to date has failed to reveal significant increases in congenital malformations.
Pregnant women with history of HSV, and no lesions or prodromal symptoms at the time of delivery, can undergo vaginal delivery; however, they should also have cultures of previously affected areas and cervix done to document possible neonatal exposure.
Risk of neonatal infection estimated to be 1/1000.
Women with genital lesions should be delivered by cesarean section as soon as possible |

(continues)

Table 1 Continued

Condition	Epidemiology/ incidence	Effects of the disease on pregnancy	Effects of pregnancy on the disease	Practice points
Herpes simplex (continued)		1/5000–1/20,000 births, especially with preterm birth. Such risk still present in absence of maternal symptoms or lesions.		after membrane rupture/onset of labor, ideally, within 4–6 hours.
Hypertensive disorders (20–22)	1–3% of all pregnancies. 70% have preeclampsia/ eclampsia, 25% essential hypertension, 5% gestational hypertension. Results in 20% of all maternal deaths.	Increased proportional to degree of hypertension: spontaneous abortion, intrauterine growth retardation and fetal death, abruptio placentae, prematurity, operative delivery, perinatal morbidity and mortality.	Incidence of chronic hypertensive complications unchanged. Acute hypertension (BP ≥ 170/110) associated with increase in maternal stroke.	BP usually decreases in first trimester (through ~20 weeks), reaching previous levels by term. Decreased maternal stroke only consequence of treating hypertension in pregnancy, other than possible decrease in fetal loss with treatment of essential hypertension in first trimester with methyldopa. BP ≥ 160/100 should be treated. Goal of treatment: diastolic BP ~90 mmHg. Methyldopa drug of choice ± hydralazine.

Condition				
Hyperthyroidism (23)	Rare, < 0.1% of pregnancies. Graves' disease most common cause.	Decreased fertility with marked hyperthyroidism. Increased: spontaneous abortion, stillbirth, low birth weight, neonatal death. Transient neonatal Graves' disease due to thyroid stimulating IgG (TSAb) occurs in 1–2% of cases, especially with history of previously affected child; however, even presence of IgG TSAb confers a low risk of neonatal Graves'.	Tendency for increased activity of disease in first trimester and postpartum. No change in natural history of ophthalmo-	TSAb may be present even after treatment for hyperthyroidism of Graves'; should be measured in all patients with history of Graves'. Treatment in pregnancy decreases risk of thyroid storm. Propothiouracil (in lowest possible doses), the drug of choice in pregnancy, is associated with slight risk of fetal goiter or hypothyroidism.
Hypothyroidism (24)	6/1000 women who carry pregnancy > 20 weeks.	Decreased fertility. Possibly increased fetal loss, adverse fetal and perinatal outcomes, with *moderate* to *severe* hypothyroidism.	20% require higher replacement dose of thyroid hormone during pregnancy.	Treatment improves fertility and probably pregnancy outcome. TSH should be repeated every trimester; a rise warrants increase in thyroid hormone.
Immune thrombocytopenia purpura (ITP) (1)	Commonly associated with, or occuring during, pregnancy. Etiology: *auto*immune or *allo*immune mechanisms.	*Maternal* If platelets <20,000 mm³, blood loss may be increased during delivery. No increase in maternal mortality	Symptoms of ITP tend to worsen. Ideally, pregnancy should be postponed until remission.	*Treatment:* as in non-pregnant state (i.e., steroids are first-line treatment, with IV IgG as second line, and splenectomy as last resort).

(continues)

Table 1 Continued

Condition	Epidemiology/ incidence	Effects of the disease on pregnancy	Effects of pregnancy on the disease	Practice points
Immune thrombocytopenia purpura (continued)		Cesarean section for obstetrical indications, since it is of unproven benefit in decreasing rate of neonatal cerebral hemorrhage. *Fetal* Increased *fetal loss* with fetal mortality of 15–25% (most common causes are spontaneous abortion and hemorrhage); 50% fetal deaths occur before the onset of labor, most due to *allo*immune mechanisms Incidence of neonatal thrombocytopenia (NATP) is 30–40%, but severe NATP (i.e., platelets $< 50/mm^3$) occurs in 10–20% at delivery or in the first 3–5 days postpartum		Maternal steroid treatment is of unproven benefit in increasing *fetal* platelet count; trials of maternal (and neonatal) IV IgG are ongoing. *Goal* of treatment: maternal platelets $> 100/mm^3$, or cessation of serious bleeding. These pregnancies best managed in a high risk obstetric center. Cordocentesis advised only in case of *allo*immune thrombocytopenia. Fetal scalp vein sampling unreliable; not recommended.

	1–4% of babies with NATP suffer from cerebral hemorrhage Women with lower platelet counts *tend* to have babies with NATP, but there are *no* reliable predictors of fetal platelet count Factors that indicate a *high risk* of NATP are controversial but include women with a previous history of ITP (especially of splenectomy), acute or chronic ITP with platelets < 100/mm^3, or a previous infant with NATP			
Inflammatory bowel disease (IBD) Crohn's disease (25–27)	Not rare in pregnancy. Prevalence of inflammatory bowel disease in the United States ranges 1–2 million people: with peak incidence at 15–30 years.	Fertility significantly reduced; reduction in fertility is proportional to the activity of Crohn's disease. If disease is quiescent, no effect on fetal outcome.	Disease not adversely affected by pregnancy per se; disease remains quiescent in about 70% of pregnant women and improves in 35% of women with active disease at time of conception.	Infertility is reversed with appropriate drug therapy resulting in remission. Management of active disease should be similar to nonpregnant patients.

(continues)

Table 1 Continued

Condition	Epidemiology/ incidence	Effects of the disease on pregnancy	Effects of pregnancy on the disease	Practice points
Inflammatory bowel disease (IBD)				
Crohn's disease (continued)		If disease active at time of conception, spontaneous abortion rates double and prematurity rate increases.	15–40% relapse rate during pregnancy if in remission at time of conception. Highest risk of exacerbation in first trimester and puerperium. Onset of Crohn's disease during pregnancy is associated with a poorer prognosis.	Safe: corticosteroids, sulfasalazine and its 5-aminosalicyclic acid component (5-ASA), and antibiotics. Should avoid 6-mercaptopurine, azothioprine, and radiological investigations.
ulcerative colitis (25–27)	Peak incidence is 20–35 years.	No effect on fertility. Incidence of live births, congenital anomalies, spontaneous abortions, and stillbirths not increased except for a high incidence of spontaneous abortions (44%) in women with severe disease requiring surgery during pregnancy.	Overall risl of exacerbation same as in nonpregnant women (50%). If disease quiescent at conception, only 33% will relapse in pregnancy. If disease active at time of conception, 40% will improve and 33% will worsen. If disease begins in pregnancy, it may be more severe with high attack rates.	In general, treatment same as in the nonpregnant patient.

Condition			
Iron deficiency anemia (IDA) (1, 28)	75–80% of pregnant women with low hemoglobin have iron IDA.	IDA associated with placenta praevia/abruptio, placental hypertrophy and pregnancy-induced hypertension, postpartum hemorrhage. Severe IDA associated with fetal growth retardation, still births.	Since demand for iron in pregnancy *cannot* be met by dietary iron alone, supplemental iron recommended (30–60 mg/day in non-IDA and 200–300 mg/day in IDA state).
Malaria (1)	~ 1000 cases of malaria in United States per year. 13 cases of congenital malaria in United States/year, but 0.3% in immune mothers and 1–4% in non-immune mothers in endemic areas.	Majority of malarial infections are caused by *Plasmodium falciparum*. Severe maternal disease causes increased fetal wastage.	Malaria can cause intrauterine infection, placental insufficiency, intrauterine growth retardation, prematurity, abortion, low birth weight, and stillbirth.	Antimalarial prophylaxis advocated for mothers living in endemic areas; may prescribe chloroquine or mefloquine.
Multiple sclerosis (MS) (1)	10–75/100,000 pregnancies (same as general population).	Uncomplicated MS has no effect on pregnancy. Exacerbations tend to occur in the first trimester and puerperium.	Relapse rate approximates that of nonpregnant state. Women with severe debilitation may experience an increase in infections, fatigue, pulmonary problems.	Rest is an important component of optimal care in pregnancy. Urinary tract infection should be treated promptly.

(continues)

Table 1 Continued

Condition	Epidemiology/ incidence	Effects of the disease on pregnancy	Effects of pregnancy on the disease	Practice points
Myasthenia gravis (1)	2–4/100,000 pregnancies (same as general population).	Neonatal myasthenia gravis occurs in 10–20% of newborns; severity proportional to maternal anti-AChreceptor autoantibody levels, but newborn may also contribute through antibody synthesis. Resolves in 2–15 weeks.	One-third improve, one-third worsen, and one-third remain stable. If diagnosed in pregnancy, mother is prone to more severe form of disease. Exacerbations tend to occur in first trimester and puerperium, with improvement in second and third trimesters.	Agents that potentiate neuromuscular blockade, such as curare, should be avoided. Magnesium sulfate, narcotics, and analgesics may lead to respiratory depression. Regional anesthesia preferred.
Renal disease (29)		Fertility decreased with chronic renal impairment. Uneventful pregnancy unusual when serum creatinine > 3.0 mg/dL (265 μM), even in absence of maternal symptoms. Outcome is usually successful when serum creatinine <1.5–2.0 mg/dL (133–177 μM), hypertension (diastolic BP > 90) is absent, and underlying renal disease is not sclero-	*Mild* renal impairment (serum creatinine < 1.4 mg/dL = 124 μM): even with preserved renal function, pregnancy termination should be considered in women with renal PAN or renal scleroderma Natural history of *other* renal diseases not affected, except possibly IgA nephropathy, focal glomerulosclerosis (FGS), membranoproliferativa-	Patients should be seen every 2–4 weeks, for: Serial 24-hour urine collections for protein and creatinine clearance BP control To rule out asymptomatic bacteriuria Criteria of hypertension and proteinuria unreliable for preeclampsia.

derma or polyarteritis nodosa (PAN).

Increased risk of pre-eclampsia and perinatal morbidity (e.g., intra-uterine growth retardation) and mortality.

tive glomerulonephritis, and reflux nephropathy

Most show *increase* in glomular filtration rate, but 15% decrease near term is permissible

Increase/appearance of proteinuria (may be nephrotic) common, up to 50% patients

Moderate renal impairment (creatinine 1.5-2.0 mg/dL = 133-265 μM):

may suffer unpredictable, and at times irreversible, loss of function during/after pregnancy

Severe renal impairment (creatinine > 3 mg/dL = 265 μM):

pregnancy should be discouraged because risk of severe maternal complications greater than that of a successful pregnancy outcome

Table 1 Continued

Condition	Epidemiology/ incidence	Effects of the disease on pregnancy	Effects of pregnancy on the disease	Practice points
Rheumatoid arthritis (RA) (1)	RA affects 1–2% of women of childbearing age and may present during pregnancy.	Anti-Ro present in 5% of women with RA, but in 50% of RA patients who also have Sjögren's syndrome; this antibody has been associated with congenital heart block, but the risk is very low. Fetal echocardiogram at 20 weeks gestation is recommended when maternal Anti-Ro is present.	75% of patients improve; most do so in the first trimester, but may not improve until the third. 25% worsen and may develop new joint lesions. Relapse *often* occurs, usually within 2 months of delivery. Course during last pregnancy is predictive of course in current pregnancy.	Many patients are able to stop nonsteroidal anti-inflammatory drugs and disease-remitting agents during pregnancy, and are often managed with analgesics. ASA is drug of choice for treatment of joint inflammation, although this may cause maternal complications (prolonged gestation and labor, ante- and postpartum hemorrhage) or neonatal pulmonary hypertension secondary to premature closure of ductus arteriosus.
Rubella infection (30)	Even with current vaccination procedures, 15–20% of young adults are susceptible.	Effects depend on gestational age at infection: first trimester: 20% congenital rubella syndrome (CRS) 85% defects at 4 years of age (e.g.,	Course of the disease is unchanged by pregnancy. Maternal disease mild.	Vaccination of seronegative women advised 48–72 hours postpartum. Vaccine virus excreted in breast milk, but no contraindication to breastfeeding.

hearing defects both peripheral and central) associated with impaired language development, subretinal neovascularization, autism, developmental defects (motor, intellectual, and behavioral, a subacute progressive panencephalitis, various endocrine abnormalities, including diabetes mellitus) second trimester: 10% defects at 4 years of age with infection after 20 weeks gestation

Maternal infection confirmed by rubella-specific IgM or fourfold rise in rubella-specific IgG (by hemagglutination) OR probably by presence of rubella-specific IgG by complement fixation technique.

Pregnancy should be deferred for 3 months after vaccination, but there is *no documented increased* risk of CRS with *inadvertent* vaccination during pregnancy.

(continues)

Table 1 Continued

Condition	Epidemiology/ incidence	Effects of the disease on pregnancy	Effects of pregnancy on the disease	Practice points
Rubella infection (continued)		In utero infection diagnosed by any rubella-specific antibody in cord blood.		
Sickle cell disease (28,31–33)	Incidence in black Americans: HβS-S, 1 in 708; HbS-C, 1 in 757; HbS-δ-Thal, 1 in 1672 (should be considered in Mediterraneans, Arabians). 80,000 deaths annually worldwide attributable to sickle cell disease.	30% overall fetal wastage with increased risk of spontaneous abortions, infertility, prematurity, intrauterine growth retardation, and perinatal death. Prior to 1970 maternal mortality was as high as 10–12% and maternal morbidity up to 80–90%. Fetal loss up to 50–60%. These figures have been markedly reduced as a result of improved obstetric and prenatal care; maternal mortality ~ 1%.	Vaso-occlusive crises increase especially in the third trimester, labor, and puerperium. Increased incidence of Congestive failure (2–20%) Pneumonia (3–15%) Pyelonephritis (5–12%) Pulmonary emboli (20–40%) Cholelithiasis (25% vs. 10 in nonpregnancy)	Sickle cell screen in early pregnancy is recommended for all black women. Prenatal diagnosis by amniocentesis, cordocentesis, or chorionic villus sampling. Early and frequent prenatal assessment of pregnant women with this condition. Supplemental folic acid useful to promote erythrocyte production. Painful crises treated as in nonpregnant states. Transfusions increase risk of *allosensitization*. Exchange transfusions by manual/erythrocytophoresis techniques

| Syphilis (34–36) | ~100,000 cases of syphilis diagnosed annually in United States. 350 cases of congenital syphilis per year. | Vertical transmission can occur in any trimester; most severe fetal disease results from syphilis in early pregnancy. 50% of percent of infants born to women with untreated primary/secondary syphilis will have congenital infection at birth. Intrauterine growth retardation, stillbirth, hepatosplenomegaly, abnormal skeletal development, and dermatitis are manifestations of congenital syphilis. Antipartum infection in the last weeks of pregnancy may be asymptomatic. | The course of syphilis is not altered by pregnancy. | may be used for specific crises; not recommended prophylactically. Pregnancy is commonly listed as an etiology for false-positive serologies, but recent studies do not show increased rates of such results in gravidas. HIV-coinfected adults show extremely high titers or paradoxically negative titers with secondary syphilis. Confirmatory tests as in nonpregnant state. A penicillin-allergic patient may be treated with erythromycin; however, penicillin should be used to treat the neonate, since fetal erythromycin levels are not adequate. Titers of VDRL don't fall rapidly enough to indicate an adequate response to treatment. |

(continues)

Table 1 Continued

Condition	Epidemiology/ incidence	Effects of the disease on pregnancy	Effects of pregnancy on the disease	Practice points
Systemic lupus erythematosus (SLE) (37–39)	1/1000, as in nonpregnant women.	Fertility unchanged. Increased fetal loss with active disease at conception and positive maternal antibodies (especially antiphospholipid). Positive anti-Ro antibody present in 20–80% of SLE patients and is associated with neonatal lupus syndrome (NLS). Risk of NLS < 5%; previously affected child is *not* predictive of outcome in current pregnancy.	With quiescent disease at conception, probably no change in frequency of flares. Exacerbations tend to occur in first trimester or postpartum (20%).	Should be followed in high risk obstetrics unit, where fetal survival > 80%. Prednisone drug of choice for therapy, but *no* prophylactic treatment or increase in dosage recommended. Decreasing C3 or C4 levels useful for distinguishing preeclampsia from SLE flare. Positive antiphospholipid Ab, in absence of clinical manifestations, does *not* require therapy.
Toxoplasmosis (40)	50–60% of women of childbearing age susceptible. Congenital infection in 1–2/1000 live births in United States.	Transmission to fetus possible at any time during pregnancy, but less likely during first trimester; overall, congenital infection in 40–60% cases. Spontaneous abortion, stillbirth, and *severe* congenital infection occur exclusively with	Pregnancy does not alter course of the disease.	Preconception serology of *high risk* women is key (i.e., women who have recently acquired cats, who handle kitty litter, eat raw/undercooked meat, or have had a recent mononucleosis-like illness). Seronegative individuals should avoid high risk

maternal infection in early pregnancy.
Asymptomatic/subclinical infection occurs in the majority of babies infected.

situations (as detailed above); serial serology should be performed throughout pregnancy. Diagnosis made by serology: rising IgM indirect fluorescent antibody titer or absolute titer of ≥1:512 is a good indicator of active recent infection; false positives do occur.
Treatment can decrease risk of congenital infection, but risk still remains substantial.
Ultrasound is not sensitive enough to diagnose all cases of congenital infection.
Cordocentesis is performed in some centers when acute infection occurs during pregnancy and therapeutic abortion is an option; treatment with spiramycin recommended while waiting for the procedure.

(continues)

Table 1 Continued

Condition	Epidemiology/ incidence	Effects of the disease on pregnancy	Effects of pregnancy on the disease	Practice points
Tuberculosis (41)	Prevalence increasing since 1985 as a result of HIV infection in population.	Intrauterine fetal infection very unusual.	No increase in risk of progression to active disease; risk of such still greatest in the 1–2 years after infection. Presentation and natural history of disease unchanged in pregnancy.	Pregnant women generally react to purified protein derivative testing in manner similar to general population. Isoniazid prophylaxis is not recommended during pregnancy unless patient was recently infected (within the last 2 years). Isoniazid, rifampin, and ethambutol have not been found to be teratogenic; prophylactic treatment of the neonate with vitamin K recommended because of possible complication of hemorrhagic disease of the newborn. Neonate born to a mother with active TB should be treated with isoniazid for the first 2–3 months of life,

| Urinary tract infections (UTI) (42,43) | Asymptomatic bacteriuria (ASB) occurs in ~5–6% of women during pregnancy, most of whom have positive urine cultures at *first* antenatal visit. Acute UTI (cystitis or pyelonephritis) complicates 2% of pregnancies; most did *not* have preceding ASB | Association of ASB with preeclampsia, anemia, prematurity, and fetal loss unproven. Acute UTI can mimic/precipitate premature labor; role in etiology of intrauterine growth retardation, fetal death, or congenital abnormalities controversial. | Pregnancy does not predispose women to ASB. However, up to 40% of women with ASB go on to develop acute symptomatic UTI during pregnancy, especially with prior history of UTI. | All women should be screened for ASB at first prenatal visit. Treatment of ASB reduces risk of acute UTI during pregnancy to 3–4%. Treatment can proceed with nitrofurantoin (for 10 days), ampicillin, or cephalexin. One-third of women treated for ASB will have persistence/recurrence of infection; suppressive therapy should be considered in such women *if* close follow-up and treatment not possible. Acute UTI usually caused by Gram-negative bacteria. |

or at least until the mother is known to be smear- and culture-negative; treatment with two drugs should be initiated if infant's skin test positive or there is evidence of clinical disease.

(continues)

Table 1 Continued

Condition	Epidemiology/ incidence	Effects of the disease on pregnancy	Effects of pregnancy on the disease	Practice points
Urolithiasis (42,43)	Complicates ~ 0.24% of pregnancies.	Increase in symptomatic urinary tract infections; otherwise, course and outcome of pregnancy unchanged.	Pregnancy has no effect on severity or progression of nephrolithiasis. Increased rate of spontaneous stone passage (70%).	Hydronephrosis (usually greater on right side) diagnosed by ultrasound is unreliable sign for urethral obstruction. Must be distinguished from acute pyelonephritis.
Varicella (1)	1–5/100,000 pregnancies.	Chickenpox pneumonia during pregnancy has a maternal mortality rate of 41% (vs. 11% in nonpregnant state). Congenital varicella syndrome is characterized by intrauterine growth retardation, limb hypoplasia, brain atrophy, cicatricial scars, mental retardation, and ocular lesions.	Clinical congenital varicella after maternal exposure to chickenpox in the first trimester ≅ 5%, probably less, and 17% in the last two weeks before birth.	Infant born 5 days prior to delivery to 2 days postpartum at greatest risk of varicella of newborn; *Varicella zoster* immunoglobulin should therefore be given also in first 3 months of life if exposed to varicella. Exposed pregnant mother should receive VZIG within 96 hours of exposure; probably no benefit beyond that time.

| Venous thromboembolism (1) | Deep venous thrombosis (DVT) of lower extremities in ~ 0.018–0.29% of pregnancies, up to 3% of patients postpartum.
Pulmonary embolism (PE) occurs in ~ 1 in 2000 pregnancies.
Increased risk associated with operative delivery, preeclampsia, and hypercoagulable states (e.g., lupus anticoagulant). | Only a problem when maternal hemodynamic integrity is compromised. | Pregnancy is a hypercoagulable state.
Diagnosis of DVT best made using combined ultrasound-Doppler techniques.
Clinical suspicion of PE should lead to V/Q scanning, since radiation exposure is far below permissible dose in pregnancy. | Warfarin should not be used between 6–12 weeks gestation; best avoided throughout pregnancy.
Prophylactic heparin (5000 U SC q12h starting at 12 weeks gestation) recommended for history of unexplained DVT in previous pregnancy, lupus anticoagulant, or other hypercoagulable state.
Heparin should be discontinued at onset of labor and restarted 2 hours postpartum (when hemostasis achieved).
Anticoagulation should be continued for 6 weeks postpartum, or until 6 months of treatment achieved when DVT occurred in index pregnancy; coumadin safe for breastfeeding. |

Vitamin deficiency: see B_{12} (above)

affected with a medical disorder safely through pregnancy and delivery. Rather, it is important to adopt a more global approach, which in an interdisciplinary fashion encompasses prepregnancy counseling and obstetrical care and, in addition, addresses the medical and social factors that might influence the well-being of the child, the mother, and the family.

MEDICAL DISEASES IN PREGNANCY

In this chapter, we have summarized the interrelationship between pregnancy outcome and a variety of maternal medical diseases. Reproductive risks associated with maternal lifestyle and various specific medical therapies are dealt with in other chapters. Table 1 addresses the two essential questions one asks when a woman with a medical disease becomes pregnant:

1. What is the effect of the disease on pregnancy?
2. What is the effect of pregnancy on the disease?

The first question deals with pregnancy loss (abortion, stillbirth, neonatal death), congenital malformations, fetal and neonatal morbidities, and maternal complications peculiar to pregnancy, such as abruptio placentae, and preeclampsia.

In the second question, we are asking whether pregnancy per se alters the course and prognosis of the disease, and to what extent and in what manner.

For the purposes of this chapter, we have limited ourselves to medical disorders that are relatively common in pregnancy and to those that are not common but are associated with specific reproductive risks. Clearly, a complete list of medical conditions in pregnancy could not be incorporated into a single chapter, and the reader is referred to the References for further information.

The final column of Table 1 is headed "Practice points." Again, the details of management and the adjustments in medical care necessary during pregnancy are numerous. We have tried to highlight a few key points for each condition that may serve as valuable clinical tips.

Answer

Women with diabetes mellitus have higher rates of fetal malformations, mainly sacral agenesis or cardiac anomalies. In addition, the baby may suffer from macrosomia, neonatal hypoglycemia, and a variety of other perinatal complications. Recent research suggests that tight glycemic control substantially decreases the risk for both malformations and perinatal complications. Some studies, however, have not shown a correlation between glycemic control and rates of major malformations. In any case, your patient's anxiety about the effects of insulin is not justified. In fact, she may end up needing more insulin during pregnancy.

REFERENCES

1. Gleicher N, ed. Principles of Medical Therapy in Pregnancy. Appleton & Lange, Norwalk, CT, 1992.
2. Pizzo PA, Butler KM. In the vertical transmission of HIV, timing may be everything. N Engl J Med 1991; 325:652-654.
3. Van der Perre P, Simonon A, Msellati P, Hitimana D, Vaira D, Bazabagira A, Van Goetem C, Stevens AM, Karita E, Sondag-Thull D, Dabis F, Lepage P. Postnatal transmission of human immunodeficiency virus type 1 from mother to infant. N Engl J Med 1991; 325:593-598.
4. Spence MR, Rebolic AC. Human immunodeficiency virus infection in women. Ann Intern Med 1991; 115(10):827-828.
5. Burrow GN, Ferris TF, ed. Medical Complications During Pregnancy, 3rd ed. Saunders, Philadelphia, 1988.
6. (a) Cherry SH, Berkowitz RL, Kase NG, eds. Medical, Surgical and Gynecological Complications of Pregnancy, 3rd ed. Baltimore, Williams & Wilkins, 1985. (b) de Swiet M, ed. Medical Disorders in Obstetric Practice. Edinburgh, Blackwell, 1985.
7. McIvor, Balter MS. Avoiding complications in the pregnancy asthmatic. Can J Diagn 1991; 87-95.
8. Drukker BH, Sauer H. Diseases of the breast. 1991. Part XVII: Chap 188:1142-1156.
9. Abrams RS, Wexler P, eds. Medical Care of the Pregnant Patient. Little, Brown, Boston, 1983.
10. Cousins L. Etiology and prevention of congenital anomalies among infants of overt diabetic women. Clin Obstet Gynecol 1991; 34:481-493.
11. Dickinson JE, Palmer SM. Semin Perinatol 1990; 14:2-11.
12. Lefkowitz CA, McLaughlin PR. Pregnancy and heart disease. Med North Am 1986; 38:5582-5587.
13. Choo Q-L, Kuo G, Weiner AJ, et al. Isolation of cDNA clone derived from a blood borne non-A, non-B viral hepatitis genome. Science 1989; 244:359.
14. Koff RS. Natural history of acute hepatitis B in adults re-examined. Gastroenterology 1987; 92:2035.
15. Wahl M, Hermodsson S, Iwarson S. Hepatitis B vaccination with short dose intervals—A possible alternative for post-exposure prophylaxis. Infection 1988; 16:229.
16. Centers for Disease Control, Immunization Practices Advisory Committee. Prevention of perinatal transmission of hepatitis B virus: Prenatal screening of all pregnant women for hepatitis B surface antigens. MMWR 1988; 37:341.
17. Lo KJ, Lee SD, Tsai YT, et al. Long-term immunogenicity and efficacy of hepatitis B vaccine in infants born to HBc Ag-positive HBsAg-carrier mothers. Hepatology 1988; 8:1647.
18. Kulhanjian JA, et al. Identification of women at unsuspected risk of primary infection with herpes simplex virus type 2 during pregnancy. N Engl J Med 1992; 916-920, 946-947.
19. Hardy DA, et al. Use of polymerase chain reaction for successful identification of asymptomatic genital infection with herpes simplex virus in pregnant women at delivery. J Infect Dis 1990; 162:1031-1035.

20. National High Blood Pressure Education Program. Working Group Report on High Blood Pressure in Pregnancy. Am J Obstet Gynecol 1990; 163:1691–1712.
21. Lindheimer MD, Katz AI. Preeclampsia: Pathophysiology, diagnosis and management. Annu Rev Med 1989; 40:233–250.
22. Ryan D, Cattran DC. Hypertensive disorders of pregnancy. Med North Am 1988; 27:5057–5064.
23. Lazarus JH, Othman S. Thyroid disease in relation to pregnancy. Clin Endocrinol 1991; 34:91–98.
24. Mandal SJ, et al. Increased need for thyroxine during pregnancy in women in primary hypothyroidism. N Engl J Med 1990; 323:91–96.
25. Kirsner JB, Shorter RG. Recent development's in non-specific inflammatory bowel disease. N Engl J Med 1982; 306:837.
26. Mayberry JF, Weterman IT. European survey of fertility in women with Crohn's disease: A case controlled study by a European collaborative group. Gut 1986; 27:821.
27. Adler DJ, Korelitz BI. Small and large bowel disease. 1991; 149:950–954.
28. Akinyanju OO, Nnatu SNN, Ogendengbe OK. Antenatal iron supplmentation in sickle cell disease. Int J Gynaecol Obstet 1987; 25:433.
29. Symposium on renal function and disease in pregnancy. Am J Kidney Dis 1987; 9:243–380.
30. Rubella vaccination during pregnancy—United States, 1971–1988. MMWR 1989; 38:289–293.
31. Schneider RG, Hightower B, Hasty TS, et al. Abnormal hemoglobins in a quarter-million people. Blood 1976; 48:629.
32. Charache S, Neibyl JR. Pregnancy in sickle cell disease. Clin Haematol 1985; 14:729.
33. Morrison JC, Schneider JM, Whybrew WD, et al. Prophylactic transfusion in pregnant patients with sickle cell disease, a randomized cooperative study. N Engl J Med 1988; 319:1447.
34. Moore JE, Mohr CF. Biologically false positive serologic tests for syphilis. JAMA 1952; 150:467.
35. Manikowska-Lesinska W, Linda B, Zajac W. Specificity of the FTA-ABS and TPHA tests during pregnancy. Br J Vener Dis 1987; 54:295.
36. Centers for Disease Control. Recommendations for diagnosing and treating syphilis in HIV-infected patients. MMWR 1988; 37:600.
37. Ramsey-Goldman R. Pregnancy in systemic lupus erythematosus. Rheum Dis Clin North Am 1988; 14:169–185.
38. Branch DW. Antiphospholipid antibodies and pregnancy: Maternal implications. Semin Perinatol 1990; 14:139–146.
39. Branch DW. Antiphospholipid syndrome: Laboratory concerns, fetal loss, and pregnancy management. Semin Perinatol 1991; 230–237.
40. Jeannel D, et al. What is known about the prevention of congenital toxoplasmosis? Lancet 1990; 336:359–361.

41. Snider DE Jr, et al. Treatment of tuberculosis during pregnancy. Am Rev Respir Dis 1980; 122:75–79.
42. Wait RB. Urinary tract infection during pregnancy. Postgrad Med 1984; 75: 153–161.
43. Coe FL, Parks JH, Lindheimer MD. Nephrolithiasis during pregnancy. N Engl J Med 1978; 288:324–326.

Part IV

Organization and Operation of Teratogen Information Services

27

Teratogen Information Services

Gideon Koren and Anne Pastuszak
The Hospital for Sick Children, Toronto, Ontario, Canada

Clinical Case

You have a patient with a potential teratogenic exposure you are not familiar with. You practice in central Florida. What should you do?

INTRODUCTION

Since the thalidomide era 30 years ago (1), perinatal medicine has been practiced by physicians and their patients as if every drug were a potential human teratogen. In reality, relatively few xenobiotics have been proven beyond doubt to pose risk to the human fetus (2), while an ever-increasing number of agents have been found to be safe. It is estimated that about half the pregnancies in North America are unplanned, and thus a very large number of women expose their fetuses to prescribed and nonprescribed agents taken for a variety of indications. Moreover, the early weeks of unplanned pregnancies are more likely to entail uncontrolled consumption of cigarettes, alcohol, and drugs of abuse by women who otherwise would try to minimize their gestational exposures.

During the last two decades, health professionals in the areas of teratology, genetics, pharmacology, toxicology, and obstetrics have been increasingly approached by pregnant women and their physicians for available information on the safety/risk of drugs, chemicals, radiation, and infections. This has led to the development of teratogen information services (TIS) in various states, provinces, and countries.

As of 1992, several dozens TIS have been operating in North America and in Europe (Table 1). This chapter reviews the structure and clinical functions of these newly formed services, their research activities, and their unprecedented potential to advance our knowledge of human teratogens. Considering both the clinical endpoint and the research potential of the endeavor, TIS offer an exciting opportunity for clinicians and scientists, as well as an inexpensive, cost-effective way of achieving dramatic improvements in patient care.

STRUCTURE AND FUNCTION OF A TERATOGEN INFORMATION SERVICE

Most TIS operate as telephone services, mainly to respond to questions from the general public and from health professionals. All TIS document the incoming calls on specially designed forms. Although various TIS have slight differences in the data collected during the telephone interview, all services aim at assessing relevant information needed to address the safety/risk of the particular case.

The TIS are manned by health professionals drawn from different medical fields, including genetic counselors, nurses, toxicologists, and pharmacists. Virtually all services are directed by physicians, most commonly geneticists, but also clinical pharmacologists-toxicologists, epidemiologists, and obstetricians. The training of health professionals for their task as teratogen information specialists varies substantially among the TIS, probably because at present there is no formal process to acquire such training.

In some programs the information given to women or health professionals over the telephone is followed by a letter. In other programs no such letters are sent, but selected patients are referred to geneticists, obstetricians, or other medical specialists. In Toronto, the Motherisk Program is presently dealing with 50–60 calls per day, which is double the load encountered 3 years ago. Women are referred to the weekly Motherisk Clinic according to criteria presented in Table 2. At the clinic, the women are seen by a physician team member who collects data on the exposure in question and any other potential risk factors before communicating with the woman the safety/risks of her exposure(s). The Motherisk physicians are pediatric pharmacologists-toxicologists, or trainees in our program, generally individuals who have already completed their specialty training in pediatrics, medicine, or emergency medicine.

SOURCES OF INFORMATION

Virtually all TIS use one or more on-line programs in reproductive toxicology, such as Reprotox or Teris. All programs obtain relevant texts in the area

Table 1 International List of Teratogen Information Services (updated 1992)

United States

Arizona
Arizona Teratogen Information Program (ATIP)
University of Arizona, Department of Pediatrics
Section of Genetics/Dysmorphology
2504 East Elm Street
Tucson AZ 85716
(602) 795-5675; in Arizona, 800-362-0101
Fax (602) 626-4884
Dee Quinn M.S., H. Eugene Hoyme M.D., Lynn Hauck M.S.

California
California Teratogen Information Service & Clinical Research Program
University of California, San Diego
Department of Pediatrics
Division of Dysmorphology & Teratology
225 Dickinson Street, #8446
San Diego CA 92103-8446
(619) 294-6084; in California, 800-532-3749
(619) 294-6217 (administrative only)
Fax (619) 291-0946
Kenneth Lyons Jones M.D., Kathleen Johnson, Christina Chambers, Lyn Dick,
Robert Felix

Colorado
TIES
The Children's Hospital
B300 Genetics
1056 East 19th Avenue
Denver CO 80218
(303) 861-6395, 800-332-2082 (Colorado), 800-525-4871 (Wyoming)
Fax (303) 861-3992
Karen Prescott M.S., David Manchester M.D., Carol Walton M.S., Cathy Marquez

Connecticut
Connecticut Pregnancy Exposure Information Service
Division of Human Genetics, Room L-5072
University of Connecticut Health Center
263 Farmington Avenue
Farmington CT 06030
(203) 679-1502; in Connecticut, 800-325-5391
Fax (203) 679-1531
Glenda Lee Spivey M.S., Sally S. Rosengren M.D., Sharon Voyer M.S.,
Robert Pilarski M.S., Joanne Brochu

(continues)

Table 1   (continued)

District of Columbia
Reproductive Toxicology Center
2440 M Street NW, Suite 217
Washington DC 20037-1404
(202) 293-5137
Fax (202) 293-7256
Anthony R. Scialli M.D., Armand Lione, Ph.D., G. Kay Padgett, Christine Colie
M.D., Greta D. Ober

Florida
Teratogen Information Services
Box 100296
University of Florida Health Science Center
Gainesville FL 32610-0296
(904) 392-3050
Fax (904) 392-3051
Donna H. Poynor M.M., Charles A. Williams M.D.

Florida Teratogen Information Service
University of Miami School of Medicine
Mailman Center
P.O. Box 016820
Miami FL 33101
(305) 547-6464
Fax (305) 547-3919
Virginia H. Carver Ph.D

Teratogen Information Service
University of South Florida
Department of Pediatrics, Box 15-G
12901 Bruce B. Downs Boulevard
Tampa FL 33613
(813) 974-2262
Fax (813) 974-4985
James K. Hartsfield D.M.D., Boris G. Kousseff M.D., Suzanne R. Sage R.N., M.S.,
Jamie L. Frias M.D.

Georgia
Centers for Disease Control
Division of Birth Defects and Genetic Diseases
Mail Stop F45
1600 Clifton Road
Atlanta GA 30333
(404) 488-4967
Fax (404) 488-4643
Muin J. Khoury M.D., Ph.D., Jose F. Cordero M.D., M.P.H.

Table 1

Illinois
Illinois Teratogen Information Service
Northwestern University
333 East Superior, Suite 1543
Chicago IL 60611
(312) 908-7441, 800-252-4847
Fax (312) 908-6643
Eugene Pergament M.D., Ph.D.

Indiana
Indiana Teratogen Information Service
Department of Medical Genetics
Indiana University Medical Center
975 West Walnut Street
Indianapolis IN 46202
(317) 274-1071
Fax (317) 274-2387
David D. Weaver M.D., Peg Davee M.S., Lola Cook M.S.

Iowa
University of Iowa Prenatal Diagnostic Unit
Department of Obstetrics and Gynecology
University of Iowa
Iowa City IA 52241
(319) 356-3561
Fax (319) 355-6728
Roger Williamson M.D., Katherine Wenstrom M.D., Susan Sipes M.D., Stanley
Grant R.N.

University of Iowa Teratogen Information Service
Department of Pediatrics/Medical Genetics
University of Iowa Hospitals & Clinics
Iowa City IA 52242
(319) 356-3347
James W. Hanson M.D., Ann Muilenburg R.N., M.A.

Kansas
Prenatal Diagnostic & Genetic Clinic
HCA Wesley Medical Center
550 North Hillside
Wichita KS 67214
(316) 688-2362
Sechin Cho M.D., Paula Floyd R.N., M.N., Richard Lutz, M.D.,
Nancy McMaster R.N., M.Ed.

(continues)

Table 1   (continued)

Massachusetts
Massachusetts Teratogen Information Service (MTIS)
National Birth Defects Center
30 Warren Street
Boston MA 02135
(617) 787-4957; in Massachusetts, 800-322-5014, (office) (617) 787-5834
Fax (617) 787-6936
Susan Rosenwasser M.Ed., Jane O'Brien M.D., Katryn Miller, M.Ed., Robin Maltz
M.P.H., Karen Treat M.S.

Embryology Teratology Unit
Warren 801
Massachusetts General Hospital
Fruit Street
Boston MA 02114
(617) 726-1742
Fax (617) 726-1866
Lewis B. Holmes M.D., Ailish M. Hayes M.D., Gerald V. Raymond M.D., Joan M.
Stoler M.D.

TERAS
c/o Dr. Fred Bieber
Department of Pathology
Brigham & Women's Hospital
75 Francis Street
Boston MA 02115
(617) 732-6507
Fax (617) 732-7513
Frederick R. Bieber Ph.D., David Genest, George Mutter, Drucilla Roberts,
Christopher Crum

Missouri
Columbia Teratogen Information Service
Department of Child Health
Medical Genetics Division
University of Missouri
1 Hospital Drive
Columbia MO 652121
(314) 882-6991
Fax (314) 882-2742
Virginia Proud M.D., Judith Miles M.D., Kathy Morris M.S.S.W.

Genetics and Environmental Information Service (GENIS)
Washington University School of Medicine
Departments of Obstetrics & Gynecology and Genetics
216 South Kings Highway
St. Louis MO 63110

Table 1

[GENIS]
(314) 454-8172
Fax (314) 454-7358
Heidi Beaver M.P.H., Sheri Babb, Laura Turlington M.S., Cindy Johnson M.S.,
James P. Crane M.D., Jeffrey M. Dicke, Jane E. Corteville, Diana L. Gray

Nebraska
Nebraska Teratogen Project
University of Nebraska Medical Center
600 South 42nd Street
Omaha NE 68198-5430
(402) 559-5071
Fax (402) 559-5737
Beth Conover R.N., M.S., Bruce Buehler M.D.

New Jersey
New Jersey Pregnancy Risk Information Service
University of Medicine and Dentistry of New Jersey-SOM
401 Haddon Avenue
Camden NJ 08103
(609) 757-7812; in New Jersey, 800-441-0025
Fax (609) 757-9792
Michael K. McCormack Ph.D., Carol Zuber M.S., Charlotte Furey B.S.N.

New York
Perinatal Environmental and Drug Consultation Service (PEDECS)
Department of Obstetrics & Gynecology
P.O. Box 668
University of Rochester Medical Center
601 Elmwood Avenue
Rochester NY 14642
(716) 275-3638
Fax (716) 244-2209
Richard K. Miller Ph.D.

Teratogen Information Service
1200 East and West Road
Building 16
West Seneca NY 14224
(716) 674-6300, x4812
Luther K. Robinson M.D., Sandra Gangell

North Dakota
John T. Martsolf M.D.
Division of Medical Genetics, Department of Pediatrics
University of North Dakota School of Medicine
501 Columbia Road

(continues)

Table 1   (continued)

[University of North Dakota]
Grand Forks ND 58203
(701) 777-4277
Fax (701) 777-3894
John T. Martsolf M.D., Mary Ebertowski R.N.

Pennsylvania
Pregnancy Healthline
Pennsylvania Hospital
Spruce Building, 7th Floor
8th and Spruce Streets
Philadelphia PA 19107
(215) 829-3601
Fax (215) 829-7423
Betsy Schick-Boschetto M.S.N., Alan E. Donnenfeld M.D., Ronald J. Librizzi D.O.

Pregnancy Safety Hotline
Department of Reproductive Genetics
School of Nursing, 2nd Floor
Western Pennsylvania Hospital
4800 Friendship Avenue
Pittsburgh PA 15224
(412) 687-SAFE
Fax (412) 578-1125
Michael J. Kerr M.S., Kathy A. Bournikos M.S., Karen Filkins M.D., Christann
Jackson M.D., Elizabeth Gettig M.S.

Department of Reproductive Genetics
Magee-Women's Hospital
300 Halket Street
Pittsburgh PA 15213
(412) 647-4168
Fax (412) 647-4343
Sandra G. Marchese M.S., Mona Penles Stadler M.S., Deanna P. Steele M.S., Luanne
Fraer M.S., Amy Niklaus M.S., Faith Callif-Daley M.S., Dolores Pegram M.Ed.

South Dakota
Teratogen and Birth Defects Information Project
School of Medicine, University of South Dakota
414 East Clark
Vermillion SD 57069
800-962-1642
Fax (605) 677-5124
Virginia P. Johnson M.D., Patricia Skorey M.N.S., B.S.N., Carol Strom M.S.

Table 1

Texas
Genetic Screening & Counseling Service
P.O. Box 2467
Denton TX 76202-2467
(817) 383-3561
Fax (817) 382-6235
Lori Wolfe M.S., Becky Althaus M.S., Donald W. Day M.D., Margaret Drummon-Borg M.D., Judith Martin M.D.

Utah
Pregnancy Riskline
44 Medical Drive
Salt Lake City UT 84113
(801) 583-2229
Fax (801) 584-8488
John Carey M.D., Marcia Feldkamp, Lynn Martinez, Marsha Leen-Mitchell

Vermont
Vermont Pregnancy Risk Information Service
Vermont Regional Genetics Center
1 Mill Street
Burlington VT 05401
(802) 658-4310
Elizabeth F. Allen Ph.D., Alan E. Guttmacher M.D.

Washington
Central Laboratory for Human Embryology
Department of Pediatrics RD-20
School of Medicine
University of Washington
Seattle WA 98195
(206) 543-3373
Fax (206) 543-3184
Tom Shepard M.D., Alan Fantel M.D., Phil Mirkes

Wisconsin
Teratogen Information Service
La Crosse Regional Genetic Services
P.O. Box 1326
La Crosse WI 54602
(608) 791-6681; for Wisconsin, Iowa, and northern Illinois, 800-362-9567
Janet Williams M.S.

(continues)

Table 1   (continued)

Great Lake Genetics
2323 North Mayfair Road, Suite 410
Milwaukee WI 53226
(414) 475-7400, (414) 475-7223
Lois Magnuson R.N., Jurgen Herrmann M.D., Bonnie-Jo Bates M.D.

Eastern Wisconsin Teratogen Service
Medical Genetics Institute, S.C.
4555 West Schroeder Drive, Suite 180
Milwaukee WI 53223
(414) 357-6555
Fax (414) 357-9394
B. Rafael Elejalde M.D., Maria M. de Elejalde M.S., R.N.

Canada

Safe Start Program
Chedoke-McMaster Medical Center
1200 Main Street West, Room 1E-1
Hamilton, Ontario L8N 3Z5
Canada
(416) 521-2100, x6788
Fax (416) 521-5008
Elizabeth Chow Tung Pharm. D.

FRAME Program (Fetal Risk Assessment from Maternal Exposure)
800 Commissioners' Road East
London, Ontario N6C 2V5
Canada
(519) 685-8293
Fax (519) 685-8156
Michael J. Rieder M.D., Carlene Morrison

Motherisk Program
Division of Clinical Pharmacology and Toxicology
The Hospital for Sick Children
555 University Avenue
Toronto, Ontario M5G 1X8
Canada
(416) 813-6780
Fax (416) 813-7562
Gideon Koren M.D., Chris Eliopoulos, Natalie Horlatsh, Sheelagh Martin, Adrianne
Einarson, Anne Pastuszak

Table 1

Department of Medical Genetics
University of British Columbia
University Hospital — Shaughnessy Site
4500 Oak Street
Vancouver, British Columbia V6H 3N1
Canada
(604) 875-2157
Fax (604) 875-2376
J. M. Friedman M.D., Ph.D., Margot Van Allen M.D., Wendy Hird M.Sc., Heidi Hogg M.Sc.

British Columbia Drug & Poison Information Centre
1081 Burrard Street
Vancouver, British Columbia V6Z 1Y6
Canada
(604) 682-2344 x2126
Fax (604) 631-5262
Janet Webb M.Sc., Bev Louis B.Sc. (Pharm), Kathy McInnes B.Sc. (Pharm)

France

Centre Regional d'Information sur les Teratogénes
Institut Europeen des Genomutations
86, rue Edmond Locard
69005 Lyon
France
33-78-25-82-10
Fax 33-78-36-61-82
Elisabeth Robert M.D.

Centre de Renseignements sur les Agents Teratogénes (CRAT)
CHU St. Antoine Laboratoire d'Embryologie
184, rue du Fauborg
75102 Paris
France
33-1-43-41-26-22, 33-1-43-41-71-00 poste 1462
Fax (33) 1-40-01-14-99
Charles Roux M.D., Elisabeth Elefant M.D., Marie Boyer M.D.

Israel

Drugs and Poisons in Pregnancy
Israel Poison Information Center

(continues)

Table 1   (continued)

[Israel Poison Information Center]
Rambam Medical Center
P.O. Box 9602
Haifa 31096
Israel
972-4-514749
Fax 972-4-534887
Yedidia Bentur M.D., Uri Taitelman M.D., Bianca Raikhlin Ph.D.

Israeli Teratological Information Service
Laboratory of Teratology
Hadassah Medical School
Jerusalem
Israel
972-2-428430
Fax 972-2-784010
Asher Ornoy M.D., Judy Arnon Ph.D., Ronit Abir M.Sc., Deganit Eini

Beilinson Teratology Information Service
c/o Prof. Paul Merlob
Department of Neonatology
Beilinson Medical Center
Petah-Tikva 49100
Israel
972-3-937-74-73/2, 922-00-68
Fax 972-3-922-96-85
Prof. Paul Merlob, Mag. Bracha Stahl, Mrs. Rachel Friedman, Mrs. Davida Shaliti

Italy

Telefono Rosso
Servizio Autonomo di Tossicologia
Policlinico Careggi
Viale Morgagni, 85
50134 Firenze
Italy
39-55-4277238
Fax 39-55-4277425
L. Caramelli M.D., B. Occupati M.D., C. Smorlesi M.D., A. Pistelli M.D.

Telefono Rosso
Ospedale San Paolo
Clinica Ostetrica Ginecologica
Via Rudini 8
20142 Milano
Italy
39-2-8910207

Table 1

[Ospedale San Paolo]
Fax 39-2-8135662
M. Buscaglia M.D., S. Dal Verme, midwife, F. Molteni M.D., P. Sulpizio M.D., G. Rognoni M.D., L. Ghisoni M.D.

Telefono Rosso
Policlinico Gemelli
Clinica Pediatrica
Servizio di Epidemiologia e Clinica dei Difetti Congeniti
Universita Cattolica del Sacro Cuore
Largo Gemelli 8
00168 Roma
Italy
39-6-3372779
Fax 39-6-3383211
Pierpaolo Mastroiacovo M.D., M. Pagano M.D., M. Valente M.D.

Telefono Rosso
c/o Icaro-ASM
Associazione Studio Malformazioni
Via Sabotino 2
00195 Roma
Italy
39-6-3701898
Fax 39-6-3701904
M.A. Serafini M.D., M. DeSantis M.D., I. Vercillo Martino M.D.

Telefono Rosso
Clinica Universitaria
Obstetrico-Ginecologica
Via Ventimiglia 3
10100 Torino
Italy
39-11-63-12-31
Fax 39-11-664-79-10 or 39-11-69-79-10
Daniela Lombardo M.D., Grazia Oberto M.D.

Spain
Servicio de Informacion Telefonica Sobre Teratogenos Español (SITTE)
Facultad de Medicina
Universidad Complutense
28040 Madrid
Spain
34-1-394-15-94
Fax 34-1-394-15-92
Dra. M.L. Martinez-Frias, E. Rodriguez Pinilla, M. Urioste Azcorra, E. Bermejo Sanchez

Table 2 Indications for Motherisk Clinic Consultation

Exposure to known or suspected teratogens
Exposure to new drugs
Exposure to drugs of abuse
Chronic maternal illness
Chronic maternal drug therapy
Occupation exposures
Any woman who wants to be seen or whose physician wishes her to be seen

of clinical teratology and related fields, such as diseases in pregnancy, drug abuse toxicology, and infectious diseases. Moreover, most services continuously review new published studies in the area of teratology for their relevance to the human exposure. In Toronto, the Motherisk team meets weekly to critically review literature and to decide whether it should be included in our "Statements." The "Statement" for each exposure is computerized to be included in all subsequent letters sent to physicians.

RESEARCH POTENTIAL

In addition to the novel clinical component introduced by the TIS, these services open new horizons for much-needed research in the area of reproductive toxicology. In the past, many scientists have stressed the need for large prospective cohorts in the area of clinical teratology; however, these were difficult and expensive to collect. For example, the Collaborative Perinatal Project, funded by the U.S. National Institutes of Health in the 1960s, prospectively collected women and their offspring. More than 5 years were spent on the collection of 50,000 cases at a cost of many millions of dollars, yet most drug cohorts were too small to prove safety/risk.

The TIS create a new reality because women call these services in real time about their exposures, thus obviating the problems of recall. Hence there are now on record hundreds of thousands of gestational exposures in North America that are a virtual gold mine for prospective research. However, there are also major issues in materializing this potential. For example, being clinical programs, many TIS do not have the infrastructure needed to conduct such research. At present, most TIS do not routinely follow up on the outcome of the pregnant women they counsel. A number of TIS follow up the outcome of a selected list of drugs of interest (e.g., new drugs, drugs for which no data exist, drugs known or suspected to be teratogenic). Yet some of the more established TIS, which by now have accumulated impressive cohorts of patients, have begun publishing their follow-up analyses. The San Diego program, headed by Dr. K. Jones, has published several peer-reviewed studies in the last few years (3,4). Similarly, the Motherisk Program in Toronto has published recently a number of prospective studies based on its follow-up (5–7).

An even more promising trend is the collaboration among TIS. We have recently published the prospective ascertainment of 149 first-trimester exposures to lithium in San Diego and Philadelphia, and in Toronto and London, Ontario (8). This study may bring about changes in the approach to this essential psychiatric drug, which was believed for decades, on the basis of retrospective studies, to be a major human teratogen.

At present, most drug companies orphan pregnant women from drug use in pregnancy by labeling their products "not proven safe" in pregnancy. Yet, in many cases these companies are reluctant to support the collection of newly available data through the TIS. Because postmarketing collection of such data is not mandatory in either the United States or Canada, many manufacturers do not feel obligated to support its collection. When this attitude is coupled with the relatively small market for most medications in pregnancy, it can be seen that the incentive for many pharmaceutical houses is negligible. Yet, half the pregnancies in North America are unplanned; the refusal of manufacturers to participate in this data collection process may potentially lead to the exclusion of all women of reproductive age from the benefit of agents whose safety has not been proven.

One author [AP] believes that only legislation will solve this example of abuse of women's rights.

FUNDING

At present TIS are funded though various sources at state, provincial, or municipal departments of health, or through private agencies. Almost invariably these important services are underfunded, mainly because of the time needed to prove their effectiveness coupled with the present difficult economic times.

EFFECTIVENESS OF THE INFORMATION COUNSELING PROCESS

To justify their functions, TIS must, like other clinical services, prove their impact on health care. This can be done in two separate dimensions:

Proving the ability of TIS to prevent unnecessary pregnancy terminations
Calculating the impact of TIS on the prevention of major birth defects

We have analyzed for this presentation data on the effectiveness of the Motherisk Program in Toronto in these two dimensions.

During the clinic visit we use a 10 cm visual analog scale (VAS) to assess each woman's tendency to continue/terminate pregnancy [(5) and Chapter 29]. Briefly, 100 denotes an absolute intention to continue pregnancy and zero an absolute tendency to terminate the pregnancy. We validated this VAS recently by showing that the vast majority of women who left our clinic with a 50% or more tendency to terminate pregnancy eventually did so (8). This questionnaire is delivered once before any information is volunteered to the woman, and again after we have explained to her what is known about her exposures.

Calculation of Cost Effectiveness of Preventing Unjustified Pregnancy Terminations

In an analysis of the first 516 VAS scores (9), we have shown that 24% of women selected to be seen in our clinic had a tendency of 50% or more or pregnancy termination prior to our intervention. Of these 24%, we reversed the tendency of 78% (18.7% of total cases) (8). For the following analysis we have used these figures to calculate the yearly rate of prevention of unnecessary terminations.

Presently we counsel in the clinic more than 600 women per year, which therefore would translate to prevention of at least 112 unnecessary pregnancy terminations. This calculation is very conservative, since it is likely that in some of the cases that are advised only by the telephone we also reverse the tendency to terminate pregnancy. However, because no VAS scores are available for these patients, we have not included them in the present analysis.

The direct medical costs of pregnancy termination have been estimated at $2000 (9). We estimated that a woman loses on average 5 days of work directly and indirectly before, during, and after an elective abortion, adding another $1000; a husband's loss was not calculated. Therefore, the cost of pregnancy termination was estimated at $3000. In some cases, first-trimester abortion may result in major complications (0.5%) and even mortality (0.03%) (10–13); however, we did not attempt to estimate these costs.

Calculation of Cost Effectiveness of Preventing Major Malformations

Table 3 presents the rates per year of Motherisk patients exposed to known teratogens and the accepted rates of drug-induced major malformations known to occur in humans with these agents (2). Our analysis reveals that almost all our patients exposed to systemic retinoids terminate their pregnancy following our counseling and that virtually all those exposed to valproic acid and carbamazepine presently undergo tests that can rule out neural tube defects. Data regarding additional teratogens are presented in Table 3.

Table 3 Estimated Number of Chemically Induced Malformations Prevented by Motherisk per Year (based only on patients seen in clinic; not including those advised over the telephone alone)

Agent	Reported major malformations (%)	Mean number of cases per year based on Motherisk data-base for 1985–1990	Estimated % preventive procedures (definitive tests or terminations)	Estimated number of malformations prevented per year
Alcohol (high dose)	10	25	80[a]	2[a]
Systemic retinoids	40	2	80[b]	0.64
Valproic acid	2	8	100[c]	0.16
Carbamazepine	1	25	100[c]	0.25
Phenytoin	8	21	40[c]	0.67
Severe carbon monoxide poisoning (grade 4–5)	50	1	100[d]	0.5
Coumadin	16	4	50[e]	0.32
Cancer chemotherapy	10	8	50	0.4
				4.94

[a]The majority of heavy drinkers seen by us have chosen to terminate following the counseling.
[b]The majority tended to terminate.
[c]The neural tube defect is detected antenatally in virtually 100%.
[d]Women with severe poisoning (loss of consciousness) have chosen to terminate.
[e]Half of cases terminate following our advice.

For the calculation of societal burden from an undiagnosed major malformation, we chose a conservative estimate of life-long costs of $1.5 million (the original figure is corrected for 1992 by adding cost of living) (14).

We included in our analysis an estimated 100 women/year above the age of 35 who were advised by us for the first time on the risk of chromosomal aberrations associated with age, most of whom subsequently underwent amniocentesis. Based on a mean risk of 1% for Down's syndrome in advanced age, this means that we counsel at least one Down's mother per year.

The annual prevention of 112 unnecessary pregnancy terminations, as a result of advising women that their exposures were not teratogenic and did not increase fetal risk (8), would result in a direct cost saving of $336,000. The rate of major complications (e.g., perforation, water intoxication, anesthetic complications) is 0.5% (10), which means that on average, every 2 years we would prevent one such case.

With an estimated minimum annual prevention of five major malformations (Table 3), a saving of $7,500,000 can be calculated. In addition, we prevent, by advising women over 35 years of age an estimated one case annually of Down's syndrome, totaling another $1,500,000 life-long costs. Summarizing all direct costs calculated above, Motherisk's preventive impact results in a direct saving of $7,836,000/year. In 1990 the operating budget of Motherisk totaled $201,395, and only $95,000 was paid by Ontario Ministry of Health, the rest being recovered mainly from research grants and fellowships.

In performing the cost-effectiveness analysis presented in this study, we have chosen only a narrow portion of our activities. Not included are the thousands of patients counseled only over the telephone. In addition we did not calculate less well-defined endpoints such as decreasing levels of anxiety and increasing levels of well-being; we do have evidence that many women tend to have a more peaceful pregnancy after being reassured they have not endangered their fetuses (see Chapter 29). In addition, we made no attempt to quantify the educational impact of Motherisk. After each consultation, we send a letter summarizing the available data to the physician caring for the mother. This information helps educate physicians and health professionals and is consequently used by them for similar cases. In addition, Motherisk team members regularly lecture to physicians and health professionals on issues of the use of drugs and chemicals in pregnancy and lactation, thus further contributing to the educational goal. Finally, the Motherisk group has been initiating and publishing prospective studies on the reproductive safety/risk of drugs and chemicals, often as the first reports on issues such as carbon monoxide poisoning (6) or chloroquine use (7) in pregnancy.

With the exponential increase in the cost of health care, the preventive role of counseling women on their teratogenic risk can decrease the load of major malformation while preventing numerous terminations of otherwise wanted pregnancies (15).

QUALITY ASSURANCE

Since TIS are novel services, it is crucial to ensure that the standard of care they deliver meets high scientific and professional standards. The newly formed Organization of Teratogen Information Services (OTIS) is presently developing guidelines for accreditation of TIS based on their ability to deliver service using careful definitions for high level of quality.

There are no similar medical areas, in which complicated information, which is very seldom clear-cut, is provided over the telephone to pregnant women who are often at high levels of anxiety. Potentially this practice exposes the TIS to medicolegal liability. Because 1–3% of children will have major malformations, many callers of TIS who have been advised over the telephone that they do not have a risk higher than the baseline of 1–3% will in fact have malformed children. This makes the documentation of all information given to the caller most crucial.

Since its inception in 1985, the Motherisk Program in Toronto has developed a quality assurance (QA) mechanism which is built into the system at various levels. We recognize that different TIS have a variety of functions; however, because Motherisk has telephone and clinic components as well as routine follow-up of pregnancy outcome and research arms, we believe our QA program may be helpful to other TIS.

The next sections describe the various functions of the Motherisk Program with special focus on the QA aspects of each step.

RECRUITMENT AND TRAINING OF COUNSELORS

The Motherisk counselors come from several sources:

1. Individuals who trained at the Pharmacology-Toxicology Specialty program at the University of Toronto and had their project course (PCL-474Y) in Motherisk. This is a whole-year, 2 days per week, exposure to the counseling experience, followed by a more intensive in-training by the pro-

gram's coordinator. It includes a formal series of lectures and mostly practical work. Prior to the project course, these students had already had structured courses in the areas of experimental and clinical pharmacology, toxicology, and teratology.
2. Registered nurses with experience either in clinical medicine or research. Their initial training, which is provided "on the job," includes reading assignments, instructions, and participation in the lectures series as in item 1 above.
3. Graduate students in pharmacology or pharmacy; their training is similar to that for registered nurses.

All counselors participate in the weekly Motherisk rounds (on Fridays), featuring discussions of cases to be seen in the coming week, new literature, and research projects. Similar to medical trainees and graduate students, each counselor makes a presentation in the "Journal club" part of these rounds. The counselors are sent to formal courses in the area of reproductive toxicology, such as the one organized by Dr. L. Holmes in Boston, and they participate in the annual meetings of OTIS.

We conduct an annual in-service examination, which includes case presentations. The test is attended by all counselors and physician-trainees serving in Motherisk and is administered without warning during one of our routine rounds.

A week later we discuss the correct answers and their basis, and the director discusses areas of deficiencies with each counselor and medical trainee.

QA OF THE COUNSELING PROCESS

All inquiries are answered first by a counselor, who decides, according to known criteria, who should be referred to a clinic consultation and who should be answered through the telephone by the physician covering the service. During the initial months of the counselors' work, both the coordinator and the assistant director of Motherisk monitor the counseling process and routinely discuss shortcomings or items that should be changed, either in style or in content.

Bimonthly, the clinical fellows review a random sample of telephone and clinical consultation forms to assess the completeness of the recorded data and the appropriateness of the advice given. The finding of this analysis are discussed in a special team meeting in which we address deficiencies and suggestions for new policies, changes in the forms, and so on. Whenever a major deviation from Motherisk policy is found (e.g., a patient was not referred to a clinic visit despite meeting the criteria) the case is discussed personally with the counselor or physician who filled out the form.

QA OF THE CLINIC CONSULTATION

Prior to counseling patients in clinic, all physician-trainees, who are already specialized in pediatrics or internal or emergency medicine, are instructed by the director about the steps and special features of this process. The forms filled out during the clinic visit are reviewed by the director when reviewing and signing the consultation letters. Any areas of deficiency are discussed with the trainee responsible.

The consultation letter includes computerized statements about the various exposures the patient experienced. A new statement is constructed by the first team physician who had to address such exposure (e.g., fluoxetine), and existing statements are revised whenever new information becomes available and has been discussed by the team in its weekly meetings. All statements are stored in a computer to be used by the medical secretary typing the letters as well as by other team members. These statements are the basis for the answers given by the counselors to patients and health professionals.

RESEARCH

While conducting follow-up of pregnancy outcome based on computerized patient data, we often identify items that should be corrected or improved either in the recording of the information or in its storage.

The area of reproductive toxicology is characterized by a very rapid growth in the body of knowledge, coupled with difficult methodological issues in conducting and interpreting data on gestational exposures. This means that health professionals dealing with these issues have to be open minded, ready to continuously learn new information and adapt new concepts. Moreover, dealing with very anxious pregnant women over the telephone calls for a combination of compassion and scientific rigor.

While it is possible that in the future a process will be created to accredit TIS counselors and maybe even programs, probably most of the burden of training and maintaining competence and quality of TIS will lie with the services themselves.

Answer

Call the Teratogen Information Service in Tampa [(813) 974-2262], one of more than 40 such services operating now in North America. The team there will give you up-to-date information and if needed will arrange for a clinic consultation.

REFERENCES

1. McBrie WG. Thalidomide and congenital abnormalities (letter). Lancet 1961; 2: 1358.
2. Koren G. This volume, Chapter 3.
3. Jones KL, Lacro RV, Johnson KA, Adams J. Pattern of malformations in the children of women treated with carbamazepine during pregnancy. N Engl J Med 1989; 320:1661–1666.
4. Jacobson S, Jones K, Johnson K, et al. Prospective multicentre study of pregnancy outcome after lithium exposure during first trimester, Lancet 1992; 339:530–533.
5. Koren G, Bologa M, Long D, Henderson K, Feldman Y, Shear N. Perception of teratogenic risk by pregnant women exposed to drugs and chemicals in early pregnancy. Am J Obstet Gynecol 1989; 160:1190–1194.
6. Koren G, et al. A multicenter, prospective study of fetal outcome following accidental carbon monoxide poisoning in pregnancy. Reprod Toxicol 1991; 5:397–403.
7. Levy M, Buskila R, Gladman D, Koren G. Pregnancy outcome following first trimester exposure to chloroquine. Am J Perinatol 1991; 8:174–178.
8. Koren G, Pastuszak A, Pellegrini E. Prevention of unnecessary pregnancy termination by counseling women on drug, chemical and radiation exposure during the first trimester. Teratology 1990; 41:657–662.
9. Hook EB. Genetic counseling and prenatal cytogenetic services: Policy implications and detailed cost-benefit analysis of programs for the prevention of Down syndrome. In Services and Education in Medical Genetics (Poster IH, Hood EB, eds). Academic Press, New York, 1979.
10. Rashbaum W. Complications of abortion. In Abortion in the Seventies (Hern WM, Andrikopoulos B, eds). National Abortion Federation, New York, 1977, pp 33–54.
11. Atrash HK, McKay T, Hogue CJ. Ectopic pregnancy concurrent with induced abortion: Incidence and mortality. Am J Obstet Gynecol 1990; 162:726–730.
12. Lawson HW, Atrash HK, Franks AL. Fatal pulmonary embolism during legal induced abortion in the United States from 1972 to 1985, Am J Obstet Gynecol 1990; 162:986–990.
13. Kaali SG, Szgetvari IA, Bartfai GS. The frequency and management of uterine perforations during first trimester abortions. Am J Obstet Gynecol 1989; 161: 406–408.

14. Schmid W. Economic aspects of prenatal genetic diagnosis. In Preventable Aspects of Genetic Morbidity, Vol II, Proceedings of the First International Conference of Preventable Aspects of Genetic Morbidity, (Hashem N, ed). Cairo, 1978, pp 168–173.
15. Koren G, MacLeod SM. Monitoring and avoiding drug and chemical teratogenicity. Can Med Assoc J 1986; 135:1079–1081.

28

Motherisk I

A New Model for Counseling in Reproductive Toxicology

Elizabeth M. Pellegrini and Gideon Koren
The Hospital for Sick Children, Toronto, Ontario, Canada

INTRODUCTION

Since the thalidomide tragedy there has been an increased awareness of the potential for drugs, chemicals, and radiation to interfere with embryogenesis and/or development of the fetus. Traditionally, women have relied on their physicians and on the media (books, magazines, and television) for answers regarding concerns about drug exposure during pregnancy. Within the past couple of years, a specialized form of information service—the teratogen information service—has appeared in a number of cities in the United States and Canada. The main function of a teratogen information service is to provide information (in all cases) and consultation (in a few cases) to health professionals and/or the general public who have concerns with respect to drug, chemical, and radiation exposure during pregnancy, to determine any potential risk to the pregnant patient and/or to her unborn child. A more detailed description of the various types of information service available can be found in Chapter 27. This chapter describes the Motherisk Program located at the Hospital for Sick Children in Toronto, Ontario, Canada, with special emphasis on its day-to-day operation. The description includes the program mandate, protocols for both the telephone information and clinic consultation components, offspring follow-up, technical support, staffing, and direction for the future.

INCEPTION

Before I knew I was pregnant I had a chest x-ray. Will this harm my baby?
I have a patient who requires therapy for UTI. Can I prescribe cephalexin?
I have Crohn's disease. What are the risks to me and my baby should I become pregnant?
Can I have my hair permed during pregnancy?

These are the types of question members of the Division of Pharmacology and Toxicology at the Hospital for Sick Children have received in the past few years, perhaps owing to increasing awareness on the part of physicians and their patients (pregnant or not) that various xenobiotics have the potential to cross the placenta and possibly to interfere with fetal development. It became apparent that a protocol should be developed to adequately assess the risk or lack of risk, and the concept of the Motherisk Program ensued. The program began operation in September 1985, first as a consultation service in a clinic setting; it has since expanded to include a telephone information service.

MANDATE

The goal of Motherisk is twofold:

1. To provide an authoritative information and consultation service to assist the pregnant patient and/or her physician in understanding fetal risk(s) that may be associated with drug, chemical, and radiation exposure(s) during pregnancy.
2. To develop and maintain an active educational and research program in the area of reproductive and developmental toxicology at the undergraduate, graduate, and postgraduate levels.

TELEPHONE INFORMATION SERVICE

The telephone information service of the Motherisk Program is available to health professionals and to the general public. Incoming calls are received by the information specialist, who at the time of the call decides whether the caller should be referred for a clinic appointment or to the physician on call, or whether the query is such that the information specialist may answer the call satisfactorily. The following criteria are used to determine whether the caller should be referred to clinic:

1. Chronic illness (e.g., epilepsy, systemic lupus erythematosus, Crohn's disease)
2. Substance abuse (e.g., cocaine, alcohol, heroin)
3. Known or suspected teratogen (e.g., phenytoin, antineoplastics)
4. Pregnancy complicated by psychosocial problems
5. Physician referral to clinic
6. Multiple exposures
7. Any woman who may not fit into the categories above but requests a clinic visit (i.e., high level of maternal anxiety)

Questions about uncomplicated single or multiple exposures (e.g., most antibiotics and analgesics) are usually answered over the telephone by the information specialist. Physicians who wish to consult with respect to various drug protocols are referred to the physician on call.

In all these queries it is essential to determine potential risk factors involving the patient, regardless of whether she is seen in the clinic or evaluated over the telephone. Not only is proper identification of the drug/chemical involved essential, but it is also very important to define the dose, time of exposure in gestation, toxicological events, underlying disease states, and other concomitant drug therapy. It is not uncommon for callers, usually physicians, to question the safety of a medication before they prescribe it. In the cases of questionable safety or lack of information, other modes of treatment may be suggested. In addition to the foregoing inquiries relating to the exposure in question, it is necessary to inquire about past medical history, since not infrequently what seems to be unimportant to the caller may influence the evaluation of risk. For example, a caller who questions paternal marijuana use and the potential effect on her unborn child may, upon questioning, reveal that she has epilepsy and is being treated with phenytoin. In this case, the caller should be provided with information regarding the potential risks with respect to phenytoin treatment and epilepsy per se, in addition to the paternal exposure to marijuana.

Callers such as the woman in the example above, whose risk is deemed to be above the baseline for malformations, are usually referred to the clinic for further consultation. When there is no apparent increase above the baseline, the caller is provided with information and an explanation of baseline risk. It is necessary to ensure that each caller understands the concept of the general population risk for having a child with a malformation and that her exposure does not increase this risk.

The Motherisk Telephone Call Report Form (Fig. 1) is completed for all calls received. All calls are entered daily into a separate database from the clinic consults and daily summary sheets are retained for quick reference and follow-up. Monthly summary sheets are used both for statistical purposes and quality assurance.

Motherisk: Telephone Call Report Form   Date_____   Time

Patient Name_____ Phone #_____   Caller_____

                                                                Address_____

Parity_____ Age_____ Referral_____   Phone#_____

PREGNANT   NOT PREG.   Phone Call Returned_____

                                                      No Answer (time & day)_____

_____wks/mos at time of expos.   Gen. Info_____   No Answer (time & day)_____

                                                 Message left _____

_____wks/mos currently   Planning_____   HEALTH -

BREASTFEEDING_____   Retro_____   General_____

       Exposure Details   ——————————————

Drug Name   **Dose/Duration**   **Route Indication   Toxicology**

1._____   _____   _____   _____   _____

2._____   _____   _____   _____   _____

3._____   _____   _____   _____   _____

4._____   _____   _____   _____   _____

         ADVISED   No increase above baseline 3%_____

Reference(s):   Baseline risk was explained_____

—————————————————   Referred for clinic appointment

—————————————————   (date/time)_____

Advised:
Other_____

_____

_____

       BREASTFEEDING   Advised: Re
                                        Breastfeeding_____

Age of Infant_____   _____

Times per day_____   _____

Follow-Up   YES___   _____

           NO___   _____

Date:_____

Comments:_____   Signature of
                                      Respondent_____

Figure 1   Motherisk telephone call report form.

Presently, the Motherisk Program receives approximately 1000 telephone queries per month, an increase of threefold since the inception of the telephone component. Long-distance calls comprise approximately 18% of the monthly total, with most calls originating outside the Toronto area code. Callers question, on average, 1.46 exposures. Of these cells, 10–15% are scheduled for clinical appointments. Twenty-five percent of the calls come from health professionals, and the majority (> 85%) are from physicians. The remainder are made up of pharmacists and public health nurses. The most common calls question the safety of various prescription medications (51%), followed by over-the-counter medications (19%), chemicals (15%), recreational substances (7%), radiation (6%), and infections (3%).

TELEPHONE FOLLOW-UP

Follow-up of pregnancy outcome is performed in all cases in which women are consulted in the clinic. In addition, the following selected cases (usually those in which information was provided over the telephone) are contacted:

1. All inquires on drugs and breastfeeding to record any medical complication
2. Cases not seen in the clinic, yet the knowledge of pregnancy outcome is desirable (such as new drugs about which no information currently exists)

The telephone follow-up is conducted either by the information specialist or by pharmacology-toxicology undergraduate students affiliated with Motherisk. A more detailed discussion of the follow-up process can be found later in this chapter.

The results of the follow-up of pregnancy outcome are added to the Motherisk database and are used to generate new data on the safety of drugs and chemicals in pregnancy. When following women not seen in clinic, a maternal data form (Fig. 2) is completed in addition to the offspring form to ensure uniformity.

CLINIC CONSULTATION

Approximately 10–15% of Motherisk callers are referred to the clinic. All patients scheduled are seen by a physician affiliated with Motherisk. Figure 2 shows the maternal data form used during the clinic interview. In addition to the primary exposure data, details on other potential risk factors are recorded. These include obstetrical and past medical history, genetic background, additional exposures other than medications, occupation, and paternal exposures.

MOTHERISK

ANTENATAL CLINIC FOR DRUG/CHEMICAL RISK COUNSELLING

THE DIVISION OF CLINICAL PHARMACOLOGY, HOSPITAL FOR SICK CHILDREN

TORONTO, ONTARIO

MOTHERISK NO._____

DATE OF CONSULTATION:_____

HSC NUMBER_____

1.   **MATERNAL DATA**

Name: _____

Address: _____

_____

Phone Number: (Home)_____   (Work)_____

Husband's Name & Work Number_____

O.H.I.P. #_____ Date of Birth _____

Race/Ethnic Background_____

Weight (dry/current):_____

Physician's name: _____   _____

Address: _____   _____

Phone Number:_____   _____

[ ] Self-Referred   [ ] Referred by her doctor

2.   **OBSTETRICAL HISTORY**

Past Obstetrical History (G-P-Ab):_____

_____

_____

_____

Birth Control Methods:_____

Duration: _____

Date stopped: _____

Figure 2   Motherisk maternal intake history form.

2

Ovulatory Drugs: _____

LMP:_____ [ ] Regular Mens. [ ] Irregular Mens. # of days_____

EDC:_____

Current Gestational Date:_____

When did she find out she was pregnant?_____
How? [ ] Blood test [ ] Urine test [ ] Ultrasound

3. PRIMARY EXPOSURE DATA

1 = DRUG, 2 = CHEMICAL, 3 = RADIATION
4 = NOT PREGNANT(PROSPECTIVE), 5 = RETROSPECTIVE
A = ADVERTANT I = INADVERTANT

Exposure type (1-5) (A or I)	Substance	Duration		Dosage	Route
		Beg. Date	**Stop Date**		

Indication for
Medication:_____

_____

More Details about Medical Condition:_____

_____

_____

3

Toxicology Events:_____

_____

_____

Side Effects of Medication:_____

_____

Ultrasound Data:_____

Ultrasound Results:_____

Amniocentesis planned for:_____ _____Reason_____

Additional Exposures:

Substance	Dates	Dosage	Rout	Indication

Ethanol:_____

Tobacco:_____

Heat:_____

Radiation:_____

Tea & Coffee:_____

Special Diet:_____

Drugs of Abuse:_____

Occupation:_____

Genetic diseases or malformations in the family:_____

_____

_____

Figure 2   (Continued)

4

Past Medical History:

Heart disease:_____

Hypertension:_____

Renal disease:_____

Diabetes:_____

Thyroid disease:_____

Epilepsy:_____

Cancer:_____

General Anaesthesia:_____

Other:_____

[ ] Married
[ ] Single

4.   **SPOUSE DATA**

Age:_____

Occupation:_____

Medication:_____

Drugs of Abuse:_____

Ethanol:_____

Tobacco:_____

Past Medical History:

_____
_____
_____
_____
_____

One of the most important pieces of information that should be gathered during the interview is the exact gestational age at the time of exposure. If a certain drug is thought to increase the incidence of cleft palate, one would not anticipate this effect if exposure to the drug occurred after fusion of the palate. When a patient is unsure of her gestational date, a sonographic examination is scheduled.

Prior to presentation of the known data concerning the exposures in question, the patient is asked to complete the visual analog scale (VAS) illustrated in Figure 3. This visual analog aids the physician in determining the patient's concept of her own risk, thus providing direction for the remainder of the interview. A study conducted by members of Motherisk has shown that women exposed to nonteratogens assign themselves, on average, a risk of 1 in 4 for having a child with a malformation. It was also shown that these women

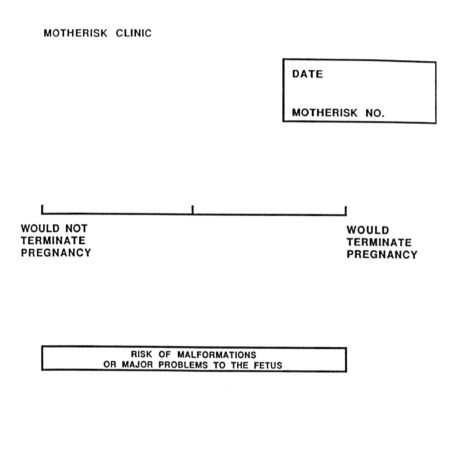

Figure 3   Maternal estimate of risk of malformed offspring.

know the baseline risk in the general population, suggesting that other factors may play a significant role in the patient's interpretation of her own risk (see Chapter 29).

Following this procedure, the physician presents to the woman the available information on her particular reproductive risk/no risk, with special focus on the teratogenic risk in the general population. Subsequently, the visual analog scale is repeated to aid the physician in determining how well the patient understands the information presented. When using the visual analog it becomes very obvious, especially in cases in which no increased teratogenic risk exists, if certain aspects need to be clarified.

In a variety of cases, additional tests may be deemed necessary by the counseling physician. These commonly include a level 2 ultrasound to rule out visible malformations, or a referral to our genetic clinic to assess, in depth, the genetic background or to arrange for an amniocentesis (e.g., age-related Down's syndrome or increased risk for neural tube defects with exposure to valproic acid).

Following the clinic visit, a letter is sent to the physician(s) caring for the woman during her pregnancy, summarizing the information presented at Motherisk. Upon request, a copy of the letter may also be sent to the patient.

FOLLOW-UP OF PREGNANCY OUTCOME

Approximately 12 months following the expected birth of the offspring, all Motherisk patients are contacted for a follow-up interview. Normally, this interview is conducted over the telephone using the Motherisk offspring form (Fig. 4). A separate form is subsequently sent to the child's pediatrician to obtain further information. The consent form for release of information, signed during the initial Motherisk interview, is used for this purpose. All data gathered are then entered into the Motherisk database for analysis.

In specific research cohorts the patient is asked to return to the clinic with her child. The intake form for this visit is identical to the one used for the telephone interview, but in addition, depending on the protocol, the child may be examined by a pediatrician/geneticist.

TECHNICAL SUPPORT

All information regarding patients and their children seen in Motherisk is stored in a database with built-in levels of security, to limit access to patient information. The hard copy of the patient interview is stored in the Motherisk office. Database management is the responsibility of the coordinator, though simple data entry may be performed by other health professionals.

MOTHERISK PROGRAM: OFFSPRING FORM

Motherisk No._____

Date of Contact_____

General Information:

Mom's Name_____   Infant's Name_____

Address   _____   D.O.B.:   _____

              _____   Pediatrician_____

Phone #   _____   Address_____

                                                  Phone:_____

Pregnancy: Termination:

Continued_____   Spontaneous_____

                                                  _____

Weight Gain_____   Elective:_____

Diseases Complicating:

Heart/Lung_____   HBP_____   UTI_____   Diabetes_____

Fever_____   Thyroid_____   Anemia_____   Polyhydramnios____

Blood Incompatibility_____   Other_____

Details_____

_____

Exposures:

Alcohol_____   Cigarettes_____

OTC_____

RX_____

_____

Other: marijuana_____

        cocaine_____

        other_____

Figure 4   One-year follow-up telephone evaluation of infant outcome.

The database program was designed at the Hospital for Sick Children using Double Helix II. Figure 5 gives examples of patient and offspring printouts using the current program.

In addition to personal computers, the Motherisk office is linked via a modem to the mainframe VAX in the hospital for more complex problem solving and for accessing Bibliographic Retrieval Services for MEDLINE

Neonatal History:

Neonatal Problems:_____

_____

_____

_____

_____

_____

_____

Special Care Required?_____

Home At _____**days**

Feeding:

Breast/bottle_____

Problems:_____

Health since discharge:_____

_____

_____

_____

_____

Visits to doctor: (reasons)_____

_____

_____

_____

Medications :List_____

_____

_____

_____

searches. The ability to perform these searches in the office rather than contracting them out provides greater flexibility within the program, since the waiting time for the information is decreased.

STAFF

The Motherisk staff is drawn from various areas of the health sciences because the evaluation of reproductive risk requires a multidisciplinary approach. Table 1 lists both the full-time and part-time staff affiliated with Motherisk.

Ultrasounds   Date   Results   Indication

_____   _____   _____   _____
_____   _____   _____   _____
_____   _____   _____   _____
_____   _____   _____   _____

**Other
tests:**_____
_____

DELIVERY
Place of Birth:_____
OB/GYN_____
Gestational Age (wks) _____   **Weight**_____
Length of Labour: 1st stage_____   **2nd stage**_____
Method:
Vaginal_____   **C/S**_____   **Complications**_____
Induction? (if yes WHY?)_____
Complications:_____
_____
_____

APGAR (if known)
One minute_____
Five minute _____

Other_____
_____
_____

Figure 4 (Continued)

Postdoctoral M.D. fellows trained at the Division of Pharmacology and Toxicology are on call for at least 1 week a month. In addition, each of the fellows participates in counseling patients in clinic and in developing new protocols for strategies for the program.

The Motherisk team meets once weekly before clinic to review recent publications, to discuss current cases, and to formulate new protocols from both research and service points of view. The protocols and strategies that ensue

Immunization   **Date**

`_____`   `_____`

`_____`   `_____`

`_____`   `_____`

Milestones: **Normal Values**

Smiled at`_____`   2 months

Lifted head`_____`   3 months

Sat unaided`_____`   6-8 months

Crawled `_____`   8-10 months

Stood`_____`   8-10 months

First word`_____`   8-12 months

Walked unaided`_____`   12-15 months

Form sent to MD: (date)`_____`
Interviewer initial`_____`

Form Received: (date)`_____`

from these meetings are stored on a word-processing document that is continuously revised and updated. The information contained therein forms the backbone for the telephone information component as well as the clinic component of Motherisk. In addition, this information is included in all letters dealing with specific exposures.

Information that is used in the consultation process is gathered from a number of sources. The medical information specialist on the team searches current journals for any new information published on drug, chemical, and radiation exposures during pregnancy in either animals or humans. These studies are then analyzed by the team to determine whether the study merits inclusion in our protocols. New textbooks are also searched for relevant information. If a question regarding an uncommon exposure or a new drug is raised, a MEDLINE search is performed to obtain any information that might be available. In the case of new agents, for which no information has

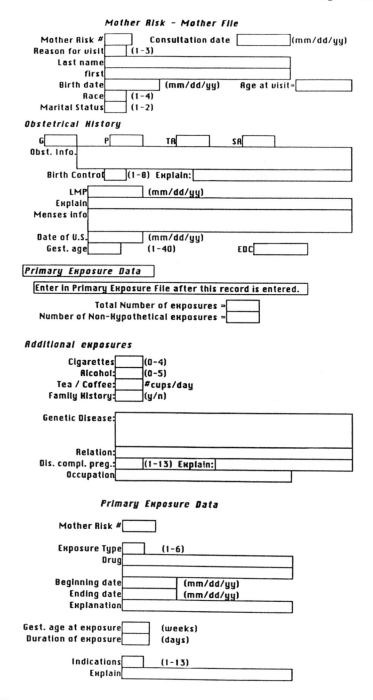

Figure 5a Motherisk database hard copy format of maternal files.

Offspring File

MotheRisk # [ ]   Mother's D of Birth [ ]

Preg. Info - termination? [ ] (1-3)
(If Yes, Explain) [ ]

Disease Compl. Pregnancy [ ] (1-13)
(If #13-Other, Explain) [ ]

Exposures During Pregnancy

Cigarettes [ ] (0-4) If 4- GA of dc'd [ ]
Alcohol [ ] (0-5) If 5- GA of dc'd [ ]
Hyperthermia [ ]
Special Diet [ ]

Drugs/Chemicals Post-consultation

Drug	Dosage	Gest Age

Full Drug Names [ ]

Delivery

Date of Birth [ ]
Weight [ ] (gms)
Age at [ ] (months)
consultation [ ] (weeks)
Gest Age at birth [ ] (1-3)

Answer Y or N: Explain:
Fetal Distress ? [ ] [ ]
Neonatal History ? [ ] [ ]
Health been good? [ ] [ ]

Outcome   Mother Risk # [ ]

Normal? [ ] (y/n) Explain [ ]
Malformation? [ ] (y/n)

Cardiac [ ] (y/n)
CNS [ ]
Ear/Eye [ ]
G.I. [ ]
Muscular [ ]
Skeletal [ ]
Skin,Teeth [ ]
Urogenital [ ]
Other [ ] Explain [ ]

Milestones

IN Months: Smiled [ ]
Lifted Head [ ]
Sat unaided [ ]
Crawled [ ]
Stood [ ]
1st Word [ ]
Walked Unaided [ ]

Figure 5b Motherisk database hard copy format of offspring files.

Table 1   The Motherisk Team

Full-time staff
1. Director — pediatrician/clinical pharmacologist/toxicologist
2. Clinical fellows — subspecializing in clinical pharmacology/toxicology
3. Coordinator — information specialist
4. Medical secretary
5. Information specialists

Part-time staff
1. Research nurse
2. Medical information specialist — pharmacist
3. Statistician, Ph.D.
4. Sonographer — physician
5. Addiction specialist — physician
6. Obstetricians and perinatologists — physicians
7. Clinical pharmacologists — physicians
8. Medical toxicologist — physician
9. Geneticist — physician
10. Prenatal genetics counselor, M.Sc.

Students
1. Graduate students (pharmacology and toxicology)
2. Undergraduate students (pharmacology and toxicology)

yet been published, the manufacturer is contacted for a summary of the voluntary reporting system adhered to and for premarketing animal studies. In certain cases, experts in a particular field may be called upon to provide insight into a particular exposure. When all the information has been gathered, it is evaluated and submitted for inclusion in protocol and strategy documents for use in future cases.

EDUCATIONAL COMPONENT

During the academic year the Motherisk programs involves undergraduate and graduate students from the Department of Pharmacology and Toxicology at the University of Toronto in various projects. This has proven to be an invaluable learning experience for the students, in addition to providing the program with more opportunity to expand research activities. The postgraduate medical fellows in clinical pharmacology participate in the educational program by supervising specific research projects.

SUPPORT

The Ministry of Health of Ontario supports the positions of the coordinator and medical secretary as well as telephone and computer expenses. All other positions are part of the educational curriculum of the involved divisions and departments. Patient consultations are billed through the Ontario Health Insurance Program (OHIP), but physician involvement in telephone information and consultation is not billed. Research protocols compete for extramural support at the appropriate agencies, and the generated funds are dedicated to answer the specific research questions (e.g., cocaine in pregnancy).

MOTHERISK SATELLITES

Programs similar to Motherisk are located throughout the Province of Ontario, including centers such as Ottawa and Hamilton. Smaller centers located in remote northern parts of Ontario consult Motherisk directly. It is hoped that by combining the data from the various centers, a strong database will be created. Such a resource is needed especially for the estimation of teratogenic risk of new compounds for which there is currently no information available.

SUMMARY

The Motherisk Program represents a new clinical approach to the problems of estimating reproductive risk following exposure to drugs, chemicals, and radiation. While the primary goal is to provide a needed service to women and their physicians, a prospective database enables us to collect information on pregnancy outcome following exposure to agents on which there are no data.

29

The Way Women Perceive Teratogenic Risk

The Decision to Terminate Pregnancy

Gideon Koren, Monica Bologa, and Anne Pastuszak
The Hospital for Sick Children, Toronto, Ontario, Canada

Clinical Case

A pregnant patient demands an abortion of an otherwise wanted pregnancy, saying that she drank three drinks per night over 3 days while on vacation, at 2 weeks postconception. You explain that this exposure is not known to increase her teratogenic risk, but she is still upset and controversial. How can you quantitate the data and provide effective counseling in this case?

INTRODUCTION

The main goal of counseling women on their teratogenic risk is to present to them an accurate, up-to-date estimate of their specific risks. However, the same data may be received and interpreted very differently by different patients, leading them to individual conclusions and finally to the decision to continue or terminate pregnancy.

Well-publicized figures from North America and Europe reveal that approximately one child is aborted for every child born (1,2), and while pregnancies are terminated for a variety of reasons, incorrect perception of a teratogenic risk may be an important factor. Most women who have been made aware of major malformations or chromosomal aberrations through ultrasound or amniocentesis choose to terminate pregnancy (3). As documented by the Greek experience after the Chernobyl disaster, even an unbased suggestion of adverse fetal outcome may prompt women to terminate pregnancy "to be on the safe side" (4).

During the first year of Motherisk, we were impressed by the number of cases of misperception and distorted information regarding the potential teratogenic risk of drugs and chemicals. In particular, we felt that many women tend to assign an unrealistically high risk to medications not known to be teratogenic. In some cases, this misperception has led to termination of pregnancy.

In an attempt to objectively quantify women's perceptions of their teratogenic risk, a 10-cm visual analog questionnaire was designed (Fig. 1). After collection of all patients' data (see Chapter 28), and before delivering our view of the apparent risk, patients are asked to assign to their potential risk for major malformations a number between 0 and 100%. We also ask what in their opinion is the risk for major malformations in the general population, because their knowledge of baseline risk is crucial for their perception of their own risk. In addition, patients are asked to quantify from 0 to 100% their tendency to terminate or continue pregnancy.

The completion of this questionnaire is followed by delivering to the patient all known information about the exposure(s) in question. Subsequently, the questionnaire is repeated. Patients are urged to express their own views and not to answer the questionnaire in a way they might think would please the interviewer.

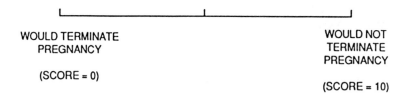

1. FEELING TOWARD TERMINATION OF PREGNANCY

WOULD TERMINATE
PREGNANCY

(SCORE = 0)

WOULD NOT
TERMINATE
PREGNANCY

(SCORE = 10)

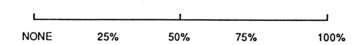

2. RISK OF MAJOR MALFORMATION

NONE   25%   50%   75%   100%

Figure 1   Visual analog scale.

Analysis of the first 80 cases on whom the visual analog scale (VAS) was used between September and December 1986 reveals the power of this tool in detecting misperception and misinformation.

Before receiving up-to-date information about the specific exposure, women exposed to nonteratogens assigned a mean risk of 24 ± 2.8% for major malformations. After the interview, however, the risk was perceived as lower (14.5 ± 3%, $p < 0.01$). The risk for major malformations in the general population was estimated as 5.6 ± 1.3%, which is comparable to the real figure in the literature. The perceived risk before and after our intervention was significantly different from that estimated by the patients for the general population (Fig. 2).

The tendency for continuation of pregnancy showed a significant change following the interview (from 7.9 ± 0.3 to 8.7 ± 0.3 in the analog scale, $p < 0.01$).

Eleven patients were exposed to medications known to be teratogenic. Their perceived teratogenic risk was unchanged (36.2 ± 11.7% before and

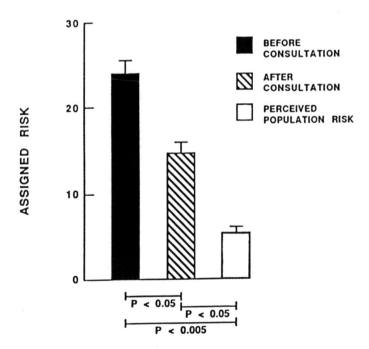

Figure 2 Patient-assigned risk of major malformation for parents not exposed to teratogens.

$36.7 \pm 15.6\%$ after the interview). Their tendency for termination/continuation of pregnancy did not change following the interview. Three of them did decide to terminate pregnancy within a few weeks of the consultation.

No correlation was found between age and perception of risk or tendency to terminate/continue pregnancy. No differences in perception of risk were detected between women referred by physicians and those who were self-referred.

Eleven of our patients were single mothers. Although they did not perceive their risk differently from married women, those who had been exposed to nonteratogens showed a significantly higher tendency to continue pregnancy before the interview (4.7 ± 1.2 on VAS units single mothers vs. 8.1 ± 0.4 married, $p < 0.05$). Following the intervention, their perception significantly changed (7.4 ± 1.2, $p < 0.05$) but was still different from married women.

No correlation was found between estimation of risk and number of preparations consumed by the woman, her age, parity, or socioeconomic status.

This analysis indicates that pregnant women exposed to nonteratogenic agents believe they have a risk of 1 in 4 of having a child with major malformations. This figure is very close to the known risk of thalidomide (5). Importantly, these women estimated the risk in the general population to be 5%, which is similar to the real figure of 4–5% (6). This means that the concept of teratogenic risk was well understood and that women were well informed about the risk in the general population. In addition, it lends clinical significance to the unrealistically high risk assigned by these women to their nonteratogenic exposures.

Two basic reasons can be put forward to explain the unrealistically high teratogenic risk assigned by pregnant women: misinformation and misperception.

Misinformation

Advisories on potential teratogenic risk appear constantly in the lay media, usually to stress risks, and very rarely to address safety of specific drugs. A recent analysis of 15 different popular magazines disclosed poor scientific standards and a clear tendency to be misleading or inaccurate (7). There was a tendency to alarm readers without justification.

In addition, popular books dealing with pregnancy often tend to assign risks to drugs not proven to be risky.

For example, the author of *Will My Baby Be Normal?* states, "Do not take any aspirin or medications that include aspirin if you think you might be pregnant. Midline body defects . . . have been attributed to this drug" (8). Such defects are not believed to be associated with salicylates in humans.

In yet another instance, J. Elkington entitled his book on reproductive toxicology *The Poisoned Womb*, although most of the data discussed do not prove poisoning in humans (9). A possible source of misinformation is the *Physicians' Desk Reference*, which includes warnings on exposures during pregnancy that are no longer correct. Reference books dealing with drug use in pregnancy have been published (6,10,11) and should be used by physicians caring for pregnant women.

Another source of misinformation is physicians. We have dealt with more than a few cases in which physicians advised women to terminate pregnancy despite nonteratogenicity (Fig. 3). This may reflect a defensive approach in the current litigious atmosphere, or the possibility that physicians themselves are misinformed. Our data indicate that women referred by physicians did not have a more accurate perception of risk than self-referred patients.

> Last December, I sought your help regarding a couple of tranquillizers I had taken within the first few weeks of my pregnancy. The prescribing doctor and a well-respected obstetrician had suggested that I abort the pregnancy.
>
> As a result of your advice, my husband and I are the ecstatic parents of a beautiful, healthy baby girl. I cannot thank you enough. The work you are doing is a wonderful necessity. If there is anything I can do for your program on a volunteer basis, I would be more than happy to be of assistance.

Figure 3 Letter of a Motherisk patient who had been advised by other physicians to terminate pregnancy.

Misperception

Our results show that even after we had advised women that medications taken by them did not increase their risk of having a malformed child, their perceived risk was significantly higher than their perception of the risk in the general population. It is conceivable that during pregnancy there is an increased sensitivity to this issue, leading to a distorted perception of risk. Of special interest is the approach of single mothers: while assigning a teratogenic risk similar to married women before receiving our advice, they were much less ready to continue pregnancy with such a risk. Single mothers may have a variety of psychological, moral, and socioeconomic reasons to discontinue pregnancy. For them, a distorted perception of teratogenic risk may be the last straw in deciding on termination of pregnancy.

Our intervention appears to have significantly changed the perception of women exposed to nonteratogenic agents in terms of estimating the risk as well as in the tendency to terminate/continue. This tendency was best documented in the subgroup of single mothers, in which some of the women who were already booked for dilatation and curettage decided to carry on the pregnancy. If postinterview assessment still reveals an unrealistically high perception of risk or tendency to terminate pregnancy, we spend additional time to explain to the woman that her apparent risk, based on current knowledge, is lower than the one perceived by her.

It may be argued that women contacting a consultative service such as Motherisk are a selected group of patients with a higher degree of concern, and therefore their perception does not accurately represent the total population of pregnant women. Yet, it is such individuals who are more likely to decide to terminate pregnancy based on wrong information. It is also possible that some women who are ambivalent about continuing their pregnancy seek a legitimate medical reason for termination. In both cases, accurate information will help the woman and her family to make a knowledgeable decision.

THE IMPACT OF RISK PERCEPTIONS ON WOMEN'S DECISIONS TO CONTINUE PREGNANCY

In an attempt to assess the relevance of the risk perception as measured by us in predicting women's apparent decision about their pregnancy, we analyzed the 123 women who expressed a tendency of 50% or more to terminate their pregnancy between September 5, 1986 (the date the VAS was first introduced) and January 29, 1988 (Table 1).

At the time of the consultation all these 123 women verbally expressed serious consideration of terminating their pregnancy in addition to filling

Table 1 Study Population

Initial Motherisk cohort (n = 516)	
Women who tended ≥50% to terminate their pregnancy prior to our information	123
Women who tended ≥ to continue their pregnancy	246
Exclusions	
Prospective cases (not yet pregnant)	5
Refusals of follow-up	3
Lost for follow-up	7
Had not reached EDC	30
Study cohort (n = 78)	
Decided to continue pregnancy (CP)	61[a]
Decided to terminate (TA)	17

[a]Outcomes as follows: 57 normal infants and 4 miscarriages.

out the VAS. Of these, the following were excluded from further analysis: 5 came for prospective advice and did not become pregnant until the analysis of the data, 3 refused to participate in the telephone follow-up, 7 could not be reached at the contact telephone numbers, and 30 had not yet reached their expected date of confinement (EDC). Thus, our study group consisted of 61 women who decided to continue their pregnancy despite their initial tendency and 17 who chose to terminate their pregnancy.

The two groups [continued pregnancy (CP), n = 61, and therapeutic abortion (TA), n = 17] did not differ statistically in their mean age, number of pregnancies, number of previous live births, therapeutic or spontaneous abortions, or number of exposures in the pregnancy in question, where "exposure" includes every medical preparation, chemical, or radiation reported during the consultation.

The tendency to terminate pregnancy before receiving the relevant medical information did not differ significantly between the CP and TA groups ($34.3 \pm 2.5\%$ vs. $24.8 \pm 5.4\%$, respectively, $p > 0.05$). Following the interview, however, there was a highly significant difference in the response of the two groups; women who eventually continued their pregnancy significantly changed their tendency: from $34.3 \pm 2.5\%$ to $84.5 \pm 3.3\%$ ($p < 0.00001$). Conversely, women who eventually terminated their pregnancies had a nonsignificant increase in the tendency to continue pregnancy and in most cases did not pass the 50% point ($24.8 \pm 5.4\%$ to $45.1 \pm 9.8\%$) ($p > 0.1$). Their tendency to terminate pregnancy after the sounseling process was significantly different from the CP group ($p < 0.0001$).

Of 61 women in the CP group, 4 had a miscarriage between 8 and 12 weeks of gestation. The other 57 women had normal pregnancy outcome, with no apparent major malformations or developmental delay up to 9 months of postnatal age.

Table 2 presents the analysis of the 17 women who chose to terminate their pregnancy. In two cases, women were exposed to drugs known to have adverse fetal outcome (BCNU for mycosis fungoides and heparin for prosthetic valve), and in a third case an amniocentesis done because of maternal age (> 35 years) tested positive for Down's syndrome.

Of interest, one woman exposed to nonteratogens claimed in the follow-up interview that her decision to terminate pregnancy was based on the information she received during the Motherisk consultation; however, the summary letter sent to her physician clearly stated that she did not have an increased teratogenic risk. One woman attributed her decision to advanced age and poor gynecological history, and another had an increased genetic risk for major malformations. In two cases, the women claimed that their obstetricians encouraged them to terminate pregnancy owing to a high teratogenic risk (up to 80%) despite our advice of no such increased risk. Eight women who perceived their teratogenic risk as high despite our advice indicated that this was their main reason for termination; four of them were unmarried.

Of the 78 evaluable pregnant patients who tended to terminate their pregnancy prior to our consultation, it is probable that we reversed the tendency in 61 (57 normal healthy babies and 4 miscarriages). Although it is impossible to prove that all these pregnancies would have been terminated with-

Table 2 Analysis of Reasons for Therapeutic Abortion as Indicated by the Women

Reason	Number of cases[a]
Exposure to drug with a potential adverse fetal effect	2
Down's syndrome detected in amniocentesis	1
Advanced age with poor gynecological history	1
Higher genetic risk for major malformations	1
Advised to terminate pregnancy by obstetricians despite exposure to nonteratogens	2
Unmarried women	4
Fears of higher teratogenic risk despite Motherisk advice	8
Claimed termination was according to Motherisk advice (not confirmed by summary letter)	1

[a]Total exceeds 17 (the number of women who chose to terminate their pregnancy) because some women had more than one reason for termination.

out our intervention, it is conceivable that this might have been the case, since most women who showed a greater than 50% tendency to terminate pregnancy after our intervention eventually did so.

The two groups (TA and CP) did not differ in a large number of characteristics and had very similar rates of drug exposures. However, most of the 17 cases in the TA group expressed obvious explanations, unrelated to the exposures in question, as factors that led them to decide to terminate their pregnancy. Four of them were unmarried; in the analysis above we have shown that single mothers, despite estimating their teratogenic risk in a similar manner to married women, have a significantly higher tendency to terminate their pregnancy.

After confirming the clinical relevance of the VAS, we now use the information collected not only for epidemiological endpoints, but also for individual cases. For example, if after the interview the woman has a tendency of termination higher than 50%, it is probable that she will not continue her pregnancy. If we are impressed that the teratogenic risk is the main reason for her tendency, and not other social, psychological, or personal reasons, we extend the interview to explain again the lack of risk associated with her exposure.

The same insight is employed to counsel women exposed to teratogenic agents, if their perception does not reflect realization of an increased risk.

Answer

Using the visual analog scale, we have shown that if the woman, before leaving your office, has a 50% or more tendency to terminate pregnancy, she will almost always carry this plan into effect. If your patient has shown such a tendency, you may wish to take more time to discuss her risk and to explain that it does not exceed the baseline. This may be the last chance.

REFERENCES

1. Macpherson AS. Health status report 1983. City of Toronto, Department of Public Health, April 1985, p 37.
2. Shairn RN. A cross-cultural history of abortion. Clin Obstet Gynecol 1986; 13: 1-17.
3. Berbie AB, Elias S. Amniocentesis for antenatal diagnosis of genetic defects. Clin Obstet Gynecol 1980; 7:5-12.
4. Trichopoulos D, Zavitsanos X, Koutis C, Drogani P, Proukakis C, Petridou E. The victims of Chernobyl in Greece: Induced abortions after the accident. Br Med J 1987; 295:1100.
5. Lenz W. Thalidomide embryopathy in Germany: 1959-1961. Prog Clin Biol Res 1985; 163c:77-83.

6. Schardein JL. Chemically Induced Birth Defects. Marcel Dekker, New York, 1985.
7. Gunderson SA, Martinez LP, Carey JC, Kochenon NK, Emergy MG. Critical review of articles regarding pregnancy exposures in popular magazines. Proceedings of the 26th Teratology Society Meeting, Boston, 1986; Abstract 88.
8. Scher J. Will My Baby Be Normal? How to Make Sure. Dial Press, New York, 1983, p 31.
9. Elkington J. The Poisoned Womb. Viking Press, London, 1985.
10. Briggs GG, Freeman RK, Yaffe SJ. Drugs in Pregnancy and Lactation, 2nd ed. Williams & Wilkins, Baltimore, 1986.
11. Shepard TH. Catalog of Teratogenic Agents, 5th ed. John Hopkins University Press, 1986.

30

Motherisk II

The First Year of Counseling on Drug, Chemical, and Radiation Exposure in Pregnancy

Gideon Koren and Yaacov Feldman
The Hospital for Sick Children, Toronto, Ontario, Canada

Stuart M. MacLeod
St. Joseph's Health Center, Hamilton, Ontario, Canada

INTRODUCTION

While hundreds of scientific papers are published every year on potential adverse reproductive effects caused by drugs, chemicals, and radiation, little has been done to crystallize a clinical approach to counseling and following up such cases. With 40–90% of pregnant women exposed to at least one medication in pregnancy (1,2), and based on the unrealistically high perception of teratogenic risk by pregnant women, as documented in Chapter 29, it is clear that the need for well-structured professional systems to counsel women and their families is crucial.

This chapter describes the characteristics of the 395 women seen by the Motherisk Program during the first year of operation and discusses the counseling process. While data will probably differ from city to city and from country to country, they do allow a fair amount of the generalization needed for rational planning of such a program.

Specifically, we have tried to identify problems typical of the general group seeking advice, as well as issues of subgroups such as women who are chronic drug users. We also identify problems resulting from drugs of abuse, alcohol drinking, and cigarette smoking.

In addition, we wished to assess whether this prospectively collected information can form a research database that will yield new knowledge on the reproductive hazards of drugs, chemicals, and radiation along with the various confounders that may affect them.

CHARACTERISTICS

The group consisted of the 395 women who were consulted at the Motherisk clinic during its first operative year (September 1985–September 1986). Among them 335 women were pregnant (84.8%) and 60 were not (15.2%), and they came either for advice about exposure in future pregnancy, or to discuss potential teratogenic risk in a previous pregnancy. In total, 65% were referred by their physicians, and 35% were self-referred.

The mean age (± SD) of the women was 29.9 ± 3 years. The pregnant women's mean age (n = 324) was 29.7 ± 0.3 years, statistically older than the mean age of women giving birth in Toronto in 1982 [n = 8068, 27.4 years ($p \leqslant 0.0001$)] (3). Marital status distribution of our population was similar to that of Toronto (1982) (Table 1).

A significant difference in distribution according to ethnicity was found, with low presentation of white and high of black women in the Motherisk group when compared to Ontario ($p < 0.0001$); however the Motherisk distribution quite accurately represents that of Toronto (with 5% black) (Table 2).

In 1982 the number of therapeutic abortions per 100 live births in Ontario was 25.1 (total number of abortions = 31,379), the highest provincial rate in Canada. No difference for the years 1979–1981 was found (4). In Toronto, a higher rate was found in 1983: 92.1 abortions per 100 live births (7428 and 8068, respectively) (3).

In the Motherisk population, a rate of 43.7 abortions per 100 live births (reported during the interview) was found, which corresponds to half the rate in Toronto ($p < 0.00001$) (Tables 3 and 4).

Table 1 Marital Status Motherisk and Toronto Populations

Marital status	Motherisk[a]		Toronto[b]		p
Single	38	(16.7%)	1085	(13.5%)	>0.2
Married	187	(82.0%)	6848	(85.4%)	>0.15
Divorced	3	(1.3%)	75	(0.9%)	>0.35
Widowed	0		7	(0.09%)	$0.1 > p > 0.05$
	228	(100%)	8015	(100%)	

[a]228 Pregnant women (out of 335).
[b]From results related to 8068 women giving birth in Toronto in 1982 (Ref. 3). Data about marital status were available about only 8015 cases.

Table 2   Ethnic Background Motherisk and Ontario Populations

	Motherisk[a]		Ontario[b]	p
White	194	(88.2)	(92.8)	$0.025 < p < 0.01$
Black	10	(4.5)	(2.54)	<0.00001
Orientals	7	(3.4)	(2.54)	>0.35
American Indians	4	(1.8)	(1.16)	>0.25
Others	4	(1.8)	(2.9)	>0.2

[a]219 Pregnant women.
[b]3,925,100 Pregnant women, from Ref. 4. Data refer to all women in the province. No subdivision according to age. No municipal information available.

Table 3   Obstetric History of Motherisk Patients

	n	Mean per woman
Pregnancies	395	2.08 ± 0.07
Births	395	0.69 ± 0.05
Therapeutic abortions	394	0.3 ± 0.03
Spontaneous abortions	394	0.23 ± 0.03

Table 4   Pregnant Women: Age, Gravidity, and Parity for Motherisk and Toronto Populations

	Motherisk[a]	Toronto[b]	p
Age $\leqslant$ 15 years	0	4 (0.05)	>0.35
Age $\leqslant$ 20 years	8 (2.5)	545 (6.8)	<0.005
Age $>$ 40 years	11 (3.4)	89 (1.1)	>0.0005
First birth $>$ 35 years[c]	22 (6.6)	295 (7.0)	>0.35
$\geqslant$ Third pregnancy	99 (29.9)	1363 (16.9)	<0.00001
P0, G1[d]	33.5%	52.23%	<0.00001

[a]335 Pregnant women.
[b]8068 Pregnant women (Ref. 3).
[c]Percent of all first births.
[d]Nullipara/multipara.

A higher representation of older women and lower one for teenagers were found in the Motherisk population when compared to Toronto ($p < 0.0001$) (Table 4).

Exposure to Medical Preparations

The women attending Motherisk were exposed to 2.04 ± 0.1 medical preparations (range 0–10). The average gestational age at the time of consultation was 12.8 ± 0.4 weeks, meaning that most exposures occurred during the first trimester.

Indications for Consultation

Exposure to drugs was reported by 278 women (70.4%); of these, 179 reported use before knowing they were pregnant (45.3%), and 127 reported use while being aware of their pregnancy (32.1%); 28 women belonged to both categories. Exposure to chemicals was reported by 61 women (15.4%) and to radiation by 61 (15.4%). Paternal exposure as the cause for the consultation occurred in two cases (0.5%) (cytotoxic drugs and retinoic acid).

ANALYSIS OF EXPOSURE TYPES IN PREGNANCY

Drugs Used by Pregnant Versus Nonpregnant Women

Table 5 presents the different types of drug and the numbers of women reporting their use ($n = 335$ and 60 pregnant and nonpregnant women, respectively). The rate of exposure to the agents in each group is expressed as a percentage.

There was a significant difference in distribution of exposures to various drug types among the two subgroups ($p < 0.0001$). More frequent use of drugs taken chronically was reported by the nonpregnant women ($p < 0.0001$), and higher use of drugs taken acutely by the pregnant women ($p = 0.083$).

No differences were found between pregnant and nonpregnant women in the following variables: age of the women and their partners, marital status, ethnic background, number of children, and numbers of spontaneous and therapeutic abortions. The proportion of nonpregnant women who worked out of the home was 92.8%, versus 74.8% ($p < 0.02$) for the pregnant women. The total number of pregnancies was higher in the latter group (2.2 ± 0.1 vs. 1.4 ± 0.2) ($p < 0.0005$).

TIMING OF EXPOSURE IN PREGNANCY

The timing of exposure was analyzed for the common types of exposure. The use of antibiotics was within the first trimester in 97% and in 63% within the first month of pregnancy. Analgesics were taken during the first trimester in 92% of the cases, and in 40% during the first month. In 4.1%, they were taken throughout pregnancy. Benzodiazepines were consumed in 92% during the first month of gestation, in 56% during the second month, and in 5% throughout pregnancy.

Table 5 Exposures to Various Agents in the Pregnant and Nonpregnant Women Attending Motherisk

Drug group	Pregnant Number	(%)	Nonpregnant Number	(%)
Drugs of abuse	45	13.4	2	3.3
Amphetamines	4	1.2	0	0
Anesthetics	24	7.2	0	0
Anesthetic gas (occupational)	4	1.2	0	0
Analgesic drugs	103	30.7	4	6.7
Anorexiants	2	0.6	0	0
Antacids	4	1.2	0	0
Antiemetics	15	4.5	1	1.7
Antibiotics	91	27.2	3	5
Anticoagulants	2	0.6	0	0
Anticonvulsants	13	3.9	11	18.3
Antidepressants	8	24	5	8.3
Antidiarrheals	3	0.9	1	1.7
Antihistamines	28	8.3	4	6.7
Antihypertensives	2	0.6	2	3.3
Antipsychotics	6	1.8	5	8.3
Antitussives	12	3.6	1	1.7
Benzodiazepines	40	11.9	2	3.3
Bronchodilators	9	2.7	9	15
HCT	5	1.5	1	1.7
Immunotherapy	5	1.5	1	1.7
Laxatives	11	3.3	0	0
Muscle relaxants	3	0.9	0	0
Nonsteroidal anti-inflammatory drugs	20	6.0	1	1.7
Ovulatory drugs	3	0.9	1	1.7
Sedatives	4	1.2	0	0
Sex steroids	11	3.3	1	1.7
Steroids	16	4.8	7	11.7
OC	27	8.06	0	0
Steroids — Total	54	16.1	8	13.3
Spermicides	7	2.1	0	0
Thyroid drugs	15	4.5	3	5.0
L-Thyroxin	11	3.3	2	3.3
PTU	4	1.2	1	1.7
Vaccination	10	3.0	1	1.7
Sulfonamides	2	0.6	2	3.3

HCT, hydrochlorothiolide; OC, oral contraceptive; PTU, propylthiouracil.

Table 6   Exposure to Confirmed or Questionable Teratogens in Pregnancy

Exposure	Number of patients[e]	Timing
Radioactive iodine	4	1st month
Cytotoxic drugs[a]	2	#1: 1st few weeks; #2: 0–14 weeks
Methyl mercury	1	1st few months
Warfarin	2	#1: 0–14 weeks; #2: throughout
Anticonvulsants	13	Throughout ($n = 6$); 1st trimester ($n = 5$)
Diphenylhydantoin	7	
Carbamazepine	5	
Pyrimidone	2	
Anesthetic gas[b]	4	Till 3rd trimester ($n = 3$); 1st trimester ($n = 1$)
Carbon monoxide[c]	7	1st trimester ($n = 2$); 2nd trimester ($n = 4$)
Tetracyclines	22	95% in 1st trimester ($n = 14$); 1st month ($n = 6$), 2nd month ($n = 2$)
Progesterone-estrogen	10	1st trimester ($n = 8$); till 2nd trimester ($n = 2$)
Cocaine	21	83% in 1st trimester
Lithium	1	Throughout
Benzodiazepines[d]	40	96% in 1st trimester
Oral contraceptives[d]	28	($n = 21$) 1st trimester. ($n = 3$) 2nd trimester
Total	155	
Alcohol (higher degrees 3 + 4)	28	
Heavy smoking		
>1 pack/day	12	
>0.5 pack/day	51	

[a]#1: at work as a nurse; #2, treatment for mycosis fungoides.
[b]Occupational exposure at work as a nurse.
[c]Gas leak, in most cases from home furnace.
[d]Suspected teratogens.
[e]A patient can be exposed to more than one teratogenic agent.

Teratogen Exposure

Exposure to known human teratogens was reported by 87 women (26%), and to suspected teratogens by 68 women (20.3%) (Table 6).

Indications and symptoms associated with the exposures are presented in Table 7. As would be expected, nonpregnant women sought advice about medications associated with chronic conditions such as epilepsy and asthma as part of planning their pregnancy.

FERTILITY PROBLEMS

Two or more spontaneous abortions were reported by 17 women (5.1%), and three or more by 5 (1.5%). Amenorrhea was reported in eight patients (2.4%), and ovulatory drugs were used by 15 patients (4.5%).

Table 7 Indications and Symptoms Related to the Various Exposures in Pregnant and Nonpregnant Women

Disease/pathology	Pregnant Number	Pregnant (%)[a]	Nonpregnant Number	Nonpregnant (%)[a]	p
Epilepsy	13	3.9	11	18.3	<0.00001
Psychiatric	26	7.8	12	20.0	<0.01
Thyroid	18	5.4	4	6.6	>0.35
Cardiovascular	28	8.3	7	11.7	>0.25
Asthma-allergies	37	11.0	17	28.3	<0.001
Inflammatory	18	5.4	7	11.7	$0.1 > p > 0.05$
Skin	16	4.8	1	1.6	>0.25
Genitourinary tract	9	2.7	0	0	$0.25 > p > 0.1$
Infectious	87	26.0	3	5.0	<0.001
Dental	15	4.5	0	0	$0.1 > p > 0.05$
Biochemical	6	0.9	0	0	>0.3
Hematologic	8	2.4	0	0	$0.25 > p > 0.1$
Infertility	17	5.1	3	5	
Operations[b]	10	3.0	0	0	
Urinary tract	2	0.6	0	0	
Symptoms					
Pain	78	23.3	5	8.3	$0.05 > p > 0.01$
Insomnia	18	6.9	0	0	$0.05 > p > 0.01$
GI symptoms	32	9.5	1	1.7	$0.25 > p > 0.1$

[a]Percent is of women in each group.
[b]General anesthesia.

Operations in pregnancy were performed under general anesthesia in 10 patients. The indications were as follows: tubal resection ($n = 1$) (ectopic pregnancy), laparoscopy ($n = 3$), extraction of kidney stones ($n = 2$), explorative laparotomy ($n = 1$), dental operation ($n = 2$), and arthroscopy ($n = 1$).

RETROSPECTIVE COUNSELING

Eleven women were concerned about exposure during a previous pregnancy and its possible effect on the outcome of the planned pregnancy. In most cases, the outcome of the previous pregnancy was adverse: there were six congenital anomalies, two stillbirths, two miscarriages, and one case of developmental delay.

PROSPECTIVE COUNSELING

Of 49 consultations dealing with a future pregnancy, the exposures were associated with chronic disease in 42 cases (85.7%), fertility problems in 3 (6.1%), and environmental or occupational exposures in 3 (6.1%).

EXPOSURES TO ALCOHOL, TOBACCO, AND DRUGS OF ABUSE

Table 8 presents our criteria for degree of alcohol consumption (5). The pregnant women seen in Motherisk tended more to abstain from drinking ($p = 0.0001$) and to drink less alcohol than the general group of pregnant women studied in Ottawa ($p = 0.0001$) (Table 9) (5). No difference was found in the heavy degrees of consumption. Comparison of alcohol consumption in the nonpregnant women of Motherisk and Ottawa reveals that the nonpregnant women seen in Motherisk had a higher tendency to abstain from

Table 8   Degree of Absolute Alcohol (AA)[a] Consumption (based on Ref. 5)

Degree	Criteria (on average)
0	Abstainers
1 Light	Consumption < 0.14 ox AA per day
2 Moderate	Consumption 0.14–0.85 oz AA per day
3 Heavy	Consumption > 0.85 oz AA per day
4 Binge drinkers[b]	Consumption > 3.0 oz AA on one occasion

[a]Absolute alcohol: 1 oz = 28.45 g.
[b]Included in the other groups.

Table 9 Degree of Alcohol Consumption During Pregnancy: Motherisk Versus Ottawa

Degree	Motherisk: $n = 332^a$		Ottawa: $n = 216^a$	p
0 Abstainers	141	(42.5%)	(18.4%)	<0.00001
1 Light	126	[37.9%]	[41.9%]	>0.25
2 Moderate	28	[8.4%]	[33.2%]	<0.0005
3 Heavy	25	[7.5%]	[6.2%]	>0.35
4 Binge drinkers	10	[3.0%]	[6.2%]	$0.1 > p > 0.05$
Drinkers	191	(57.5%)	(81.6%)	<0.00001
0 + 1 + 2	295	(88.9%)	(90.7%)	>0.35
3 + 4	25	(7.5%)	(9.3%)	>0.35

[a]Numbers in brackets represent % of the total.
Source: Modified from Ref. 5.

Table 10 Degree of Alcohol Consumption by Nonpregnant Women: Motherisk Versus Ottawa

Degree	Motherisk: $n = 56$		Ottawa: $n = 216$	p
0 Abstainers	17	(30.4%)	(4.6%)	<0.00001
1 Light	33	(58.9%)	(24.5%)	<0.00001
2 Moderate	5	(8.9%)	(52.8%)	<0.00001
3 Heavy	1	(1.8%)	(18.0%)	<0.001
4 Binge drinkers	0	(0%)	(30.1%)	<0.00001
Drinkers	39	(69.6%)	(95.4%)	<0.00001
0 + 1 + 2	55	(98.2%)	(81.9%)	<0.005
3 + 4	1	(1.8%)	(18.1%)	<0.005

Source: From Ref. 5.

Table 11 Degree of Smoking

Degree	Criteria (on average)
0	Abstainers
1 Light	Consumption < 0.5 pack/day
2 Moderate	Consumption 0.5–1.0 pack/day
3 Heavy	Consumption > 1.0 pack/day

Source: From Ref. 5, used with permission.

drinking ($p = 0.0001$), tended to drink less alcohol ($p = 0.0001$), and had lower proportions of heavy degrees of consumption ($p = 0.0022$) (Table 10).

Smoking

Table 11 presents our criteria for degrees of smoking (5). The degrees of use of cigarettes during pregnancy in the Motherisk group and in Ottawa and comparison of results of study performed in California (6) are shown in Table 12. The percentage of smokers in the Motherisk group was similar to that in Ottawa. Our nonpregnant patients had a lower percentage of smokers than Ottawa study groups ($p = 0.042$).

Abuse of Drugs

Fifty-seven women consumed drugs of abuse (12.0%). Forty-five were pregnant (13.4%) and two nonpregnant (3.3%). Cannabinoids and cocaine by far exceeded all other drugs (Table 13). Some women used more than one drug.

Exposure to Radiation

Sixty-two women were exposed to radiation: 6 (9.8%) at their workplace (diagnostic or security equipment) and 53 during diagnostic tests (86.9%). Two women requested information about video display terminals. The dosage of the radiation was calculated in each case according to standard tables. No case of dosage above the teratogenic level (fetal exposure > 10 rad) was found. Table 14 shows the distribution according to different diagnostic tests.

Table 12 Degree of Smoking During Pregnancy: Motherisk Versus Ottawa and Motherisk Versus California

Degree	Motherisk: $n = 330$		Ottawa: $n = 217$	p
Abstainers	221	(67.0%)	(75.5%)	>0.25
Smokers	109	(33.0%)	(24.4%)	>0.25

Degree[a]	Motherisk: $n = 330$[b]		California: $n = 12,349$	p
Abstainers	228	(66.7%)	8027 (65.0%)	
Light (< 1 ppd)	60	(18.2%)	2766 (22.4%)	$0.1 > p > 0.05$
Heavy (≥ 1 ppd)	47	(14.2%)	1556 (12.6%)	>0.25

[a]ppd, pack per day.
[b]Smoker information not available for all 300.
Source: From Refs. 5 and 6.

Table 13 Abuse of Drugs During Pregnancy

Drug	Number of users[a]
Cannabinoids	29
Cocaine	21
Heroin	3
Hallucinogens	2
Others[b]	2

[a]Some women used more than one drug.
[b]Prolonged use of codeine, and use of benzodiazepines.

In most cases the exposure to radiation occurred during the first trimester (52 women; 86.7%), with only two women exposed during the second trimester (3.3%). The mean time of acute exposures was 4.8 ± 0.5 gestational weeks.

Exposure to Chemicals

Sixty-two women were exposed to various chemicals; 26 (42.6%) from environmental sources (pollution, pesticides, insecticides) and 27 (44.2%) as a part of their occupation. Two women were exposed to the agents inadvertently (3.3%). Six women requested counseling about exposures to cosmetics, sweeteners, or herbal preparations (9.9%). The mean time of exposure to chemicals was 12.1 ± 2.2 gestational weeks (range 2–32).

Table 14 Diagnostic Radiation During Pregnancy[a]

System	Number of women	%
Dental	18	30.0
Digestive system	13	21.6
Skeletal	10	16.6
Respiratory	7	11.6
Renal	5	8.3
Thyroid	4	6.6
Genital	2	3.3
Other	3	5.0
		103

[a]One woman had 2 radiodiagnostic tests.

Table 15 Degree of Smoking: Pregnant Versus Nonpregnant

Degree	Pregnant ($n = 330^a$)		Nonpregnant ($n = 56$)		p
	Number	%	Number	%	
Abstained	223	67.8	47	84.0	$p < 0.05$
<1 pack/day	60	18.2	6	10.7	>0.15
≥1 pack/day	3	5.3	8	14.2	$0.1 < p < 0.05$

[a]Smoker information not available for all 330.

Use of Alcohol and Tobacco

A higher percent of smokers was found among the pregnant women than among the nonpregnant ones (Table 15).

Significant differences were detected in the distribution of consumption of alcohol between the pregnant and nonpre;gnant women ($p = 0.028$), with more abstainers in the former, but with a higher rate of heavy users (degrees 3 + 4) ($p = 0.072$) (Table 16). Abuse of drugs was reported in 47 cases: by 45 pregnant (13.4%), and 2 nonpregnant women (3.3%). Use of two or more drugs was reported by 17 pregnant women (5.1%) and by none of the nonpregnant women ($p < 0.05$). Comparison of drug abusers in pregnancy ($n = 46$) to the other pregnant women ($n = 284$) reveals that the abusers were younger, more likely to be single or divorced, and with fewer pregnancies, but significantly more elected abortions (Table 17).

The distribution of degrees of alcohol use differed between the drug abusers and the nonabusers (Table 18). None of the cocaine users abstained from

Table 16 Degree of Alcohol Consumption: Pregnant Versus Nonpregnant[a]

Degree	Pregnant ($n = 332$)		Nonpregnant ($n = 57$)		p
	Number	(%)	Number	(%)	
0 Abstained	141	42.5	17	30.4	NS
1 Light	126	37.9	33	58.9	$0.005 < p < 0.01$
2 Moderate	29	8.4	5	8.9	NS
3 Heavy	25	7.5	1	1.8	NS
4 Binge drinker	10	3.0	0	0	NS
3 + 4	29	8.7	1	1.8	NS

[a]Alcohol use information not available for all women.

Table 17 Drug Abusers Versus Nonabusers

Variables	Nonabusers	Abusers	p
Age, years			
Woman	30.1 ± 0.3	27.2 ± 0.9	<0.0005
Partner	32.1 ± 0.3	29.5 ± 1.1	0.01 < p < 0.025
Marital status			
Single	10.6%	54.8%	<0.00001
Married	88.8%	38.7%	<0.00001
Divorced	0.6%	6.5%	<0.01
Race			
White	87.6%	100%	p < 0.05
Nonwhite	12.4%	0	p < 0.05
Employment			
Out of home	25.8%	21.4%	p < 0.05
At home	74.2%	78.6%	p < 0.05
Obstetric history			
Gravida	2.23	1.98	NS
Parity	0.74	0.36	<0.005
Abortion	0.26	0.53	<0.005
Miscarriage	0.09	0.23	NS
Referral			
Self	64.4%	76.5%	NS
Physician	35.6%	23.5%	NS
Number exposures	2.0 ± 1.1	1.9 ± 0.3	NS

Table 18 Degree of Alcohol Consumption According to Abuse of Drugs

Degree	Nonabusers		Abusers		p
0 Abstained	132	(46.0%)	9	(20.0%)	<0.005
1 Light	114	(39.7%)	12	(26.7%)	<0.1
2 Moderate	17	(5.9%)	11	(24.4%)	<0.0001
3 Heavy	14	(14.9%)	11	(24.4%)	<0.00001
4 Binge drinkers	7	(2.4%)	3	(6.6%)	<0.2

Table 19 Degree of Smoking According to Abuse of Drugs

Degree	Nonabusers		Abusers		p
0 Abstained	208	(72.7%)	13	(29.4%)	<0.00001
1 Light	37	(12.9%)	19	(43.2%)	<0.00001
2 Moderate	28	(9.8%)	11	(25.0%)	<0.01
3 Heavy	11	(3.8%)	1	(2.3%)	>0.35

Table 20   Degree of Smoking: Women Versus Partners

Degree	Partners		Women		p
0 Abstained	235	(64.0%)	225	(69.5%)	<0.2
1 Light	45	(12.3%)	57	(15.5%)	<0.2
2 Moderate	55	(15.0%)	41	(11.2%)	<0.2
3 Heavy	26	(7.1%)	12	(3.3%)	<0.05

alcohol, and they had a higher tendency to binge drinking than abusers of other drugs.

The frequency of smoking, and particularly the light and moderate degrees, was higher among drug abusers than among nonabusers ($p = 0.0001$) (Table 19).

DATA ABOUT THE PARTNERS

Partners' mean age was 32.0 ± 0.3 years ($n = 381$); 363 men were employed (96.8%) and only 12 did not work (3.2%). Eight of those who did not work were students. Chronic disease states or medical conditions were reported in 88 cases (23.1%), and genetic diseases or malformations were reported in 10 (2.6%). Exposure to drugs was reported in 35 cases only (9.2%).

Comparison of alcohol and smoking degrees among the women and their spouses reveals a very close pattern (Tables 20 and 21). There was a highly significant correlation between the degrees of alcohol use, cigarette smoking, and drug consumption (Table 22).

ANALYSIS OF THE APPROACH TO THE COUNSELING

At the end of the interview and the collection of possible risk factors, the counseling physician presents to the woman or family an estimation of the

Table 21   Degree of Alcohol Consumption: Women Versus Partners

Degree	Partners		Women		p
0 Abstained	120	(32.5%)	151	(40.9%)	<0.1
1 Light	156	(42.3%)	150	(40.6%)	>0.35
2 Moderate	44	(11.9%)	31	(6.5%)	<0.05
3 Heavy	36	(9.7%)	26	(8.4%)	>0.3
4 Binge drinking	6	(1.6%)	10	(2.7%)	>0.2

Table 22 Correlation Between Maternal and Paternal Use of Alcohol, Cigarettes, and Drugs of Abuse

	Abstained[a]	Users[a]	Total	p
Alcohol				
abstained[b]	73	78	151	
users[b]	47	171	218	<0.001
	120	249	369	
Smoking				
abstained[b]	192	63	255	
users[b]	43	69	112	<0.001
	235	132	367	
Abuse of drugs				
abstained[b]	299	25	324	
users[c]	21	24	45	<0.001
	320	49	369	

	<Moderate use[a,d]	Heavy use[a,e]		p
Alcohol[c]				
⩽moderate use[b,d]	307	33	340	
heavy use[b,e]	25	4	29	>0.4
	332	37	369	

[a]Spouse.
[b]Women.
[c]Degrees 0 + 1 + 2 vs. 3 + 4.
[d]Degrees 0 + 1 + 2.
[e]Degrees 3 + 4.

Table 23 Recommendations of the Service

Recommendations	Number of women	%[a]
Ultrasound	102	30.4
Amniocentesis	41	12.2
Other tests	32	9.5
Avoid exposure	94	28.1
Continue treatment	56	16.7
Elevated risk	22	6.6
Termination	5	1.5
Total[b]	242	72.2

[a]Out of all pregnant women ($n = 335$).
[b]More than one recommendation was offered in several cases.

risk to the offspring. In many cases, the risk equals that of the general population. In certain cases, additional recommendations are given (Table 23):

1. Ultrasonographic examination, to determine the exact gestational age and the accurate timing of exposure and to rule out detectable malformations. In addition, ultrasound is recommended in cases of high maternal anxiety, or when a new drug with no literature available is involved.
2. Amniocentesis when maternal age is higher than 35 years, when familial history indicates a risk for neural tube defect or chromosomal aberrations, or when a woman has been exposed to drugs causing meningomyelocele (e.g., valproic acid).
3. Other tests, such as serum α-fetoprotein in cases of higher risk for open neural tube defects (e.g., in exposure to valproic acid). Genetic counseling is offered whenever a history of genetic problems is revealed, or whenever amniocentesis has to be scheduled. Sometimes measurement of antibody titers is recommended in cases of suspected viral infection.
4. Recommendation to avoid further exposure to a teratogen or suspected teratogen.
5. Recommendation to continue use of a medication needed to control a chronic illness. In cases of possible harmful effect to the offspring, alternative therapy is discussed.

RESULTS OF TESTS IN PREGNANCY

Positive results obtained in ultrasound were reported in three cases: severe encephalocele, vertebral anomaly, and two placentas with one normal fetus. Only the first case resulted in pregnancy termination. Amniocentesis was performed in 41 of 50 cases of women 35 years and older (81%). Comparing the rate of performance of this test in Manitoba (1985) and by us reveals 2.0 and 12.2%, respectively (7).

Termination of pregnancy as a result of information delivered by the Motherisk physicians occurred in five cases (1.5%). One case was decided upon following the sonographic result (encephalocele). In the other cases, women were exposed to drugs or chemicals as follows:

1. Carbon monoxide with evidence of severe maternal intoxication (levels in air 800 ppm).
2. Laetril use (exposure to cyanide).
3. Long dermal exposure to BCNU for mycosis fungoides during 1–5 gestational weeks.
4. Valproic acid use.
5. Phenytoin use in a case of an unplanned pregnancy.

SUMMARY

During the first year of Motherisk most women contacting us were asked to come for a consultation. Subsequently, after gaining experience, and following a substantial increase in the number of calls (currently 40–60 per day), only selected cases are scheduled for appointment, the rest being answered by the telephone by the information specialist or by the attending physician (see details in Chap. 28).

Several characteristics in our cohort indicate that the women counseled by us are a selected group who consider seriously risks associated with pregnancy: they are significantly older than pregnant women in Toronto in general, they tend to electively abort significantly less often than the average woman in Toronto, and they drink less alcohol than the amount reported for pregnant women in other studies. These facts indicate that it is unlikely that women use the Motherisk program to legitimize a desire to terminate pregnancy. These women, as a group, take the pregnancy in question very seriously and try to avoid preventable risks such as alcohol consumption.

The ethnic distribution of Motherisk patients closely reflects that of Greater Toronto, suggesting that the service is equally known and accessible to the various groups. Of concern is whether women of lower socioeconomic status, who may often have a cluster of risk factors, have been informed about this new service; however, our data deliberately omit certain details on education and income, since we feel that questions about these details may offend some distressed women who come for consultation about reproductive risks.

Our analysis reveals that about half of our patients seek advice soon after an inadvertent exposure in early pregnancy, and about one-third take medications knowing they are pregnant. One-sixth of our patients were not pregnant at the time of consultation, seeking advice about future use of a medication, generally for a chronic condition. A unique group of patients are those who had experienced adverse outcome in a previous pregnancy and wish to know whether the ill effect can be associated with drug/chemical exposure. In many such cases, litigation against a physician or drug company is being considered by the family, and the counselor should be extremely careful in assuring that his or her advice is well understood by the family.

There are clear differences between women who were exposed inadvertently before realizing they were pregnant and those who plan pregnancy, generally while being treated with a drug. The women in the former group are characterized by high levels of anxiety, since in addition to consuming up to 10 preparations they also did not reduce their alcohol intake and often did not quit taking recreational drugs. Those in the latter group, while planning pregnancy, try to avoid any unnecessary exposure, including other drugs, chemicals, or radiation. While the consultation process is essentially similar, it is important to counsel women with inadvertent exposures during the week they contact the clinic, since these women may consider termination of their pregnancy, whereas the prospective counseling is generally performed at more leisure.

Of our patients, about half were exposed to known or questionable teratogens. Clearly, in such cases the counseling process is essential in furnishing the family with up-to-date, accurate information about the patient's risk. In our opinion, it is not enough to state that a drug is teratogenic; the physician should quote an accurate figure of risk: we have found that often women believe that exposure to any "teratogen" is consistent with a very high percentage of adverse effects (see Chapter 29).

Of special interest is the woman who abuses recreational drugs. Typically, she is young, often unmarried, uses cannabinoids or cocaine as part of her lifestyle, and has found she is pregnant 2–3 months after conception. As shown by our data, such a woman tends to consume more alcohol and cigarettes, and her lifestyle correlates avidly with that of her spouse. We find that in most cases such patients, terrified by potential adverse effects to the unborn baby, have no problems in quitting drugs, cigarettes, and alcohol. The main task is to estimate their drug/alcohol dose prior to the time they found they were pregnant, and in most cases to reassure them that if the use of these substances is discontinued, risk is low, since at nonabusive levels of ingestion, the substances are not known to be human teratogens. The exceptions are heavy drinkers, who may have consumed alcohol in doses associated with fetal alcohol syndrome, and drug addicts.

It is essential to try to ascertain that the woman is not addicted to the drugs in question. If addiction is suspected or confirmed, the patient should be referred to an addiction specialist (see Chapter 7).

Exposure to nonmedical chemicals stresses the need for a strong background in medical toxicology. A group dealing with such issues should have a toxicologist as a team member or as a resource. Most major cities have a poison information center, and both parties will certainly benefit from such a collaboration.

More and more women are concerned about potential adverse effects of chemical exposure in the workplace. As documented in Chapter 19, relatively few occupational exposures have been proven to adversely affect reproductive outcome. Before suggesting that a woman quit her job, the counselor should be able to back such a decision with scientific evidence. Several manufacturers of metal products (e.g., lead, nickel) have tried to exclude from the production line all women of reproductive age. It took women centuries to get where they are today in the workplace; it may be quite easy to remove them if scientific evidence is eschewed in favor of unsubstantiated beliefs. Practically speaking, a letter suggesting removal of a pregnant woman from work is likely to end at the desk of a compensation board, which probably will wish to see the evidence the decision was based on.

Radiation in pregnancy occurs mostly before pregnancy was evidenced and becomes a very stressful event because of the connotation of teratogenic effects stemming from the Hiroshima and Nagasaki experiences. Enough evidence has been accumulated to indicate that diagnostic x-ray with a fetal radiation dose of less than 5 rad is not associated with measurable adverse effects in humans (see Chapter 22). While the same is true for most radioisotopes, the sad experience in half of the pregnant women in Athens, Greece following the Chernobyl nuclear accident illuminates the severity of the misinformation and misperception: it has been estimated that about half the women in early pregnancy chose to terminate it because of their fears of teratogenic risks associated with radioisotopes emitted during the Chernobyl disaster (8).

Finally, we turn to the research advantages and shortcomings of a prospectively collected database such as Motherisk. Being a clinical service, our information may not include items that might be deemed important for the analysis of such data. For example, most women come to us with high levels of anxiety following an exposure in pregnancy; we feel that it is unethical to ask them about their education and income, even though these factors are essential for identification of socioeconomic status. This restraint may hamper attempts to assess neurobehavioral development, which is known to be affected by maternal education. One way to solve this problem is to ask such questions postnatally, at the time of the follow-up interview. As shown in our data, Motherisk patients represent a selected group of women who are concerned enough to call in and come for a consultation. Clinically this is exactly the group one should support, since members may decide to terminate pregnancy on the basis of misinformation and a high degree of anxiety. However, in conducting research with this group, the scientist will have to account for differences between these patients and the population at large before generalizations can be made.

Every prospective study is a lengthy process, and the generated numbers may be too small to prove or rule out an increased teratogenic risk. Yet, this is a scientifically sound mechanism of collecting data on new drugs and chemicals on which no reproductive information exists.

For example, no data have been published on the safety of H_2 blockers in pregnancy, even though cimetidine and ranitidine are among the most widely prescribed drugs in North America. We have already ascertained the outcome of 20 pregnancies associated with these agents, collected prospectively through Motherisk.

A key problem in studies in teratology is ascertaining the exposure in question. Many studies rely on patients' recall; as shown by us recently, recall is incomplete, inaccurate, and often biased (9). Studies relying on medical charts assume that the pregnant women took the prescribed medication. Moreover, these charts will not disclose over-the-counter medications, alcohol drinking, smoking, or drugs of abuse. In Motherisk, patients are interviewed during or within a few days after the time of exposure, and this timing yields a high level of confidence about the time, dose, and indications of the exposure.

We feel that this meticulously collected information can create an important database for research of reproductive effects in pregnancy. The identified shortcomings should be accounted for in the evaluation of the data, and because of the numerous potential variables involved, the planning and execution of such analysis should be supervised by a medical epidemiologist or statistician.

REFERENCES

1. Harbison RD. Teratogens. In Cassarett and Doull's Toxicology (Doull J, Gaum K, Sumner D, eds). New York, Macmillan, 1980, pp 158–175.
2. Rubrin PC, Craig GF, et al. Prospective survey of use of therapeutic drugs, alcohol and cigarettes during pregnancy. Br Med J 1986; 292:81–85.
3. MacPherson AS. Health Status Report 1983. City of Toronto Department of Public Health, 1985, pp 20–41.
4. Grossman L. Ontario Statistics 1984. Ministry of Treasury and Economics of Ontario, 1984.
5. Fried PA, Watkinson B, Grant A, Knights RM. Changing patterns of soft drug use prior and during pregnancy: A prospective study. Drugs Alcohol Depend 1980; 6:323–343.
6. Weiner L, Rosett HL, Edelin KC, Alpert JJ, Zuckerman B. Alcohol consumption by pregnant women. Obstet Gynecol 1983; 61:6–12.
7. Oliver TK, Lange JR. Congenital anomalies: Detection and strategies for management. Semin Perinatol 1985; 9:154.
8. Trichopoulos D, Zavitsanos X, Koutis C, Drogari P, Proukakis C, Petridou E, et al. The victims of Chernobyl in Greece: Induced abortions after the accident. Br Med J 1987; 295:1100.
9. Feldman Y, Koren G, Matiace D, Shear N, MacLeod SM. Determinants of recall and recall bias in studies of drug exposure in pregnancy. Teratology.

31

Evaluating the Effects of Drugs in Pregnancy

A Guide to Critical Assessment of the Literature

Thomas R. Einarson
The Hospital for Sick Children, Toronto, Ontario, Canada

INTRODUCTION

Sir William Osler stated that "the desire to take medicine is perhaps the greatest feature which distinguishes man from the animals." That desire has resulted in the production and consumption of vast quantities of pharmaceutical entities. In fact, the use of drugs in Western society has increased to the point that virtually every person has been exposed to them.

Unfortunately, some of the drugs that are being consumed are not completely innocuous. In particular, the adverse effects of drugs in pregnancy have become the focus of considerable concern to the public subsequent to the thalidomide disaster that occurred during the 1950s.

In prescribing medication, particularly for the pregnant patient, the benefits of drug therapy must be weighed against the costs. In addition to direct costs, adverse events and their sequelae as well as economic consequences must be considered. The prudent practitioner wishes to provide patients with optimal care while avoiding problems.

To accomplish this goal, it is imperative that an appropriate level of current knowledge be maintained. Drug information is presently being provided by a host of sources that vary widely in quality, credibility, validity, and usefulness. Information on drugs in pregnancy is most often meager at best, and it is not unusual to find conflicting reports. Thus the individual practitioner must be able to read the literature critically and know how to assess the value of an article.

METHODS OF BECOMING INFORMED

Methods for acquisition of drug-related knowledge include primary literature (medical journals), secondary literature (textbooks, drug compendia), professional meetings, colleagues, other health professionals, drug information centers, product monographs, and manufacturers' sales representatives. Depending on the information required, these sources vary widely in their ability to provide the practitioner with adequate information with which to make informed decisions.

Weston (1) reported that physicians most frequently utilized medical journals for drug information, followed closely by consultation with colleagues. Third was attendance at professional meetings. Stinson and Mueller (2) produced similar results in a survey of 402 physicians. Medical literature was the prime source of drug information, and 99% of the respondents claimed that they regularly consulted medical journals.

Others have found differing results. Utilizing primary medical literature ranked fourth in a survey by Nickman and coworkers (3), and fifth by Covell et al. (4). Thus, original research reports are not being read by all practitioners.

WHY READ THE LITERATURE?

Keeping Up

Patient care is rapidly advancing as research provides newer and more efficacious agents. If these new agents are indeed better, then they should be used. In addition to learning about improvements in therapy, it is essential to read the literature to be knowledgeable about adverse events. To provide optimal patient care, reading the primary literature is essential.

There are also less altruistic reasons for maintaining current knowledge. In cases of litigation, courts often decide on the basis of what is "normal" or "standard practice," or what the "the prudent practitioner" would do. To know what is considered appropriate, one must constantly read.

The Issue of Bias

Information supplied by manufacturers is provided in several forms: product monographs, advertising, and verbally through sales representatives.

Monographs are prepared as leaflets, and also may appear in texts such as the *Physician's Desk Reference* (PDR) (5) in the United States, or the *Compendium of Pharmaceuticals and Specialties* (CPS) (6) in Canada. Although the monographs must comply with federal regulations, they are not complete in their disclosure of information. Descriptions of adverse events are usually limited to a listing of possible or documented occurrences. Obviously, information on unauthorized uses of drugs is omitted.

Manufacturers have a vested interest in promoting their products, which can be a source of bias. It is the function of sales representatives to generate revenue through increased sales of their own products. The profit incentive could encourage major bias in providing information. The PDR is published by the manufacturers of the pharmaceutical products it describes, and inclusion is voluntary. The CPS is published by the Canadian Pharmaceutical Association and may therefore be less prone to bias. However, the main purpose of these books is to present product monographs; PDR and CPS are not intended to be texts for therapeutics or pharmacology. Thus, despite widespread use, they do have some limitations.

Books often take years to prepare and publish, and thus may contain information that is incomplete or outdated. Most often, books are not peer reviewed. As a result, they may contain flaws and may reflect personal opinions rather than generally accepted scientific knowledge.

In addition to editorials and commentaries, journals present abstracts, articles, and reviews, which provide information that may be used in clinical decision making. Abstracts are often incomplete and final versions may never be published for a number of reasons. Reviews can sometimes be biased, with two reviewers arriving at opposite conclusions. Research articles are reports made by researchers who describe their work firsthand. Thus, research articles appear to be the best source of information for the practitioner.

Because most of the primary literature is peer reviewed, it is less prone to bias and thus is to be preferred as a source of information concerning drugs and their effects. Peer-reviewed articles are often given more credence than those that have not been peer reviewed. Therefore, clinical decision makers should be able to read and evaluate the primary literature and apply the information to their patients.

EVALUATING THE JOURNAL

The journal in which an article is published may have a great influence on the article's perceived value. A journal may be the official publication of a professional society; it may be owned by a large publisher, or even by drug manufacturers. Obviously, ownership could influence the content of the journal. Another factor not often considered is the source of revenue for the journal. Some are financed through subscriptions; others receive funding from the dues paid to the professional society that publishes them. Some are totally financed by drug companies; others are financed through the sale of advertising. It is best to determine the ownership and publication policy of the journal when considering an article. An article that is interspersed with commercial advertisements may not be as free from bias as one from a journal having no commercial ads, or having them confined to a separate section.

Most journals receive unsolicited manuscripts from authors who receive no remuneration. These are considered to be highest in quality. Some journals pay authors to write papers for them; others require a fee to have the papers published. In such cases, there is a conflict of interest, and less credibility is often given to paid articles. This information is often contained in the "Requirements for Authors" section. Perhaps the gold standard in journals is the *New England Journal of Medicine*, which contains little commercial advertising, is peer reviewed, has a panel of experts available to critique most subjects, and is funded through subscriptions.

PROPERTIES OF GOOD STUDIES

To evaluate the literature properly, the practitioner must understand the organization of an article as well as concepts of research design, statistical analysis, and logic. He or she must be able to identify strengths and weaknesses of different designs and to use judgment to determine the credibility or importance of the results.

Studies may be classified as correlational or experimental. Correlational studies include surveys and simple observations. Experimental studies involve the manipulation of a variable while all else is held constant, thus proving that the intervention caused the result. Studies of the latter type are to be preferred because they eliminate competing explanations for the obtained results. Campbell and Stanley (7) present a thorough discussion of the advantages of experimental design.

Scientific papers must be organized in a manner that allows the reader to be able to fully understand exactly what took place and to evaluate the results. Generally, articles are arranged as follows: introduction, methods, results, discussion, and conclusions.

Introduction

The introduction should be brief and to the point. Its purpose is to present the *statement of purpose*. The purpose must be stated explicitly; if not, it is impossible for the reader to determine whether the research achieved its goal. The introduction may contain background information to support the undertaking of the study. Such background should contain only pertinent references and factual information. Some writers will state not only the purpose of the study but also the hypotheses they tested. That practice is commendable and should be encouraged.

At the heart of the research lies the purpose of the study (and the hypotheses, if stated). The remainder of the paper should be constructed to demonstrate how the research addressed the problem at hand and what resulted from it. In other words, all other parts must relate to the purpose. For that reason, it is crucial that the purpose of the paper be stated explicitly.

Methods

The methods section should be so explicit that the reader could duplicate the study. It is important to know *exactly* how the study was carried out. The methods section should include information about the sample collection and testing, instrument validation and use, procedures involved, data collection and analysis, and criteria for judging results.

Sample

Ideally, researchers would identify an entire population of interest and randomly select subjects for inclusion in their study. However, in reality, such a situation never occurs; convenience samples are always used. To be truly random, every member of the population of interest must have an equal chance of being selected.

What is important is that the sample be representative of the population to which results will be extrapolated. In general, the larger the sample, the more representative it will be. The problems with large samples are the cost involved, the time needed for processing, and the logistics of analysis. Researchers thus try to use as small a sample as possible while obtaining significant results that may be generalized to other people.

To minimize problems associated with sampling, several techniques are used. A sample may be selected and subjects then randomly assigned to treatment or control groups. Random assignment, although it does not totally correct for lack of random selection, serves to limit bias through minimizing differences between groups. Thus, differences in outcome may be attributed to the intervention with a greater degree of certainty.

To help assure that groups being investigated are similar, it is preferable for researchers to compare groups with respect to all variables that could affect outcome. For example, age and socioeconomic status (SES) of the mother have been known to affect fetal outcomes. If adverse outcomes on the fetus were of interest, groups of subjects must be compared to detect any differences. If differences were found, they would have to be dealt with either through stratification (i.e., compare only offspring of mothers of a similar age or SES) or through statistical analysis (i.e., holding age as a covariate).

It is important to note that statistical tests only detect differences that may exist; they do not guarantee sameness. Only when groups are significantly different do tests indicate a problem. To gauge the degree of difference, exact statistics should be presented (e.g., $p = 0.067$ rather than $p > 0.05$), as suggested by Bailar and Mosteller (8).

Independent Variables

An independent variable is one that is manipulated in an experimental study, such as the dose of a drug or the length of time of a treatment. Variables that cannot be manipulated, such as sex or race, are called moderator variables or grouping variables. These variables must be described explicitly in the methods section so that the reader knows exactly what has been done. The choice of independent variables must reflect the purpose of the study.

Dependent Variables

The dependent variables is that which is measured. It could be the presence of a teratogenic outcome after exposure to a drug, or the measure of systolic blood pressure after consumption of an antihypertensive medication. One needs to ask whether the dependent variable being measured is, in fact, a valid measure for the purpose of the study.

Instrument

The instrument, the device used for measuring the results, may be a survey questionnaire, a blood pressure cuff, or an expert who judges whether a child is normal or abnormal.

It is critical that the validity of the instrument be verified for the purpose of the study. Validity may be equated with accuracy of measurement. In other words, it is the degree to which an instrument measures what it is intended to measure. As stated above, validity is assured for a specific purpose; if the instrument were used for more than one purpose, it would have to be validated for each.

Most often, face validity is determined by having experts or knowledgeable persons read and evaluate a questionnaire. A pretest should be done to detect flaws and to improve questions. New laboratory test results are usually compared with those from standard procedures. If so, a correlation coefficient may be reported.

Validity is most important to determine; however, it is very often subjective and difficult to measure. As a result, reliability coefficients are often presented in an attempt to provide some indirect evidence that the instrument may be valid. Reliability coefficients measure consistency and, in contrast to popular misconception, are a property of the data, not of the instrument. If an instrument is valid, it will produce reliable data (i.e., $r \geq 0.80$); however, the reverse may not be true. For example, an instrument could reliably measure invalid data (i.e., by producing the same wrong answer time after time, it would show itself to be consistent but not accurate). Thus, high reliability is no guarantee of what is really desired, validity. However, if the reliability coefficient is low (i.e., < 0.4), then the instrument is most likely not valid and research results should be suspect.

Raters

When judgments are made by different individuals concerning a variable of interest (e.g., a diagnosis of an adverse drug reaction), it is preferable to have the individuals judge independently and then compare the judgments. Several statistical methods have been developed for determining the degree of agreement among judges. If the variable being judged is measured on a continuous scale (i.e., at interval level), Pearson's r is often calculated. Rosenthal (9) presents a method for adjusting r among several judges. For ranked data, Kendall's tau may be calculated between two judges, or Kendall's W for three or more (10). For categorical data, such as diagnosis, kappa (11, 12) may be used. Tests of statistical significance should be presented for each coefficient.

Statistical Tests

The methods section should state the statistical test used for verifying each hypothesis. Authors should not simply list the tests without context; it should be made clear how each will be applied.

The preferred format is to present the hypotheses to be tested, which are derived from the purpose of the study. Ideally, they would be stated in the same order as in the introduction.

The error level that will be tolerated should be stated explicitly. Perhaps the most commonly selected alpha level is 0.05. However, there is nothing magic about that number; it is quite arbitrary. Many researchers would accept 0.10 as an acceptable level, especially with exploratory work such as in a pilot study.

Parametric statistics, such as Student's t-test and analysis of variance, are most commonly seen. However, their use is predicated on the assumption that the variable under study is normally distributed in the population being studied, that measurement is at least interval level, and that samples are randomly selected. Most researchers are willing to allow the first two assumptions, but the third is never achieved. As a result, nonparametric (also called distribution-free) statistics may be preferred, especially with small sample sizes.

Statement of Limitations

A good study will state its limitations as well as its delimitations. No study can look at all possible patients or types of patient, all types of adverse reaction, or all drugs. As a result, each study will have its limitations. If these are stated, the reader can better judge the importance of the study findings and to place them in their proper context.

Results

Results should be presented systematically in the same order as the stated objectives. Tables may be used to present data, but should not duplicate the text. Frequencies should be accompanied by percentages for the reader's convenience. Statistical tests should state the test used, the value of the test, the degrees of freedom, and the significance value. For example, one should say that no difference between groups are detected with respect to SES [χ^2 = 1.22, degrees of freedom (df) = 2, p = 0.543] rather than simply stating there was no difference.

It is appropriate to describe the sample of subjects and to compare groups with respect to variables that could affect outcomes. Any pilot test results should then be presented, followed by a presentation of data from each hypothesis test. Any finding that was incidental may be mentioned, but conclusions may not be drawn if the researchers did not plan to investigate those findings.

Discussion

Often, the discussion section may be combined with results or conclusions, or both. The purpose is to elaborate on results to bring them to a conclusion. Reference should be made to other similar work, and justification presented for differing results.

Conclusions

The statements made from research should be of prime concern to the reader. It is the validity of these statements that is subject to threats as described by Campbell and Stanley (7). The reader should examine them carefully and determine whether the study design, sample selection, and methods support statements made.

In addition, the generalizability of the statements is limited by the sample selected and by the nature of the experiment. The authors should state the limitations of the applicability of the findings. Only a randomly selected sample is truly representative of the population, and that is virtually impossible to achieve.

Perhaps the most common misuse of research results is the conclusion that correlation demonstrates causation. If two events occur at the same time, or in sequence, it does not prove that one caused the other. The reader should beware of conclusions that overstep the data. To prove causation, one must use rigid experimental design, and even that has limitations. A good rule is to be skeptical.

A common error is to take evidence from a cross-sectional study, such as a survey, and make longitudinal statements from it. For example, if one did a survey that compared opinions of young people with those of old people and found a difference, one could not conclude that as people age, their opinions change. Conclusions must be based on the research performed. To make a conclusion about changes associated with aging, one would have to conduct a longitudinal study on a group of people and measure their opinions at different ages.

PROBLEMS OF RESEARCH IN PREGNANCY

Several difficulties arise in evaluating drugs for use in pregnant patients. Perhaps the greatest problem is that no drugs are tested in pregnant women. All pharmaceutical products approved for marketing must be tested on animal models, but such models are not always appropriate. In fact, thalidomide was tested on rats and mice, but failed to produce teratogenic outcomes. As a result, information regarding the use of drugs in pregnancy must be generated by alternate methods. These methods include editorials, case reports, anecdotal letters to the editor, and epidemiological studies.

However, such reports have shortcomings. They most often focus on possible adverse effects of a drug in pregnancy; rarely do they address the issue of safety in pregnancy. Such information would also be useful for clinical decision making.

Case Reports

Case reports are submitted to journals by clinicians and researchers, usually on a volunteer basis. The quality of the reports varies with the authors and situations. Ideally, a patient would be rechallenged with the drug to determine whether the same reaction would be repeated. However, such a practice may be impractical, impossible, or unethical.

A major benefit of case reports is the identification of rare events. These events include effects due to a rarely used drug, a rare disease, a rare combination of drugs, or a rare or unusual occurrence of an adverse effect. Examples: the identification of aplastic anemia following chloramphenicol administration to children and observations of the development of phocomelia after maternal thalidomide ingestion. These reports alerted authorities to major problems, of which we are all now aware.

The disadvantage is that causation cannot be established from case reports. Consider the case of Bendectin (a combination of doxylamine succinate and pyridoxine hydrochloride), an antinauseant used in pregnancy. Case reports associated a supposed syndrome of birth defects and maternal consumption of Bendectin during pregnancy. Law suits followed, and researchers began to analyze mountains of data. As a result, the only drug indicated for nausea of pregnancy was removed from the market owing to adverse publicity. However, a recent meta-analysis (13) has demonstrated that the statistical combination of all published data on Bendectin shows it not to be associated with abnormal fetal outcomes. Thus, case reports should be evaluated with the fact in mind that they do not prove causation.

Often, case reports will alert clinicians to new indications for drugs. For researchers, they suggest new areas of study and hypotheses to be tested. Another useful function is to verify the effectiveness of a treatment in groups that have not been clinically tested. For example, drug trials rarely include neonates or pregnant women.

What are particularly lacking are case reports of drugs that have been safely used in pregnancy. Such information would be as valuable as reports of adverse events. Such reports are now being collected by the Motherisk team at the Hospital for Sick Children in Toronto and are shared with interested practitioners.

Editorials

An editorial is usually an opinion expressed by a learned author or a small group of experts. Most often, these opinions are supported by clinical data and experience (14). Editorials are most useful for describing the state of the art for a particular topic, for identifying clinical problem areas, or for describing what may be expected in "normal" therapeutics. Nonetheless, editorials are opinions, subject to personal biases.

Letters

Letters to the editor are unsolicited accounts that may contain case reports, brief experiments, or preliminary research data. They are usually not peer reviewed and may contain opinion and personal bias. Some journals, such as the Lancet and the New England Journal of Medicine, publish many letters that are often given great credence. They have similar drawbacks to case reports and should be given similar consideration.

Correlational Studies

Since experimental studies are not commonly performed on pregnant women, researchers have developed correlational methods that may be applied to establish facts about drug use. Three main types that use correlational methods are surveys, case control studies, and cohort studies.

Surveys are cross-sectional and provide important information. The nature of a survey, however, does not permit longitudinal conclusions. Surveys do identify areas that require further study. Readers should note that surveys cannot establish causation, as discussed above.

When large bases of information are available, it is possible to perform epidemiological studies on the data (15). In such cases, huge sample sizes may be achieved. Therefore, results are more likely to converge on the truth.

Epidemiological studies may be either prospective or retrospective. Prospective studies begin on a specified date and follow cases through time to note the occurrence of a specified outcome. Retrospective studies look back into records to detect evidence for exposure to a drug or for adverse reactions. The latter may be subject to bias from the researcher, who often must make judgments. As a result, prospective studies may be considered to be of higher quality than retrospective studies. However, the former require large numbers of subjects and tend to be very time-consuming and costly.

Case control studies begin with a particular outcome and search the records for evidence of exposure to a drug. A comparison group of nonaffected subjects is selected and records are searched to determine the rate of exposure in normals. Rates are compared to arrive at an odds ratio for a drug producing a specific adverse effect. A ratio of unity (i.e., 1) indicates no drug effect, but higher values may signify a relationship. Confidence intervals should be presented to indicate whether a relationship is statistically significant. If unity is within the interval, there is no association between the drug and an adverse effect. Conversely, if the interval excludes unity, there is a relationship.

The presence of a relationship does not prove absolutely that the drug caused the event. One must weigh all the available evidence, including animal models, case reports, and theories of mechanisms behind the reaction.

Cohort studies are opposite to case control studies. They begin with a group of subjects exposed to a drug and a comparison group of nonexposed subjects and follow the subjects prospectively (or retrospectively in a chart review) to determine the frequency of adverse events. A risk ratio is calculated, which is very similar to the odds ratio of case control studies.

Prospective cohort studies are ideal in that they measure incidence of adverse events. However, cohort studies require a very large number of subjects, especially if the adverse event under study is rare. Case control studies can produce similar data with fewer subjects, hence they are more often employed.

META-ANALYSIS

When reading the literature, one may be presented with a number of studies producing varied results. The problem is how to analyze the data to arrive at an overall conclusion concerning the relationship of a drug and a given outcome. In the past, reviews were done, but these were subject to much bias. A mathematical method has been developed to help overcome bias and arrive at a single overall value that describes the drug-outcome relationship; namely, meta-analysis.

Glass (16) coined the term *meta-analysis* to refer to the statistical combination of research from independent studies. Since that time, meta-analysis has become increasingly popular as a method for summarizing the literature (17). The prefix *meta* is used in the sense of secondary, in that results of completed studies may be aggregated to arrive at an overall summary estimate of the true effect of a drug.

For epidemiological studies, meta-analysis gives an overall odds ratio that describes the relationship between a drug and an outcome. Einarson et al. (13) have presented a method for meta-analysis of epidemiological studies. Other methods have been presented for clinical trials (18,19).

Meta-analysis is to be preferred as a method for aggregation of results from individual studies because it is systematic, thorough, quantitative, and less prone to bias. Studies that vary in quality may be given more weight than those of lower quality throughout (20,21). Similarly, studies having larger sample sizes may be given more weight. Readers are encouraged to consult meta-analyses for reviews of specific drugs.

Presently, the Motherisk team at the Hospital for Sick Children in Toronto is collecting meta-analyses of drugs in pregnancy. These analyses will be used to assist clinicians and pregnant patients in their decision-making process.

REFERENCES

1. Weston K. Sources of drug and other biomedical information. Drug Inf J 1979; 13:11–14.
2. Stinson ER, Mueller DA. Survey of health professionals' information habits and needs. JAMA 1980; 243:140–143.
3. Nickman NA, Hadsall RS, Wertheimer AI. Pharmacist not yet a drug advisor. Drug Intell Clin Pharm 1988; 22:174–175.

4. Covell DG, Uman GC, Manning PR. Information needs in office practice: Are they being met? Ann Intern Med 1985; 103:596–599.
5. Baker CE (publ). Physician's Desk Reference, 47th ed. Medical Economics Data, Oradell, NJ, 1993.
6. Krogh CME, ed. Compendium of Pharmaceuticals and Specialties, 22nd ed. Canadian Pharmaceutical Association, Ottawa, Ontario, 1987.
7. Campbell DT, Stanley JC. Experimental and Quasi-Experimental Designs for Research. Houghton Mifflin, Boston, 1963.
8. Bailar JC, Mosteller F. Guidelines for statistical reporting in articles for medical journals. Ann Intern Med 1988; 108:266–273.
9. Rosenthal R. Meta-Analytic Procedures for Social Research. Sage, Beverly Hills, CA, 1984.
10. Siegel S. Nonparametric Statistics for the Behavioral Sciences. McGraw-Hill, New York, 1956.
11. Cohen J. A coefficient of agreement for nominal scales. Educ Psychol Meas 1960; 20:37–46.
12. Fleiss JL. Measuring nominal scale agreement among many raters. Psychol Bull 1971; 76:378–382.
13. Einarson TR, Leeder JS, Koren G. A method for meta-analysis of epidemiologic studies. Drug Intell Clin Pharm 1988; 22:813–824.
14. Leeder JS, Spielberg SP, MacLeod SM. Bendectin: The wrong way to regulate drug availability. Can Med Assoc J 1983; 129:1085–1087.
15. Kleinbaum DG, Kupper LL, Morgenstern H. Epidemiologic Research: Principles and Quantitative Methods. Van Nostrand Reinhold, New York, 1982.
16. Glass GV. Primary, secondary, and meta-analysis of research. Educ Res 1976; 5:3–8.
17. Wolf FM. Meta-analysis. N Engl J Med 1987; 317:576.
18. DerSimonian R, Laird N. Meta-analysis in clinical trials. Controlled Clin Trials 1986; 7:177–188.
19. L'Abbé KA, Detsky AS, O'Rourke K. Meta-analysis in clinical research. Ann Intern Med 1987; 107:224–233.
20. Chalmers TC, Smith H. Blackburn B. A method for assessing the quality of a randomized controlled trial. Controlled Clin Trials 1981; 2:31–49.
21. Sacks HS, Berrier J, Reitman D, Ancona-Berk VA, Chalmers TC. Meta-analyses of randomized controlled trials. N Engl J Med 1987; 316:450–455.

32

Teratogenicity and Litigation

J. Steven Leeder
The Hospital for Sick Children, Toronto, Ontario, Canada

Stephen P. Spielberg
Merck Research Laboratories, West Point, Pennsylvania

Clinical Case

One of your patients comes to your office with her baby boy, who has a large ventricular septal defect. The woman took Bendectin (doxylamine and vitamin B₆) for morning sickness, and she wants to know whether the drug caused the VSD.

INTRODUCTION

In mid-1983, Merrell Pharmaceuticals, Inc. announced the decision to cease production of the doxylamine-pyridoxine combination marketed in North America as Bendectin (Debendox in Great Britain and Lenotan in West Germany), which was used in the treatment of nausea and vomiting in pregnancy. This decision originated from negative publicity and financial concerns, which were based on numerous lawsuits launched in the United States as well as on the resulting increase in insurance premiums. Of major concern was the impact on the general public of widespread and misinformed coverage. Shortly after Merrell's announcement, a spokesman for the Public Citizen Health Research Group in Washington, DC, said that the action of the company in removing Bendectin from the market meant that "hundreds of thousands of pregnant women and their unborn offspring will be spared the risk of exposure" (*The Globe and Mail*, Toronto, Ontario, June 10, 1983, 2).

The contradiction between concerns in the lay press (and debates in courts of law leading to withdrawal of the drug) and the evidence obtained from numerous epidemiological studies prompted the appearance of several editorials and reviews objecting to the high level of public concern that stemmed from considerable negative publicity (1–4). A common theme in these articles was the apparent injustice of having the availability of perhaps the best-studied drug in pregnancy regulated by public hysteria fueled by the sensationalistic press and the media attention given to the litigation cases under way. The Bendectin saga forces the pharmaceutical industry, health care professionals, and the scientific community to face a number of important issues related to drug exposure in pregnancy, teratogenicity, and litigation.

The thalidomide experience of the 1960s increased the realization by the public and the legal profession that some human malformations may be caused by nongenetic environmental factors (e.g., exposure to drugs, toxicants, radiation). This awareness, accompanied by the philosophy of some individuals, at least, that someone must be responsible for the damages incurred, and thus is obliged to provide compensation, has resulted in an increase in litigation involving malformed infants, the most publicized cases of which continue to involve Bendectin. The medicolegal issues related to the field of teratology are very complex, encompassing, among others, the legal rights of the unborn fetus, the etiology of the congenital malformation, the temporal association between ingestion (exposure) and causality, the definition of an expert witness, and the necessity of demonstrating negligence and causality. One problem with respect to the latter point is that causality is taken to be an extension of negligence, however illogical this may seem to the scientific community. An additional problem is that legal proof requires only 51% certainty, whereas the scientific criterion for a causal relationship is considerably higher (95%). Brent provides a very comprehensive review of the issues involved in litigation on congenital malformations, including a discussion of the adverse effects of the litigation process on the families of malformed infants (5). This chapter examines the possible consequences of litigation on the already complicated issues related to drug use in pregnancy, using the Bendectin experience for illustrative purposes.

HISTORY OF BENDECTIN

Bendectin was introduced in 1956 as a formulation of doxylamine succinate, an antihistamine with antinauseant properties; dicyclomine hydrochloride (Bentylol), an antispasmodic; and pyridoxine hydrochloride (vitamin B_6). It was the only agent approved by the U.S. Food and Drug Administration (FDA) for control of morning sickness, but not until the 1970s was there any scientific documentation of its efficacy. A randomized, double-blind, multicenter study comparing the effects of the three components alone and in combination versus placebo concluded that doxylamine-pyridoxine was an effective combination, whereas dicyclomine made no significant contribution to the overall effectiveness of the product (6). Therefore dicyclomine was removed from the formulation in the United States in 1976, and in July 1978, Bendectin was licensed in Canada as the two-ingredient product.

Concerns about the possible teratogenic effects of Bendectin were first raised in 1969 when Paterson described congenital limb deformities in an infant whose mother had allegedly taken Bendectin during pregnancy (7). Also included were descriptions of four similar cases reported to the Canadian Food and Drug Directorate of the Department of National Health and Welfare. An additional infant with "similar deformities" was reported in 1977, leading Paterson to conclude, on the basis of these 6 cases and 80 more reported to the FDA, that "Bendectin may not be safely used in pregnancy . . ." (8). The scientific validity of this conclusion is very questionable without an estimate of the total number of exposures to Bendectin during pregnancy for use as a denominator. In addition, the dubious merit of evidence presented as a case report is obvious, since there are no suitable controls, the dosage of medications ingested is often not quantified, and patient characteristics (e.g., smoking and drinking history, caffeine use, illnesses during pregnancy, parity, and the presence of chronic disorders such as epilepsy and diabetes mellitus) are often not mentioned. Attempts to establish a causal relationship are further confounded by the use of other drugs during the first trimester of pregnancy.

An epidemiological study by Rothman and colleagues (9) found a weak association between Bendectin (and a number of other drugs) and some congenital heart defects. This study was not designed to assess Bendectin, but rather to investigate the relationship between hormones taken during pregnancy and congenital heart disease in the offspring. Several drugs were reportedly taken more frequently by the mothers of affected children, including ampicillin, acetylsalicyclic acid, and codeine, drugs not usually noted for their teratogenic potential. Information concerning Bendectin and other nonhormonal drugs was obtained by an open-ended question that may have permitted major recall bias, as was noted by the authors: the mothers with malformed babies were more likely to be concerned and presumably better able to remember the events of the pregnancy (including drug use) than women whose offspring were unaffected. This study was unable to distinguish associations between the underlying indication for drug use and congenital heart disease from direct associations between the drugs themselves and congenital heart disease. In addition, the numbers of affected infants for each drug were small. The authors did not consider any of the weak associations to be significant and indicated that their findings should be considered as exploratory.

Coinciding with these anecdotal reports was the initial, well-publicized legal action launched in Florida by Michael and Elizabeth Makdeci against Richardson-Merrell, Inc. (now Merrell-Dow Pharmaceuticals, Inc.). The Makdecis sued for $12 million on behalf of their son David, who was born with limb deformities. His mother had taken Bendectin during the pregnancy. In a seemingly contradictory decision, reached in May 1980, the Florida jury concluded that nothing should be awarded to the boy or to his parents for damages but stated that the parents should receive $20,000 for medical expenses (10). Because of this contradiction, the case was retried in early 1981. The jury ruled in favor of Merrell-Dow, thereby exonerating Bendectin from any responsibility for the malformation. In a second case, a Washington jury awarded $750,000 to the family of a 12-year-old girl born with an incompletely formed right hand. The girl's mother had taken Bendectin during pregnancy. Two weeks later, on June 9, 1983, the company decided to cease production of the product worldwide because the cost of trial attorneys and insurance premiums was approaching the U.S. dollar sales of the drug. Subsequent legal action in both these cases concluded in favor of the defendant, with the U.S. Court of Appeals upholding the 1981 jury decision in the Makdeci trial on August 15, 1983. The award in the Washington trial was canceled on September 1, 1983, when the judge overturned the jury's decision in a judgment notwithstanding the jury's verdict. Despite successful defense of these two cases, Merrell-Dow had no intention of resuming production of Bendectin.

Four years after withdrawal of the drug, litigation cases alleging teratogenic effects from Bendectin taken during pregnancy were still being tried. In January 1987, a Pennsylvania state court jury awarded $2 million to a 6-year-old boy born with club feet, and half of this amount was for punitive damages. In July of the same year, a Washington, DC, jury awarded $95 million to a plaintiff born with malformed arms and hands, $75 million of which was for punitive damages. In both these cases, Merrell-Dow filed posttrial motions to seek a judgment notwithstanding the verdict or a new trial as well as a reduction of the $95 million award (11).

By late 1987, a total of 17 trials involving Bendectin had taken place, 13 of which ended in favor of Merrell-Dow. From a purely scientific perspective, it is difficult to understand the basis for this litigiousness. Even in 1983, at the time of Bendectin's removal from the market, there were available considerable epidemiological data from large prospective trials (12–19) and from retrospective analyses of patient data (20–29) which provided evidence against a causal relationship between Bendectin use in pregnancy and teratogenic effects in the offspring of those pregnancies. Despite the different study designs employed and the inherent strengths and weaknesses of the individual studies, almost all were unable to demonstrate any statistical association between Bendectin use and subsequent malformations. One exception was the Rothman study (9) discussed previously. Mitchell and colleagues (23) compared Bendectin exposure in groups of infants with isolated cleft palate, cleft lip with or without cleft palate, heart defects, and other malformed infants who served as controls. Their data suggested that early exposure to Bendectin in utero did not appreciably increase the risk of any of these malformations, directly contradicting the association noted in the Rothman study. The lack of association between Bendectin exposure and congenital heart disease was also confirmed by a follow-up study by Zierler and Rothman (30), which sought to evaluate and remove the possible bias resulting from differential recall of exposure history by obtaining such information from two sources. Jick et al. (24) had found more infants with atresia of the intestine among the Bendectin-exposed group than among the control group (4 vs. 2, respectively) in a total cohort of 2255 exposed and 4582 unexposed controls. Since the 95% confidence interval included unity, a causal association was considered unlikely.

Eskenazi and Bracken (28) found that mothers of infants with congenital malformations had an increased likelihood of having used Bendectin during pregnancy than the mothers of unaffected control infants. In particular, there was a statistically significant association between Bendectin exposure and pyloric stenosis, although the open-ended questionnaire used to ascertain drug exposure during pregnancy may have produced recall bias. In addition, the association with pyloric stenosis was based on 6 exposed cases, whereas a study by Mitchell et al. (31) found no relationship between Bendectin exposure and this particular malformation based on 56 exposed cases. The latter study also reduced the effect of recall bias by using two control groups of malformed infants. A study by Aselton and colleagues (32) also minimized the possibility of recall bias by obtaining exposure data from prescription records. These investigators found that the association between Bendectin exposure and pyloric stenosis was most pronounced in mothers who had filled five or more prescriptions for the drug during their pregnancy. The authors concluded that their data provided additional evidence for a relationship between continuous Bendectin use during pregnancy *or* severe nausea of pregnancy (necessitating prolonged Bendectin use) and pyloric stenosis, but chose, on the basis of the conflicting data and the absence of a biologically plausible explanation for the association, not to interpret these findings as causal.

Cordero and associates (14) interviewed parents whose infants had selected malformations and were unable to demonstrate any stastically significant differences in exposure to Bendectin for any of 12 defect categories studied. Among the six subgroups of infants with limb reduction defects, only those with amniotic bands had had a significantly increased exposure to Bendectin.

When time stratification was performed, a weak statistical association was found between exposure to the three-component formulation and esophageal atresia, and between the two-ingredient formulation and encephalocele. The association between exposure and amniotic bands was observed only when the data were not stratified for time. There were three weak statistical associations, but the authors concluded that these did not constitute a causal relationship between exposure to Bendectin and these particular categories of birth defects. The press, on the other hand, emphasized the associations without qualification, thus contributing to widespread misinformation.

Review of the literature, therefore, suggests that on the basis of available epidemiological data, there is little evidence, if any, to justify the number of lawsuits filed against the manufacturer of Bendectin in the past few years. If there is any association between Bendectin exposure and a specific malformation, the most likely candidate on the basis of available information would be pyloric stenosis. Since this outcome does not develop until several weeks after birth, it is debatable whether it can be considered a congenital birth defect. From a mechanistic perspective, any relationship between Bendectin and pyloric stenosis is tenuous, since this condition affects males three to four times more frequently than females, occurs in firstborns in approximately half the cases, and may be associated with a genetic predisposition.

To be fair, it is unlikely that any litigation has been initiated with the sole intention of forcing the manufacturer to remove Bendectin from the market. Nor is it safe to assume that lawyers for the plaintiffs are arguing that Bendectin should not be used under any circumstances. One explanation for the legal action has been presented in this manner: the information given to prescribing physicians was not adequate to allow them to make an appropriate risk/benefit analysis of the risks of using the drug. In addition, some legal actions may have proceeded on the premise that the manufacturer's literature should have narrowed the indications for Bendectin rather than promoting it for routine use in minor nausea of pregnancy (33). One could argue that if the epidemiological data are unable to demonstrate an increased risk of malformations with Bendectin exposure, then, strictly speaking, it is difficult to inform practitioners of the risks associated with its use. Discussions of the justifiability of the Bendectin litigation are moot, since Merrell-Dow has already been forced to make a decision concerning the availability of Bendectin and has no plans to reintroduce the drug, despite successful defense in the majority of cases that went to trial. Rather, addressing the implications of having drug availability determined by the mass media and the litigation process will be more productive.

IMPLICATIONS OF THE BENDECTIN CASE

The implications of excessive litigation in the absence of scientific justification for a causal relationship between drug exposure and subsequent malformation are severalfold. Perhaps the most obvious is the likelihood that efficacious agents will be withdrawn from general use, leaving (at least in the case of Bendectin) a void in the drug therapy of hyperemesis gravidarum. The net effect is that physicians must now make a decision either not to treat the nausea or to prescribe alternative antinauseants for which there is considerably less information on the risk of malformations. A decline in Bendectin use from 32% in 1980 to 17% in 1982 was attributed to adverse publicity around the time of the first litigation cases (32), whereas Jick and Garrison (34) report that the use of the drug decreased from 17% in 1982 to 0.6% in 1984. The use of other emetics was low by comparison and did not appreciably increase over the same 2-year period (3.1 and 3.8%, respectively). Within the group of other emetics, the use of prochlorperazine and promethazine increased slightly from 11 to 22 users, and 25 to 53 users, respectively, in 1982 and 1984. Thus, initial data suggest that physicians are choosing to avoid pharmacological treatment of nausea and vomiting of pregnancy rather than risk the consequences of exposure to less-studied alternatives. This trend provides an opportunity to focus attention on the effects of untreated nausea and vomiting in pregnancy.

The symptomology of nausea and vomiting of pregnancy has been associated with a lower incidence of spontaneous abortion than occurs in women without these symptoms (12,35), and in this respect may be considered as a favorable sign. On the other hand, there are animal data demonstrating that maternal nutritional deficiencies during gestation may result in an increased incidence of malformations in the offspring (36,37). The data in humans are less clear. Hyperemesis gravidarum has been associated with a 2.1-fold increased risk of central nervous system malformations, a 4-fold increase in eye/ear malformations, and a 4.7-fold increase in the risk of Down's syndrome in the offspring (38). Vomiting, on the other hand, was not associated with any such increased risks. Further complicating the issue is the finding that at all stages of pregnancy, vomiting was related to the number of products taken. When hyperemesis was recorded, drug usage in the first 4 months of pregnancy was more than double compared to its absence. Regardless of the relationship between hyperemesis and fetal malformations, it is not unreasonable to surmise that discontinuation of Bendectin may be associated with an increase in untreated nausea and vomiting in pregnant women, possibly accompanied by an increase in the number of hospitalizations required to correct nutritional imbalances and hydration status. This appears to be the case, since a recent review has revealed a dramatic increase in hospitalizations of pregnant women for treatment of hyperemesis gravidarum coinciding with the removal of Bendectin from the market (Stephen Lam, M.D., personal communication). The economic cost in terms of hospitalization costs and loss of work time has yet to be determined. Perhaps of more concern is the increased risk of exposure to multiple medications and increased risk of some form of iatrogenic disease that can accompany hospitalization.

We have noted that Bendectin is perhaps the best-studied drug in pregnancy. Yet even with the available data, it is difficult to remove all residual uncertainty that a given exposure is not harmful, and it is unlikely that having even more epidemiological data will appreciably resolve this uncertainty, let alone substantially affect future litigation cases involving Bendectin. Holmes has stated that ". . . in view of the extensive data . . . on Bendectin and the limited data available on many other commonly used drugs, one can argue that well-designed studies of other drugs would be of greater value to the public at this time" (2). The major question is, Who will pay for these studies? The Bendectin experience will no doubt serve as a deterrent to even the most altruistic pharmaceutical firms, since there is little, if any, incentive to develop and market future agents for use in pregnancy. This may seriously hamper the development of new pharmacological agents for use in pregnancy-unique disorders.

In a general sense, the negative publicity accorded the Bendectin debate may adversely affect a pregnant woman's perception of the risk associated with any drug ingestion during pregnancy. One should not underestimate the influence of the lay press in modifying the behavior of the general public. As evidence of this, one expert in the field related personal knowledge of seven pregnancies that were terminated in response to a 1979 headline of a supermarket tabloid (3). That headline referred to "a monstrous scandal that could be far larger than the thalidomide horror. . . ." It is unfortunate that the analogy to the thalidomide story has engendered so much hysteria in the public, since the limb deformities presented in the lay press do not represent the full phenotypic effect of the drug. While there is good reason for therapeutic nihilism during pregnancy, in some instances the benefit/risk ratio favors continuation of drug therapy: for example, most antibiotic therapy, and treatment of seizure disorders. It is therefore important that the risks of any drug exposure during pregnancy be placed in the proper perspective and that the concerned, pregnant patient be made fully aware of the background malformation rate so that any decisions regarding continuation of the pregnancy will be fully informed decisions (see Chapter 29).

Perhaps the most serious litigation-related consequence of drug use during pregnancy is that any pharmacological agent widely used at the time of conception or during pregnancy may become the target of unjustified (on a scientific basis) litigation. Using Bendectin as an example, Brent has presented the potential magnitude of this problem (3). With an estimated 30 million infants exposed to Bendectin early in gestation and a background malformation rate of 3%, chance alone would account for 900,000 malformed infants whose mothers had taken Bendectin during pregnancy. Similarly, if the rate of spontaneous occurrence of limb reduction defects is considered to be one in 3000, then 10,000 such defects would have occurred by chance alone among the offspring exposed to Bendectin. Thus, chance alone could account for thousands of malformations in a population exposed to a commonly used pharmacological intervention. The recent controversy surrounding pre- and periconceptional spermicide use and outcome of pregnancy, and the subsequent initiation of litigation proceedings, may be the most recent manifestation of this phenomenon. As in the case of Bendectin, the weight of epidemiological evidence does not appear to favor any association between maternal spermicide use and pregnancy outcome despite initial reports to the contrary (39,40). The reality of the matter is that many more similar situations could present in the future.

POSSIBLE SOLUTIONS

Recommendations to decrease the number of malpractice lawsuits in general have been directed toward the litigation process itself through education of the patient, improving the health care system, making awards more realistic by various means, decreasing lawyer representation in legislative bodies seeking to enact tort reforms, and eliminating the contingency fee system (5). Recommendations made specifically to decrease the number of nonmeritorious congenital malformation lawsuits included establishing authoritative sources of information to assist the court (with the intent of providing unbiased scientific opinions on the issues of interest), introducing the concept of medicolegal workup for preliminary determination of the merit of a particular case, and creating new laws to define responsibility and rights of fetus, parents, and physician, as well as the pharmaceutical or other industries (5). These are as pertinent today as they were when first presented 25 years ago. The goals of both the legal and medical communities should be the protection of pregnant patients while assuring the continuing availability of safe medications for these patients. These goals may be achieved in several ways. One possibility is the application of meta-analysis to epidemiological studies for determining a quantitative test statistic from published teratogenicity data, particularly when existing data are contradicting and were generated by different study methodologies (41). In addition, a better mechanistic understanding of, and the ability to assess individual susceptibilities to, drug-induced birth defects (42) would help determine the likelihood of a causal relationship between drug exposure and malformations in any given case. Finally, the onus is on both the legal and medical communities to assure continual improvement in expert testimony to the level of peer-review quality.

Alternatively, since a legal decision is dependent on the merits and arguments particular to an individual case, perhaps the most effective intervention in an epidemic that is rapidly becoming out of control is education of the patient on an individual basis. This is best achieved through specialty clinics established solely to educate the patient by presenting the most up-to-date information on the risk(s) of a given compound in a completely unbiased manner so as to ensure that the patient is aware of the background malformation rate *and* any inherent risks of the exposure in question. Information of this type would serve to minimize the patient's perception of the risk involved with a given exposure and would ensure that any related decisions during the course of pregnancy were fully informed. In addition, the data obtained prospectively from a multicenter network of such services would be important in increasing the number of exposures to less widely used agents, thus improving the accuracy of the risk assessments. The ultimate impact of this type of intervention on the current and potential litigation problem will become apparent only with the passage of time.

Answer

Meta-analysis of a large number of studies has failed to show association between the drug and any major malformation.

REFERENCES

1. Leeder JS, Spielberg SP, MacLeod SM. Bendectin: The wrong way to regulate drug availability. Can Med Assoc J 1983; 129:1085–1087.
2. Holmes LB. Teratogen update: Bendectin. Teratology 1983; 27:277–281.
3. Brent RL. The Bendectin saga: Another American tragedy. Teratology 1983; 27: 283–286.
4. Hays DP. Bendectin: A case of mourning sickness. Drug Intell Clin Pharm 1983; 17:826–827.
5. Brent RL. The law and congenital malformations. Clin Perinatol 1986; 13:505–544.
6. Advisory Committee, Food and Drug Administration. The Bendectin Peer Group Report (NDA 10-598). US Department of Health, Education and Welfare, Washington DC, April 1975.
7. Paterson DC, Congenital deformities. Can Med Assoc J 1969; 101:175–176.
8. Paterson DC. Congenital deformities associated with Bendectin. Can Med Assoc J 1977; 116:1348.

9. Rothman KJ, Fyler DC, Goldblatt A, Kriedberg MB. Exogenous hormones and other drug exposures of children with congenital heart disease. Am J Epidemiol 1979; 109:433–439.

10. Kolata GB. How safe is Bendectin? Science 1980; 210:518–519.

11. Moss DC. Bendectin tide turning? Am Bar Assoc J Nov 1, 1987, pp 18–19.

12. Milkovich L, van den Berg BJ. An evaluation of the teratogenicity of certain antinauseant drugs. Am J Obstet Gynecol 1976; 125:244–248.

13. Shapiro S, Heinonen OP, Siskind V, Kaufman DW, Monson RR, Slone D. Antenatal exposure to doxylamine succinate and dicyclomine hydrochloride (Bendectin) in relation to congenital malformations, perinatal mortality rate, birth rate, and intelligence quotient score. Am J Obstet Gynecol 1977; 128:480–485.

14. Cordero JF, Oakley GP, Greenberg F, James LF. Is Bendectin a teratogen? JAMA 1981; 245:2307–2310.

15. Fleming DM, Knox JDE, Crombie DL. Debendox in early pregnancy and fetal malformation. Br Med J 1981; 283:99–101.

16. Morelock S, Hingson R, Kayne H, Dooling E, Zuckerman B, Day N, Alpert JJ, Flowerdew G. Bendectin and fetal development. A study at Boston City Hospital. Am J Obstet Gynecol 1982; 142:209–213.

17. Gibson GT, Colley DP, McMichael AJ, Hartshorne JM. Congenital anomalies in relation to the use of doxylamine/dicyclomine and other antenatal factors. Med J Aust 1981; 1:410–414.

18. General Practitioner Clinical Trials. Drugs in pregnancy survey. Practitioner 1963; 191:775–780.

19. Michaelis J, Michaelis H, Glück E, Koller S. Prospective study of suspected associations between certain drugs administered during early pregnancy and congenital malformations. Teratology 1983; 27:57–64.

20. Bunde CA, Bowles DM. A technique for controlled survey of case records. Curr Ther Res 1963; 5:245–248.

21. Smithells RW, Sheppard S. Teratogenicity testing in humans: A method demonstrating safety of Bendectin. Teratology 1978; 17:31–35.

22. Harron DWG, Griffiths K, Shanks RG. Debendox and congenital malformations in Northern Ireland. Br Med J 1980; 281:1379–1381.

23. Mitchell AA, Rosenberg L, Shapiro S, Slone D. Birth defects related to Bendectin use in pregnancy. I. Oral clefts and cardiac defects. JAMA 1981; 245:2311–2314.

24. Jick H, Holmes LB, Hunter JR, Madsen S, Stergachis A. First trimester drug use and congenital disorders. JAMA 1981; 246:343–346.

25. Newman NM, Correy JF, Dudgeon GI. A survey of congenital abnormalities and drugs in private practice. Aust NZ J Obstet Gynaecol 1977; 17:156–159.

26. Greenberg G, Inman WHW, Weathereall JAC, Adalstein AM, Haskey JC. Maternal drug histories and congenital malformations. Br Med J 1977; 2:853–856.

27. Golding J, Vivian S, Baldwin JA. Maternal anti-nauseants and clefts of lip and palate. Hum Toxicol 1983; 2:63–73.

28. Eskenazi B, Bracken M. Bendectin (Debendox) as a risk factor for pyloric stenosis. Am J Obstet Gynecol 1982; 144:919–924.

29. Aselton PJ, Jick H. Additional follow-up of congenital limb disorders in relation to Bendectin use (letter). JAMA 1983; 250:33–34.
30. Zierler S, Rothman KJ. Congenital heart disease in relation to maternal use of Bendectin and other drugs in early pregnancy. N Engl J Med 1985; 313:347–352.
31. Mitchell AA, Schwingl PJ, Rosenberg L, Louik C, Shapiro S. Birth defects in relation to Bendectin use in pregnancy. II. Pyloric stenosis. Am J Obstet Gynecol 1983; 147:737–742.
32. Aselton P, Jick H, Chentow SJ, Perera DR, Hunter JR, Rothman KJ. Pyloric stenosis and maternal Bendectin exposure. Am J Epidemiol 1984; 120:251–256.
33. Brushwood DB. Two legal issues: Expert witness and Bendectin case (letter). Drug Intell Clin Pharm 1983; 17:848–849.
34. Jick SS, Garrison JM. Discontinuation of Bendectin (letter). Am J Public Health 1988; 78:322–323.
35. Kullander S, Kallen B. A prospective study of drugs and pregnancy. II. Antiemetic drugs. Acta Obstet Gynecol Scand 1976; 55:105–111.
36. Rosenzweig S, Blaustein FM. Cleft palate in A/J mice resulting from restraint and deprivation of food and water. Teratology 1971; 3:47–51.
37. Warkany J, Petering H. Congenital malformations of the brain caused by short zinc deficiencies in rats. Am J Ment Defic 1973; 77:645–653.
38. Heinonen OP, Slone D, Shapiro S. Birth Defects and Drugs in Pregnancy. Publishing Sciences Group, Littleton, MA, 1977.
39. Anon. Data do not support association between spermicides, birth defects. FDA Drug Bull 1986; 16:21.
40. Schlesselman JJ. "Proof" of cause and effect in epidemiologic studies: Criteria for judgment. Prev Med 1987; 16:195–210.
41. Einarson TR, Leeder JS, Koren G. A method for meta-analysis of epidemiologic studies. Drug Intell Clin Pharm 1988; 22:813–824.
42. Strickler SM, Miller MA, Andermann E, Dansky LV, Seni M-V, Spielberg SP. Genetic predisposition to phenytoin-induced birth defects. Lancet 1985; 2:746–750.

Index